The Wound Management Manual

Notice

Medicine is an ever-changing science. As new research and clinical experience broaden our knowledge, changes in treatment and drug therapy are required. The authors and the publisher of this work have checked with sources believed to be reliable in their efforts to provide information that is complete and generally in accord with the standards accepted at the time of publication. However, in view of the possibility of human error or changes in medical sciences, neither the authors nor the publisher nor any other party who has been involved in the preparation or publication of this work warrants that the information contained herein is in every respect accurate or complete, and they disclaim all responsibility for any errors or omissions or for the results obtained from use of the information contained in this work. Readers are encouraged to confirm the information contained herein with other sources. For example and in particular, readers are advised to check the product information sheet included in the package of each drug they plan to administer to be certain that the information contained in this work is accurate and that changes have not been made in the recommended dose or in the contraindications for administration. This recommendation is of particular importance in connection with new or infrequently used drugs.

The Wound Management Manual

Edited by

Bok Y. Lee, MD, FACS
Professor of Surgery
New York Medical College
Attending Physician, Department of Surgery—Cardiovascular and Thoracic Surgery
Westchester Medical Center
Valhalla, New York
Director of Surgical Research
Sound Shore Medical Center of Westchester
New Rochelle, New York
Adjunct Professor, Center for Biomedical Engineering
Rensselaer Polytechnic Insititute
Troy, New York

McGraw-Hill
Medical Publishing Division

New York   Chicago   San Francisco   Lisbon   London   Madrid   Mexico City
Milan   New Delhi   San Juan   Seoul   Singapore   Sydney   Toronto

The Wound Management Manual

Copyright © 2005 by The McGraw-Hill Companies, Inc. All rights reserved. Printed in the United States of America. Except as permitted under the United States Copyright Act of 1976, no part of this publication may be reproduced or distributed in any form or by any means, or stored in a data base or retrieval system, without the prior written permission of the publisher.

1 2 3 4 5 6 7 8 9 0 KGPKGP 0 9 8 7 6 5 4

ISBN: 0-07-143203-5

This book was set in Garamond by GTS.
The editor was Marc Strauss; the editorial assistant was Marsha Loeb.
The production supervisor was Richard Ruzycka.
Project management was provided by TechBooks.
Quebecor World Kingsport was printer and binder.

This book is printed on acid-free paper.

Library of Congress Cataloging-in-Publication Data

The wound management manual / [edited by] Bok Y. Lee.
     p. ; cm.
   ISBN 0-07-143203-5
   1. Wound healing—Handbooks, manuals, etc.   2. Skin—Ulcers—Treatment—Handbooks,
manuals, etc.   3. Bedsores—Prevention—Handbooks, manuals, etc.   4. Wounds and
injuries—Treatment—Handbooks, manuals, etc. I. Lee, Bok Y., 1928
   [DNLM: 1. Decubitus Ulcer—prevention & control.   2. Skin Ulcer—prevention & control.
3. Decubitus Ulcer—surgery.   4. Skin Ulcer—surgery. WR 598 W938 2004]
   RD94.W698 2004
   616.5'45—dc22

                                                                                    2004040344

I dedicate this book to my wife, Dr. Taihee Lee,
in grateful appreciation for the support she has given me.
She has been and continues to be a driving force and inspiration.

Contents

Contributors IX

Preface. XIII

1. Etiology and Management of Foot Ulcerations 1
   Bauer E. Sumpio, Stephen M. Schroeder, and Peter A. Blume

2. Molecular Therapies for Wounds: Modalities for Stimulating Angiogenesis and Granulation 17
   Vincent W. Li, Elaine F. Kung, and William W. Li

3. Theoretical and Practical Aspects of Oxygen in Wound Healing 44
   Thomas K. Hunt and Stefan Beckert

4. Topical Oxygen Therapy as an Adjunctive Modality in Wound Healing 55
   Francis Rossi, Eric S. Baskin, Shail N. Patel, and Adam J. Teichman

5. Negative–Pressure Wound Therapy (Vacuum–Assisted Closure). 65
   Jeffrey A. Niezgoda and Barbara Schibly

6. Historical Aspects of Wound Healing. 72
   Bok Y. Lee and Marcelo C. DaSilva

7. Electrical Stimulation in Wound Repair. 80
   Joseph McCulloch

8. Antioxidant Effects of Ultra-Low Microcurrents in Wound Healing 90
   Bok Y. Lee, Alfred J. Koonin, Keith Wendell, and John Hillard

9. Lymphedema and Wound Healing: A Case for Codependence. 104
   John M. Macdonald

10. Role of Matrix Macromolecules in the Etiology and Treatment of Chronic Ulcers 109
    Seth L. Schor, Ana M. Schor, Robert P. Keatch, and Jill Belch

11. Management of Acute Wounds 122
    Zahid B. M. Niazi and Justin Sacks

12. Noninvasive Evaluation of the Cutaneous Circulation 131
    Bok Y. Lee and Lee E. Ostrander

13. Pathophysiology of Diabetic Foot Lesions and Their Treatment with the Circulator Boot 141
    Richard S. Dillon

14. Intermittent Pneumatic Compression Devices in Critical Limb Ischemia 212
    George Louridas

15. Dermagraft: Living, Bioengineered, Human Dermis for Healing Chronic Wounds 219
    Gary D. Gentzkow

16. Management of Complex and Pathologic Wounds with Integra. 226
    Marc E. Gottlieb

17. Biomaterial Wound Matrix from Small Intestine Submucosa:
    Review and Efficacy in Diabetic Wound Healing 290
    Robert G. Frykberg and Jason P. Hodde

18. Skin Substitutes in Acute and Chronic Wounds. 298
    Kevin G. Donohue and Vincent Falanga

19. Wound Closure by External Tissue Expansion. 309
    Ralph Ger and Eli S. Schessel

20. The Diabetic Foot: A Comprehensive Approach 339
    Bok Y. Lee, Phyllis Berkowitz–Smith, V. J.Guerra, and Robert E. Madden

21. Foot Compartment Syndrome—Modified Plantar Medial Approach Fasciotomy 367
    Bok Y. Lee, Phyllis Berkowitz–Smith, V. J. Guerra, and Irfan M. Jameel

Index 373

Contributors

Eric S. Baskin, DPM
Chief Resident of Podiatric Surgery
Bon Secours New Jersey Health System
Hoboken, New Jersey
Topical Hyperbaric Oxygen as an Adjunctive Modality in Wound Healing

Stefan Beckert, MD
Department of General Surgery
Klinik fur Allgemeine Chirurgie
Tubingen, Germany
Theoretical and Practical Aspects of Oxygen in Wound Healing

Jill Belch, PhD
Consultant in Vascular Medicine
Vascular Diseases Research Unit
Ninewells Hospital and Medical School
Dundee, Scotland
Role of Matrix Macromolecules in the Etiology and Treatment of Chronic Ulcers

Phyllis Berkowitz-Smith, BA, RVT
Chief
Medical Technology
Veterans Administration Medical Center
Castle Point, New York
The Diabetic Foot: A Comprehensive Approach; Foot Compartment Syndrome: Modified Plantar Medial Approach Fasciotomy

Peter A. Blume
DPM
Podiatrist Yale School of Medicine
New Haven, Connecticut

Marcelo C. DaSilva, MD, FACS
Department of Thoracic and Cardiovascular Surgery
Loyola University Chicago—Stritch School of Medicine
Maywood, Illinois
Historical Aspects of Wound Healing

Richard S. Dillon, MD, FAPWC, FACE, FACP, FACA, FSVMB
Assistant Clinical Professor of Medicine
Jefferson Medical School
Former Chief of Endocrinology
Philadelphia General Hospital
Philadelphia, Pennsylvania
Bryn Mawr Hospital
Bryn Mawr, Pennsylvania
Emeritus Staff and Medical Consultant
Circulator Boot Corporation
Malvern, Pennsylvania
The Pathophysiology of Peripheral Vascular Disease and its Treatment with the End-Diastolic Pneumatic Boot (Circulator Boot)

Kevin G. Donohue, MD
Department of Dermatology and Skin Surgery
Roger Williams Medical Center
Providence, Rhode Island
Boston University School of Medicine
Boston, Massachusetts
The Use of Skin Substitutes in Acute and Chronic Wounds

Vincent Falanga, MD
Chairman
Department of Dermatology and Skin Surgery
Roger Williams Medical Center
Providence, Rhode Island
Professor
Departments of Dermatology and Biochemistry
Boston University School of Medicine
Boston, Massachusetts
The Use of Skin Substitutes in Acute and Chronic Wounds

Robert G. Frykberg, DPM, MPH
College of Podiatric Medicine
Des Moines University
Des Moines, Iowa
Biomaterial Wound Matrix from Small Intestine Submucosa: Review and Efficacy in Diabetic Wound Healing

Gary D. Gentzkow, MD
Consultant
Medical Advisor to Smith & Nephew Wound
    Management
Rancho Santa Fe, California
*Dermagraft, Living, Bioengineered, Human Dermis for
    Healing Chronic Wounds*

Ralph Ger, MD
Professor of Surgery
State University of New York at Stonybrook
Stonybrook, New York
Professor of Anatomy
Albert Einstein College of Medicine
Bronx, New York
Wound Closure by External Tissue Expansion

Marc E. Gottlieb, MD, FACS
Plastic Surgeon
Plastic & Reconstructive Surgery
Pheonix, Arizona
*Integra Tissue Regeneration Matrix: Its Use for Managing
    Chronic Wounds*

V. J. Guerra, MD
Formerly Surgical Resident
    Sound Shore Medical Center
    Westchester, New York
*The Diabetic Foot: A Comprehensive Approach; Foot
    Compartment Syndrome: Modified Plantar Medial
    Approach Fasciotomy*

John Hillard, RN
Formerly Wound Care Specialist
    Northeast Center for Special Care
    Lake Katrine, New York
*Antioxidant Effects of Ultra-Low Microcurrents in
    Wound Healing*

Jason P. Hodde, MS
Cook Biotech Incorporated
West Lafayette, Indiana
*Biomaterial Wound Matrix from Small Intestine
    Submucosa: Review and Efficacy in Diabetic
    Wound Healing*

Thomas K. Hunt, MD
Professor Emeritus
Department of Surgery
Director, Wound Healing Laboratory

University of California, San Francisco
San Francisco, California
*Theoretical and Practical Aspects of Oxygen in Wound
    Healing*

Irfan M. Jameel, MD
Formerly Surgical Resident
    Sound Shore Medical Center
    Westchester, New York
*Foot Compartment Syndrome: Modified Plantar Medial
    Approach Fasciotomy*

Robert P. Keatch, PhD
Microengineering and Biomaterials Group
Faculty of Engineering and Physical Sciences
University of Dundee
Dundee, Scotland
*Role of Matrix Macromolecules in the Etiology and
    Treatment of Chronic Ulcer*

Alfred J. Koonin, MB, CHB, PhD, FRCS
Formerly Medical Director American Institute
    of Degeneration Pacific Polisadrs, California
*Antioxidant Effects of Ultra-Low Microcurrents in
    Wound Healing*

Elaine F. Kung, MD
Yale School of Medicine
New Haven, Connecticut
The Angiogenesis Foundation
Cambridge, Massachusetts
*Molecular Therapy for Wounds: Modalities
    for Stimulating Angiogenesis and Granulation*

Vincent W. Li, MD, MBA
Scientific Director
The Angiogenesis Foundation
Cambridge, Massachusetts
Director, Angiogenesis Clinic
Department of Dermatology
Brigham and Women's Hospital
Boston, Massachusetts
*Molecular Therapy for Wounds: Modalities
    for Stimulating Angiogenesis and Granulation*

William W. Li, MD
President and Medical Director
The Angiogenesis Foundation
Cambridge, MA
*Molecular Therapy for Wounds: Modalities for
    Stimulating Angiogenesis and Granulation*

Bok Y. Lee, MD, FACS
Professor of Surgery
New York Medical College
Attending Physician, Department of Surgery—
    Cardiovascular and Thoracic Surgery
Westchester Medical Center
Valhalla, New York
Director of Surgical Research
Sound Shore Medical Center of Westchester
New Rochelle, New York
Adjunct Professor, Center for Biomedical Engineering
Rensselaer Polytechnic Institute
Troy, New York
Historical Aspects of Wound Healing
*Antioxidant Effects of Ultra-low Microcurrents in
    Wound Healing*
Noninvasive Evaluation of the Cutaneous Circulation
The Diabetic Foot: A Comprehensive Approach
*Foot Compartment Syndrome: A New Approach to an
    Old Problem*

**George Louridas, MBBCh, FCS (SA), Mmed
    (Surg), Wits., FACS**
Section Head, Vascular Surgery
Department of Surgery
St. Boniface General Hospital and Health Sciences
    Center
University of Manitoba
Manitoba, Canada
*Intermittent Pneumatic Compression Devices in Critical
    Limb*

John M. Macdonald, MD, FACS
Department of Dermatology and Cutaneous Surgery
University of Miami School of Medicine
Miami, Florida
*Lymphedema and Wound Healing: A Case for
    Codependence*

Robert E. Madden, MD, FACS
Professor of Surgery
Department of Vascular Surgery
Westchester Medical Center
Valhalla, New York
The Diabetic Foot: A Comprehensive Approach

Joseph McCulloch, Ph.D, PT, FAPTA, CSW
Dean
School of Allied Health Professions
Louisiana State University Health Sciences Center
Shreveport, Louisiana
Electrical Stimulation in Wound Repair

**Zahid B. M. Niazi, MD, FRCSI, FACS, FICS,
    CHT Plast (UK)**
Attending Plastic Surgeon
Westchester Medical Center
Valhalla, New York
St. Agnes Hospital
White Plains, New York
Community Hospital
Dobbs Ferry, New York
Our Lady of Mercy Hospital
Bronx, New York
Blythedale Children's Hospital
Valhalla, New York
Chief of Craniofacial Surgery
Director of Microsurgical Reconstruction
Director of Research and Education
Director of Quality Assurance, Division of Plastic
    Surgery
Fellow, New York Academy of Medicine
Assistant Professor of Surgery and
Assistant Professor of Otolaryngology
New York Medical College
Valhalla, New York
Management of Acute Wounds

Jeffrey A. Niezgoda, MD, FACEP
Medical Director
Center for Comprehensive Wound Care and
    Hyperbaric Oxygen Therapy
St. Luke's Medical Center, Aurora Healthcare
President, Hyperbaric & Wound Care Associates
Milwaukee, Wisconsin
*Negative Pressure Wound Therapy (Vacuum Assisted
    Closure)*

Lee E. Ostrander, PhD
Department of Biomedical Engineering
Jonsson Engineering Center
Rensselaer Polytechnic Institute
Troy, New York
*Noninvasive Evaluation of the Cutaneous
    Circulation*

Shail N. Patel, DPM
Co-Chief Podiatric Surgical Resident
Department of Surgery
St. Mary Hospital—Bon Secours and Canterbury
    Partnership for Care
Hoboken, New Jersey
*Topical Oxygen Therapy as an Adjunctive Modality in
    Wound Healing*

Francis Rossi, DPM, FACFAOM, CWS
Medical Director
Bon Secours Wound Healing Center
Jersey City, New Jersey
Topical Oxygen Therapy as an Adjunctive Modality in Wound Healing

Justin Sacks, MD
Chief Resident
Division of Plastic Surgery
Mount Sinai Medical Center
New York, New York
Management of Acute Wounds

Eli S. Schessel, MD
Chief, Division of Plastic Surgery
Catholic Medical Center
Queens, New York
Wound Closure by External Tissue Expansion

Barbara Schibly, MD, MPH
Staff Physician
Center for Comprehensive Wound Care and
    Hyperbaric Oxygen Therapy
St. Luke's Medical Center, Aurora Healthcare
Milwaukee, Wisconsin
Negative Pressure Wound Therapy (Vacuum Assisted Closure)

Ana M. Schor, PhD
Reader in Experimental Pathology
Unit of Cell and Molecular Biology
Dental School
University of Dundee
Dundee, Scotland
Role of Matrix Macromolecules in the Etiology and Treatment of Chronic Ulcers

Seth L. Schor, PhD
Professor of Cell and Molecular Biology
Dental School

University of Dundee
Dundee, Scotland
Role of Matrix Macromolecules in the Etiology and Treatment of Chronic Ulcers

Stephen M. Schroeder, DPM
Chief, Podiatric Surgery
The Vancouver Clinic
Department of Surgery
Southwest Washington Medical Center
Vancouver, Washington
Etiology and Management of Foot Ulcerations

Bauer E. Sumpio, MD, PhD
Professor of Surgery and Radiology
Chief of Vascular Surgery
Director, Yale Center for Vascular Disease
Yale University School of Medicine
New Haven, Connecticut
Etiology and Management of Foot Ulcerations

Adam J. Teichman, DPM
Co-Chief Podiatric Surgical Resident
Department of Surgery
St. Mary Hospital—Bon Secours and Canterbury
    Partnership for Care
Hoboken, New Jersey
Topical Oxygen Therapy as an Adjunctive Modality in Wound Healing

Keith Wendell, PhD
University of Metaphysics
Sedona, Arizona
Royal Melbourne Institute of Technology
Melbourne, Australia
Research Director
American Institute of Regeneration, Inc.
Simi Valley, California
Antioxidant Effects of Ultra-Low Microcurrents in Wound Healing

Preface

Chronic ulceration of the skin can lead to significant morbidity and mortality in disabled and bedridden patients and is notoriously difficult to manage. These ulcers have a low frequency of spontaneous healing and, when spontaneous healing does occur, it often produces poor results. The magnitude of the problem of pressure ulcers increases when one considers the growing population of elderly patients who will develop skin ulcers secondary to arterial and venous disease. With ever increasing cost of health care, physicians face the dilemma of providing expensive and prolonged care to those who suffer from the consequences of illness, injury, or aging. Pressure ulcers have a tremendous impact on a patient's overall well being, prolong their hospitalization, and increase treatment costs and time.

Between 600,000 and 2.5 million persons in the United States have chronic leg or foot ulcers. The cost of treating these wounds is estimated at $5–9 billion a year. Throughout the world, there are many clinicians, surgeons, scientists, and molecular biologists (to name but a few disciplines) devoting their careers to the understanding and treatment of chronic ulcers and pressure sores. This book is intended to bring this new work together to stimulate the interest of physicians, surgeons, and wound care professionals faced with the management and care of their patient's who present with chronic ulcers and pressure sores. Recent advances and significant developments in understanding on the cellular level of the process of wound healing and modalities including growth factors, angiogenesis, oxygen therapy, and electrical stimulation in wound care and tissue repair and engineering are just a few topics that are explored in this book, along with surgical management

I wish to thank all the contributors who accepted the invitation to join in this work with enthusiasm and fervor. A special note of gratitude must be extended to Marc Strauss, Executive Editor, McGraw-Hill Medical Publishing Division, Marsha Loeb, Editorial Assistant, and to Teresa Schaffner and Phyllis Berkowitz-Smith.

Bok Y. Lee

The Wound Management Manual

1 Etiology and Management of Foot Ulcerations

Bauer E. Sumpio, Stephen M. Schroeder, and Peter A. Blume

Introduction
Biomechanics of Walking and Ulcer Formation
Etiology of Foot Ulcers
   Vascular Insufficiency
   Neuropathy
   Musculoskeletal Deformities
   Diabetes

Wound Assessment and Management
Vascular Assessment and Management
Neuropathy and Musculoskeltal Assessment and Management
Summary
References

INTRODUCTION

An ulcer is a focal loss of epidermal and dermal skin layers resulting from breaks in the dermal barrier with subsequent erosion of the underlying subcutaneous tissues.[1] In severe cases that go untreated, the breach may extend deep, involving muscle and bone. Simple cutaneous breakdown is not uncommon in the foot due to shearing forces and direct trauma. These lesions typically heal unless the wound repair mechanisms are suboptimal because of impaired perfusion, infection, or repeated, continuous traumatic insults. Lack of sensation in the foot allows these simple breaks to cascade to ulceration. Diminished perfusion decreases the resilience of skin and subcutaneous tissue leading to their rapid death with resultant ulceration. Vascular insufficiency impedes wound healing by reducing the supply of oxygen, nutrients, and soluble mediators important for tissue repair. Therefore, the progression from dermal breakdown to foot ulceration can be attributed to impaired arterial supply, peripheral neuropathy, musculoskeletal deformities, or a combination of these factors (Table 1–1).[2]

The etiology of most foot ulcers can be ascertained quite accurately by a careful problem-focused history and physical examination. Early recognition of the etiology of these foot lesions and prompt management of the ulcer is essential for good functional outcome. In many cases, successful salvage of an extremity is dependent upon a multidisciplinary team of specialists; timely consultation is warranted.

The cost of treating lower-extremity ulcers is staggering. Items factored into the equation include physician visits, hospital admissions, home health care, wound care supplies, rehabilitation, time lost from work, and jobs lost. Adding to the cost is the chronic nature of these wounds, high rate of recurrence, and propensity to become infected. In the United States, the annual cost of ulcer treatment is upward of $2.5 billion per year.[3,4] An England-based study estimated that the cost of 4 months of outpatient treatment for venous ulcers varied between $250 and $2500.[5] One recent study looked at 78 patients presenting to the Cleveland Clinic with venous ulcers and showed that the average total medical cost per patient was $9685 with a mean follow-up of 119 days.[6]

The social cost of these lesions becomes a factor by affecting a patient's lifestyle as well as attitude. It adds to the total cost by reducing their working capacity. The ability to perform on the job may be temporarily or permanently affected by the condition.[7] Extrapolating from previously reported figures,[8,9] there is an estimated 10 million work days lost in the United States annually from lower-extremity ulcers and this figure may be low. A 1994 report focused on the financial, social, and psychological implications of lower-extremity lesions in 73 patients.[10] It was concluded that they accounted for a

Table 1–1. Risk Factors for the Development and Nonhealing of Foot Ulcers

---

1. **Arterial insufficiency (Atherosclerosis, Vasculitis)**
   $TcPO_2 \leq 30$ mm Hg
   Ankle pressure ≤ 40 mm Hg, toe pressure ≤ 30 mm Hg

2. **Venous hypertension**

3. **Sensorimotor neuropathy**

4. **High plantar pressure**
   History of prior ulceration
   Prior surgery involving metatarsal heads
   Callus, blister, or macerated skin

5. **Altered biomechanics**
   Limited joint mobility
   Limited toe dorsiflexion

6. **Musculoskeletal deformity**
   Severe nail pathology
   Prominent metatarsal heads; claw toes
   Charcot foot
   Other plantar bony prominences

8. **Infections**

9. **Trauma**

10. **Diabetes**

---

substantial threat to a patient's quality of life. Their interviews revealed interesting statistics. Of the study patients, 68% reported feelings of fear, social isolation, anger, depression, and negative self-image because of the ulcers; 81% of the patients felt that their mobility was adversely affected. Within the younger population that was still actively working, there was a correlation between lower-extremity ulceration and adverse effects on finances, time lost from work, and job loss. In addition, there was a strong correlation between time spent on ulcer care and feelings of anger and resentment. These factors combined to have a negative emotional impact on their lives.

BIOMECHANICS OF WALKING AND ULCER FORMATION

The human foot is a complicated biological masterpiece containing 26 bones, numerous joints, and a network of ligaments, muscles, and blood vessels. Before understanding common etiologies for foot ulcers, an appreciation of the biomechanics required for locomotion is essential. Gait is a complex set of events that requires triplanar foot motion and control of multiple axes in order for complete bipedal ambulation (Fig. 1–1A).[11] When the heel hits the ground, its outer edge touches first. The foot is in a supinated position, which makes it very firm and rigid. Soft-tissue structures (muscles, tendons, and ligaments) then relax allowing the foot to pronate. It becomes less rigid and is able to flatten, absorb the shock of touchdown, and adapt to uneven surfaces. During midstance, the heel lies below the ankle joint complex. The front and back of the foot are aligned and the foot easily bears weight. Toward the end of midstance, the soft tissue structures begin to tighten; the foot resupinates and regains its arch. It is again very firm, acting as a rigid lever for propulsion. The heel lifts off the ground, swings slightly to the inside, and the toes push weight off the ground.

Sensory input from the visual and vestibular systems, as well as proprioceptive information from the lower extremities, is necessary to modify learned motor patterns and muscular output to execute the desired action. There are a variety of external and internal forces[2] that can have an impact on foot function. The combination of body weight pushing down and ground reactive force pushing up create friction and compressive forces. Shear results from the bones of the foot sliding parallel to their plane of contact during pronation and supination. Foot deformities or ill-fitting footwear will enhance pressure points since they focus the forces on a smaller area. When the foot flattens too much, or over pronates, the ankle and heel do not align during midstance and some bones are forced to support more weight. The foot strains under the body's weight causing the muscles to pull harder on these areas, making it more difficult for tendons and ligaments to hold bones and joints in proper alignment. Over time, swelling and pain on the bottom of the foot or near the heel may occur. Bunions can form at the great toe joint and hammertoe deformities can form at the lesser toes. Abnormal foot biomechanics resulting from limited joint mobility and foot deformities will magnify shearing forces resulting in increased plantar pressure on the foot during ambulation. This can represent critical causes for tissue breakdown.

■ ETIOLOGY OF FOOT ULCERS
Vascular Insufficiency

Arterial insufficiency is suggested by a history of underlying cardiac or cerebrovascular disease, complaints of leg claudication or impotence, or pain in the distal foot when supine (rest pain). Findings of diminished or absent pulses, pallor on elevation, dependent rubor, sluggish capillary toe refill, absence of toe hair, and

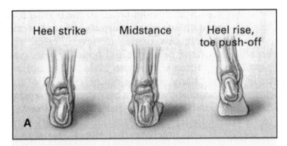

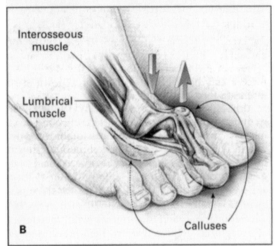

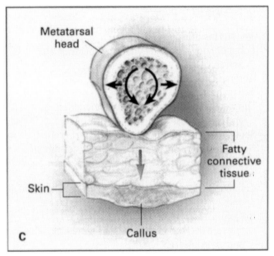

Figure 1–1. A. Biomechanics of gait. The normal mechanics of the foot and ankle are the combined effects of muscle, tendon, ligament, and bone function. Gait is classically divided into four distinct segments: (1) heel strike, where the lateral calcaneus makes contact with the groud and the muscles, tendons, and ligaments relax, allowing for optimal energy absorption: (2) midstance, where the foot is flat and is able to adapt to uneven terrain, maintain equilibrium, and absorb the shock of touchdown. The calcaneus is just below the ankle, keeping the front and back of the foot aligned for optimum weight bearing; (3) heel rise, where the calcaneus lifts off, the foot pronates, and the muscles, tendons, and ligaments tighten and the foot regains its arch; (4) toe push off. **B.** Forces on the foot. Friction and compressive forces are produced by the body weight pushing down and ground reactive forces pushing up. Friction and pressure combine as a shear force during dynamic walking as a result of the bones of the foot sliding relative to each other in a direction parallel to their plane of contact during pronation and supination. Wasting of intrinsic muscles of the foot results in an imbalance in the forces acting on the bony structures. This can lead to toe deformities, prominent metatarsal heads, equinus deformity, varus position of the hind foot, and proximal malalignment. **C.** Consequences of callus formation. Inadequate distribution of the forces of weight bearing or the presence of foot deformities can lead to abnormal movement which produces excessive stress and results in breakdown of connective tissue and muscle. Copied with permission from: Habershaw G, Chzran J. Biomechanical considerations of the diabetic foot. In: Kozak GP, Campbell DR, Frykberg RG, Habershaw GM, eds. *Management of Diabetic Foot Problems.* 2nd ed. Philadelphia: Saunders; 1995:53–65.

thickened nails are consistent with impaired arterial perfusion to the foot. Ischemic ulcers are characterized by absence of bleeding, pain and a precipitating trauma or underlying foot deformity (Table 1–2). They often develop on the dorsum of the foot (Fig. 1–2*A*), and over the first (Fig. 1–2*B*) and fifth metatarsal heads (Fig. 1–2*C*). Ischemic ulcers are uncommon on the plantar surface, as the pressure is usually less sustained

and perfusion better. A heel ulcer can develop from constant pressure applied while the heel is in a dependent position or during prolonged immobilization and bed rest (Fig. 1–2*D*). It should not be a surprise that a patient with relatively mild symptoms of arterial insufficiency develop limb-threatening extremity ulcers. This is due to the fact that once an ulcer is present, the blood supply necessary to heal the wound is greater than that

Table 1–2. Characteristics of Common Ulcers

---

1. Arterial

Commonly located on toes, plantar foot, and
    pressure points

Severely painful

Black, gray, or white base without granulation tissue

Shallow with sharply demarcated and irregularly
    shaped borders

Foot is cold to touch

Dependent rubor present

2. Venous insufficiency

Commonly located on medial aspect of lower leg
    and ankle

Absent or mild pain

Red granular base

Surrounding tissues are pigmented, indurated,
    and edematous

Foot is warm to touch

No dependent rubor, however, cellulites is common

3. Neuropathic

Commonly located under metatarsal heads, on top and at
    ends of digits, and at posterior and plantar heal

No pain

Lesions are deep, commonly covered with thick callus,
    and often infected

Ischemia and/or venous insufficiency may be present

---

needed to maintain intact skin. A chronic ulcer will develop unless the blood supply is improved.

Elevated venous pressures due to perforator or deep vein incompetency or venous thrombosis reduce the pressure gradient for perfusion and results in inadequate tissue perfusion because the elevated venous pressures and the venous stasis hinders clearance of breakdown products. However, venous ulcers rarely present in the foot and are commonly located in the "gaiter" distribution of the leg, around the medial malleolus, where the venous pressures are highest, and are associated with a swollen leg with a distinctive skin appearance (Fig. 1–3; Table 1–2).

Four foot-related risk factors have been identified in the genesis of pedal ulceration: peripheral neuropathy, evidence of increased pressure, altered biomechanics, limited joint mobility, bony deformity, and/or severe nail pathology.[2]

Neuropathy

Neuropathy is the most common underlying etiology of foot ulceration and frequently involves the somatic and autonomic fibers. Although there are many causes of peripheral neuropathy, diabetes mellitus is by far the most common (Table 1–3).

Neurotrophic ulcers typically form on the plantar aspect of the foot at areas of excessive focal pressures, which are most commonly encountered over the bony prominences of the metatarsal heads and the forefoot region due to the requirements of midstance and heel off during the gait cycle (Fig. 1–4). Loss of protective sensation in the foot can rapidly lead to ulceration if patient education and preventative measures are not taken.

Type-A sensory fibers are responsible for light-touch sensation, vibratory sensation, pressure, proprioception, and motor innervation to the intrinsic muscles of the foot. The muscles showing early involvement are the flexor digitorum brevis, lumbricals, and interosseous muscles.

Type-C sensory fibers detect painful stimuli, noxious stimuli, and temperature. When these fibers are affected, protective sensation is lost. This manifests as a distal, symmetric loss of sensation described in a "stocking" distribution and proves to be the primary factor predisposing patients to ulcers and infection.[12] Patients are unable to detect increased loads, repeated trauma, or pain from shearing forces. Injuries such as fractures, ulceration, and foot deformities will, therefore, go unrecognized. Repeat stress to high-pressure areas or bone prominences that would be interpreted as pain in the nonneuropathic patient, also go unrecognized. Sensory dysfunction results in increased shearing forces and repeated trauma to the foot. Patients have inadequate protective sensation during all phases of gait; therefore, high loads are undetected due to loss of pain threshold, which results in prolonged and increased forces.[13,14] These problems manifest as abnormal pressure points, increased shearing, and greater friction to the foot. Because all of this goes unrecognized in the insensate foot, gait patterns go unchanged and the stresses eventually cause tissue breakdown and ulceration.

Autonomic involvement causes an interruption of normal sweating at the epidermal level and causes arteriovenous shunting at the subcutaneous and dermal level. Hypohydrosis leads to a noncompliant epidermis that increases the risk of cracking and fissuring. AV shunting diminishes the delivery of nutrients and oxygen to tissue regions and skin and subcutaneous tissues become more susceptible to breakdown.[15]

Musculoskeletal Deformities

Atrophy of the small muscles within the foot results in nonfunctioning intrinsic foot muscles referred to as an "intrinsic minus foot" (Fig. 1–1B).[16] The muscles showing early involvement are the flexor digitorum brevis, lumbricals, and interosseous muscles. These groups act

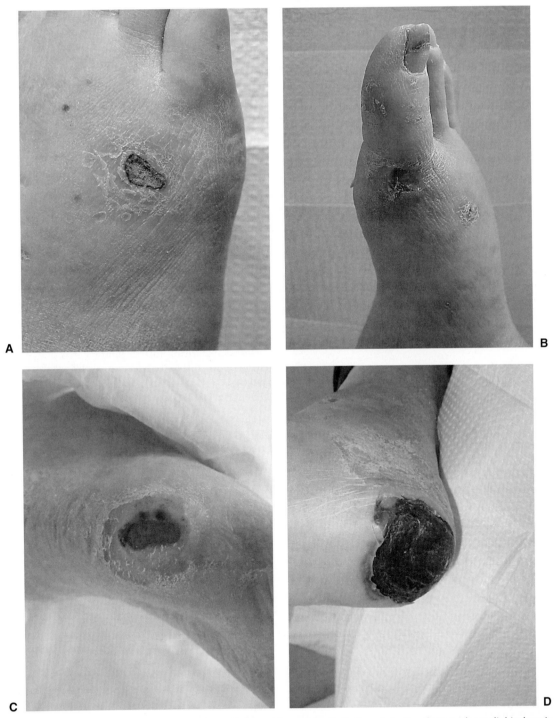

Figure 1-2. Common ischemic ulcerations. ***A.*** Dorsal foot ulcer. ***B.*** Hallux abductovalgus with medial ischemic ulcer. ***C.*** Necrotic fifth metatarsal head ulcer. ***D.*** Heel ulcer.

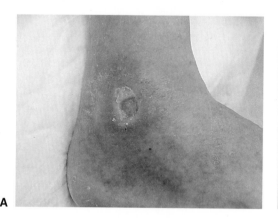
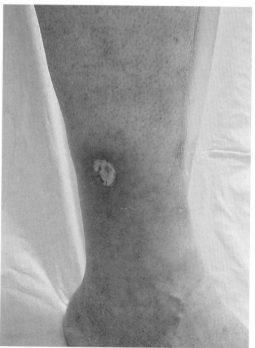

A

B

Figure 1–3. Example of venous stasis ulcer. **A.** Note the typical location in the "gaiter" region of the leg. **B.** Stasis ulcers may also occur on the lateral leg. Note the chronic inflammation, varicosities, and telangectasias.

to stabilize the proximal phalanx against the metatarsal head preventing dorsiflexion at the metatarsal phalangeal joint (MTPJ) during midstance in the gait cycle. With progression of the neuropathy, these muscles atrophy and fail to function properly. This causes the MTPJs to become unstable allowing the long flexors (flexor digitorum longus and flexor hallucis longus) and extensors (extensor digitorum longus and extensor hallucis longus) to act unchecked on the digits. Dorsal contractures develop at the MTPJs with development of hammer digit syndrome, also known as "intrinsic minus disease." The deformity acts to plantarflex the metatarsals, making the heads more prominent and increasing the plantar pressure created beneath them (Fig. 1–4). It also acts to decrease the amount of toe weight bearing during the gait cycle, which also increases pressure on the metatarsal heads. Normal anatomy consists of a metatarsal fat pad located plantar to the MTPJs. This structure helps to dissipate pressures on the metatarsal heads from the ground. When the hammer digit deformity occurs, the fat pad migrates distally and becomes nonfunctional. This results in elevated planter pressures that increase the risk of skin breakdown and ulceration due to shearing forces.[1]

Overpowering by the extrinsic foot muscles also leads to an equinus deformity at the ankle and a varus hind foot. A cavovarus foot type can develop leading to decreased range of motion of the pedal joints, an inability to adapt to terrain, and low tolerance to shock (Fig. 1–5). In essence, a mobile adapter is converted to a rigid lever. Pressure is equal to body weight divided by surface area, thus decreasing surface area below a metatarsal head with concomitant rigid deformities leads to increased forces or pressure to the sole of the foot. When neuropathic foot disease is associated with congenital foot deformities, such as long or short metatarsals, a plantar-flexed metatarsal, abnormalities in the metatarsal parabola, or a Charcot foot (Fig. 1–6), there is a higher propensity toward breakdown as a result of increased and abnormal plantar foot pressures.

Increasing body weight and decreasing the surface area of contact of the foot components with the ground will increase pressure. A low pressure but constant insult over an extended period can have the same ulcerogenic effect as high pressure over a shorter period. This is typical of the effect of tight-fitting shoes. If the magnitude of these forces in a given area is large enough, either skin loss or hypertrophy of the stratum corneum (callus) occurs (Fig. 1–1C). The presence of callus in patients with neuropathy should raise a red flag since the risk of ulceration in a callused area is increased by two orders of magnitude. Clinical findings predictive of high plantar pressure are summarized in Table 1–1.

Table 1–3. Etiologies of Peripheral Neuropathy

1. **Acquired**

Diabetes Mellitus	Hypothyroidism
Guillain-Barré Syndrome	Sarcoidosis
Alcoholism	Myeloma
Malignancy	Collagen Vascular Disease(s)
Uremia	Acromegaly
Cryoglobulinemia	Spinal Cord Disorders

2. **Hereditatry**

Charcot–Marie–Tooth Disease	Tangier Disease
Dejerines-Sottas Disease	Fabry's Disease
Refsum's Syndrome	Friedreich's Ataxia

3. **Toxic**

Chloramphenicol	Lithium
Isoniazid	Pyridoxine
Nitrofurantoin	Disulfuram
Dapsone	Ethionamide
Cisplatin	Vincristine
Metronidazole	Gold
Hydralazine	Amiodarone
Phenytoin	Colchicine
Lead	Arsenic
Cyanide	Mercury
Thallium	Trichloroethylene

4. **Infection**

Leprosy	Herpes Zoster
Diptheria	Lyme Disease
HIV	

5. **Entrapment**

Carpal Tunnel Syndrome	Tarsal Tunnel Syndrome

Diabetes

Diabetic patients are particularly prone to foot ulcers. Approximately 16 million people, comprising 6% of the U.S. population is estimated to have diabetes.[17] In 1996 alone, there were 798,000 new cases of diabetes diagnosed. This becomes even more significant with increasing age as the prevalence of diabetes increases to 18% in the population over age 65.[17] Of the U.S. diabetic population, it is estimated that 15% will develop manifestations of diabetic foot disease in their lifetime.[18] In addition, diabetics have an annual incidence of 2 to 3% for developing a foot ulceration.[18] Although representing only 6% of the population, diabetics account for 46% of the 162,000 hospital admissions for foot ulcers annually.[18] This prevalence of foot disease in the diabetic population results in significant clinical and economic impact. Data from the National Hospital Discharge Survey demonstrates that approximately 51% of nontraumatic lower extremity amputations are performed on diabetics.[19] The age-adjusted amputation rate is between 15–40% higher in diabetics than nondiabetics.[19]

The American Diabetes Association consensus group found that for patients with diabetes, the risk of ulceration was increased among males, patients with poor glucose control, those with the disease for more than 10 years, or those with cardiovascular, retinal, or renal complications.[2] Diabetics are prone to atherosclerotic disease as well as neuropathy. As the disease process progresses, alterations in distal perfusion can be experienced and a

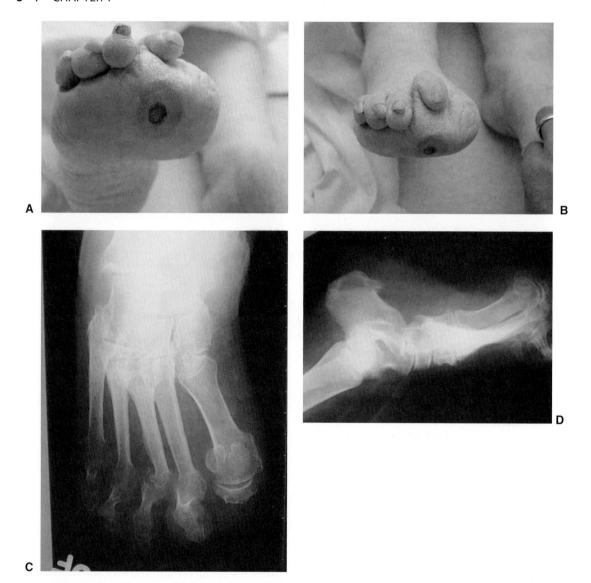

Figure 1–4. Example of neurotropic ulcer. ***A.*** Plantar second metatarsal head ulcer, well perfused, but neurotropic. Pressures often increase in this area after hallux amputations. ***B.*** Note the hammertoe deformity of the second digit. ***C.*** Corresponding foot x-ray showing subluxation at the second MTP joint. ***D.*** Lateral view of same patient.

neuropathic component may become apparent. Atherosclerotic complications are seen at a younger age in diabetics and tend to involve the tibioperoneal vessels with sparing of the pedal vasculature.[20] The relative sparing of pedal vessels becomes relevant as they facilitate and become excellent targets for distal bypass. Neuropathy is shown to be present in 42% of diabetics after 20 years.[21] and is usually a distal symmetric sensorimotor polyneuropathy affecting both myelinated type-A fibers and unmyelinated type-C fibers. Diabetic neuropathy manifests with reduced or absent reflexes, sensory loss in a stocking and glove distribution, and intrinsic muscle wasting. Furthermore, the ability of diabetic patients to ward off even superficial infections is impaired. Purely ischemic diabetic foot ulcers are uncommon, representing between 10–15% of ulcers.[22] More commonly, ulcers have a mixed ischemic and neuropathic origin representing 33% (Table 1–2).[22]

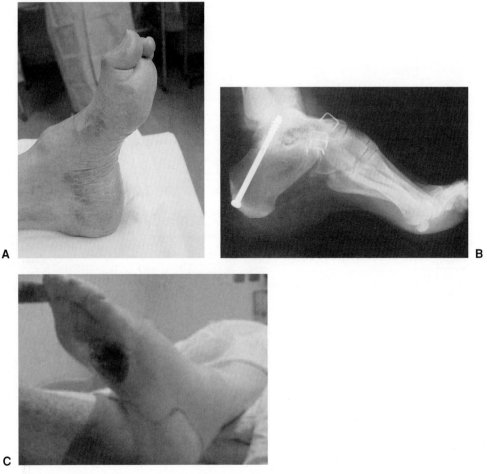

Figure 1–5. Patient with an equinovarus deformity of foot, secondary to resection of the peroneal complex. ***A.*** Picture of the leg. ***B.*** X-ray of the leg. ***C.*** Foot wound along the lateral edge due to equinovarus.

WOUND ASSESSMENT AND MANAGEMENT

Successful management of foot ulcers involves recognition and correction of the underlying etiology, as well as appropriate wound care and prevention of recurrence. Assessment of the ulcer consists of determining the size and depth of the wound and inspection of the surrounding area for local signs of infection or gangrene. Several classification systems have been devised for descriptive purposes and to act as prognostic indicators (Table 1–4).[23]

The absence of systemic manifestations, such as fever, chills, or leukocytosis is an unreliable indicator of underlying infection, especially in the diabetic immunocompromised population and the use of plain films to rule out osteomyelitis, or deep culture of the wound are

frequently needed. Aggressive mechanical débridement, systemic antibiotic therapy, and strict nonweight bearing are the cornerstones for effective wound care. Sharp débridement in the operating room or at the bedside, when applicable, allows for thorough removal of all necrotic material and optimizes the wound environment. Foot soaks, whirlpool therapy, or enzymatic débridement have a use but are rarely effective and may lead to further skin maceration or wound breakdown. There are no prospective randomized studies demonstrating the superiority of dressing products compared to standard saline wet to dry sterile gauze in establishing a granulation bed. Use of moist dressings in clean, granulating wounds has been recommended to enhance the wound environment. In cases of gross wound infections and rampant cellulitis, use of a silver containing medication, such as Silvadene, may be necessary in the initial

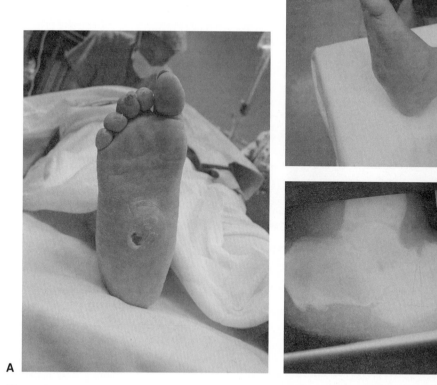

Figure 1–6. Example of an ulcer occurring in a patient with a Charcot foot deformity. **A.** Plantar view of the ulcer. **B.** Medial view of the ulcer. Note the severe equinous deformity and the rockerbottom foot. **C.** X-ray of the foot demonstrating the subluxed midfoot.

setting to reduce the bacterial load. Oral antimicrobial therapy should be instituted based on the suspected pathogen and clinical findings. Intravenous antimicrobials should be administered for severe infections. Future advances, such as use of bioactive drugs (eg, Recombinant PDGF, Regranex) or skin substitutes (eg, Apligraf, Dermagraft) are showing promising results and have proved useful under specific circumstances.

VASCULAR ASSESSMENT AND MANAGEMENT

Once a wound has been evaluated and initially managed, the emphasis turns to early accurate assessment of possible impaired perfusion. In the majority of patients, the presence of a palpable pedal pulse is a good indicator of adequate vascular supply for wound healing. In patients with weak or absent pulses, however, adequacy of perfusion and healing potential are assessed initially by noninvasive physiological studies.[24] These include

measurement of segmental limb pressures, pulse volume waveform assessment, and transcutaneous oxygen measurements. It must be emphasized that any given patient may require only selected tests.

Segmental limb pressures are an extension of the bedside ankle–brachial index (ABI) (Table 1–5).[25,26] They are indicated in any patient whose history and physical examination is suggestive of peripheral vascular disease. By obtaining pressures at successive levels on the extremity, the area of disease can typically be localized. Measurement of an ankle pressure <40 mm Hg suggests a low likelihood of healing (Table 1–1). Diabetics with medial sclerosis and patients with chronic renal insufficiency often have nonocclusive calcified vessels, showing ABIs >1.3, and limiting the utility of segmental limb pressures in the vascular evaluation. It may be necessary, therefore, to look at toe pressure measurements, transcutaneous oximetry, or waveform analysis.

The toe–brachial index (TBI) is a more reliable indicator of foot perfusion in diabetics because the small vessels

Table 1–4. Common Wound Classification Systems

Meggitt/Wagner classification of foot ulcers	
Grade 0:	Cellulitis present with no open lesions
Grade 1:	Superficial ulcer
Grade 2:	Deep ulcer involving tendon, bone, or joint capsule
Grade 3:	Localized infection (abscess or osteomyelitis)
Grade 4:	Forefoot gangrene
Grade 5:	Gangrene to the majority of the foot

University of Texas diabetic wound classification system	
Grade 0:	Preulcerative or site of healed ulcer
Grade 1:	Superficial wounds through the epidermis or dermis, but not to tendon, capsule, or bone
Grade 2:	Deep wounds penetrating to tendon or capsule but not bone
Grade 3:	Deep wounds penetrating to bone or into a joint
	Stage A: Clean wound without infection
	Stage B: Nonischemic infected wound
	Stage C: Ischemic noninfected wound
	Stage D: Infected ischemic wounds

Yale University diabetic foot wound classification system	
Stage 0:	Preulcerative lesion
	A. Without sign of necrosis or soft tissue infection
	B. With necrosis
	C. Tissue infection with or without necrosis
Stage 1:	Superficial ulcer extending into dermis
	A. Without sign of necrosis or soft tissue infection
	B. With necrosis
	C. Tissue infection with or without necrosis
Stage 2:	Deep ulcer extending into subcutaneous fat
	A. Without sign of necrosis or soft tissue infection
	B. With necrosis
	C. Tissue infection with or without necrosis
Stage 3:	Deep ulcer involving tendon, ligament, or joint capsule
	A. Without sign of necrosis or soft tissue infection
	B. With necrosis
	C. Tissue infection with or without necrosis
Stage 4:	Deep ulcer involving bone
	A. Without sign of necrosis or soft tissue infection
	B. With necrosis
	C. Tissue infection with or without necrosis

Table 1–5. ABI and TBI Values: Normal and Various Clinical Presentations

	ABI	TBI
Normal	1.11 ± 0.10	$>0.60 \pm 0.17$
Claudication	0.59 ± 0.15	0.35 ± 0.15
Rest Pain	0.26 ± 0.13	0.11 ± 0.10
Tissue Loss	0.05 ± 0.08	0.11 ± 0.10

of the toes are often spared of medial calcification (Table 1–5). The absolute toe pressures are valuable in the estimation of ulcer healing potential with a pressure >30 mm Hg being favorable for wound healing (Table 1–1).[27]

An adjunctive method for establishing the disease level is through waveform analysis using pulse volume recordings (PVR) (Table 1–6).[28] PVRs are obtained through the application of sequential blood pressure cuffs with an air pleythysmographic technique. The normal PVR waveform has a sharp upstroke and peak with a reflected wave present before returning to baseline (Fig. 1–7A). With mild obstruction, the reflected wave is lost, the up-stroke delayed, and the peak blunted (Fig. 1–7B). Moderate to severe obstruction produces a bowing of the down-stroke away from the baseline (Fig. 1–7C). A flat PVR is irregular with low amplitude and indicates severe obstruction (Fig. 1–7D).

Segmental blood pressure testing, TBI measurements, and waveform analysis can be performed before and after exercise to unmask occlusive disease not apparent on resting studies. With exercise, blood flow normally increases three- to fivefold to meet the increased demand and resistance in the muscular bed. The presence of significant stenosis limits this compensatory response and magnifies the pressure gradient across the lesion. A normal response to exercise is a slight increase, or no change, in the ankle systolic pressure compared to baseline and rules out vascular insufficiency as the cause of symptoms. A fall in ankle pressure by more than 20% of baseline, or below an absolute pressure of 60 mm Hg requiring more than 3 minutes to recover, is considered abnormal.[29] Single-level disease is inferred with a recovery time less than 6 minutes and multilevel disease is

Table 1–6. Normal Velocity Values in the Lower Extremity

	Velocity (cm/s)
Aorta	100 ± 20
CIA/EIA	119 ± 22
CFA	114 ± 25
SFA	94 ± 14
Pop	69 ± 14

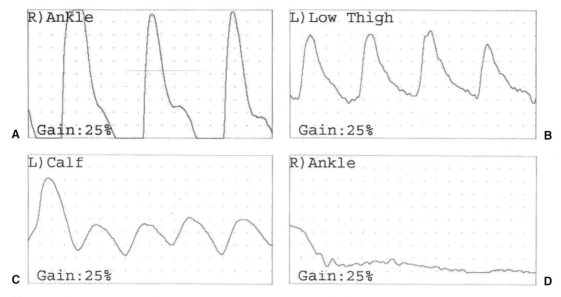

Figure 1-7. Examples of PVR waveforms. **A.** Normal Waveforms. Note the sharp upstroke and peak with a reflected wave. **B.** Mild obstruction. Reflected wave is lost, up-stroke is delayed, and peak is blunted. **C.** Moderate to severe disease. Note how the down-stroke is bowed away from the baseline. **D.** Severe obstruction; waveform is flat.

inferred with a recovery time greater than 6 minutes. The administration of pharmacological agents, such as Priscoline, or the induction of reactive hyperemia can be performed in place of exercise testing in patients with limited exercise ability due to cardiopulmonary disease or musculoskeletal problems.

Transcutaneous oxygen measurement ($TcPO_2$) may provide supplemental information regarding local tissue perfusion. Platinum oxygen electrodes are placed on the chest wall, as well as the legs or feet. The absolute value of oxygen tension at the foot or leg can be determined and a ratio of this value to that of the chest wall may be evaluated. A normal value at the foot is 60 mm Hg and a normal chest/foot ratio is 0.9.[30] Controversy exists regarding the optimal level for tissue healing. It is generally accepted that wounds are likely to heal if oxygen tension is greater than 40 mm Hg (foot/chest ratio >0.5) and that healing is not likely with a value less than 20 mm Hg. $TcPO_2$ measurements can also be obtained in conjunction with exercise testing. Normally, the value will not diminish, however, in the patient with arterial occlusive disease, the value will fall. It should be noted that factors such as excessive lower extremity edema could alter the $TcPO_2$ measurement and lead to inaccurate readings.

Magnetic resonance angiography (MRA) has rapidly come to the forefront as a noninvasive vascular imaging modality and serves as a supplemental method for closely assessing the vasculature in patients with severe IV con-

trast allergy, contrast-induced nephropathy, or severe inflow disease and slow distal flow. MRA can display reconstructed images as a conventional arteriogram with excellent demonstration from the infrainguinal arteries to the small vessels of the foot. It is particularly useful for visualization of the distal vessels of the leg and foot in patients with severe proximal occlusive disease. MRA has been shown to be more sensitive in identifying patent vessels at all levels in patients with severe disease with the greatest difference seen in the distal vasculature.[31] It can be used to quantitate the degree of arterial stenosis with a reasonable degree of correlation to conventional angiography[32] and has been used to measure blood flow velocities. However, MRA is still expensive and is not used as an initial vascular assessment tool, but is most appropriate when more detailed studies are needed in patients who are poor candidates for invasive testing.

IV contrast angiography continues to be the gold standard for imaging of the blood vessels and is traditionally reserved for anatomic assessment prior to a planned intervention. The procedure is performed in the angiography suite by interventional radiologists usually utilizing a femoral puncture for access. Following completion of the procedure and removal of the sheath, the access area must be observed for the development of hematoma and the extremity evaluated for any evidence for peripheral embolization.

The arteriographic appearance of the vessels can distinguish the level and severity of disease as well as suggest an etiology. Atherosclerosis produces segmental or diffuse plaques with varying degrees of stenosis. Because atherosclerotic plaques are often asymmetric and eccentric, multiple planner views are necessary for an accurate assessment. The formation of collateral vessels is seen in patients with chronic disease and abrupt contrast cut-offs without collateralization suggests arterial embolization. Aneurysms might be inferred from an enlarged lumen, however, when partially thrombosed they may be difficult to visualize. Arterial wall medial calcification can be demonstrated on scout films prior to injection with IV contrast and the severity estimated. One of the main advantages of contrast angiography over noninvasive methods is the potential for intervention at the time of the study by performing percutaneous transluminal angioplasty (PTA) or stenting procedures.

In summary, the assessment of a patient with foot ulcers stemming from peripheral vascular disease encompasses a thorough history and physical examination with the adjunctive use of the noninvasive vascular laboratory to confirm, localize, and grade lesions. While multiple noninvasive and invasive methods are available to assess the peripheral vasculature, it should be obvious that not every patient requires an exhaustive battery of tests in order to evaluate their vascular status. In general, only those tests likely to provide information that alters the course of action should be performed. Differing clinical syndromes mandate the extent of peripheral vascular testing. It is imperative that flow-limiting arterial lesions are evaluated and reconstructed or bypassed if ischemic foot ulcers are to heal.

NEUROPATHY AND MUSCULOSKELETAL ASSESSMENT AND MANAGEMENT

Cutaneous pressure perception measured by Semmes–Weinstein monofilaments is widely considered to be an ideal screening instrument for neuropathy and potential for ulceration, because of its simplicity, sensitivity, and low cost.[33–35] People with normal foot sensation can usually feel a 4.17 filament, which is equivalent to 1 g of linear pressure. Patients who cannot detect a 5.07 monofilament when it buckles (equivalent to 10 g of linear pressure) are considered to have lost protective sensation.[36] Several cross-sectional studies have indicated that foot ulceration is strongly associated with elevated cutaneous pressure perception thresholds. Magnitudes of association, however, were provided in a case-control study by McNeely et al.,[37] who reported an unadjusted sevenfold risk of ulceration in those patients (97% male) with insensitivity to the 5.07 monofilament. Abnormal mechanical forces that can result in ulcerations should be addressed with the use of off-loading devices or other modalities in order to assist in wound healing.

The presence of neuropathy mandates attention to the biomechanics of the foot. The role of the podiatrist or foot surgeon in evaluation of these patients cannot be underscored enough. Use of F scan to assess abnormally high pressure areas has led to greater use of orthotic devices in the prevention of skin breakdown. This computerized gait analysis system uses an ultrathin Tekscan sensor consisting of 960 sensor cells (5 mm^2 each). The sensor is used in a floor mat system designed to measure barefoot or stocking-foot dynamic plantar pressures indicating those subjects with pressures $\geq$6 kg/cm^2. Off-loading strategies, such as total contact casting or removable walkers, has resulted in significant decreases in healing times. The stresses placed upon the foot can be intrinsic in nature, as was previously described with respect to digital contractures, or extrinsic in nature. These external forces can result from inappropriate footwear, traumatic injury, and/or foreign bodies. Shoes that are too tight or too shallow are a frequent, yet preventable, component to the development of neuropathic ulcers. Boulton, et al.[13] and Veves et al.[14] demonstrated that there is an increase in both static and dynamic foot pressures when evaluating the neuropathic foot. To date, high pressures alone have not been shown to cause foot ulceration. Masson et al.[38] evaluated high plantar foot pressures in rheumatoid patients with no sensitivity deficit and noted that there was no evidence of foot ulceration. A variety of shoe modifications, such as rocker sole design and different types of insoles, have shown that it is possible to reduce plantar foot pressures, thus decreasing risks of ulceration.[39–41]

Reconstructive foot surgery may often become the conservative treatment in order to avoid major amputations in these chronic neuropathic wounds. The endpoint for chronic diabetic foot wounds should include reduction in the number of major amputations, prevention of infection, decrease probability of ulceration, maintaining skin integrity, and improvement of function. Successful outcomes for diabetic foot reconstruction should result in less intrinsic pressures via minor amputations, arthroplasties, osteotomies, chondylectomies, exostectomies, tendon procedures, and joint arthodesis. Open wounds can be treated in one stage and are primarily closed with premorbid tissue using local flap reconstruction and soft tissue repair.[42] Plastic surgical repair of these wounds can help avoid the production of inelastic scar tissue over weight-bearing surfaces. Extrinsic pressures and intrinsic pressures can be further neutralized with postop accommodative shoe gear. Prophylactic diabetic foot surgery may prevent recurrent ulceration and decrease the risk of major amputations.[43,44] Surgical biomechanics, plastic and soft-tissue reconstruction, as well as appropriate off loading are all essential to creating a stable platform from which to keep these difficult patients free from tissue breakdown and as functional as possible.

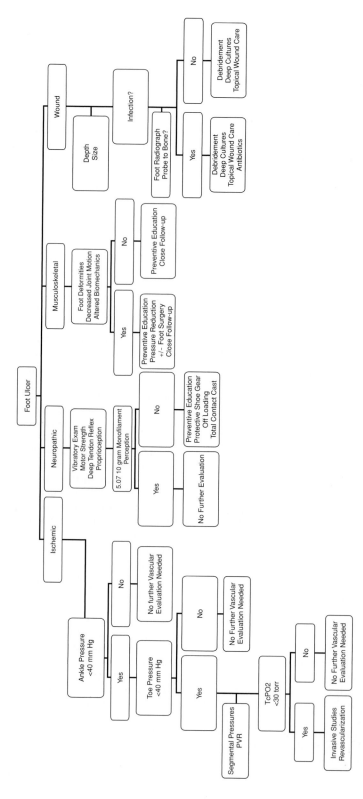

Figure 1–8. Algorithm for assessment and management of foot ulcers.

SUMMARY

It was shown in 1986 that, "chronic skin ulcers" added up to significant costs.[19] The average cost of a lower extremity amputation in the 1990s was calculated to be between $24,000 and $40,000.[45] In 1990, $600 million was spent on the 54,000 lower-extremity amputations performed that year.[19] The role of the vascular surgeon in the evaluation, diagnosis, and management of foot ulcers is critical.[46] Foot disease is a common complication of diabetes that can have tragic consequences. For the majority of patients with foot ulcers, adherence to the principles outlined above will suffice for optimum treatment of these wounds (Fig. 1–8).

Tight glucose control can reduce microvascular diabetic complications, including peripheral sensory neuropathy and thus development of foot ulcers. Patient education is essential for risk-factor reduction and early recognition of foot complications (Table 1–7).

Table 1–7. SIX P's of Prevention

Podiatric care
- Regular visits, examinations and foot care
- Risk Assessment
- Early detection and aggressive treatment of new lesions

Pulse examination
- Evaluation for claudication and rest pain
- Assessment of foot pulses; non-invasive vascular testing when indicated

Protective shoes
- Adequate room to protect from injury; well cushioned
- Walking sneakers, extra depth, custom-molded shoes
- Special modifications as necessary

Pressure reduction
- Pressure measurements
- Cushioned insoles, custom orthoses, padded hosiery

Prophylactic surgery
- Correct structural deformities—hammertoes, bunions, Charcot
- Prevent recurrent ulcers over deformities
- Intervene at opportune time

Preventive education
- Patient education-need for daily inspection and necessity for early intervention
- Physician education for significance of foot lesions, importance of regular foot examinations and current concepts in diabetic foot management

---

Awareness and training of healthcare providers in diagnosing and treating diabetic foot disease is paramount and may begin with such simple measures as adding a wall poster or chart reminder to conduct foot examinations on all diabetic patients at every office visit.

The population affected by foot disease represents a significant portion of the elderly and diabetic communities. The major areas of influence include neuropathy, arterial vascular disease, and infection. Special attention is required in an attempt to limit morbidity and extend limb life in the diabetic patient. These include patient education and frequent inspection of the neuropathic foot. Careful assessment of vascular disease leading to bypass surgery when indicated, evaluation and management of biomechanical abnormalities, and aggressive treatment of any infections is also required to affect the natural history of this disease.[47] The multidisciplinary approach to limb salvage will enable us to provide a comprehensive treatment protocol yielding greater long-term viability of the lower extremity.

Advances in telemedicine will allow both the patient and care provider greater opportunity for interaction, which will hopefully improve patient management. The Internet will allow for real-time evaluation of wounds from the home setting decreasing transportation needs and costs. Last, with advances digital photography, it is probable that diabetic patients and their physicians will be able to access ulcer history and progression from a diskette that forms part of the medical record. Such systems require a way for the care providers to categorize and share critical data, which is simple to use, yet powerful enough to communicate management options.

ACKNOWLEDGMENTS

The authors wish to acknowledge the use of an unrestricted grant from the North American Foundation for Limb Preservation in the preparation of this manuscript.

REFERENCES

1. Sumpio B. Foot ulcers. *New Engl J Med.* 2000;343(11): 787–793.
2. American Diabetes Association. Preventive foot care in people with diabetes [position statement]. *Diabetes Care Suppl. 1.* 1999;22.
3. Simon DA, McCollum CN. Approaches to venus leg ulcers within the community: Compression, pinch grafts and simple venus surgery. *Ostomy Wound Manage.* 1996;42:34–40.
4. Lazarus GS, Cooper DM, Knighton DR, et al. Definitions and guidelines for assessment and evaluation of healing. *Arch Dermatol.* 1994;130:489–493.
5. Harkiss KJ. Cost analysis of dressing material used in venus leg ulcers. *Pharm J (August).* 1985;268–279.
6. Olin JW, Beusterien KM, Childs MB, et al. Medical costs of treating venus stasis ulcers: Evidence from a retrospective cohort study. *Vasc Med.* 1999;4:1–7.

7. Phillips TJ, Dover JS. Leg ulcers. *J Am Acad Dermatol.* 1991;25:965–987.

8. Browse NL, Burnand KG. The postphlebitic syndrome: A new look. In: Bergan JJ, Tao JST, eds. *Venous Problems.* Chicago, Ill: Year Book, 1978;395–404.

9. Dewolfe VG. The prevention and management of chronic venous insufficiency. *Pract Cardiol.* 1980;6:197–202.

10. Phillips TJ, Stanton B, Provan A, et al. A study of the impact of leg ulcers on quality of life: Financial, social, and psychological implications. *J Am Acad Dermatol.* 1994;31:49–53.

11. Hutton W, Stokes I. The mechanics of the foot. In: Klenerman L, ed. *The Foot and Its Disorders.* Oxford: Blackwell Scientific; 1991;11–25.

12. Levin ME: Preventing amputation in the patient with diabetes. *Diabetes Care.* 1995;18:1383.

13. Boulton A, Hardisty C, Betts R, Franks C, Worth R, Ward J, et al. Dynamic foot pressure and other studies as diagnostic and management aids in diabetic neuropathy. *Diabetes Care.* 1983;6:26–33.

14. Veves A, Fernando D, Walewski P, et al. A study of plantar pressures in a diabetic clinic population. *Foot.* 1991;2:89–92.

15. Saltzman CL, Pedowitz WJ: Diabetic foot infection. In *AAOS Instructional Course Lectures,* Vol. 48. 1999:317.

16. Habershaw G, Chzran J. Biomechanical considerations of the diabetic foot. *Management of Diabetic Foot Problems.* 2nd ed Philadelphia: Saunders; 1995:53–65.

17. U.S. Department of Health and Human Services National Diabetes Fact Sheet; 1998.

18. Reiber G, Lipsky B, Gibbons G. The burden of diabetic foot ulcers. *Am J Surg.* 1998;176:5S–10S.

19. Reiber G, EJ B, Smith D. Lower extremity foot ulcers and amputations in diabetes. In: Harris, ed. *Diabetes in America.* 2nd ed. Bethesda, MD: National Institutes of Health Publication; 1995:409–427.

20. Kamal K, Powell RJ, Sumpio BE. The pathobiology of diabetes mellitus: Implications for surgeons. *J Am Coll Surg.* 1996;186:271–289.

21. O'Brien I, Corrall R. Epidemiology of diabetes and its complications. *N Eng J Med.* 1988;318(24):1619–1623.

22. Laing P. The development and complications of diabetic foot ulcers. *Am J Surg.* 1998;176:11S–19S.

23. Frangos S, Kilaru S, Blume P, Shin J, Sumpio B. Classification of diabetic foot ulcers: Improving communication. *Int J Angiol.* 2002;11:1–7.

24. Collins K, Sumpio B. Vascular Assessment. In: Blume P, ed. *Clinics in Podiatric Medicine and Surgery.* Philadelphia: Saunders; 2000.

25. Yao JST. Hemodynamic studies in peripheral arterial disease. *Br J Surg.* 1970;57:761.

26. Carter S, Lezack JD. Digital systolic pressures in the lower limbs in arterial disease. *Circulation.* 1971;43:905–914.

27. Orchard T, Strandness DJ. Assessment of peripheral vascular disease in diabetes: report and recommendation of an international workshop sponsored by the American Diabetes Association and the American Heart Association, September 18–20, 1992 New Orleans, Louisiana. *Circulation.* 1993;88:819–832.

28. Strandness DE, Jr. Peripheral arterial system. *Duplex Scanning in Vascular Disorders.* 2nd ed. New York: Raven Press; 1993;159.

29. Weitz J, Bynre J, Clagett P. Diagnosis and treatment of chronic arterial insuffiiciency of the lower extremites: A critical review. *Circulation.* 1996;94:3026–3033.

30. Byrne P, Provan J, Ameli F, et al. The use of transcutaneous oxygen tension measurements in the diagnosis of peripheral vascular insufficiency. *Ann Surg.* 1984;200:159–167.

31. Carpenter JP, Owen RS, Baum RA, et al. Magnetic resonance angiography of peripheral runoff vessels. *J Vasc Surg.* 1992;16:807.

32. Hertz SM, Baum RA, Owen RS, et al. Peripheral arterial stenosis: Comparison of magnetic resonance and contrast arteriography. *Am J Surg.* 1993;166:112.

33. Lavery L, Armstrong D, Vela S. Practical criteria for screening patients at high risk for diabetic foot ulceration. *Arch Intern Med.* 1998;158(2):157–162.

34. Kumar S, Fernando D, Veves A, Knowles E, Young M, AJM B. Semmes–Weinstein monofilaments: a simple, effective and inexpensive screening device for identifying diabetic patients at risk of foot ulceration. *Diabetes Res Clin Pract.* 1991;13:63–68.

35. Simeone L, Veves A. Screening techniques to identify the diabetic patient at risk of ulceration. *J Am Podiatr Med Assoc.* 1997;87:313–317.

36. Birke J, Sims D. Plantar sensory threshold in the ulcerative foot. *Leprosy Rev.* 1986;57:261–267.

37. McNeely M, Boyko E, Ahroni J, Stensel V, Reiber G, Smith D, et al. The independent contributions of diabetic neuropathy and vasculopathy in foot ulceration: how great are the risks? *Diabetes Care.* 1995;18:216–219.

38. Masson E, Hay E, Stockley I, Veves A, Betts R, Boulton A. Abnormal foot pressures alone may not cause ulceration. *Diabetic Med.* 1989;6:426–428.

39. Barrow J, Hughes J, Clark P, et al. A study of the effect of wear on the pressure-relieving properties of foot orthosis. *Foot.* 1992;1:195–199.

40. Boulton A, Franks C, Betts R, Duckworth T, Ward J. Reduction of abnormal foot pressures in diabetic neuropathy using new polymer insole material. *Diabetes Care.* 1984;7:42–46.

41. Nawoczenski D, Birke J, Coleman W. Effect of rocker sole design on plantar forefoot pressures. *J Am Podiatr Med Assoc.* 1988;78:455–460.

42. Blume P, Partagas L, Sumpio B, Attinger C. Single stage surgical treatment of noninfected diabetic foot ulcers. *J. Plastic Reconst Surg.* 2002;109:601–609.

43. Armstrong D, Lavery L, Stern S, Harkless L. Is prophylactic diabetic foot surgery dangerous? *J Foot Ankle Surg.* 1996;35(6):585–589.

44. Catanzariti A, Blitch E, Karlock L. Elective foot and ankle surgery in the diabetic patient. *J Foot Ankle Surg.* 1995;34(1):23–41.

45. Ollendorf D, Kotsanos J, Wishner W, Friedman M, Cooper T, Bittoni M, et al. Potential economic benefits of lower extremity amputation prevention strategies in diabetes. *Diabetes Care.* 1998;21:1240–1245.

46. Knox R, Dutch W, Blume P, Sumpio B. Diabetic Foot Disease. *Int J Angiol.* 2000;1(1):1–6.

47. Yeager R, Moneta G, Edwards J, Williamson W, McConnell D, Taylor L, et al. Predictors of outcome of forefoot surgery for ulceration and gangrene. *Am J Surg.* 1998;175(5):388–390.

2 Molecular Therapy for Wounds: Modalities for Stimulating Angiogenesis and Granulation

Vincent W. Li, Elaine F. Kung, and William W. Li

Introduction
Differences between Acute Versus Chronic Wounds
Wound Healing at the Molecular Level
Angiogenesis and Granulation
  Overview of Wound Angiogenesis
  Angiogenic Growth Factors in Wounds
  Wound Extracellular Matrix as Infrastructure for Angiogenesis
  Bone Marrow-Derived Stem Cells
Prerequisites for the Use of Advanced Therapies
Targeting Wound Healing at the Molecular Level
  Growth Factor Therapy for Wound Healing
  Gene Transfer
Tissue-Engineered Skin Constructs for Wound Healing
  Epidermal Substitutes

  Dermal Substitutes
  Extracellular Matrices (Nonliving)
  Bilayered Skin Substitutes
  Next Generation of Tissue Engineering
Stem Cells for Wound Angiogenesis and Wound Healing
  Bone Marrow-Derived Cells
  Endothelial Progenitor Cells
Devices that Facilitate Wound Healing and Their Role in Wound Neovascularization
  Hyperbaric Oxygen Therapy (HBO)
  Vacuum-Assisted Closure
  Electrical Stimulation
  Laser and Optical Stimulation
  Radiofrequency Ablation
Future Directions for Wound Angiogenesis and Wound Healing
References

INTRODUCTION

Chronic wounds cause significant morbidity and impairment to quality of life in more than 4 million patients each year in the United States.[1] Common poorly healing wounds include diabetic or neuropathic ulcers, venous or arterial insufficiency ulcers, and pressure ulcers. Conventional wound care has primarily consisted of passive interventions, such as dressings, antimicrobial agents, and off-loading devices. Recent advancements over the past decade, however, have brought into clinical use new therapeutic technologies that actively stimulate healing at the molecular level.

Successful wound healing depends upon angiogenesis—the growth of new capillary blood vessels. Clinically, new capillaries first become visible in the wound bed 3 to 5 days after injury and their appearance is synonymous with granulation, the creation of a provisional matrix comprised of proliferating blood vessels, migrating fibroblasts, and new collagen.[2] Impaired granulation is a classic hallmark of the chronic wounds encountered with diabetes and venous or arterial insufficiency. Wound angiogenesis has thus become a major focus of study and therapeutic development. Because angiogenesis is required for healing all wounds, its induction is clinically beneficial in many situations where rapid wound closure is required. The advent of therapeutic growth factors, gene therapy, tissue-engineered constructs, stem cell therapy, and other drugs and devices that act through cellular and molecular-based mechanisms, is enabling the modern surgeon and wound-care provider to actively promote wound angiogenesis to accelerate healing. This chapter reviews the basis for therapeutic angiogenesis in wound care and describes both the biological principles and clinical applications of current and emerging angiogenic treatment modalities.

DIFFERENCES BETWEEN ACUTE VERSUS CHRONIC WOUNDS

Acute wounds heal in a well-orchestrated multistep process, involving a series of interrelated cellular and molecular events. A modern interpretation of the wound healing cascade can be most simply described as involving: hemostasis, inflammation, angiogenesis, epithelialization, and remodeling.[3] This process assists in restoring the integrity and function of the damaged tissue.

By contrast, a *chronic nonhealing wound* has been defined as a wound that fails to proceed through the orderly and timely series of events required to produce a durable structural, functional, and cosmetically acceptable closure.[4] Wound specialists commonly define a chronic wound as one that has failed to heal after 4 to 6 weeks of conservative management. Chronic wounds are also characterized by cellular senescence. In such wounds, a fraction of critical cells are incapable of dividing, and have only a muted ability to respond to growth factor stimulation. Studies of venous stasis ulcers have shown that a marker for "difficult to heal" ulcers is if the percentage of cell populations that are senescent is >15%.[5] Cells from biopsy specimens obtained from the margins of chronic wounds are significantly less capable of proliferating in response to exogenous growth factors than corresponding cells from acute wounds.[6,7] In addition, growth factor levels in the chronic wound appear to be insufficient to sustain cell proliferation. In contrast to normally healing wounds that have a high level of mitogenic activity, wound fluid collected from chronic wounds stimulates lower levels DNA synthesis.[8] Epithelial cells from chronic wounds have a reduced capacity for migration. Wounds that do not close (epithelialize) faster than 0.5 mm/week are not likely to heal. Furthermore, while wound proteases—matrix metalloproteinases (MMPs) that enzymatically degrade proteins in damaged cells and matrix—are required for normal wound healing, excessive levels of MMPs in chronic wound fluid can adversely degrade protein growth factors, matrix, and granulation tissue.[9–11] Hence, early

intervention, proper wound bed preparation, and advanced therapies are now used to halt and reverse the progression of chronic wounds.[12]

WOUND HEALING AT THE MOLECULAR LEVEL

Initially following injury, a network of fibrin, thrombin, red blood cells, and platelets serves to tamponade injured capillaries and ensure hemostasis. Thrombin stimulates angiogenesis by a variety of mechanisms including: promoting the detachment of endothelial cells from the basement membrane of existing blood vessels; promoting endothelial cell migration through the $\alpha_v\beta_3$ integrin, a cell surface adhesion molecule; stimulating the release of vascular endothelial growth factor (VEGF) from platelets and smooth muscle cells; and enhancing vascular survival through interactions with the $\alpha_v\beta_3$ integrin.[13] Activated platelets release growth factors, such as VEGF, platelet-derived growth factor (PDGF), basic fibroblast growth factor (bFGF), transforming growth factor beta (TGF-β), hepatocyte growth factor (HGF), and angiopoietin-1 (Ang-1).[14–18] The fibrin clot becomes a temporary scaffold upon which inflammatory cells, fibroblasts, and endothelial cells invade during tissue repair.[19] Cytokines and growth factors chemotactically attract neutrophils, monocytes, and macrophages into the wound bed, leading to the inflammatory phase of healing. Inflammatory cells kill microorganisms and release matrix metalloproteinases (MMPs) necessary to remove damaged extracellular matrix components. In addition, activated macrophages secrete PDGF, bFGF, VEGF, TGF-β, HGF, angiopoietin-1, and insulin-like growth factor-1.[20] Furthermore, tumor necrosis factor-alpha (TNF-α) and interleukin-1-alpha (IL-1α) secreted by monocytes and macrophages induce endothelial cells to produce cell adhesion molecules. In response, the endothelial cells express interleukin-8 (IL-8), which stimulates adhesion molecules on inflammatory cells. This facilitates binding of inflammatory cells to the blood vessel wall, and then margination into wound bed tissue. TNF-α and IL-1α stimulate fibroblast proliferation and collagen synthesis, as well as up-regulate MMP production. These cytokines also down-regulate tissue inhibitor of metalloproteinases (TIMPs) and interferon gamma (IFN-γ), which inhibit fibroblasts migration and collagen synthesis.

As the inflammatory phase of wound healing wanes, the fibroblasts and endothelial cells continue producing growth factors and maintain high levels of cell proliferation. This stage is known as the proliferative phase of wound healing. Fibroblasts secrete IGF-1, FGF-2, TGF-β, PDGF, VEGF, and keratinocyte growth factor (KGF); endothelial cells produce VEGF, FGF-2, TGF-β, and PDGF; and keratinocytes generate TGF-α, TGF-β, and VEGF. These cytokines and growth factors stimulate cell proliferation, extracellular matrix production, and new capillary formation, all vital to new tissue formation.[21] Endothelial cells release collagenase and plasminogen activators, which degrade vascular basement membranes and fibrin clot, allowing invasion of endothelial capillary beds into the wound. The fibroblasts produce extracellular matrix molecules, such as proteoglycans, glycosaminoglycans, and fibronectins, which reinforce the provisional matrix onto which tissue proliferation can occur.

After epithelialization and the formation of an initial scar, the wound undergoes a remodeling phase, which may last for months. During this phase, equilibrium is achieved between the synthesis of new scar matrix and its degradation. Fibroblasts synthesize extracellular matrix components, such as, collagen, elastin, and proteoglycans, but also produce MMPs and TIMPs. Fibroblasts also produce lysyl oxidase, which cross-links extracellular matrix components. During this phase, angiogenesis ceases and the density of capillaries also decreases in the wound site.

Normally, wound healing occurs rapidly in a dynamic molecular environment suitable for the hemostasis, inflammatory, proliferative, and remodeling phases. Chronic wounds are deficient in granulation tissue, which is essential for establishing the nutritional network needed to support regenerative tissue. Chronic wounds also show delayed epithelialization as a result of decreased cellular proliferative and migratory capacity.[22,23] Defective formation of the supporting stroma occurs in the chronic wound as well. Excessive protease production can lead to growth factor degradation and diminution of the proliferative capacity of the wound.[24,25] Coupled with cellular senescence, these complex, multifactorial forces contribute to impaired wound healing.[26]

ANGIOGENESIS AND GRANULATION

Overview of Wound Angiogenesis

Because granulation is a vital process in wound healing, understanding the molecular mechanisms that regulate wound angiogenesis is useful in treating chronic wounds. Although granulation is often assigned to the proliferative stage in the classic wound-healing model, angiogenesis is actually initiated immediately upon wounding and is mediated throughout the entire healing process. We have proposed an "angiogenesis model of wound healing" to fully describe the role of wound neovascularization:

Step 1. **Angiogenesis Initiation.** Tissue damage leads to the release of bFGF normally sequestered within intact cells and the extracellular matrix.[27] Bleeding and hemostasis in a wound also initiates angiogenesis. The first clot element present in a wound, thrombin, is a potent stimulator of endothelial cells. Thrombin up-regulates cellular receptors for VEGF and potentiates the effect of this growth factor.[28] Endothelial cells exposed to thrombin also release gelatinase A, which promotes the local dissolution of basement membrane, an essential early step of angiogenesis.[29]

The first cell to reach an acute wound is the platelet. Platelets contain multiple growth factors, including PDGF, VEGF, TGF-α, TGF-β, bFGF, platelet-derived endothelial cell growth factor (PD-ECGF), and Ang-1. These factors stimulate endothelial proliferation, migration, and tube formation.[30,31]

Step 2. **Angiogenesis Amplification.** Wound angiogenesis is amplified by inflammation. Macrophages and monocytes release a myriad of angiogenic factors as they marginate into the wound bed, including PDGF, VEGF, Ang-1, TGF-β, bFGF, IL-8, and TNF-α.[32] Several growth factors (PDGF, VEGF, bFGF) synergize in their ability to vascularize tissues.[33]

Proteases that break down damaged tissues further release matrix-bound angiogenic stimulators. Enzymatic cleavage of fibrin in wounds yields fibrin fragment E (FnE). This fragment stimulates angiogenesis directly and also enhances the effects of VEGF and bFGF.[34] Expression of the inducible COX-2 enzyme in the inflammatory stage of healing also leads to the production of VEGF and other promoters of angiogenesis.[35]

Step 3. **Vascular Proliferation.** As angiogenesis is maintained, granulation becomes clinically evident in the wound bed. Hypoxia is an important driving force for sustaining wound angiogenesis. The hypoxic gradient between injured and healthy tissue leads to gene expression of hypoxia-inducible factor alpha (HIF-1α) and production of VEGF.[36] VEGF, present in both wound tissue and wound fluid, triggers endothelial cell proliferation.[37] Another property of VEGF is its ability to induce edema through hyperpermeability, hence its alternate name, vascular permeability factor (VPF).[38] Hypoxia also leads to endothelial cell production of

Step 4. **Vascular Stabilization.** Newly formed blood vessels must be stabilized before blood flow can begin. Vascular stabilization is governed by Ang-1, its receptor Tie2, and the interactions between smooth muscle cells and pericytes with endothelial cells. Binding of Ang-1 to Tie2 on angiogenic endothelial cells leads to the production of PDGF and the recruitment of smooth muscle cells and pericytes to the newly forming vasculature.[40–42] A deficiency in PDGF leads to abnormal, poorly formed blood vessels.[43]

Step 5. **Angiogenesis Suppression.** Angiogenesis is suppressed at the terminal stages of healing.[44] Levels of growth factors decline as tissue normoxia is restored and inflammation subsides. At the same time, endogenous angiogenesis inhibition becomes a dominant force. Pericytes that stabilize endothelial cells secrete an inhibitory form of activated TGF-β that impedes vascular proliferation.[45] Epidermal production of interferon-beta also inhibits angiogenesis.[46] Endostatin, a cleavage product of collagen XVIII, surrounding the vascular basement membrane, and vasostatin, another endogenous inhibitor, may suppress wound vascularity.[47,48]

Angiogenic Growth Factors in Wounds

A number of molecules have been identified as proangiogenic factors. These include thrombin, fibrinogen fragments, thymosin beta 4, and numerous peptide growth factors. Angiogenic growth factors are important physiological proteins that circulate in the bloodstream, are stored in platelets and inflammatory cells, and are sequestered within the extracellular matrix. More than 20 distinct angiogenic growth factors have been identified, including VEGF/VPF, acidic fibroblast growth factor (FGF-1), FGF-2, PDGF, TGF-β, progranulin, and leptin.

Folkman and Klagsbrun first identified FGF-1 and FGF-2 as angiogenic growth factors. FGF can be recovered from activated macrophages and the epidermis and soft tissue of wounds. FGF-1 and FGF-2 demonstrate potent angiogenic activity by standard angiogenesis experimental models, such as the rabbit cornea and chorioallantoic membrane assays. Although FGF-1 and FGF-2 are not secreted because they lack a transmembrane signal peptide, they may be released from injured cells or liberated by other mechanisms.[49]

VEGF potently induces granulation tissue formation. It also stimulates angiogenesis and vasopermeability. Cellular injury and tissue hypoxia, both hallmarks of tissue injury, are potent inducers of VEGF secretion and VEGF receptor expression in a wound. Angiopoietins also belong to the family of growth factors that act upon vascular endothelium. Angiopoietin-1, a naturally occurring angiogenesis agonist, and angiopoietin-2, an angiogenesis antagonist, act via the Tie-2 receptor.[49]

Wound Extracellular Matrix as Infrastructure for Angiogenesis

In addition to growth factors and chemotactic factors, the extracellular matrix is required for wound angiogenesis. The extracellular matrix of a healing wound transforms from fibrin to fibronectin, and hyaluronan to Type I and III collagen. Fibroblasts that invade the fibrin clot lyse and deposit fibronectin and hyaluronan, both ingredients for early granulation tissue. The granulation tissue begins at the periphery of the clot and grows centrally as it moves into the wound space.[49] The extracellular environment regulates wound angiogenesis, in part, by modulating endothelial cells receptor expression. For example, endothelial cells plated on fibronectin or fibrin gel express higher levels of the $\alpha_v \beta_3$ integrin than those plated on collagen or collagen gels. In an *in vitro* model of wound angiogenesis, three-dimensional fibrin gel stimulates early wound clot, whereas, three-dimensional collagen gel stimulates granulation tissue.[49]

Bone Marrow Derived-Stem Cells

Stem cells harbored within adult bone marrow contribute to wound angiogenesis. These cells, called endothelial progenitor cells (EPCs), can also be isolated in small numbers in the peripheral circulation of normal healthy adults.[50,51] Following trauma or surgery, EPCs are mobilized into the circulation and home to sites of neovascularization, where they differentiate into adult endothelial cells. Placental growth factor (PGF), a member of the VEGF family, and its receptor flt-1 (VEGF-R1) have been identified as critical mediators for EPC recruitment in angiogenesis, although other, as yet, unidentified factors may also play a role.[52]

PREREQUISITES FOR THE USE OF ADVANCED THERAPIES

Prior to initiation of advanced therapies, a number of issues must be considered. These include: (1) correct diagnosis of the underlying condition; (2) need for sharp debridement; (3) maintaining a moist wound environment; (4) infection control; (5) appropriate off loading; and (6) maintaining adequate nutritional status. Proper

nitric oxide (NO), which improves local blood flow by promoting vasodilation and angiogenesis.[39]

wound healing cannot take place without appropriate wound bed preparation, regardless of the wound etiology.

An important step in wound management is preventing accumulation of devitalized, necrotic tissue. Devitalized tissues are both physical and chemical impediments to granulation and epithelialization. Sharp debridement, an essential component of chronic wound management, removes foreign bodies, callus, and necrotic, infected, or avascular tissue. This can be accomplished with a scalpel blade, iris scissors and forceps, or a dermatologic curette. Proper debridement converts the chronic wound into an acute wound, allowing for resumption of the normal healing process. Removing wound eschar and fibrinous debris helps re-epithelialization since keratinocytes cannot migrate on fibrin.[53] Débridement also eliminates senescent cells at wound periphery that are unresponsive to growth factors.[54] In addition, the controlled tissue trauma achieved by sharp debridement liberates growth factors normally stored in the extracellular matrix.[55] The mild bleeding from debridement brings thrombin—a potent angiogenic factor—and platelets—which release endogenous PDGF and other growth factors into the wound bed, as well as a mild inflammatory infiltrate.[56] Débridement also appears to recruit bone marrow-derived endothelial progenitor cells into the circulation and contributes to angiogenesis in the wound bed.[57]

A seminal study published in 1996 by Steed and colleagues showed that sharp debridement alone can improve the incidence of complete wound healing in a clinical trial studying diabetic neuropathic ulcers. With the addition of a therapeutic growth factor (rhPDGF-BB) to sharp debridement, the incidence of completely healed wounds is nearly tripled (>80%), compared with débridement alone (25%).[58]

In addition to surgical débridement, autolytic interactive dressings, enzymes, and mechanical methods may be used adjunctively. The autolytic interactive dressings liquefy slough. Enzymatic débridement using papain-urea is appropriate for thick, adherent eschar, while collagenase is more appropriate for removing fibrinous debris or for maintenance débridement. Mechanical débridement includes saline wet-to-dry dressings, irrigation or pulsatile lavage, and whirlpool therapy. Saline wet-to-dry dressings, which may be painful for patients, are not advocated by most wound specialists. Whirlpool therapy liquefies debris, but may introduce bacteria into other immersed sites and macerate intact skin. The wound should be re-evaluated periodically, since management should change as it progresses through the various stages of healing.[59]

Another component of wound bed preparation is infection control. Bacteria impair the healing process by: (1) competing with cells of the wound bed for oxygen and nutrients; (2) releasing toxins into the wound tissue; and (3) stimulating the prolonged release of inflammatory cytokines and proteolytic enzymes that degrade granulation tissue and wound stroma. Although all chronic wounds contain bacteria, not all show signs of infection. Colonization differs from contamination in that it refers to replicating organisms on the wound surface. Wounds that contain nonviable tissue (slough, eschar) offer a hospitable environment for colonization. In contrast, true tissue infection occurs when bacteria have invaded healthy tissues to such a depth and extent that their presence is obviously deleterious, which invokes an immune response from the patient.

The concept of "critical colonization" refers to the presence of bacteria on the surface of the wound to such an extent that the build-up of their secreted toxins, cytokines, and proteases results in impaired healing progress. Wounds that are critically colonized may present as bright-red friable granulation tissue with malodor and increased drainage. However, the only sign of critical colonization may be simply a stalling of the healing process.[60] A number of sustained-release antiseptic drugs (Iodosorb, Healthpoint) and silver dressings (Acticoat, Smith & Nephew; Actisorb, Johnson & Johnson Wound Management; Silverlon, Argentum Medical; SilvaSorb gel, AcryMed/Medline) are now commercially available. Silver dressings like Acticoat have been shown to have a 99.9999% bacterial kill rate within 30 minutes, without harming the wound bed or causing bacterial resistance.[61]

Other considerations that must be kept in mind when using advanced modality therapy includes reducing the physical pressure, friction, and shear forces on a wound through off-loading. In diabetic patients, this can be accomplished by means of appropriate orthotics and weight-alleviating devices to off-load the weight-bearing surfaces of the foot. Maintaining adequate nutrition is essential, as is the avoidance of repeated mechanical and chemical trauma is vital for proper healing. Appropriate management of underlying concomitant medical conditions is vital.

TARGETING WOUND HEALING AT THE MOLECULAR LEVEL

Growth Factor Therapy for Wound Healing

Using recombinant biotechnology, human growth factor genes inserted into yeast cells produce growth factors, proteins that can be harvested, purified, and formulated into pharmaceutical-grade products. The high purity, yield, and the reliability of production are major advantages of recombinant growth factors. Limitations include the short half-life and temperature sensitivity of protein drugs. At present, recombinant human PDGF-BB is the only therapeutic growth factor that has received FDA approval for wound healing. Although not approved for wound healing, granulocyte-macrophage colony-stimulating factor (GM-CSF) is available and has been studied for healing diabetic foot ulcers.

Recombinant Human Platelet-Derived Growth Factor-BB (rhPDGF-BB)

Platelet-derived growth factor (PDGF) is a potent angiogenic factor essential for normal wound healing. PDGF is a pluripotent peptide secreted by platelets, as well as, monocytes, macrophages, fibroblasts, and endothelial cells. PDGF stimulates endothelial cells to proliferate forming functional blood vessels, stabilizing the neovasculature by recruiting smooth muscle cells and pericytes.[62,63] PDGFs represent a family of growth factors consisting of two polypeptide chains (A and B) that form dimers: PDGF-AA, -AB, and -BB. All three PDGF isoforms are present in human platelets. The PDGF receptor has a transmembrane structure with extracellular ligand-binding domains and intracellular tyrosine kinase domains. Two PDGF receptors exist, named Rα or Rβ, with each possessing different specificities for their ligands. The B subunit of PDGF can affiliate with either the PDGF-Rα or PDGF-Rβ subunit, while the A subunit of PDGF can interact only with the PDGF-Rα.[64] PDGF-BB can activate any PDGF receptor homodimer or heterodimer; therefore, therapeutic application of PDGF-BB can activate both configurations of its receptor.

Although all isoforms of PDGF stimulate angiogenesis, the PDGF-BB isoform is more potently angiogenic than PDGF-AA. The mechanisms of PDGF-driven angiogenesis are multifold.[65,66] When PDGF-BB binds to the PDGF-β receptor (PDGF-Rβ) on endothelial cells, only cells from microvessels, and not larger vessels, undergo increased DNA synthesis.[67,68] PDGF-BB is also a potent chemotactic factor that induces endothelial migration, an effect not seen with PDGF-AA.[65,69] Experiments using time-lapse video microscopy have shown that PDGF-BB elicits not only the migration of single endothelial cells, but also the movement of entire vascular cord-like structures.[30] This vascular migration contributes to the repair response when confluent endothelial cell monolayers are wounded in tissue culture. Vascular migration is also facilitated by matrix metalloproteinases (MMPs) and angiogenic integrins ($\alpha_v\beta_3, \alpha_v\beta_5, \alpha_5\beta_1$).[70] The integrin $\alpha_v\beta_3$ is detected in proliferating microvessels in the periwound stroma at day 3 after injury, but disappears after granulation tissue is matured.[71] PDGF-BB induces integrin expression in a differential fashion, depending on whether the extracellular matrix is primarily collagen or fibronectin.[72]

Vascular tube formation is promoted by PDGF-BB via blockade of the cell cycle's transition from G0 to G1. This blockade facilitates a three-dimensional conforma-

tional change to occur in newly forming blood vessels.[73] Importantly, PDGF-BB promotes vascular maturation by mediating the recruitment and differentiation of mesenchymal stem cells into mural cells (pericytes and smooth muscle cells).[41–43] The PDGF-Rβ is expressed in pericytes, which require the growth factor ligand for normal development.[43] In PDGF-B knock-out mice, angiogenic capillaries are devoid of pericytes. However, in PDGF-intact systems, PDGF-Rβ-expressing pericyte progenitor cells proliferate and migrate along PDGF-B-expressing endothelial sprouts. PDGF-BB is, therefore, a pluripotent growth factor. Studies of cultured bovine aortic endothelial cells grown in tissue culture have shown that the addition of PDGF induces a dose-dependent increase in endothelial cell migration, compared to cells grown in a serum-free control system.[30] Endothelial cells originally taken from the rat thoracic aorta were grown on top of a collagen gel in tissue culture. This substrate allows endothelial cells to undergo tubulogenesis and form vascular tubes. When macrophage-conditioned medium was incubated with endothelial cells, an increase in vascular tube formation occurred in a dose-dependent fashion with respect to glucose. The addition of a monoclonal antibody to PDGF-BB markedly suppressed tubulogenesis. This shows that the stimulatory effect seen was specifically due to PDGF and not another factor. Therefore, inflammatory infiltrates releasing PDGF stimulate vascular tube formation.[74] PDGF also stimulates angiogenesis in the mouse corneal micropocket assay, following implantation of a sustained-release polymer pellet containing the growth factor.[62] The effects of PDGF-BB in vascular stabilization have also been observed in studies of brain capillaries in wild-type versus PDGF knock-out mice. Brain capillaries from PDGF knock-out mice were distorted and showed heterogenous thickness and swelling of the endothelial cell, indicative of less than optimal functional flow.[75]

An early version of growth factor therapy was the autologous formulation called Procuren (Curative Health Services), a platelet-releasate developed in the 1980s. Blood was drawn from the patient and platelets isolated and treated with thrombin to release their contents. The resulting releasate was supplied to patients in 10-cc tubes and applied to their wound. Such autologous formulations had certain drawbacks related to manufacturing, lack of standardization, patient heterogeneity, lack of characterized components, and cost (~$5000). Although a prospective clinical trial was never conducted, a retrospective chart review of 3830 patients showed a statistically significant increase in wound closure rate in 1475 diabetic patients, although the time to healing was unknown.[76]

In the 1990s, a pure recombinant human PDGF was successfully developed. rhPDGF-BB was produced by genetically engineered yeast cells into which the gene for the PDGF B chain is inserted. Recombinant PDGF-BB became commercially available as Becaplermin (Regranex 0.01% gel; Johnson and Johnson Wound Management) following its FDA approval for the treatment of chronic diabetic ulcers in December 1997. Clinical trials have shown that becaplermin is safe and effective for increasing the incidence of complete wound closure when used in conjunction with good standard wound care.[77]

A Phase 2 double-blind, placebo-controlled, multi-center clinical trial of 118 patients with full-thickness diabetic foot ulcers present for at least 8 weeks demonstrated clinical efficacy of becaplermin. Becaplermin (rhPDGF, 0.003%) resulted in doubling the incidence of complete healing compared to placebo with difference between the groups evident as early as 6 weeks after initiation of therapy. The same incidence of healing achieved by placebo group at 20 weeks was observed in becaplermin groups at 10 weeks.[77] Subsequently, a Phase 3 multicenter, randomized, parallel group clinical trial evaluated effects of once-daily topical becaplermin gel (rhPDGF-BB 0.01%) in 922 patients with nonhealing diabetic foot ulcers. Based on an analysis of patients with a baseline ulcer area of ≥ 10 cm^2 common to all trials (representing 95% of all patients), the study demonstrated the growth factor-treated group had 50% incidence of complete wound closure at 20 weeks as opposed to 35% with placebo gel-treated group.[78,79] These data fulfilled the criteria for FDA approval, where the only acceptable clinical endpoint is complete wound closure defined as 100% epithelialization with no drainage.

Reduced time-to-healing and diminished overall healthcare costs are also important considerations in modern wound management. Reduced healing time lessens risk of infectious complications, decreases overall costs, and improves quality of life for patients. In clinical trials, becaplermin (0.01%) gel significantly decreased the overall time to complete wound closure compared to placebo gel. A retrospective analysis of cases from the Phase 3 clinical trials of becaplermin indicated a cost savings of as much as $1127 compared to the costs of good wound care alone, whereby slower healing led to increased expenditures.[80]

Although the package insert of becaplermin recommends twice-daily changes of saline-moistened dressings, as were performed in the clinical trials, in actual clinical practice, once-daily dressing change is efficacious, requiring less visiting nurse assistance, improving patient compliance, and reducing trauma to the wound site. An open-label study was conducted in 124 patients with full-thickness, lower-extremity diabetic foot ulcer, receiving becaplermin and once-daily dressing change. The study demonstrated that once-daily dressing change

was as efficacious as twice-daily dressing changes, with complete healing in 57.5% of patients with a mean time of closure of 63 days.[81]

Therapeutic angiogenesis using becaplermin is now been considered as part of the standard of care for diabetic foot ulcers. In the first 4 years following its FDA approval, the drug has been used to treat over 250,000 chronic ulcers. Because angiogenesis is required for healing all types of wounds, becaplermin is also useful intervention in nondiabetic wounds. Becaplermin is commonly prescribed in off-label fashion and has successfully healed venous stasis ulcers, arterial insufficiency ulcers, pressure ulcers, ischemic ulcers, burns, traumatic wounds, and dehisced surgical wounds.[82]

Becaplermin has been studied in the treatment of pressure ulcers, a heterogeneous and challenging group of wounds. The initial clinical trials showed that becaplermin may be useful in treating pressure ulcers, especially prior to surgical closure. In a multicenter, double-blind Phase 2 study of 124 patients with chronic, full-thickness pressure ulcers, 58% of patients in the becaplermin (rhPDGF-BB 0.01%)-treated group achieved $>90\%$ closure at 16 weeks compared to 29% of the placebo group.[84] Measurement of microvessels present in these wounds showed significantly ($p = 0.025$) increased angiogenesis, compared to wound biopsies from patients receiving the placebo gel.[83,84] Although becaplermin has not yet been approved for the treatment of pressure ulcers, it is used as adjunctive therapy for wound care in nursing homes, wound care facilities, and neurological units where pressure ulcers commonly develop.

Venous insufficiency ulceration is another condition successfully treated by becaplermin, in combination with standard compression. Venous ulcers result from incompetent valves in lower-extremity veins, leading to venous reflux and hypertension, edema with inflammation, and eventual skin breakdown. The vasculature within the venous ulcer is abnormal in structure and is hyperpermeable, causing the leakage of macromolecules and fibrin that form cuffs around microvessels. Endogenous growth factors are thought to be trapped within these cuffs, rendering them unavailable to stimulate tissue repair.[85] Delivery of becaplermin may replenish growth factors in the wound bed. From a mechanistic point of view, this growth factor may stimulate wound angiogenesis to generate new capillaries with a normal phenotype.[86] Two randomized, placebo-controlled studies were performed using daily or twice-weekly becaplermin gel for 16 weeks, along with sharp débridement and compression wraps. An intent-to-treat analysis of the data demonstrated a higher incidence of complete healing with becaplermin compared to placebo for wounds ≥ 5 cm^2.[85] An intent-to-treat analysis of data from the two clinical trials found a higher incidence of complete healing with becaplermin

(0.01%) compared to placebo for wounds ≥ 5 cm^2 (46 vs. 7% in study 1; and 38 vs. 23% in study 2). Although the studies were not powered for statistical significance, these findings are consistent with the clinical experience in wound care centers where becaplermin is used adjunctively for venous ulcer management.

With appropriate use, topical growth factor therapy can significantly accelerate the healing of chronic wounds. From the experience of the Angiogenesis Clinic at Brigham & Women's Hospital, proper wound care that optimizes the efficacy of becaplermin include:

- properly executed sharp débridement
- control of microbial bioburden
- control of excessive protease activity
- off-loading (for diabetic foot ulcers or pressure ulcers)
- adequate compression (for venous ulcers)
- adequate nutrition
- management of macrovascular disease
- patient compliance
- minimization of antiangiogenic medications[82]

Other Growth Factors

Growth factors beside rhPDGF-BB has been studied in clinical trials. Thus far, most studies have yielded disappointing results. This may be, in part, due to the complexity of the target wound, suboptimal clinical trial design, and limitations in the choice of trial endpoints. A brief discussion of several important growth factor trials follows.

Keratinocyte Growth Factor-2 (KGF-2)—Keratinocyte growth factor-2 (KGF-2) also known as FGF-10, stimulates epithelialization and granulation and protects endothelial cells from VEGF-induced vascular permeability.[87,88] A topical form of recombinant KGF-2 (repifermin; Human Genome Sciences) has completed Phase 2 study in venous insufficiency ulcers. In this randomized, double-blind, parallel group, placebo-controlled multicenter study of topical repifermin at 20 and 60 μg/cm^3, 94 patients with venous insufficiency ulcers were enrolled. Repifermin was administered twice weekly for 12 weeks as a topical spray with standard compression dressing. Higher incidence of achieving 75% wound closure was observed in repifermin-treated group (71% for low dose and 63% for high dose) as compared to placebo group (45%). Following application of repifermin, 90% closure was achieved in wounds ≤ 15 cm^2 and ≤ 18 months duration. The repifermin spray was well-tolerated and demonstrated minimal immunogenicity. However, analysis of all the Phase 2 data did not show statistical differences, in part because the control group healed extremely well. An important limiting factor in the trial may have been the absence of débridement in the study protocol.

Fibroblast Growth Factor 2 (FGF-2)—Fibroblast growth factor-2 (FGF-2, or basic FGF) was the first identified angiogenic growth factor with potent *in vitro* and *in vivo* activity. A topical formulation of recombinant bovine FGF-2 (rbFGF) has been reported in the successful treatment of burns, donor site wounds, and chronic dermal wounds, with daily applications, in a randomized, placebo-controlled trial of 1665 patients in Beijing.[89,90] Of 654 patients enrolled in the burn group, healing time was faster with rbFGF-treated patients for second-degree burns compared to the control group. Histological evaluation of the rbFGF-healed wounds showed substantially more capillary sprouts and tubes in growth factor-treated patients compared to controls. In addition, the regenerated epidermis and dermis were thicker in the rbFGF-treated group compared to controls. No major adverse effects were observed, including the development of hypertrophic scars.

Since 2001, recombinant human FGF-2 (Trafermin, Kaken Pharmaceutical) has been commercially available in Japan as a topical spray (Fiblast), which is applied daily to intractable skin ulcers. Fiblast is also being studied in Japan for gum regeneration in periodontal disease. Although various developers have explored recombinant FGF-2 in preliminary wound studies in the United States, clinical trials were never completed to enable submission for consideration of FDA approval.

Granulocyte-Macrophage Colony-Stimulating Factor (GM-CSF)—Granulocyte-macrophage colony-stimulating factor (GM-CSF) is an angiogenic growth factor that exerts its influence throughout the whole wound healing process. Besides stimulating bone marrow to produce more granulocytes and macrophages, it also regulates the proliferation and differentiation of fibroblasts, endothelial cells, and keratinocytes. GM-CSF enhances granulation tissue and wound contraction and prevents bacterial contamination from obstructing the healing process. In a study involving 70 patients, rhu-GM-CSF (Leucomax, Molgranostim, Novartis) was applied in a 10 μg/mL saline solution over venous leg ulcers covered by nonadhesive wound compression dressing. The average healing time for all venous ulcers treated with rhu-GM-CSF was 18 weeks with complete closure in 97% of the patients.[91] Of patients with ulcers >10 cm^2 treated with rhu-GM-CSF, 92% achieved complete closure after 28 weeks. The recurrence rate at 3-year follow-up of patients treated with rhu-GM-CSF plus compression was 18.2 compared to 44% treated with compression alone or 26% treated with vein stripping. There were no reported local or systemic side effects from the topical rhu-GM-CSF therapy. This growth factor is commercially available for use in the support of hematological disorders, but is currently not approved for use in wound care.

Transforming Growth Factor-Beta (TGF-β)— Transforming growth factor-β (TGF-β) is a cytokine released by a variety of cells, such as platelets and macrophages, during wound repair. TGF-β is known to be deficient in poorly healing wounds, such as diabetic ulcers and venous leg ulcers. The role of TGF-β in wound healing has been the subject of debate, because, while it stimulates fibroblasts and endothelial cells, under certain experimental conditions, it can also inhibit vascular endothelial cells. There are at least five isoforms of TGF-β, encoded by-different genes.

A bioresorbable collagen sponge containing TGF-β2 (BetKine, Celtrix/Genzyme Tissue Repair) releases the growth factor into the wounds. It has been studied in Phase 2 clinical trials for diabetic foot ulcers. In a multicenter, double-blind, randomized, placebo-controlled trial involving 177 diabetic patients, the high dose (5 μg/cm^2) TGF-β2-treated patients showed statistically significant healing compared to controls, in terms of frequency of complete closure and time to closure. In the study, 61% of twice-weekly TGF-β-treated patients achieved complete closure within 21 weeks, compared to 32% of patients receiving placebo sponge.[92]

Another form of TGF-β, TGF-β3 (Novartis), has also shown encouraging results. A pilot randomized, blinded, placebo-controlled trial enrolling 270 patients with pressure ulcers studied the effect of daily topical use of TGF-β3.[93] TGF-β3 treatment led to statistically significant improvement only at the higher dose of 2.5 μg/cm^2 as compared to placebo control and only during the initial 8 weeks of therapy. This pilot study was notably hindered by a high rate (43%) of patient drop-out. A larger, multicenter, blinded study of TGF-β has not yet been conducted.

Other Stimulatory Peptides

Thymosin β4—Not a true growth factor, thymosin β4 is a naturally occurring 43-amino acid peptide found in high concentrations in platelets, which promotes endothelial and keratinocytes migration. As a low-molecular weight peptide, it has the ability to diffuse long distances through tissue. A therapeutic version of thymosin β4 has been developed (Tβ4, RegeneRx Biopharmaceuticals licensed from NIH). Tβ4 increases proliferation and tube formation of human umbilical vein endothelial cells (HUVECs) and enhances vascular sprouting.[94] In preclinical studies, Tβ4 accelerated healing of diabetic and aged mice with poorly healing wounds.[95] A Phase 1 safety study of Tβ4 with 20 normal healthy volunteers found no adverse effects related to the

drug. Further clinical trials in different types of chronic wounds are planned for the future.

A related molecule, thymosin α1 (Tα1, Zadaxin, SciClone) is an immunomodulatory factor and may also have potential for accelerating wound healing. It is currently approved in Asia for the treatment of Hepatitis B and C and is under investigation as an an adjuvant therapy for the treatment of metastatic melanoma. *In vitro* and *in vivo* studies of Tα1 suggest that it enhances tube-like structure formation of (HUVEC) on Matrigels and stimulates HUVEC migration in chemoattractant assays. Hence, Tα1 may be useful in angiogenesis and wound repair.[96]

ACT—Synthetic peptides cleaved from thymosin, ACT 1 and 2 (Activor Corporation), have been developed to stimulate wound angiogenesis. In the Boyden chamber chemotactic assay, ACT 1 and 2 stimulated endothelial cell migration in a dose-response manner. In the scratch-wound closure assay, endothelial cell migration to the wounded area increased by fourfold with ACT 1 and by threefold with ACT 2 compared to cells growing in control media. Topical application of ACT 1 in rodents with full-thickness skin biopsy wounds resulted in 15% greater re-epithelialization after 7 days compared to saline-treated control. Intraperitoneal injections of ACT 1 showed 42% greater re-epithelialization after 4 days and 67% greater re-epithelialization after 7 days. These findings led to an IRB-approved clinical trial of ACT 1 on wound healing in humans.[97]

TP-508—Thrombin is a potent angiogenic stimulator and a synthetically manufactured 23-amino acid peptide fragment, TP-508 (Chrysalin, Chrysalis Biotechnology), is being developed to accelerate wound healing. TP-508 binds to high-affinity thrombin receptors and mimics cellular effects of thrombin at sites of tissue injury. A variety of studies have shown that TP-508 stimulates angiogenesis.[98] When tested in the chick embryo chorioallantoic membrane (CAM) assay, TP-508 increases the density and size of CAM blood vessels relative to controls. TP–508 also stimulates chemokinesis and chemotaxis in a dose-dependent fashion in cultured human aortic and human microvascular endothelial cells. Treatment of full-thickness excisional wounds in rats with a single topical application of 0.1 μg of TP-508 accelerated wound closure by 39%, on average, compared to controls by day 7 ($p < 0.001$). Histologic examination revealed larger functional vessels in the granulation tissue.[99] Breaking strength after complete closure was also greater in wounds treated with TP-508.

A four-center, randomized, double-blind, placebo-controlled Phase 1/2 study evaluated TP-508 in 59 patients with chronic diabetic foot ulcers. TP-508 was administered twice weekly in conjunction with good standard wound care practices, including débridement and off-loading. The drug was well-tolerated with no significant adverse events noted. Preliminary efficacy analysis showed positive trends for 100% epithelialization and time-to-closure in the TP-508-treated groups. Additional clinical studies of TP-508 are planned.

Angiogenic Growth Factor Combinations for Wound Healing

During wound healing, multiple growth factors are expressed in a well-orchestrated temporal fashion. For example, PDGF is expressed on vascular endothelium of injured skin 1 day after wounding. VEGF expression peaks between 3 to 7 days after wounding, corresponding to the appearance of granulation tissue. bFGF expression peaks 5 days after wounding but returns to baseline by day 7.[100]

Multiple growth factors collaborate and synergize with one another during angiogenesis. For example, several growth factors (FGF-2, TGF-β, and PDGF) can independently stimulate the production of VEGF.[101,102] VEGF interacts with the growth factors angiopoietin-1 (Ang-1) and PDGF to stabilize vessels and enhance vascular survival.[103,104] An interplay occurs between many growth factors to guide the initiation and maturation of blood vessels in the granulation bed.[103] A study using polymers for controlled delivery of growth factors in subcutaneous tissue compared vascular formation with VEGF alone and PDGF combined with VEGF. Sustained release of VEGF alone resulted in small, immature microvessel formation. However, when PDGF and VEGF were coreleased, smooth muscle cells and pericytes were recruited, forming more mature vessels. In another study with ischemic limb injury to nonobese diabetic mice, dual delivery of both PDGF and VEGF resulted in statistically significant increase in mature blood vessel density compared to either growth factors delivered alone.[105] PDGF and FGF-2 may also collaborate to promote a higher quantity of more durable blood vessels in both ischemic and nonischemic tissue. Combinatorial growth factor therapy has not yet been clinically studied for wound healing.

Optimizing Growth Factor Therapy

During wound healing, proteases are transiently expressed at the growing tips of new capillary blood vessels. Proteases exert enzymatic activity that promotes vascular invasion, digests extracellular matrix, and facilitates tissue remodeling and the removal of necrotic tissue.[70] Chronic wounds and chronic wound fluid express excessive protease activity. Studies of diabetic wound drainage show that protease levels range widely from 0 to 400 relative units of MMPs, 60–2000 relative units of plas-

min, to 13–49,000 relative units of elastase.[106] Diabetic patients also have elevated circulating systemic levels of MMP-2, -8, and -9.[107] Such protease elevation may destroy growth factors, inhibit angiogenesis, and digest newly formed granulation tissue. For these reasons, control of excessive protease activity is essential for wound management and the promotion of therapeutic angiogenesis.

ORC/Collagen (Promogran; Johnson & Johnson Wound Management) is a bioactive dressing that neutralizes destructive proteases in chronic wound fluid. ORC/Collagen also has been shown to directly bind growth factors and sustain-releasing them over time. An *in vitro* study showed that ORC/Collagen protected the biological activity of several angiogenic growth factors, such as PDGF, VEGF, and bFGF, despite the presence of plasmin. In another study, the activity of exogenous PDGF in chronic wound fluid was recovered after incubation with ORC/Collagen as compared to standard gauze dressing.[108] Based on this activity, ORC/Collagen is clinically used to promote wound healing in the presence of excessive protease activity.

The ORC/Collagen dressing should be cut to the size of the wound. It is rapidly absorbed after placement over the wound bed. A secondary dressing should cover the site to maintain a moist wound environment. Over a period of time, the ORC/Collagen dissolves and resorbs completely into the wound.[65] ORC/Collagen can be combined with becaplermin to augment the exposure of wounds to angiogenic growth factor stimulation. We have proposed a "bilayer sandwich technique" to coadminister becaplermin and ORC/Collagen. After sharp débridement to remove necrotic tissue and fibrinous slough, becaplermin gel is thinly spread over the wound surface using a cottontipped applicator. A piece of ORC/ Collagen is then layered on top of the becaplermin in the wound bed. Third, a final layer of becaplermin is carefully applied to the top of the ORC/Collagen dressing. The bilayer of becaplermin sandwiching the ORC/Collagen allows sustained-release of growth factors to chronic wounds over time. A secondary dressing, such as a hydrogel, gauze, film hydrocolloid alginate, or foam dressings can be placed over the bilayer to maintain a moist wound environment.

Gene Transfer

Gene-based therapies offer the theoretical advantage of delivering sustained local expression of growth factors to target tissues.[109,110] Human genes encoding growth factors can be engineered into plasmids to create so-called "naked DNA" for gene transfer to tissues. Alternatively, the genes can be incorporated into nonpathogenic viral vectors. Genes encoding PDGF have been transferred into and induced in wounds both in animal models and in patients with chronic wounds. Furthermore, gene therapy may allow the modification of cells, such as fibroblasts, in skin equivalents to enhance their engraftment.[110]

Because the epidermal barrier is disrupted in cutaneous wounds, gene transfer to the wound bed is possible with nonintegrative viral vectors or nonviral transfection methods. For example, gene-gun delivery, direct application of naked DNA, liposomal or electroporative transfer, intraulcer injection, microvascular transfection, or wound bed implantation of genetically modified cells are all feasible options for treating chronic wounds. Besides upregulating expression of cytokines and growth factors at the wound site, antisense oligonucleotides have been used to regulate the activity of collagen genes in the hope of controlling fibrosis. Some important caveats, however, should be considered with local gene delivery to resident cells in a chronic wound. Necrotic tissue may be a physical barrier for gene delivery. The wound exudate may degrade the genetic material through proteolytic activity. Wound dermal cells, such as fibroblasts and endothelial cells, may be more difficult to target than epidermal cells. As with all gene therapies, there is risk of immunologic or toxic side effects. Overall, current clinical studies of gene therapy and gene transfer support the safety and promise of this molecular-based approach to wound care.

Ex Vivo Gene Transfer

Ex vivo gene transfer involves the transfection of cells outside the patient's body. Cells, such as keratinocytes or fibroblasts, can be harvested from skin biopsy samples for gene insertion in culture. The patient can then be regrafted with the transfected cells. This method allows confirmation of gene transfer into targeted cells before delivery to the patient and avoids direct administration of vectors of patients. Therefore, *ex vivo* cutaneous gene transfer has been a major area of focus and has produced all the published examples of corrective cutaneous gene delivery to date.[110]

In Vivo Gene Transfer

In vivo gene transfer involves the transfection of cells inside the patient's body. Direct administration of genetic material has been attempted with both nonviral and viral vectors via topical application, direct injection, application to wounded skin surfaces, electroporation, and bioplastic particle insertion. Topical application has primarily been tried using nonviral plasmid vectors with follicular predominance in uptake and expression, but demonstrated low efficiency. Direct injection into intact skin has achieved epidermal, dermal, and subcutaneous gene transfer using nonviral and viral vectors. Retroviral vectors applied to wounded skin offer another means of stable cutaneous gene transfer,

achieving prolonged gene transfer to cells of the epidermis and appendages. Electroporation following direct injection targets multiple cell types in the skin. Bioplastic particle acceleration or the gene gun bombardment of vector-coated microparticles has been used for wound healing.[110]

Nonviral Fibroblast Growth Factor-1 (NV1FGF)— NV1FGF-(GenCell/Aventis) is a nonviral gene transfer therapy in which a plasmid encodes the gene for human FGF-1 (acidic FGF). A multicenter Phase 1 study was performed enrolling 51 patients with severe, unreconstructible lower-extremity ischemia with rest pain or leg ulcers.[111] NV1FGF was injected directly into thigh and calf muscle at various single (0.5, 1, 2, 4, 8, and 16 mg) and repeat (2×0.5, 2×4, 2×8 mg) doses. Patients were followed for 6 months. NV1FGF was well-tolerated with no serious adverse events reported attributable to the treatment. No increase in serum FGF-1 was observed, suggesting that gene expression remained localized. Arteriography was performed at 12 weeks and clearly showed visible new collateral blood vessels in the limbs of 33% of patients, when compared to their pretreatment angiograms. NV1FGF led to a significant reduction in ischemic pain ($p < 0.001$), an increase in $TcPO_2$ ($p < 0.01$), and improved ankle-brachial index (ABI) scores ($p < 0.01$) at 6 months. Healing of ischemic leg ulcers was observed in most patients, and aggregate ulcer size decreased significantly compared to pretreatment values ($p < 0.01$). At the study's conclusion, 4 (7.8%) patients had died, 8 (15.7%) were alive with amputation required, and 39 (76.5%) were alive without requiring amputation. Historical comparison of 6-month outcomes in similar PAD patients under standard care showed a death rate of 20%, a rate of patients alive with amputation of 35%, and patients alive without amputation of 45%. Further studies of NV1FGF are continuing.

Vascular Endothelial Growth Factor (VEGF)— VEGF has multiple family members (VEGF-A, VEGF-B, VEGF-C, and VEGF-D). VEGFs interact with high-affinity tyrosine kinase receptors, of which the best known are VEGF-R1 (or fms-like tyrosine kinase, flt-1) and VEGF-R2 (or human kinase insert domain-containing receptor, KDR, and its mouse homolog, flk-1). These two receptors are selectively expressed on angiogenic endothelial cells.[112] VEGF-R2 (KDR/flk-1) is thought to be primarily responsible for transducing the signal for endothelial proliferation and chemotaxis during VEGF-driven angiogenesis. VEGF binding to KDR/Flk-1 is mediated by a coreceptor called neuropilin-1 (Nrp-1). Neuropilin-1 is abundantly expressed in the wound neovasculature. Antagonism of Nrp-1, a non-tyrosine kinase that potentiates VEGF–KDR binding, inhibits VEGF-driven endothelial cell migration.[113] Treatment of wounds with antibodies directed against Nrp-1 led to a 67% decrease in vascular density ($p = 0.0132$). These findings suggest that Nrp-1 and VEGF play an important role in regulating wound angiogenesis. VEGF directly mediates angiogenesis by stimulating cell proliferation, vascular hyperpermeability, and vascular survival.[114] Immediately after wounding, exposure of the endothelium to thrombin causes up-regulation of the receptors VEGF-R1 and VEGF-R2.[13,115] VEGF initiates angiogenesis by causing perivascular mural cells (pericytes and smooth muscle cells) to detach from the endothelium of parent vessels. This vascular destabilization, requiring the coordinated action of another growth factor, angiopoeitin-2 (Ang-2), allows the formation of numerous new "daughter" vessels from a single parent venule.[116] Vascular sprouting and endothelial migration is facilitated by angiogenic integrins and the secretion of matrix metalloproteinases.[117] VEGF, also known as vascular permeability factor (VPF), also renders microvascular endothelial cells hyperpermeable to plasma proteins and circulating macromolecules. These VEGF-mediated effects may be the cause of wound edema and excessive exudation.[118]

Plasmid human $VEGF_{165}$ is a nonviral form of gene therapy using a plasmid encoding the gene for human $VEGF_{165}$. This naked DNA approach was first used by Isner and colleagues[119] in Boston to demonstrate "proof of concept" of therapeutic angiogenesis in a patient with critical limb ischemia. A follow-up study delivered $phVEGF_{165}$ to 10 limbs in 9 patients with severe peripheral arterial disease, ischemic ulcers, and/or rest pain.[120] All patients had baseline ankle–brachial index (ABI) measurements <0.6 and/or toe–brachial index (TBI) <0.3. The $phVEGF_{165}$ (2000 g) was injected into the calf or distal thigh at entry into the study, followed by a second identical injection 4 weeks later. VEGF gene expression was observed by transient rises in serum VEGF and this correlated with the development of new collateral vessels (200- to >800-μm diameter) in the limb demonstrated by digital subtraction angiography. Serial magnetic resonance angiography was performed and showed improved distal blood flow in 8 of 10 limbs. The ABI improved significantly from 0.33 to 0.48 ($p = 0.02$). Exercise tolerance increased in 5/5 patients who were able to perform a graded treadmill test and pain-free walking time at 13 weeks improved by 152% from baseline measurements following gene therapy ($p = 0.43$). Ischemic ulcers healed or were clinically improved in 4 of 7 limbs, leading to limb salvage in 3 patients who had previously been recommended for below-the-knee amputation. Overall, $phVEGF_{165}$ was well tolerated, with side effects limited to lower-extremity edema, consistent with the hyperpermeability activity of VEGF. Further studies of $phVEGF_{165}$ are planned.

TISSUE-ENGINEERED SKIN CONSTRUCTS FOR WOUND HEALING

Wound repair requires cellular and molecular interactions among inflammatory, vascular, connective tissue, and epithelial cells amidst a suitable extracellular matrix. Prior to the advent of tissue engineering, the gold standard for closure of tissue defects was autologous skin grafts, tissue flaps, or free-tissue transfers. This creates donor sites, which can increase pain, scarring, infection, and add additional healthcare costs. Tissue-engineered skin substitutes can provide the cellular substrate and molecular components necessary for accelerating healing. These engineered products can stimulate angiogenesis by elaborating growth factors in the wound bed and by providing a three-dimensional scaffold for the in growth of new capillaries. The persistence of allogeneic cells weeks to months after implantation is a topic of active investigation. Early pilot studies led to the conclusion that cells did not persist weeks to months after implantation.[121] More recent work is revealing that cells from tissue engineered living skin equivalents such as Apligraf can persist at the wound site. Theoretically, this may permit deficient or corrupt tissue to be replaced by functional neonatal-derived cells.

The Tissue Reference Group was established by the FDA in February, 1997 to assist in defining which tissue-based products should be regulated as medical devices or as biologic products. A medical device is defined, in part, by its not achieving its purpose through chemical action within or on the body and is not dependent upon being metabolized.[122] A biologic product includes cells or tissue for repair or replacement. A so-called "combination product" is one combining the categories of device and/or biologic and/or drug.[123] The primary mode of action determines which FDA Center has lead responsibility. It should be noted that for devices there are three types of marketing applicatons to the FDA:

1. A Premarket Approval Application (PMA) requires controlled clinical trials in humans to evaluate safety and efficacy;

2. A 510(k) premarketing notification requires only that a product demonstrate "substantial equivalence" to a legally marketed device. The 510(k) approval does not require controlled clinical trials and, therefore, has substantially less or no evidence-based data to indicate clinical efficacy.

3. Humanitarian Device Exemption (HDE) is an expedited approval to market, aimed at a limited patient population (<4000 patients in the U.S.) for which no alternatives are marketed.[124] Such products are exempt from extensive clinical studies, but still require data to show evidence of safety.

An exemption from marketing approval during human studies may also be accomplished through an Investigational Device Exemption (IDE), which gives access of promising products to patients with serious illnesses at select clinical centers under an approved clinical protocol.

Tissue-engineered constructs can be classified according to which skin compartment for which the construct substitutes and from which compartment the cells or constituents are derived.

Epidermal Substitutes

Cultured Epidermal Autograft

Cultured epidermal autograft (Epicel; Genzyme Biosurgery) emerged from the pioneering work of Green and Rheinwald, who first described methods for culturing human epidermal cells.[125] Epicel is derived from an autologous skin biopsy. The epidermis is enzymatically disaggregated and suspended with irradiated 3T3 murine fibroblasts. The cell suspension is fed with a specialized growth media containing cholera toxin, epidermal growth factor, and hydrocortisone, among other components. After the cell colonies become confluent, the keratinocytes are released with the enzyme dispase, which cleaves basement membrane attachments, such as fibronectin, collagen IV, and, to a lesser extent, laminin. The detached keratinocytes are then transferred onto a nonadherent gauze dressing.[126] This culture procedure can amplify the initial biopsy size by 1,000–10,000 times within a few weeks.[127]

Since the early 1980s, Epicel or its predecessor manufactured by Biosurface Technologies has been used to treat burns, chronic leg ulcers, pressure ulcers, epidermolysis bullosa, and cutaneous wounds from excisions. Epicel is FDA approved through a HDE for patients who have deep dermal or full-thickness burns comprising 30% or more of total body surface area, and in patients who have surgical removal of large congenital nevi. It has the advantages of being an autologous permanent wound dressing not requiring a donor site. However, it requires 2–3 weeks of graft cultivation before use. It is also sensitive to bacterial infections and antiseptic toxins and is somewhat difficult to handle due to its fragility. Epicel lacks a dermal component, which may contribute to scarring and permits unstable attachment to wound bed.[128] It has been speculated that the absence of dermis may contribute to lower percentage of graft take. Hence, cultured epidermal autografts have also been combined with dermal components.

Cultured Epidermal Allograft

Cultured epidermal allografts are derived from unrelated donors, such as neonatal foreskin. Unlike Epicel, cultured epidermal allografts can be grown in advance and are ready for use without a 2 to 3-week incubation period. These allografts release growth factors that stimulate granulation and epithelialization from wound edges and adnexal structures. Wound healing appears to occur by stimulation of host keratinocytes, rather than by permanent acceptance of the allogeneic cells.[129] These allografts lack dermal components; hence, wound contracture, graft blistering, and inadequate cosmesis occur with use. A randomized clinical trial of 9 elderly patients studied cultured epidermal allografts versus nonadherent dressings in the healing of split-thickness skin graft donor sites.[130] The mean time-to-complete healing was 8.4 days in allografted sites compared with 15.3 days in control sites. Biopsy specimens taken from allografted areas 2 months postengraftment showed no evidence of survival of cultured allogeneic cells by multilocus DNA analysis.

The requirement for graft cryopreservation at −70 to −120°C circumvents difficulties in obtaining fresh cultured epidermal allografts with patient visits.[131] These grafts may be thawed at room temperature prior to use. A cryopreserved allogeneic epidermal construct (CryoCeal, XCELLentis/Innogenetics) has been developed with a 6-month shelf-life. Although cultured epidermal allografts are not yet available in the United States, they have been used to treat burns, chronic leg ulcers, donor sites, facial dermabrasion wounds, and epidermolysis bullosa in other countries. Large, randomized, placebo-controlled trials are needed to determine the efficacy of these grafts.

Dermal Substitutes

Cryopreserved Dermal Substitute

Dermagraft (Advanced Tissue Sciences/Smith & Nephew) is made of cultured human fibroblasts grown on a polyglactin. Dermal fibroblasts from neonatal foreskin are seeded on a polyglactin bioabsorbable mesh and cultured with circulating nutrients in a sterile, closed bioreactor system to control culture conditions and to maintain sterility. These living cells attach, proliferate, secrete growth factors and cytokines, and produce human collagen. Hence, the dermal extracellular matrix is self-generated without the need for additional exogenous human or bovine collagen. A unique characteristic of Dermagraft is that it is cryopreserved and stored at −75°C ± 10°C. By thawing in a water bath at 34–37°C for 2 to 3 minutes, Dermagraft can be brought back to metabolic activity, as measured by the MTT assay. The product, which is 5 × 7.5 cm, should be cut to fit the size of the wound and inserted into the defect. A mesh primary dressing and a bolster should be placed over the Dermagraft. Because the mesh is covered on both sides with cells and matrix, either side may face the wound bed. Dermagraft has a 6-month shelf-life in a −20°C freezer and is resistant to tearing and easy to handle due to the polyglactin mesh. Furthermore, there is no evidence that the product is rejected.[132]

Metabolically active human fibroblasts in Dermagraft facilitate healing of chronic wounds.[133] This occurs by the recapitulation of the normal role of fibroblasts in the wound bed, which proliferate and generate matrix components and cytokines. Moreover, fibroblasts in Dermagraft serve to deposit normal neonatal fibroblasts in a chronic wound environment in which there may be defective or "corrupt" cellular elements.

The angiogenic properties of fibroblast-based engineered tissues were demonstrated via standard experimental angiogenesis assays, such as the chick chorioallantoic membrane assay, the rat aortic ring assay, and cultured endothelial cells. Such studies have shown that Dermagraft induces endothelial cell migration as well as vascular tube formation. These activities may be inhibited by neutralizing antibodies to HGF/SF and VEGF illustrating the key role of these growth factors in Dermagraft behavior.[133]

In the initial pivotal clinical trial of 281 patients, Dermagraft plus standard therapy (sharp debridement, saline-moistened gauze, and pressure-reducing footwear) was compared to standard therapy alone for the treatment of diabetic foot ulcers of at least 6 weeks duration.[134] It was initially found that at the 12-week endpoint, there was no statistically significant difference in complete healing between the treatment versus control groups (38.5 versus 31.7%, respectively). Patients received one Dermagraft weekly for up to 8 weeks. However, further scientific analysis revealed that metabolic activity was heterogeneous and that many patients received Dermagraft with a high proportion of nonviable cells. Through retrospective analysis, 50.8% of the patients who received Dermagraft with viable cells within a specified therapeutic range achieved complete wound closure compared to 31.7% of patients treated with standard therapy.[135] In January 1998, an FDA advisory panel recommended approval of Dermagraft with the condition that the company perform a postmarketing study to confirm efficacy. Nevertheless, the FDA did not approve the PMA and requested a repeat multicenter, randomized, clinical trial of 314 patients, using metabolically active Dermagraft plus standard therapy compared to standard therapy alone.[136] Separately, Dermagraft was permitted to be available to patients through a Treatment IDE through select clinical centers. Effectiveness data subsequently submitted to the FDA on the 245 patients in the supplemental study showed that 30.0% of the Dermagraft-treated group achieved the primary endpoint of 100% wound closure compared to 18.3% of the control group at 12 weeks. A Bayesian statistical analysis was required in order to permit analysis of patients before and after a midterm modification to analyze only ulcers greater than 6 weeks

duration. Furthermore, the median wound closure for the Dermagraft group was 91% compared to 78% for the control group ($p = 0.044$). Ulcers treated with Dermagraft healed significantly faster than ulcers treated with standard therapy ($p = 0.04$). Patients treated with Dermagraft were 1.7 times more likely to heal than the control patients at any given time ($p = 0.044$). After the repeat trial, in September, 2001 Dermagraft received FDA approval through a PMA for the treatment of diabetic foot ulcers greater than 6 weeks duration extending through the dermis. In July, 2003 Dermagraft also received FDA approval through a HDE for the treatment of wounds in dystrophic epidermolysis bullosa. Similar to the clinical trial protocol, we have found that the use of the product weekly or every other week for the first 3 to 6 weeks is better than less frequent (such an monthly) implantations.

Extracellular Matrices (Nonliving)

Extracellular matrix products are generally derived from devitalized tissue to produce an immunologically inert acellular dermal matrix.

Allogeneic Acellular Dermal Matrix

Alloderm (LifeCell Corporation) is an acellular dermal matrix derived from fresh donated cadaver skin and is regulated by the FDA as human tissue for transplantation. The cadaver skin is processed with high salt to remove the epidermis and a solution to extract the cellular material, resulting in an immunologically inert acellular dermal matrix with an intact basement membrane. The lyophilization process minimizes damage to the tissue structure. Hence, this allogeneic devitalized cadaver skin can be used as nonimmunogenic synthetic dressing, with a shelf-life of 2 years. It can be cryopreserved, glycerol preserved, or lyophilized. Besides providing a dermal matrix for tissue regeneration, it allows the use of thinner split-thickness autografts. In a study of 12 cases of clinical application of AlloDerm plus an ultrathin (0.004–0.006 inch) autograft to full-thickness burn wounds, the average skin graft take rate was 91.5%, with mean time of donor site re-epithelization of 6 days.[137] All patients had a nearly normal range of joint motion (average 95% of normal) after a 1-year follow-up. Alloderm has also been used in soft-tissue defects and scarring on the face. Transplantation of this acellular dermal matrix followed by autografting avoids scarring and contracture. Ultrastructural analysis shows that the implanted matrix becomes populated with viable blood vessels and recipient host cells over time.[138]

Dermal Regeneration Template

Integra (Integra Life Sciences Corporation/Johnson & Johnson Wound Management) was FDA approved through a 510(k) in 1996 for full- or partial-thickness thermal injury where sufficient autograft is not available or not desirable due to the condition of patient. The advantage of Integra is that it is readily available to cover the large surface areas involved with severe third-degree burns. The synthetic epidermal layer is a disposable polysiloxane sheet and the matrix beneath is comprised of bovine collagen, chondroitin-6-sulfate, and shark-derived glycosaminoglycan. The porous dermal scaffold allows for the migration and integration of host fibroblasts and endothelial cells. Integra is used in acute burn wounds via a two-step process: it is first applied to the wound, which is followed by placement of split-thickness skin graft or cultured epidermal sheets a few weeks later. Disadvantages of this product include: its opaque quality, which precludes visualization of the wound bed; the relative ease of product slippage on the wound bed, which requires suturing the product in place; and the potential for trapping fluid drainage. Fluid collecting under Integra poses a risk for infection, hematoma formation, and premature separation of matrix from wound.

Single-step methods are also being investigated to treat chronic wounds with matrix products. For example, cultured autologous keratinocytes have been seeded directly to the wound bed beneath the Integra in porcine wound models. Integra absorbed the keratinocyte suspension more readily than did the wound bed. In fact, the keratinocytes migrated through the Integra and formed a confluent surface epithelium. In addition, keratinocytes seeded directly onto the Integra and, to a lesser extent, onto the wound bed, accelerated remodeling of the Integra matrix when compared to controls without keratinocytes. Therefore, the concept of combining cultured epidermal cells with Integra may ultimately prove to be more clinically efficacious and practical than the use of the product alone or with the current two-step method.[139]

Matrix of Human Dermal Fibroblasts

TransCyte (Advanced Tissue Sciences/Smith & Nephew) is made from fibroblasts seeded onto a nylon scaffold attached to a silastic membrane. The product was FDA approved through a PMA in March, 1997 for second- and third-degree burns. Prior to October 1998, TransCyte was marketed as Dermagraft-TC. Neonatal fibroblasts are cultured on nylon fibers embedded in a silastic layer for 4 to 6 weeks in a closed bioreactor system that supports the natural deposition of matrix proteins. During this time, fibroblasts secrete matrix components, including collagen, forming a dense cellular tissue. Freezing the construct renders the fibroblasts nonviable, but leaves behind a solid product of human matrix proteins, glycosaminoglycans, and growth factors. One advantage of TransCyte is that it provides a semitransparent dressing, allowing inspection of the wound site prior to autografting. In clinical studies, TransCyte has been found to

be as effective in preparing the wound bed for autografting as control cryopreserved human cadaveric skin. A multicenter, randomized, control study of 132 excised burn wounds demonstrated that TransCyte is as effective as human cadaveric skin in the healing of burns.[140] In addition, TransCyte has the benefits of permitting immediate closure of clean middermal burn wounds, rapid adherence to the wound surface, and enhancement of wound healing. Analysis by enzyme-linked immunoabsorbent assay (ELISA), Western blot, immunohistochemistry, and PCR has identified multiple matrix components in TransCyte including: collagen I, III, and VI, fibronectin, tenascin, thrombospondin-2, elastin, and proteoglycans.[141]

Porcine Small Intestine Submucosa

Oasis (Cook Biotech/HealthPoint) is a wound dressing made from porcine small intestinal submucosa (SIS). The product was FDA approved for marketing through a 510(k) in January, 2000 for the coverage of wounds. The serosa, smooth muscle, and mucosa of porcine small intestines are removed, leaving an acellular matrix composed of Types I, III, and V collagen and growth factors, such as TGF-β and FGF-2.[142] Therefore, the product serves as a three-dimensional extracellular structure for cytokines and adhesion molecules and a scaffold for tissue growth. The cell-free matrix does not generate immune-mediated inflammatory reactions, in part, because it suppresses human helper T-cell activation and differentiation.[143] When human microvascular endothelial cells (HMECs) were seeded onto SIS, the HMECs grew to single-layer confluence and penetrated the SIS.[144] In addition, *in vitro* studies showed SIS can support epidermal cell and fibroblast attachment, migration, and proliferation with deposition of basement membrane.[145] In an *in vitro* study, SIS induced tube formation by HMEC in a three-dimensional fibrin-based angiogenesis assay. Addition of anti-VEGF neutralizing antibody blocked tube formation. Western blot and ELISA analysis has revealed that SIS has up to 0.77 ng VEGF/g of product.[146] Based on these mechanisms of action, the clinical uses of SIS has ranged from the healing of chronic wounds to surgical repair abdominal wall, urinary bladder, tendons, vessels, and dura mater.

Bilayered Skin Substitutes (Living cells)

Bilayered Skin Equivalent (BSE)

Apligraf (Graftskin, Organogenesis) is a living bilayered (both dermis and epidermis) skin substitute. Apligraf was FDA approved through PMA in 1998 for the treatment of venous insufficiency ulcers and through a supplemental PMA in 2000 for the treatment of diabetic foot ulcers. The dermal layer is made of live allogeneic fibroblasts grown on Type I bovine collagen matrix. The epidermal layer is composed of live allogeneic human neonatal keratinocytes exposed to an air–liquid interface in order to form a stratum corneum. The product resembles human skin histologically, produces matrix proteins, and secretes growth factors. Ancillary cells such as, melanocytes, endothelial cells, and Langerhans cells, are missing from Apligraf. The absence of antigen-presenting Langerhans cell may explain why clinical rejection has not been observed with Apligraf. The patient's own melanocytes appear to migrate into the Apligraf as they do during normal wound healing.[147] The product is contraindicated in patients who are allergic to bovine collagen, or have hypersensitivity reactions to Apligraf–agarose shipping medium.[147]

Apligraf does not behave like an autologous skin graft. Rather, it replaces cells or growth factors that are either deficient, not actively synthesized, or nonfunctional. Apligraf, which measures 7.5 cm, is easy to apply in an outpatient setting, and has a shelf-life of only 5 days. It is shipped to a practitioner's office in a sealed and sterile agarose-filled plastic container. Generally, surgical wound bed preparation is performed a few days before Apligraf implantation. Most commonly, Apligraf is meshed or fenestrated before placement. Formerly, it was believed that this would allow for fluid drainage, but since the product is not a permanent wound covering, fluid retention is not the issue. The meshing or fenestration process likely forces cells out of quiescence and induces up-regulation of cytokines. Unlike other tissue-engineered constructs, Apligraf is commonly implanted with a 1 cm overlap over the wound margins. There is no need to suture the product to the wound. One attachment technique utilizes cyanoacrylate to bond the overlapping edges to the wound periphery. Recommended dressings include Mepitel (Molynycke) a silicon hydrophobic reusable primary dressing or a nonadhesive petrolatum gauze dressing such as Xeroform, and a bolster dressing. Compression devices should be added for venous leg ulcer, and off-loading should be used for diabetic neuropathic ulcers. At 1-week follow-up, if there are no signs of infection, the primary dressing should not be removed. After 1- to 2-week follow-up, the primary dressing should be removed gently and changed and the wound gingerly irrigated with saline, but not debrided. Residual visible Apligraf material should not be removed. Although the product was implanted weekly in clinical trials, in actual clinical practice, Apligraf is generally reapplied after 4 to 6 weeks.

The FDA approved Apligraf for venous ulcers based on a randomized, controlled, multicenter study in 297 patients with venous ulcers.[148] In patients treated with Apligraf and compression, 57% of patients had complete healing at 24 weeks, compared with 40% of patients treated with compression alone. At 6 months, 56% of patients had complete closure

with Apligraf compared to only 49% of the control group. The Apligraf group also healed three times more rapidly than the compression alone group, which was a median of 61 days compared to 181 days. In a retrospective analysis of this trial, the cost of Apligraf plus compression was $20,257 for an average of 3.3 applications per patient compared to $27,493 for the cost of weekly treatments of Unna boots.[149] In a subgroup analysis of 120 patients with venous leg ulcers over 1-year duration, Apligraf plus compression led to complete healing in 47% of patients compared to only 19% of control patients treated with compression alone ($p = 0.002$). Over a 12-month follow-up period, ulcers recurred in 22.2% of patients in the control group and in 18.1% of those patients who healed with Apligraf.

Apligraf was approved for diabetic foot ulcers based on a prospective, randomized, controlled, mulicenter study of 208 patients.[150] The product was applied at the beginning of the study and weekly thereafter for a maximum of 4 weeks. The control group received standard care including, surgical debridement, off-loading devices, and saline-moistened dressings. At a 12-week follow-up, 56% of the Apligraf-treated patients had achieved complete wound healing compared to 38% of the control group($p = 0.0082$). The median time-to-complete closure was 65 days for the Apligraf-treated group compared to 90 days for the control group. Furthermore, there was a significantly lower incidence of osteomyelitis at the treatment site in the Apligraf group compared to control (2.7 versus 10.4%, $p = 0/04$). At 6 months, Apligraf-treated ulcers also had a lower frequency of recurrence compared to ulcers treated with standard care (5.9 versus 12.9%)

Efficacy of Apligraf on difficult-to-heal wounds can be attributable to the new cells and the associated growth factors and matrix materials introduced into the wound bed. In this fashion, the skin construct acts as a "solid state delivery vehicle." It also promotes healing by secondary intention or a graft that allows tissue remodeling over time. In over 80,000 applications, there has never been a reported rejection.[151]

Cultured Composite Skin (CCS)

OrCel Bilayered Cellular Matrix (Cultured Composite Skin, Ortec International Inc./Cambrex Bio Science) is a collagen sponge composed of cocultured allogeneic donor keratinocytes and fibroblasts derived from foreskin tissue. OrCel received FDA approval through a PMA in August, 2001 for the treatment of split-thickness skin donor sites in burn patients. The allogeneic keratinocytes and fibroblasts secrete cytokines and growth factors, such as VEGF, GM-CSF, and TGF-α to the wound bed. Fibroblasts also deposit extracellular matrix components. The porous sponge absorbs wound fluid and acts as a scaffold for in-migration of patient's own fibroblasts and endothelial cells. OrCel differs from Apligraf in that the cells in OrCel are not as densely populated nor allowed to fully differentiate with a stratum corneum. On the one hand, this may result in cells that are in a replicative growth phase rather than quiescent. Preliminary studies indicated that OrCel may express enhanced levels of VEGF (twofold) and GM-CSF (tenfold) compared to Apligraf.[152] On the other hand, cells that are only partially differentiated in OrCel are unlikely to express the full range of molecular mediators found in a fully differentiated living skin equivalent such as Apligraf. As the tissue is repaired, the donor cells in the OrCel are thought to be resorbed and the patient's own cells repopulate the wound bed. Within 2 weeks, OrCel is essentially completely resorbed and a new epithelium is formed with patient's own cells.[153] The pivotal clinical trial was a prospective, randomized, controlled study of 82 patients to examine the efficacy of OrCel in facilitating wound closure of split-thickness skin donor sites in burn patients compared to Biobrane-L, a standard-of-care dressing. Mean and median time to 100% wound closure by photographic, planimetric, and investigator assessments were all significantly shorter ($p < 0.05$) for OrCel-treated patients compared to control group.[153] There was also significantly less scarring, rate of infection, and accelerated recropping. OrCel received FDA approval under a Humanitarian Device Exemption in February 2001 for the treatment of surgical donor sites created during the release-of-hand contractures in patients with recessive dystrophic epidermolysis bullosa. In another controlled study, the efficacy of OrCel plus conventional therapy (hydroactive foam with compression system) was compared to conventional therapy alone for 40 patients with venous leg ulcers. At 12-week follow-up, 53% of patients treated with OrCel achieved 100% wound closure compared to 26% of patients in control group.[153]

Next Generation of Tissue Engineering

Autologous Precursor Cells

Precursor cells show promise in generating engineered autologous skin substitutes. Precursor cells for epidermal keratinocytes are easily obtainable from the outer root sheath of anagen hair follicle.[154] EpiDex (Modex / IsoTis) is an autologous epidermal equivalent generated from the patient's hair follicle that is commercially available in Europe. In the United States, EpiDex received a Humanitarian Use Device designation from the FDA in October 2002 in anticipation for a Humanitarian Device Exemption. Six weeks after a simple hair pluck, EpiDex can be generated in 1-cm discs on a silicone membrane.

Because current skin substitutes do not have capillary networks, the incorporation of microvessels in skin substitutes is under investigation. Black and colleagues have developed a vascular network embedded within a skin equivalent by culturing keratinocytes, dermal fibroblasts, and umbilical vein endothelial cells in a chitosan-linked collagen-glycosaminoglycan sponge.[155] Schechner and colleagues have described conditions that allow for the formation of microvessels in a three-dimensional collagen/fibronectin matrix gel with human umbilical vein endothelial cells.[156] Endogenous stem or progenitor cells can also be grown *ex vivo* within a matrix scaffold. The construct can be transplanted and resorbed, leaving a neo-organ of transplanted cells and stroma. Supp and colleagues have cultivated a fully human skin equivalent with complete pilosebaceous units and histologic, immunologic, and ultrastructural properties similar to healthy human skin.[157]

Gene-Activated Matrix

In vivo local gene transfer can be combined with tissue engineering. Gene-activated matrix (GAM) consists of plasmid DNA and a biodegradable matrix in the form of a lyophilized implant or sponge, injectable gel or paste, and medical device coating. The GAM carrier serves as a lattice for the DNA until endogenous fibroblasts arrive at the wound site. Once fibroblasts become transfected, they can secrete plasmid-encoded proteins to amplify signals for tissue regeneration. This system allows the *in vivo* genetic manipulation of fibroblasts. An *in vivo* study with rat skin dermis demonstrated that plasmid-encoded PDGF-BB led to a three- to fourfold increase of granulation tissue at the implantation site, compared to direct injection of PDGF-B plasmid.[158]

STEM CELLS FOR WOUND ANGIOGENESIS AND WOUND HEALING

Bone Marrow-Derived Cells

The bone marrow is a reservoir for progenitor cells that can be recruited to a wounded site for nonhematopoietic tissue regeneration. Transplantation of green fluorescent protein (GFP)-labeled bone marrow into non-GFP mice was used to study the participation of bone marrow stem cells in cutaneous wound healing. GFP+ cells were found deposited in blood vessels, hair follicles, striated muscle, sebaceous glands, and epidermis of wounded recipient mice. Hence, wounding stimulates the bone marrow to release progenitor cells into the circulation that home to the injured site.[159] Furthermore, autologous bone marrow cells have been reported in the successful closure of chronic wounds in three patients, who failed standard and advanced therapies, including skin substitutes.[160] Bone marrow aspirates were directly injected into the wounds and their edges after wound bed preparation. Histologic comparison of pre- and posttreatment biopsies suggests engraftment of bone marrow cells. Specifically, there was increased cellularity and immature cells present. Clinically, the autologous bone marrow treatment resulted in increased vascularity of the wound bed and increased skin thickness.[159]

In Japan, clinical trials have been conducted using bone marrow-derived mononuclear cells autologously transplanted into ischemic limbs by direct injection of bone marrow aspirate into the gastrocnemius muscle. In the study, limbs injected with bone marrow-derived mononuclear cells improved in ischemic status compared to saline injected ones, as well as those treated with peripheral blood-derived mononuclear cells.[161] In the patients studied, 18% of the CD34+ cells were characteristic of endothelial cells. In addition to supplying endothelial progenitor cells, bone marrow-derived cells also provide a source for angiogenic factors. The CD34− cells expressed mRNAs for bFGF, VEGF, and angiopoietin-1, whereas the CD34+ cells expressed their receptors. Ischemia improved and was maintained after 24 weeks follow-up in patients treated with bone marrow-derived mononuclear cells. In all 45 legs injected with bone marrow-derived mononuclear cells, the ankle–brachial index (ABI) improved from a mean of 0.35 to 0.42 at week 4 and 0.46 at week 24 ($p < 0.0001$). The transcutaneous oxygen level increased from 28 to 46 mm Hg at week 4 and 45 mm Hg at week 24 ($p < 0.0001$). Also, pain-free walking time increased from 1.3 to 3.6 minutes at week 4 and 3.7 minutes at week 24 ($p < 0/0001$). Angiography demonstrated a striking increase in collateral vessels in 27 out of 45 patients. Besides ischemic status, approximately half of the patients experienced improvement in leg ulcers, including those with toe salvage.[161]

CD34+ progenitor cells may also be separated and collected from peripheral blood using a system (Isolex 300i, Baxter) of monoclonal antibodies, immunomagnetic beads, and a stem cell-releasing agent PR34+. This system is in current clinical use for hematopoietic reconstitution of CD34 cells after myeloablative therapy in CD34-negative tumors (high-dose chemotherapy and autologous progenitor cell rescue). Preliminary studies are underway using these methods to collect progenitor cells for wound-healing applications.

Endothelial Progenitor Cells

Recent advances in vascular biology and developmental biology have led to cell-mediated vascular regeneration as a new paradigm for therapeutic neovascularization. This concept was rapidly introduced after the discovery of circulating endothelial progenitor cells (EPC) in adult peripheral blood by Asahara and colleagues in 1997.[162]

EPCs have also been identified in adult peripheral blood, bone marrow, and human umbilical cord blood.[50,163] Transplantation of *ex vivo* or culture-expanded EPCs have been shown to effectively enhance angiogenesis in ischemic tissues.[164,165]

The *in situ* formation of blood vessels from EPCs or angioblasts is termed vasculogenesis. The process begins with the formation of cell clusters or blood islands, which fuse to capillary networks in the embryo. With blood circulation, the capillary network differentiates into an arteriovenous vascular system. EPCs are located at the periphery, while hematopoietic stem cells (HSCs) are located in the center of the blood islands. EPCs differentiate into vascular endothelial cells (EC), whereas, HSCs differentiate into mature blood cells. Since EPCs and HSCs share several surface antigens, such as, flk-1, Tie-2, and CD34, they are thought to derive from a common precursor, the hemangioblast.[50] This is in contrast to angiogenesis, which is the sprouting of new capillaries from preexisting mature ECs. Until recently, vasculogenesis was considered limited to early embryogenesis and angiogenesis was credited for postnatal neovascularization. Recent studies discovered the presence of endothelial progenitor cells in the systemic circulation, suggesting that undifferentiated precursors mobilized from the bone marrow contribute to postnatal neovascularization. *In vitro*, these circulating EPCs differentiate into mature ECs.[162,166]

In addition, circulating EPCs may have implications for therapeutic vasculogenesis, such as the enhancement of collateral vessel growth and angiogenesis in ischemic tissues. Circulating EPCs may play a role in the delivery of anti- or proangiogenic agents to sites of pathologic or utilitarian angiogenesis, respectively. EPCs have been mobilized from bone marrow into peripheral blood in response to ischemic stimuli in adult animals.[50] In animal models, transplantation of heterogeneous, homologous, and autologous culture-expanded EPCs have been shown to improve collateral vessel formation, incorporate into new capillaries, and increase the levels of angiogenic growth factors, such as bFGF, VEGF, angiopoietin-1, and IL-1α, in sites of active angiogenesis such as ischemic tissues.[161,163,164] These findings suggest that naturally circulating EPCs or exogenously transplanted EPCs may contribute to neovascularization in adults.

DEVICES THAT FACILITATE WOUND HEALING AND THEIR ROLE IN WOUND NEOVASCULARIZATION

Hyperbaric Oxygen Therapy (HBO)

Chronic wounds are often hypoxic. Adequate tissue oxygen tension is essential in infection control and wound healing. Hyperbaric oxygen therapy (HBO) is defined as a modality in which the entire body is exposed to oxygen under increased atmospheric pressure to cause tissue hyperoxia up to ten times the usual levels by elevating oxygen tension (PO_2) in the wound bed during treatment. Generally the patient breathes 100% oxygen inside a pressurized treatment chamber at two to three times atmospheric pressure for a session lasting 60 to 90 minutes. The average duration of HBO therapy is 2 to 4 weeks, although the range depends on the response of the patient.

At such high oxygen saturation, cellular oxygen requirements are met without employing circulating hemoglobin. At such doses, the oxygen acts like a drug producing biochemical and physiologic benefits.[167] HBO is clearly useful for reducing reperfusion injury. It improves infection control by enhancing leukocyte mobility. HBO stimulates fibroblast proliferation and collagen synthesis, both of which are important in granulation. It enhances microcirculation by reducing edema and stimulating angiogenesis.[168] Using HBO allows switching between hyperoxic and hypoxic conditions, thereby, inducing angiogenesis.[167]

HBO enhances *in vitro* epidermopoiesis, the formation of a stratified epithelium. This has important implications for epidermal regeneration during cutaneous wound healing. Normal human fibroblasts, keratinocytes, melanocytes, and dermal and skin equivalents were exposed to a HBO regimen (up to 3 atm, up to 10 consecutive daily treatments, lasting 90 minutes), consistent with protocols in practice for wound healing therapy. Fibroblast proliferation, keratinocyte differentiation, and epidermopoiesis in skin equivalents occurred after HBO treatments.[169]

HBO promotes angiogenesis and wound healing in part by increasing VEGF expression. In a Japanese study, 10 patients with chronic ulcers were treated with 20 sessions of 100% O_2 at 3 times atmospheric pressure. Six of the ten patients had detectable plasma VEGF levels after 20 treatments with HBO. Interestingly, these patients experienced ulcer healing. By contrast, 4 patients with unhealed ulcers had no detectable plasma levels of VEGF after HBO.[170] In another study with 40 patients, topical HBO at 1.004 to 1.013 atm was used to treat necrotic gangrenous wounds over the course of 12 months. Of wounds treated with topical HBO, 90% healed compared to 22% treated with standard wound care. Capillary density per high-power field was significantly higher in patients treated with topical HBO compared to those treated with standard wound care.[171]

The majority of published reports on HBO consist of review articles, case reports, and uncontrolled studies with small sample size. Despite the dearth in well-designed clinical trials, HBO therapy has become adjunctive therapy for wound care in deep and superficial, infected and noninfected, ischemic and well-perfused wounds.

Despite the scientific data on hyperbaric oxygen on wound healing, randomized placebo-controlled multicenter clinical trials in large populations, such as diabetic patients, will help elucidate criteria for selecting patients for HBO therapy and give credibility to accelerated wound healing using this type of treatment.

The Hyperbaric Oxygen Therapy Committee of the Undersea and Hyperbaric Medical Society recommends HBO for clostridial myonecrosis, acute traumatic ischemia, improved healing in problem wounds, necrotizing soft tissue infections, refractory osteomyelitis, compromised skin grafts and flaps, and thermal burns.[172] Of note, the U.S. Centers for Medicare and Medicaid Services' (CMS) national coverage policy limits reimbursement only to therapy administered in a chamber and only for the following conditions: acute carbon monoxide intoxication, decompression illness, gas embolism, gas gangrene, acute traumatic peripheral ischemia, acute peripheral arterial insufficiency, crush injuries, progressive necrotizing infections, preparation and preservation of compromised skin graft, chronic refractory osteomyelitis, osteoradionecrosis, soft tissue radionecrosis, cyanide poisoning, and actinomycosis. As of April 2003, coverage extends to diabetic leg ulcers of Wagner grade III or higher, that has failed standard wound therapy with no signs of healing for at least 30 days. However, many types of common chronic ulcerations are not covered, including decubitus and stasis ulcers, chronic peripheral vascular insufficiency, and thermal burns.

Vacuum-Assisted Closure

Vacuum-Assisted Closure (VAC; Kinetic Concepts, Inc.) consists of an open-cell polyurethane ether foam sponge and noncollapsible suction tubing with an adjustable vacuum pump. The VAC is secured to the wound with an occlusive adhesive dressing that acts as a sealant and can be changed several times a week. Negative pressure therapy by VAC, pioneered by Argenta and Morykwas, was FDA approved through a 510(k) in 1995 to promote wound healing in acute and chronic wounds and through an additional 510(k) in December 2002 for an additional indication of partial-thickness burns.[173] VAC applies sustained negative pressure to the wound bed. As a result, it reduces third-space edema allowing better oxygen and nutrient delivery to and toxin elimination from the wound. It also removes debris and exudate, thereby, decreasing bacterial colonization and promoting granulation.[174] Negative pressure induces changes in the cytoskeletal shape of endothelial cells within a wound, that likely induces angiogenic gene expression.[82] From the perspective of microbial control, the VAC decreases bacteria count from 10^7 to 10^2–10^3/g of tissue between day 4 and 5, which is the result achieved by saline dressing changes three times a day for 11 days.[174]

The VAC converts an open wound into a controlled, closed environment. The typical range of pressure applied is between 50 to 125 mm Hg. The pore size of the foam sponge ranges from 400 to 600 μm, which allows maximal in-growth of granulation tissue. The foam sponge dressing is cut to fit the wound and placed into the deepest portion of the wound. A plastic adhesive drape should be placed over the sponge, overlapping the wound margins by at least 5 cm to obtain an airtight seal.[175]

VAC is generally well-tolerated by patients. Some manageable issues associated with the VAC include excessive granulation tissue in-growth into the sponge, bleeding during dressing changes, transient pain occurring when the sponge is first connected to the suction and subatmospheric pressure is transmitted to the wound. Often a distinctive odor, not representative of infection, is present, which is associated with the interaction of the sponge and exudates.[175]

The VAC has been reported to be superior to normal saline dressing in the management of chronic wounds. In a prospective randomized study of chronic full-thickness ulcers, the efficacy of 6-week treatment with VAC was compared to several gel products made by Healthpoint (HP), including Iodosorb gel, an antiseptic containing dextran beads with 0.9% Iodosorb (cadexomer iodine), and/or Panafil (papain–urea–chlorophyllin–copper) débriding ointment.[174] In the study, increased rate of wound healing was observed in the VAC group compared to the HP group. The mean number of PMNs and lymphocytes decreased in the VAC group, but increased in the HP group; hence, VAC appeared to be better at reducing inflammation at wound sites. In addition, more capillaries were present in the soft tissue of VAC treated wounds compared to HP-treated wounds. In particular, the VAC improves skin graft survival because it provides constant negative pressure under occlusive dressing. The negative pressure allows the graft and the wound bed to become well apposed despite surface contour irregularities. It also removes wound fluid, preventing the accumulation of hematoma or seroma. The VAC dressing maintains a moist environment, preventing dessication. In addition, it stabilizes the graft, minimizing shear stress. Last, it is associated with lower bacterial counts at wounds sites. In a retrospective study of 61 patients that underwent split-thickness skin grafts (STSG), 34 were managed with VAC and 27 with bolster dressings.[176] Only 3% of patients managed with VAC required repeated STSG compared to 19% managed with bolster dressings. However, the study did not control for the etiology of wounds between the VAC and bolster dressing groups.[176] VAC has also been used concomitantly with tissue-engineered products and becaplermin. In the case of tissue-engineered products. VAC therapy should not

be used after the first week of product implantation so as to avoid removal of soluble molecular wound-healing mediators released by the implanted constructs.

Electrical Stimulation

For over 40 years, it has been postulated that the skin has a positive electrical potential, whereas, the tissue beneath has a negative electrical potential. This charge distribution becomes disturbed when a wound is present and generates what is referred to as the "current of injury," which persists until the tissue defect is repaired. The flow of current can be measured during the wound-healing process. Macrophages, mast cells, or granulocytes travel along a voltage gradient to the positive potential or cathode.[177] Animal models and human studies have demonstrated blood flow improvement near a positive potential.[178] However, the charge ceases in a dry ulcer, since a moist wound environment is necessary for the bioelectric system to function, or when the wound is completely healed. One theory involving current of injury postulates that healing becomes arrested if the current does not flow. The main rationale for electrical stimulation is to mimic the natural current of injury to "jump start" or accelerate the healing process.[179]

Electrical stimulation is defined as the use of an electric current to transfer energy to a wound.[179] This intervention has been used by the physiotherapist since the early 1960s and has been investigated in at least 15 controlled studies.[180] Capacitively coupled electrical stimulation transfers electrical current through two electrodes over wet conductive media, such as a hydrogel-impregnated gauze placed in the wound bed and on the skin at a distance from the wound. The most extensively tested waveform has been the monophasic twin-peaked high voltage-pulsed current (HVPC), with a pulse width ranging from 20 to 200 μsec. Electrical stimulation is generally applied for 45 to 60 minutes, 5 to 7 times per week. An *in vivo* study has been conducted on the effect of electrical stimulation on the healing of full-thickness excisional wounds in diabetic mice. Of the mice treated with electrical stimulation, 36% experienced wound closure compared to 12.5% of the sham-treated mice. In addition, wounds treated with 12.5 volts achieved significant decrease in surface area and change in the shapes of wounds compared to sham-treated controls.[177]

The Dermapulse (GerroMed, Hamburg, Germany) is an example of a battery-powered device that delivers pulsed electrical stimulation. A study of Dermapulse on chronic venous ulcers showed that capillary density in the ulcer increased by 43.5%, oxygen level at the ulcer margin improved by 80%, and ulcer size decreased in a short period of time.[177] This suggests that electric stimulation has positive effects on wound angiogenesis and healing. Mechanistic studies on Dermapulse on growth factor and receptor expression are underway.[177] Of note, the U.S. Centers for Medicare and Medicaid Services (CMS) issued a national coverage decision in April, 2003 that covers reimbursement using electrical stimulation for chronic Stage III and IV pressure ulcers, arterial ulcers, diabetic ulcers, and venous stasis ulcers only after standard wound therapy has failed for at least 30 days. Electrical stimulation for wound healing is not covered by insurance for use in the home setting.

Laser and Optical Stimulation

Laser biostimulation was introduced over 20 years ago in the Soviet Union, Hungary, and Austria as a means of irradiating areas of the skin to accelerate wound healing. Since then, low-level laser therapy of less than 10 J/cm^2 has been used by some wound specialists to treat chronic ulcers with primarily anecdotal results and a few published studies.[181,182] Laser biostimulation for wound healing has not been formally FDA approved because its efficacy has not been well documented.[183]

It has been hypothesized that cellular proliferation or regeneration occurs by exposing cells in a wound to photon energy. Direct or indirect interference of visible and infrared wavelengths on mitochondrial components of the respiratory chain may affect signal transduction in cellular proliferation. Certain types of lasers, particularly the HeNe, when used at proper wavelengths, have shown to affect fibroblast proliferation, attachment, and procollagen, as well as, collagen production in vitro.[183] An *in vivo* study compared the mechanical and chemical properties of wounds treated with helium/neon (HeNe) lasers and nontreated wounds in a diabetic rat model. The laser-treated wounds had 84% greater tensile strength than the nontreated wounds. In addition, the total collagen of laser-treated wounds were significantly greater than nontreated wounds, but pepsin-soluble collagen was appreciably less, indicating laser-treated wounds were more resistant to proteolytic degradation.[184] An *in vitro* study of low-intensity laser irradiation on human umbilical vein endothelial cell (HUVEC) demonstrated that doses between 2 and 8 J/cm^2 and at intensities between 20 and 65 mW/cm^2 caused a significant increase in HUVEC proliferation compared to nonirradiated cells.[185] Thus far, data suggest that low-intensity laser may facilitate angiogenesis and tissue repair by stimulating endothelial cell proliferation. A number of mechanisms for biostimulation have been proposed, including increasing transmembrane proton gradient and an increase in adenosine triphosphate (ATP) synthesis (by up to 70%) within mitochondria.[186] In addition, low-intensity laser exposure has induced proangiogenic factors in cell lines other than endothelial cells.[185] For example, low-level laser therapy stimulates human T lymphocytes in suspension *in vitro* to release angiogenic growth factors into the media, which then have the ability to stimulate endothelial cell proliferation.[187] Yu and colleagues found that Argon laser biostimulation for 4–8 minutes can cause the release of the angiogenic factors TGF-β and PDGF from fibroblasts, as determined by ELISA.[188] Furthermore, at macrovascular levels, low-level laser irradiation modulates calcium influx in vascular smooth muscle cells in an *in vivo* rat mesenteric model.[189] By causing potent dilation in arterioles, low-level laser irradiation may increase flow in the microcirculation.

As an alternative to laser irradiation, light-emitting diodes and their effects on cells have also been studied. When cultured fibroblasts were exposed to LEDs of varying wavelengths, there was a higher rate of proliferation ($p \leq 0.001$) than control.[190] The National Aeronautics and Space Administration (NASA) has a LED medical program using wavelengths of 680, 730, and 880 nm, which has been shown to increase DNA synthesis in fibroblasts by fourfold at 4 J/cm^2.[191] The advantages of LEDs are that they can be arranged in large, flat arrays allowing the treatment of large wounds. NASA's LED-light therapy, developed by Quantum Devices Inc., is currently in clinical trial for diabetic leg ulcers.

Several well-controlled animal studies show beneficial effects from laser biostimulation of wounds in loose-skinned animals.[183] There are only case reports in humans that attest to the efficacy of helium/neon (HeNe) and gallium arsenide (GaAs) lasers for wound healing.[19] One problem in interpreting the results of different studies is the use of different kinds of lasers, energy setting, time exposures, wound types, and cell types.

Radiofrequency Ablation

Radiofrequency (RF) treatment of chronic wounds release endogenous growth factors, which triggers cell proliferation and accelerated wound healing. RF-based devices have been used in cardiac catheterization and ablation, bone and wound healing therapies, decompression of herniated discs, and arthroscopic procedures. Coblation technology, like most conventional RF-based devices, performs tissue remodeling functions, such as, ablation, coagulation, desiccation, or excision. Coblation-treated tendons demonstrated increased expression of α_v integrin subunit and VEGF expression at 9 days compared to controls, but returned to a level consistent with normal tendon tissue at 90 days.[192] RF plasma-based micropuncture appears to stimulate a beneficial angiogenic wound healing response in chronically injured tissue.

FUTURE DIRECTIONS FOR WOUND ANGIOGENESIS AND WOUND HEALING

A variety of molecular-based therapies are available or under development to accelerate wound healing. Novel growth factor delivery systems, such as angiogenic gene sutures, autologous stem cell transplantation, genetically modified tissue-engineered constructs, and growth factor-impregnated dressings or sprays, are now under clinical investigation.[161,193–195] In the future, combinatorial therapies of growth factors, growth factors with tissue-engineered constructs, sequential use of tissue-engineered skin substitutes, and the use of biological agents and tissue engineered skin constructs with HBO, the VAC, or other methods to deliver energy, such as electrical stimulation or lasers, may prove to be additive or even synergistic in their actions on wound healing. The tools of genomics and proteomics may eventually be used to help profile wounds to tailor therapy in individual patients. Well-controlled clinical trials are required to distinguish advanced modalities with true efficacy from mass-marketed wound care products that have no data to support their use. As wound research and technology development continues, there will undoubtedly be new insights into, and technologies for, accelerating wound angiogenesis to promote improved healing in patients.

REFERENCES

1. Frost & Sullivan U.S. Advanced Wound Management Product Report, 2000, San Jose, CA.

2. Li WW, Li VW, Tsakayannis D. Angiogenesis: a control point for normal and delayed wound healing. *Contemp Surg Suppl.* 2003;3–10.

3. Clark RAF. Wound repair: Overview and general considerations. In: Clark RAF (ed.). *The Molecular and Cellular Biology of Wound Repair,* 2nd Ed. New York: Plenum Press, 1995:3–37.

4. Lazarus GS, Cooper DM, Nighton DR, et al. Definitions and guidelines for assessment of wounds and evaluation of healing. *Arch Dermtol.* 1994;130:489–493.

5. Stanley A, Osler T. Senescence and the healing rates of venous ulcers. *J Vasc Surg.* 2001;33(6):1206–1211.

6. Vande Berg JS, Rudolph R, Hollan C, Haywood-Reid PL. Fibroblast senescence in pressure ulcers. *Wound Repair Regen.* 1998;6(1):38–49.

7. Mendez MV, Stanley A, Menzoian JO, et al. Fibroblasts cultured from venous ulcers display cellular characteristics of senescence. *J Vasc Surg.* 1998;28(5):876–883.

8. Trengove NJ, Bielefeldt-Ohmann H, Stacey MC. Mitogenic activity and cytokine levels in nonhealing and healing chronic leg ulcers. *Wound Repair Regen.* 2000;8(1):13–25.

9. Hasan A, Murata H, Badiavas E, et al. Dermal fibroblasts from venous ulcers are unresponsive to the action of transforming growth factor-beta 1. *J Dermatol Sci.* 1997;16:59–66.

10. Stanley AC, Park HY, Menzoian JO, et al. Reduced growth of dermal fibroblasts from chronic venous ulcers can be eliminated with growth factors. *J Vasc Surg.* 1997;26:994–999.

11. Harding KG, Morris HL, Patel GK. Science, medicine and the future: healing chronic wounds. *Brit Med J.* 2002; 324(7330):160–163.

12. Brem H. Specific paradigm for wound bed preparation in chronic wounds. *Proc Sympo Sponsored by the European Tissue Repair Soc,* November 24–25. 2000:33–38.

13. Maragoudakis ME, Tsopanoglou NE. On the mechanism(s) of thrombin induced angiogenesis. *Adv Exp Med Biol.* 2000; 476:47–55.

14. Page CP. The involvement of platelets in non-thrombotic processes. *Trends Pharmacol Sci.* 1988;9:66–71.

15. Liu Y, Kalen A, Risto O, Wahlstrom O. Time- and pH-dependent release of PDGF and TGF-beta from platelets *in vitro. Platelets.* 2003;14(4):223–237.

16. Pintucci G, Froum S, Green D, et al. Trophic effect of platelets on cultured endothelial cells are mediated by platelet-associated fibroblast growth factor-2 (FGF-2) and vascular endothelial growth factor (VEGF). *Thromb Haemost.* 2002; 88(5):834–842.

17. Nakamura T, Nawa K, Nishino T, et al. Purification and subunit structure of hepatocyte growth factor from rat platelets. *FEBS Lett.* 1987;224(2):311–316.

18. Li JJ, Huang YQ, Basch R, Karpatkin S. Thrombin induces the release of angiopoietin-1 from platelets. *Thromb Haemost.* 2001;85(2):204–206.

19. Natarajan S, Williamson D, Stiltz AJ, et al. Advances in wound care and healing technology. *Amer J Clin Dermatol.* 2000; 5:269–275.

20. Polverini PJ, Leibovich SJ. Induction of neovascularization in vivo and endothelial proliferation in vitro by tumor-associated macrophages. *Lab Invest.* 1984;51:635–642.

21. Schultz GS, Mast BA. Molecular analysis of the environment of healing and chronic wounds: cytokines, proteases, and growth factors. *Wounds 10 Suppl F.* 1998;1F-9F.

22. Teixeira AS, Andrade SP. Glucose-induced inhibition of angiogenesis in the rat sponge granuloma is prevented by aminoguanidine. *Life Sci.* 1999;64:655–662.

23. Blakytny R, Jude EB, Ferguson MW, et al. Lack of insulin-like growth factor 1 (IGF1) in the basal keratinocyte layer of diabetic skin and diabetic foot ulcers. *J Pathol.* 2000;190: 589–594.

24. Cechowska-Pasko M, Palka J, Bankowski E. Alterations in glycosaminoglycans in wounded skin of diabetic rats. A possible role of IGF-I, IGF-binding proteins and proteolytic activity. *Acta Biochim Polon.* 1996;43:557–565.

25. Barrick B, Campbell EJ, Owen CA. Leukocyte proteinases in wound healing: roles in physiologic and pathologic processes. *Wound Repair Regen.* 1999;7:410–422.

26. Agren MS, Steenfos HH, Dabelsteen E, et al. Proliferation and mitogenic response to PDGF-BB of fibroblasts isolated from chronic venous leg ulcers is ulcer-age dependent. *J Invest Dermatol.* 1999;112:463–469.

27. Vlodavsky I, Fuks Z, Ishai-Michaeli R, et al. Extracellular matrix resident basic fibroblast growth factor: implications for the control of angiogenesis. *J Cell Biochem.* 1991;45:167–176.

28. Tsopanoglou NE, Maragoudakis ME. On the mechanism of thrombin-induced angiogenesis. Potentiation of vascular endothelial growth factor activity on endothelial cells by up-regulation of its receptors. *J Cell Biochem.* 1999;274: 23969–23976.

29. Nguyen M, Arkell Jackson CJ. Human endothelial gelatinases and angiogenesis. *Int J Biochem Cell Biol.* 2001;33:960–970.

30. Thommen R, Humar R, Misevic G, et al. PDGF-BB increases endothelial migration on cord movements during angiogenesis *in vitro. J Cell Biochem.* 1997;64:403–413.

31. Folkman J, Klagsbrun M: Angiogenic factors. *Science.* 1987; 235:442–447.

32. Koch AE, Polverini PJ, Leibovich SJ. Induction of neovascularization by actived human monocytes. *J Leukoc Biol.* 1996; 39:233–238.

33. Crowther M, Brown NJ, Lewis CE, et al. Microenvironmental influence on macrophage regulation of angiogenesis in wounds and malignant tumor. *J Leukoc Biol.* 2001;70:478–490.

34. Bootle-Wilbraham CA, Tazzyman S, Lewis CE, et al. Fibrin fragment E stimulates the proliferation, migration, and differentiation of human microvascular endothelial cells *in vitro.* *Angiogenesis.* 2001;4:269–275.

35. Amano H, Hayashi I, Majima M. Cyclooxygenase-2 and adenylate cyclase/protein kinase A signaling pathway enhances angiogenesis through induction of vascular endothelial growth factor in rat sponge implants. *Human Cell.* 2002;15:13–24.

36. Giordano FJ, Johnson RS. Angiogenesis: the role of the microenvironment in flipping the switch. *Curr Opin Genet Devel.* 2001;11:35–40.

37. Howdieshell TR, Riegner C, Sathyanarayana McNeil PL. Normotoxic wound fluid contains high levels of vascular endothelial growth factor. *Ann Surg.* 1998;228:707–715.

38. Dvorak HF, Brown LF, Dvorak AM. Vascular permeability factor/vascular endothelial growth factor, microvascular hyperpermeability, and angiogenesis. *Am J Pathol.* 1995;146: 1029–1039.

39. Smith RS Jr, Lin KF, Chao J. Human endothelial nitric oxide synthase gene delivery promotes angiogenesis in a rat model of hindlimb ischemia. *Arterioscler Thromb Vasc Biol.* 1995;22: 1279–1295.

40. Darland DC, D'Amore PA. Blood vessel maturation. *J Clin Invest.* 1999;103:157–158.

41. Korff R, Kimmina S, Augustin HG, et al. Blood vessel maturation in a 3-dimensional spheroidal coculture model direct contact with smooth muscle cells regulates endothelial cell quiescence and abrogates VEGF responsiveness. *FASEB J.* 2001;15:447–457.

42. Hirschi KK, Rohovsky SA, D'Amore PA, et al. Endothelial cells modulate the proliferation of mural cell precursors via platelet-derived growth factor-BB and heterotypic cell contact. *Circ Res.* 1999;84:298–305.

43. Lindahl P, Johansson BR, Betsholtz C, et al. Pericyte loss and microaneurysm formation in PDGF-B-deficient mice. *Science.* 1997;277:242–245.

44. Brown NH, Smyth EA, Reed MW. Angiogenesis induction and regression in human surgical wounds. *Wound Repair Regen.* 2002;10:245–251.

45. Antonelli-Orlidge A, Saunders KB, D'Amore PA, et al. An activated form of transforming growth factor beta is produced by cocultures of endothelial cells and pericytes. *Proc Natl Acad Sci U S A.* 1989;86:4544–4548.

46. Beienberg DR, Bucana CD, Fidler IJ. Progressive growth of infantile cutaneous hemangiomas is directly correlated with hyperplasia and angiogenesis of adjacent opidermis and inversely correlated with expression of the endogenous angiogenesis inhibitor IFN-beta. *Int J Oncol.* 1999;14:401–408.

47. Bloch W. Hoggel K, Werner S, et al. The angiogenesis inhibitor endostatin impairs blood vessel maturation during wound healing. *FASEB J.* 2000;14:2373–2376.

48. Lange-Asschenfeldt B, Velasco P, Detmar M. The angiogenesis inhibitor vasostatin does not impair wound healing at tumor-inhibiting doses. *J Invest Dermatol.* 2001;117:1036–1041.

49. Tonnesen MG, Feng X, Clark RAF. Angiogenesis in wound healing. *J Invest Dermatol Symp Proc.* 2000;5:40–46.

50. Asahara T, Masuda H, Takahashi T, et al. Bone marrow origin of endothelial progenitor cells for postnatal vasculogenesis in physiological and pathological neovascularization. *Circ Res.* 1999;85:221–228.

51. Carmeliet P, Luttun A: The emerging role of the bone marrow-derived stem cells in (therapeutic) angiogenesis. *Thromb Haemost.* 2001;86:289–297.

52. Hattori K, Heissig B, Wu Y, et al. Placental growth factor reconstitutes hematopoiesis by recruiting VEGFR1(+) stem cells from bone-marrow microenvironment. *Nat Med.* 2002; 8:841–849,2002.

53. Kudo M, Van de Water K, Plantefaber LC, et al. Fibrinogen and fibrin are antiadhesive for keratinocytes: a mechanism for fibrin eschar slough during wound repair. *J Invest Deramatol.* 2001;117:1369–1381.

54. Mendez MV, Stanley A, Park HY, et al. Fibroblasts cultured from venous ulcers display cellular characteristics of senescence. *J Vasc Surg.* 1998;28:876–883.

55. Vlodavsky I, Bar-Shavit R, Ishai-Michaeli R, et al. Extracellular sequestration and release of fibroblast growth factor: a regulatory mechanism? *Trends Biochm Sci.* 1991;16:268–271.

56. Antoniades HN, Galanopoulos T, Neville-Golden J, et al. Injury induces *in vivo* expression of platelet-derived growth factor (PDGF) and PDGF receptor mRNAs in skin epithelial cells and PDGF mRNA in connective tissue fibroblasts. *Proc Natl Acad Sci U S A.* 1991;88:565–569.

57. Condon ET, Wang JH, Redmond HF, et al. Lipopolysaccharide and surgery induces mobilization of bone marrow-derived endothelial progenitor cells. Poster 140: Presented at the annual meeting of the American Association for Cancer Research Annual Meeting; April 6–10, 2002; San Francisco, CA.

58. Steed DL, Donohoe D, Lindsley L, et al. Effect of extensive débridement and treatment on the healing of diabetic foot ulcers. Diabetic Ulcer Study Group. *J Am Coll Surg.* 1996; 183:61–64.

59. Sibbald RG. What is the bacterial burden of the wound bed and does it matter? *Proc. a Symp. Sponsored by the European Tissue Repair Soc, November.* 24–25, 2000:41–46.

60. Gilchrist B. Infection and culturing. In: Krasner D, Kane D, Eds. *Chronic wound care: A clinical source book for healthcare professionals.* 2nd ed. Wayne, PA: Health Management Publications, 1997:109–114.

61. Wright JB, Lam K, Burrell RE. Wound management in an era of increasing bacterial antibiotic resistance: A rate for topical silver treatment. *Am J Infect Control.* 1998;26:572–577.

62. Cao R, Brakenhielm E, Pawliuk R, et al. Angiogenic synergism, vascular stability and improvement of hindlimb ischemia by a combination of PDGF-BB and FGF-2. *Nature Med.* 2003;5(9):604–613.

63. Doxey DL, Ng MC, Iacopino AM, et al. Platelet-derived growth factor levels in wounds of diabetic rats. *Life Sci.* 1995;57:1111–1123.

64. Sellen RA, Hart CE, Phillips PE, et al. Two different subunits associate to create isoform-specific platelet derived growth factor receptor. *J Biol Chem.* 1989;264:8871–8778.

65. Li WW, Li VW. Therapeutic angiogenesis for wound healing. *Wounds.* 2003;15:2–12S.

66. Risau W, Drexler H, Mironov V, et al. Platelet-derived growth factor is angiogenic in vivo. *Growth Factors.* 1992;7(4): 261–265.

67. Battegay EJ, Rupp J, Iruela-Arispe L, et al. PDGF-BB modulates endothelial proliferation and angiogenesis *in vitro* via PDGF beta-receptors. *J Cell Biol.* 1994;125:917–928.

68. Bar RS, Boes M, Han MN, et al. The effects of platelet-derived growth factor in cultured microvessel endothelial cells. *Endocrinology.* 1989;124:1841–1848.

69. Koyama N, Watanabe, Tezuka M, et al. Migratory and proliferative effect of platelet-derived growth factor in rabbit retinal endothelial cells: Evidence of an autocrine pathway of platelet-derived growth factor. *J Cell Physiol.* 1994;158:1–6.

70. Zhu WH, Guo X, Francesco Nicosia R. Regulation of vascular growth and regression by matrix metalloproteinases in the rat aorta model of angiogenesis. *Lab Invest.* 2000;80:545–555.

71. Clark RAF, Tonnesen MG, Cheresh DA, et al. Transient functional expression of alpha v beta 3 on vascular cells during wound repair. *Am J Pathol.* 1996;148:1407–1421.

72. Xu J, Clark RAF. Extracellular matrix alters PDGF regulation of fibroblast integrins. *J Cell Biol.* 1996;132:239–249.

73. Kimura I, Tsuneki H, Ogasawara M, et al. Platelet-derived growth factor blocks the cell-cycle transition from the G0 to G1 phase in sub-cultured angiogenic endothelial cells in rat thoracic aorta. *Jpn J Pharmacol.* 1997;74:303–311.

74. Kobayashi S, Kimura I, Kimura M. Diabetic state-modified macrophages in GK rat release platelet-derived growth factor-BB for tube formation of endothelial cells in rat aorta. *Immunopharmacology.* 1996;35:171.

75. Hellstrom M, Gaqrhardt H, Betsholtz C, et al. Lack of pericytes leads to endothelial hyperplasia and abnormal vascular morphogenesis. *J Cell Biol.* 2001;153(3):543–553.

76. Glover JL, Weingarten MS, Buchbinder DS, et al. A 4-year outcome-based retrospective study of wound healing and limb salvage in patients with chronic wounds. *Adv Wound Care.* 1997;10:33–38.

77. Steed DL. The Diabetic Ulcer Study Group. Clinical evaluation of recombinant human platelet-derived growth factor for the treatment of lower extremity diabetic ulcers. *J Vasc Surg.* 1995;21:71–81.

78. Smiell JM, Wieman TJ, Steed DL, et al. Efficacy and safety of becaplermin (recombinant human platelet-derived growth factor-BB) in patients with nonhealing, lower extremity diabetic ulcers: A combined analysis of four randomized studies. *Wound Repair Regen.* 1999;7:333–346.

79. Wieman TJ, Smiell JM, Su Y. Efficacy and safety of a topical gel formulation of recombinant human platelet-derived growth factor-BB (becaplermin) in patients with chronic neuropathic diabetic ulcers. A phase III randomized placebo-controlled double blind study. *Diabetes Care.* 1998;21:822–827.

80. Zagari M, Martens L, Wieman T, et al. Treatment of diabetic foot ulcers with topical recombinant growth factor gel achieves higher healing rates and results in lower protected costs of care. Poster presented at Clinical Symposium on Wound Care; October 8–11, 1998; Atlanta. GA.

81. Embil JM, Papp K, Sibbald G, et al. Recombinant human platelet-derived growth factor-BB (becaplermin) for healing chronic lower extremity diabetic ulcers: An open-label clinical evaluation of efficacy. *Wound Repair Regen.* 2000;8: 162–168.

82. Li VW, Li WW. Angiogenic therapy for chronic wounds: The clinical experience with becaplermin. *Contemporary Surg. (Nov Suppl)* 2003;26–32S.

83. Pierce GF, Tarpley JE, Vande Berg J, et al. Tissue repair processes in healing chronic pressure ulcers treated with recombinant platelet-derived growth factor BB. *Am J Pathol.* 1994;145:399–410.

84. Rees RS, Robson MC, Perry BH, et al. Becaplermin gel in the treatment of pressure ulcers. A phase II randomized, double-blind, placebo-controlled study. *Wound Repair Regen.* 1999; 7:141–147.

85. Wieman TJ. Efficacy and safety of recombinant human platelet-derived growth factor-BB (becaplermin) in patients with chronic venous ulcers: A pilot study. *Wounds.* 2003; 15(8):257–264.

86. Li WW, Tsakayannis D, Li VW. Angiogenesis: A control point for normal and delayed wound healing. *Contemp Surg. (Nov Suppl)* 2003;5–11S.

87. Xiu YP, Zhao Y, Marcus J, et al. Effects of keratinocyte growth factor-2 (KGF-2) on wound healing in an ischaemia-impaired rabbit ear model and on scar formation. *J Pathol.* 1999; 188:431–438.

88. Gillis P, Savla U, Volpen OV, et al. Keratinocyte growth factor induces angiogenesis and protects endothelial barrier function. *J Cell Biochem.* 1997;64:403–415.

89. Fu X, Shen Z, Chen Y, et al. Randomized placebo-controlled trial of use of topical recombinant bovine basic fibroblast growth factor for secondary burns. *Lancet.* 1998;352: 1661–1664.

90. Fu X, Shin Z, Chen Y, et al. Recombinant bovine basic fibroblast growth factor accelerates wound healing in patients with burns, donor sites, and chronic dermal ulcers. *Chin Med J (Engl.)* 2000;113:367–371.

91. Jaschke E, Zabernigg A, Gattringer C. Recombinant human granulocyte-macrophage colony-stimulating factor applied locally in low doses enhances healing and prevents recurrence of chornic venous ulcers. Poster. Wound Healing Society Meeting 2001, Baltimore, Maryland.

92. Robson MC, Steed DL, McPherson JM, et al. Effects of transforming growth factor β2 on wound healing in diabetic foot ulcers: a randomized controlled safety and dose-ranging trial. *J App Res.* 2002;2.

93. Hirschberg J, Coleman J, Rees RS, et al. TGF-β3 in the treatment of pressure ulcers: a preliminary report. *Advan Skin Wound Care.* March/April 2001;91–95.

94. Grant DS, Rose W, Yaen C, et al. Thymosin beta4 enhances endothelial cell differentiation and angiogenesis. *Angiogenesis.* 1999;3:125–135.

95. Philp D, Badamchian M, Schermeta, et al. Thymosin Tβ4 and a synthetic peptide containing its actin-binding domain promote dermal wound repair in db/db diabetic mice and in aged mice. *Wound Rep Regen.* 2003;11:19–24.

96. Malinda KM, Sidhu GS, Banaudha KK, et al. *J Immunol.* 1998;160:1001–1006.

97. Lee WL. Pro-angiogenic synthetic peptides may expedite wound healing. *Dermatol Times* December 2001:31.

98. Norfleet AM, Bergmann JS, Carney DH. Thrombin peptide, TP508, stimulates angiogenic responses in animal models of dermal wound healing, in chick chorloallatoic membranes, and in cultured human aortic and microvascular endothelial cells. *Gen Pharmacol.* 2000;35:249–254.

99. Stiernberg J, Norfleet AM, Redin WR, et al. Acceleration of full-thickness wound healing in normal rats by the synthetic thrombin peptide, TP508. *Wound Repair Regen.* 2000; 8:204–215.

100. Li WW, Li VW. Therapeutic angiogenesis for wound healing. *Wounds.* 2003;15(9 *Suppl.*):25–125.

101. Pertovaara L, Kaspainen A, Mustonen T, et al. Vascular endothelial growth factor is induced in response to transforming growth factor-beta in fibroblasts and endothelial cells. *J Biol Chem.* 1994;269:6271–6274.

102. Dolecki GJ, Connolly DT. Effects on a variety of cytokines and inducing agents on vascular permeability factor mRNA levels in U937 cells. *Biochem Biophys Res Commun.* 1991;180: 572–578.

103. Folkman J, D' Amore PA. Blood vessel formation: what is its molecular basis? *Cell.* 1996;87(7):1153–1155.

104. Thurston G, Suri C, Smith K, et al. Leakage-resistant blood vessels in mice transgenically overexpressing angiopoietin-1. *Science.* 1999;286:2511–2514.

105. Richardson TP, Peters MC, Mooney DJ, et al. Polymeric system for dual growth factor delivery. *Nature Biotechnol.* 2001;19:1029–1034.

106. Cullen B, Smith R, Morrison L, et al. Mechanism of action of PROMOGRAN, a protease modulating matrix, for the treatment of diabetic foot ulcers. *Wound Repair Regen.* 2002;10: 16–25.

107. Lobman R, Ambrosch A, Schultz AG, et al. Expression of matrix-metalloproteinases and their inhibitors in the wounds of diabetic and nondiabetic patients. *Diabetologia.* 2002; 45:1011–1016.

108. Ovington L, Cullen B. Matrix metalloprotease modulation and growth factor protection. *Wounds.* 2003;14(5 *Suppl.*):2–13.

109. Hammond HK, McKirnan MD. Angiogenic gene therapy for heart disease: A review of animal studies and clinical trials. *Cardiovasc Res.* 2001;49:561–567.

110. Khavari PA, Rollman O, Vahlquist A. Cutaneous gene transfer for skin and systemic diseases. *J Int Med.* 2002;252:1–10.

111. Comerota AJ, Throm RC, Pilsudski R, et al. Naked plasmid DNA encoding fibroblast growth factor type 1 for the treatment of end-stage unconstructible lower extremity ischemia: preliminary results of a phase I trial. *J Vasc Surg May.* 2002; 35(5):930–936.

112. Dormandy JA, Rutherford RB. Management of peripheral arterial disease (PAD). TransAtlantic Inter-Society Consensus (TASC). *J Vasc Surg.* 2000;31(1): S1–S296.

113. Zachary I, Gliki G. Signaling transduction mechanisms mediating biological actions of the vascular endothelial growth factor family. *Cardiovasc Res.* 2001;49:568–581.

114. Matthies AM, Low QE, DiPietro LA, et al. Neuropilin-1 participates in wound angiogenesis. *Am J Pathol.* 2002;160: 289–296.

115. Maragoudakis ME, Tsopanoglou NE, Andriopoulou P, et al. Effects of thrombin/thrombosis in angiogenesis and tumour progression. *Matrix Biol.* 2000;19:345–351.

116. Dvorak HF: VPF/VEGF and the angiogenic response. *Sem Perinatol.* 2000;24:75–78.

117. Nissen NN, Polverini PJ, Koch AE, et al. Vascular endothelial growth factor mediates angiogenic activity during the proliferative phase of wound healing. *Am J Pathol.* 1998;152: 1445–1452.

118. Dvorak HF, Nagy JA, Feng D, et al. Vascular permeability factor/vascular endothelial growth factor and the significance of microvascular hyperpermeability in angiogenesis. *Curr Top Microbiol Immunol.* 1999;237:97–132.

119. Isner JM, Pieczek A, Symes J, et al. Clinical evidence of angiogenesis following arterial gene transfer of ph $VEGF_{165}$. *Lancet.* 1996;348:370–374.

120. Baumgartner I, Pieczek A, Isner JM, et al. Constitutive expression of ph $VEGF_{165}$ after intramuscular gene transfer promotes collateral vessel development in patients with critical limb ischemia. *Circulation.* 1998;97:1114–1123.

121. Phillips TJ, Manzoor J, Falanga V, et al. The longevity of a bilayered skin substitute after application to venous ulcers. *Arch Dermatol.* 2002;138(8):1079–1081.

122. www.fda.gov/cber/summaries/melkersontrg.htm

123. www.fda.gov/cber/summaries/weber100300.htm

124. www.fda.gov/fdac/features/2002/302_heal.html

125. Rheinwald J, Green H. Serial cultivation of strains of human epidermal keratinocytes: formation of keratinizing colonies from single cells. *Cell.* 1975;6:331–344.

126. Bello YM, Falabella AF, Eaglestein WH. Tissue-engineered skin: current status in wound healing. *Am J Clin Dermatol.* 2001;2(5):305–313.

127. Rusczcak Z, Schwartz RA. Modern aspects of wound healing: an update. *Dermatol Surg.* 2000;26(3):219–229.

128. Compton C, et al. Skin regenerated from cultured epithelial autografts on full-thickness burn wounds from 6 days to 5 years after grafting. *Lab Invest.* 1989;60:5.

129. Phillips TJ, Kehinde O, Green H, Gilchrest BA. Treatment of skin ulcers with cultured epidermal allografts. *J Am Acad Dermatol.* 1989;21:191–199.

130. Phillips TJ, Provan A, Colbert D, et al. A randomized single-blind controlled study of cultured epidermal allografts in the treatment of split-thickness skin graft donor sites. *Arch Dermatol.* 1993;129:879–882.

131. Hiroko T, Yukihiro U, Toshihiko Y, et al. Cryopreserved cultured epidermal allografts achieved early closure of wounds and reduced scar formation in deep partial-thickness burn wounds (DDB) and split-thickness skin donor sites of pediatric patients. *Burns.* 2001;27:689–698.

132. Naughton G, Mansbridge J, Gentzkow G. A metabolically active human dermal replacement for the treatment of diabetic foot ulcers. *Artif Organs.* 1997;21:1203–1210.

133. Martin TA, Harding KG, Jiang WG. Regulation of angiogenesis and endothelial cell motility by matrix bound fibroblasts. *Angiogenesis.* 1999;3:69–76.

134. Gentzkow GD, Iwasaki SD, Lipkin S, et. al. Use of Dermagraft, a cultured human dermis, to treat diabetic foot ulcers. *Diabetes Care.* 1996;19(4):350–354.

135. Eaglestein WH, Falanga V: Tissue-engineering for skin: an update. *J Am Acad Dermatol.* 1999;39:1007–1010.

136. Data on file with Smith & Nephew.

137. Tsai CC, Lin SD, Lai CS, Lin TM. The use of composite acellular allodermis-ultrathin autograft on joint area in major burn patients—one year follow-up. *Kaohsiung J Med Sci.* 1999; 15:651–658.

138. Wainwright DJ. Use of an acellular allograft dermal matrix (AlloDerm) in the management of full-thickness burns. *Burns.* 1995;21:243–248.

139. Jones I, James SE, Martin R, et al. Upward migration of cultured autologous keratinocytes in Integra™ artificial skin: a preliminary report. *Wound Repair Regen.* 2003;11:132–138.

140. Purdue GF, Hunt JL, Still JM, et al. A multicenter clinical trial of a biosynthetic skin replacement, Dermagraft-TC, compared with cryopreserved human cadaver skin for temporary coverage of excised burn wounds. *J Burn Care Rehab.* 1997;18:52–57.

141. Naughton GK, Mansbridge JN. Human-based tissue-engineered implants for plastic and reconstructive surgery. *Clinics Plastic Surg.* 1999;26(4):579–586.

142. Voytik-Harbin SL, Brightman AO, Kraine MR, et al. Identification of extractable growth factors from small intestinal submucosa. *J Cell Biochem.* 1997;67:478–491,1997.

143. Palmer EM, Beilfuss BA, van Seventer GA, et al. Human helper T-cell activation and differentiation is suppressed by porcine small intestine submucosa. *Tissue Eng.* 2002;8(5):893–900.

144. Hodde JP, Record RD, Badylak SF, et al. Retention of endothelial cell adherence to porcine derived extracellular matrix after disfection and sterilization. *Tissue Eng.* 2002;8(2):225–234.

145. Lindberg K, Badylak SF. Porcine small intestine submucosa (SIS): A bioscaffold supporting in vitro primary human epidermal cell differentiation and synthesis of basement proteins. *Burn.* 2001;27(3):254–266.

146. Hodde JP, Record RD, Badylak SF, et al. Vascular endothelial growth factor in porcine–derived extracellular matrix. *Endothelium.* 2001;8(1):11–24.

147. Falanga V: How to use Apligraf to treat venous ulcers. *Skin Aging* February 1999;30–36.

148. Falanga V, Sabolinski M. A bilayered living skin construct (Apligraf) accelerates complete closure of hard-to-heal venous ulcers. *Wound Repair Regen.* 1999;7:201–207.

149. Kirsner R, Falanga V, Fiverson D, et al. Clinical experience with a human skin equivalent for the treatment of venous leg ulcers: process and outcomes. *Wounds.* 1999;11(6):137–144.

150. Veves A, Falanga V, Sabolinski ML, et al. Apligraf diabetic foot ulcer study. Graftskin, a human skin equivalent, is effective in the management of noninfected neuropathic diabetic foot ulcers: A prospective randomized multicenter clinical trial. *Diabetes Care.* 2001;24(2):290–295.

151. Data on file with Organogenesis.

152. Silberklang M. *Presentation Advanced Wound Care Sympo* April 29, 2002.

153. Data on file with Ortec.

154. Michel M, L' Heureux N, Pouliot R, et al. Characterization of a new tissue-engineered human skin equivalent with hair: *In Vitro Cell Develop Biol Anim.* 1999;35(6):318–326.

155. Black AF, Berthod F, L'Heureux N, et al. In vitro reconstruction of a human capillary-like network in a tissue-engineered skin equivalent. *FASEB J.* 1998;12(13):1331–1340.

156. Schechner J, Nath A, Zheng L, et al. In vivo formation of complex microvessels lined by human endothelial cells in a immunodeficient mouse. *Proc. Natl Acad Sci U S A.* 2000;97(16):9191–9196.

157. Supp DM, Bell SM, Morgan JR, et al. Genetic modification of cultured skin substitutes by transduction of human keratinocytes and fibroblasts with platelet-derived growth factor-A. *Wound Repair Regen.* 2000;8(1):26–35.

158. Bonadio J. Tissue engineering via local gene delivery. *J Mol Med.* 2000;78:303–311.

159. Badiavas EV, Abedi M, Butmarc J, et al. Participation of bone marrow derived cells in cutaneous wound healing. *J Cell Physiol.* 2003;196:245–250.

160. Badiavas EV, Falanga V. Treatment of chronic wounds with bone marrow-derived cells. *Arch Dermatol.* 2003;139:510–516.

161. Tateishi-Yuyama E, Matsubara H, Murohara T, et al. Therapeutic angiogenesis for patients with limb ischemia by autologous transplantation of bone marrow cells: A pilot study and a randomized controlled trial. *Lancet.* 2002;360: 427–435.

162. Asahara T, Murohara T, Sullivan A, et al. Isolation of putative endothelial progenitor cells for angiogenesis. *Science.* 1997; 275:964–967.

163. Murohara T, Ikeda H, Duan J, et al. Transplanted cord blood derived endothelial progenitor cells augment postnatal neovascularization. *J Clin Invest.* 2000;105:1527–1536.

164. Kalka C, Masuda H, Asahara T, et al. Transplantation of *ex vivo* expanded endothelial progenitor cells for therapeutic neovascularization. *Proc Natl Acad Sci U S A.* 2000;97:3422–3427.

165. Shintani S, Murohara T, Ikeda H, et al. Mobilization of endothelial progenitor cells in patients with acute myocardial infarction. *Circulation.* 2001;103:2776–2779.

166. Peichev M, Naiyer AJ, Pereira D, et al. Expression of VEGFR-2 and AC133 by circulating human CD34(+) cells identifies a population of functional endothelial precursors. *Blood.* 2000;95:952–958.

167. Fulton JE: The use of hyperbaric oxygen (HBO) to accelerate wound healing. *Dermatol Surg.* 2000;26(12):1170–1172.

168. Kalani M, Jorneskog G, Brismar K, et al. Hyperbaric oxygen (HBO) therapy in treatment of diabetic foot ulcers. *J. Diabetes Complications.* 2002;16:153–158.

169. Dimitrlievich SD, Paranjape S, Mills JG, et al. Effect of hyperbaric oxygen on human skin cells in culture and in human dermal and skin equivalents. *Wound Repair Regen.* 1999;7: 53–64.

170. Tokunaga A, et al. Hyperbaric oxygen (HBO) increases plasma VEGF levels. *Wound Healing Symp.* 2002.

171. Heng MC, Harker J, Csathy G, et al. Angiogenesis in necrotic ulcers treated with hyperbaric oxygen. *Ostomy Wound Manage.* 2000;46(9);18–28,30–32.

172. Wunderlich RP, Peters EJG, Lavery LA. Systemic hyperbaric oxygen therapy: Lower extremity wound healing and diabetic foot. *Diabetes Care.* 2000;23(10):1551–1555.

173. Argenta LC, Morykwas MJ. Vacuum-assisted closure: A new method for wound control and treatment. *Ann Plastic Surg.* 1997;38:563.

174. Ford CN, Reinhard ER, Yeh D, et al. Interim analysis of a prospective randomized trial of vacuum-assisted closure versus the health point system in the management of pressure ulcers. *Ann Plastic Surg.* 2002;49(1):55–61.

175. DeFranzo AJ, Argenta LC, Marks MW, et al. The use of vacuum-assisted closure therapy for the treatment of lower-extremity wounds with exposed bone. *Plastic Reconstr Surg.* 2001;108(5):1184–1191.

176. Scherer LA, Shiver S, Owings JT, et al. The vacuum assisted closure device: A method of securing skin grafts and improving graft survival. *Arch Surg.* 2002;137:930–934.

177. Braddock M, Campbell CJ, Zuder D. Current therapies for wound healing: electrical stimulation, biological therapeutics, and the potential for gene therapy. *Int J Dermatol.* 1999; 38:808–817.

178. Thawer HA, Houghton PE, Butryn A, et al. Effects of electrical stimulation on wound closure in mice with experimental diabetes mellitus. *Wounds.* 2000;12(6):159–169.

179. Sussman, C. Electrical stimulation for wound healing. In: Sussman C, and Jensen BB, eds. *Wound Care: A Collaborative Practice Manual for Physical Therapists and Nurses.* Aspen Publications, 1997.

180. Clark M: What happens when we disagree about the quality of the "evidence" in evidence based practice? *Europ Tissue Repair Soc.,* 2001. www.etrs.org/bulletin7_1?section4b.html.

181. Schindl A, Schindl M, Schindl L, et al. Low intensity laser irradiation improves skin circulation in patients with diabetic microangiopathy. *Diabetic Care.* 1998;21(4):580–584.

182. Schindl A, Schindl M, Schindl L, et al. Diabetic neuropathic foot ulcer: successful treatment by low intensity laser therapy. *Dermatology.* 1999;198:314–316.

183. Conian MJ, Rapley JW, Cobb CM. Biostimulation of wound healing by low-energy laser irradiation. *J Clin Periodontol.* 1996;23:492–496.

184. Reddy K, Stehno-Bittel L, Enwemeka CS. Laser photostimulation accelerates wound healing in diabetic rats. *Wound Repair Regen.* 2001;9:248–255.

185. Schindl A, Merwald H, Schindl L, et al. Direct stimulatory effect of low-intensity 670 nm laser irradiation on human endothelial cell proliferation. *Brit J Dermatol.* 2003;148:334–336.

186. Passarella S, Casamassima E, Cingolani A, et al. Increase of proton electrochemical potential and ATP synthesis in rat liver mitochondia irradiated in vitro by helium-neon laser. *Fed Eur Biochem Soc.* 1984;175:95–99.

187. Agaiby AD, Ghali LR, Dyson M, et al. Laser modulation of angiogenic factor production by T-lymphocytes. *Laser Surg Med.* 2000;26(4):357–363.

188. Yu W, Naim JO, Lanzafame RJ. The effects of photo-irradiation on the secretion of TGF and PDGF from fibroblasts in vitro. *Laser Surg Med Suppl.* 1994;6, 8.

189. Maegawa Y, Itoh T, Nishi M, et al. Effects of near-infrared low-level laser irradiation on microcirculation. *Laser Surg Med.* 2000;27(5):427–437.

190. Vinvk EM, Cagnie BJ, Cambier DC, et al. Increased firboblast proliferation induced by light emitting diode and lower power laser irradiation. *Lasers Med Sci.* 2003;18(2):95–99.

191. http://www.dermavista.com/NASA.html

192. Tasto JP, Cummings J, Amiel D, et al. Radiofrequency-based micro-tenotomy for treating chronic tendinosis. White paper.

193. Jeschke MG, Herndon DN, Baer W, et al. Possibilities of non-viral gene transfer to improve cutaneous wound healing. *Curr Gene Ther.* 2001;1:267–278.

194. Supp DM, Supp AP, Bell SM, Boyce ST. Enhanced vascularization of cultured skin substitutes genetically modified to overexpress vascular endothelial growth factor. *J Invest Dermatol.* 2000;114:5–13.

195. Breitbart AS, Grande DA, Laser J, et al. Treatment of ischemic wounds using cultured dermal fibroblasts transduced retrovirally with PDGF-B and VEGF121 genes. *Ann Plast Surg.* 2001;46:555–562.

Theoretical and Practical Aspects of Oxygen in Wound Healing

Thomas K. Hunt and Stefan Beckert

Introduction and History
Oxygen in Tissue
Oxygen in Injured Tissue
Mechanisms
    Immunity to Infection
    Collagen Sythesis and Infection
    Angiogenesis
    Oxidants

Chronic Wounds
Clinical Strategies
Hyperbaric Oxygen
Conclusions
References

INTRODUCTION AND HISTORY

Oxygen is as important to wounds as it is to life itself. Lack of oxygen is the most common cause of clinical wound problems.[1] Simple therapies based on new knowledge of oxygen supply and delivery can restore healing that has failed, can accelerate healing that is slow, and can prevent wound complications.[2] Unfortunately, these simple solutions have not been eagerly received and, in many cases, particularly with regard to hyperbaric oxygen, are still needlessly controversial.

Data indicating the importance of oxygen in wound healing goes back many years. Surgeons have noted for centuries that wounds in poorly perfused tissues heal poorly and are excessively prone to infection.[3] In Andean agricultural lore, descending to the lower, winter habitat is the appropriate therapy for wounds that fail to heal in the high summer pastures. Experimental evidence of inadequate epithelization at high altitude was recorded more than 60 years ago.

Medical interest in oxygen therapy for problem wounds rose quickly in the 1960s, instigated by the serendipitous observation by Jaques Cousteau's divers that their work wounds healed most rapidly when they lived for weeks at a time in a "habitat" 30 feet under water.[4] Shortly thereafter, clinicians working with hyperbaric oxygen (HBO) observed that it stimulated growth of granulation tissue in ischemic and irradiated wounds.[5]

However, medical people had been taught for many decades that only additional circulating hemoglobin and not arterial tissue concentration (PO_2) could influence tissue oxygen content and, for that reason, if none other, HBO was slow to gain acceptance.

Although, for most purposes, the belief in hemoglobin is well placed, it is not true of wounds in which inflammation and the diffusion barrier induced by injury are the most important obstacles to local oxygen transport and cell function. These obstacles can be overcome only by means of supporting local perfusion and maintaining a high arterial PO_2.[6] Unfortunately, the primacy of hemoglobin is still taught and the issues of wound healing are not recognized as exceptions to the rule. Many physicians have taken a categorical opinion that hyperbaric oxygen has to prove its advantages and the hyperbaric community has not been aggressive about proving it.

Nevertheless, the advantages to wound healing of increasing arterial, and thus tissue and intracellular PO_2, are well documented in animal and human cells, wounds, and subcellular preparations.[2] Furthermore, once the technology to measure tissue PO_2 was established, physiologists confirmed that wound PO_2 is (1) low,[7] (2) can be raised by oxygen supplementation (ie, raising arterial PO_2), and (3) is relatively insensitive to blood hemoglobin levels.[8] Furthermore, healing and resistance to infection are demonstrably enhanced when hypoxia in wounds is corrected or even raised to above normal.

OXYGEN IN TISSUE

The route that oxygen takes from air to the capillary membrane is well known.[9, 10] The remainder of its journey to its point of use is not so well understood. The most important point, generally ignored, is that oxygen diffuses through capillary membranes and across the extracellular space driven only by the force of the arterial PO_2 gradient. It also enters cells in proportion to its PO_2 (concentration) and is consumed there. In normal tissues, the diffusion distances between capillary and mitochondrion are so short that only a small gradient is necessary to conquer the distance and that gradient is maintained because hemoglobin releases oxygen and supports PO_2 as the oxygen is consumed.[11]

"Tissue PO_2," is limited by arterial PO_2 (can never rise above it) and is a measure of oxygen *concentration* in a given tissue. In other words, it is an expression of oxygen "availability".[12] For present purposes, PO_2 is expressed as millimeters of mercury.

Oxygen "concentration" is important because oxygen is not only a source of energy. It is also a substrate of a number of enzymes that are important in healing. They include prolyl hydroxylase (an "oxygenase" that controls the rate of collagen deposition) and the phagocytic oxygenase (that produces oxidants for bacterial killing and oxidant-signaling purposes). As always, the substrate concentration(s) (the PO_2, in this instance) in enzymatic reactions, controls the *rate* of product formation.

How much oxygen a given "oxygenase" uses at a given substrate concentration depends, to a degree, upon the avidity, the "passion," with which the enzyme and the substrate combine. The avidity is expressed as the K_m for that enzyme. K_m (the Michaelis Menton constant) is the concentration of the substrate (molecular oxygen in this case) that allows the enzyme to produce its end product at half the maximal rate (see later, Fig. 3–1). Cytochrome oxidase ($2H^+ + O_2 \rightarrow H_2O$), perhaps the most avid for oxygen, produces its product at half-maximal rate, even when PO_2 is less than 1 mm Hg. It is so avid for oxygen that PO_2 must fall to lethal levels before its rate is affected. On the other hand, collagen prolyl hydroxylase that is essential to collagen deposition has a K_m of about 25 mm Hg.[13] The production rate of its product, hydroxylated collagen proline, depends on PO_2 throughout the entire physiologic range, from 0 to 250 mm Hg. Bactericidal oxidant production has a higher K_m and is even more vulnerable to hypoxia.

Providing oxygen to a wound is not the same as providing it to a working muscle that extracts large amounts of oxygen, but has a plentiful microcirculation with a short distance between the mitochondria and capillaries. At low PO_2, arterial blood can deliver considerable oxygen to working muscle over a short distance provided there is enough hemoglobin. However, wounds are another problem. Lacking concentration (ie, a high partial pressure), oxygen can penetrate only short distances, too short to be of much help to all but minor wounds.[6] On the other hand, high local tissue concentrations can be reached even in anemic subjects if arterial PO_2 and blood flow are high and oxygen consumption is relatively low, as it is in most wounds. Although the time-honored belief is that anemia is detrimental to wound healing, the fact is that low hemoglobin becomes important to healing only

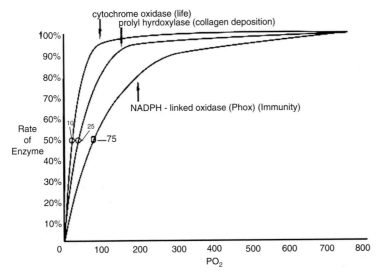

Fig. 3–1. Kinetics curves for prolyl hydroxylases and cytochrome oxidase showing that as oxygen concentration falls (right to left), collagen deposition due to prolyl hydroxylation and bactericidal oxidant production will fall long before cell viability is threatened.

Oxidant Signaling

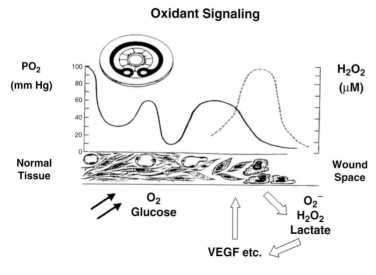

Fig. 3–2. Oxygen is consumed in the signaling zone, next to the wound space, by conversion to oxidants. Oxidants (dashed line) are quickly used. Note the lack of quantification. Hydrogen peroxide level in the wound space is 2 to 6 μmol. Molecular oxygen and glucose, neither angiogenic, are converted to oxidants, lactate, and hypoxia, all angiogenic. Molecular oxygen, however, supports vessel growth at the response zone where the new vessels grow. Other growth factors that emanate from the macrophages and are omitted for clarity also converge on the response zone, the sum total increasing cell replication, collagen production, etc.

at quite low levels, about 6 g or hct 15—however, anemia and poor perfusion together is a serious problem.[14,15]

The rapidity of perfusion is dependent upon blood pressure and the resistance to flow in the capillary network in question. Resistance to flow is mainly a function of arteriolar muscle tone. Normally, arterioles dilate to increase flow as a response to oxygen demand, but this response is easily overcome as a result of low blood volume, dehydration, cold, pain, and sympathomimetic drugs.[16–18] All these conditions are common impediments to wounds. Vasoconstriction prolongs the time that blood flows through any tissue. At low flow, PO_2 drops further than at higher flow during the passage of blood.

OXYGEN IN INJURED TISSUE

Tissue injury diminishes perfusion and oxygen delivery by damaging local microvasculature. Subsequent coagulation deepens the injury and further reduces perfusion. Inflammatory cells, primed and activated on entering the wound, begin to consume large amounts of oxygen by converting it to oxidants. The energy for the conversion comes from aerobic glycolysis (ie, not from oxygen). Lactate is produced as a by-product. The result is hypoxia in a highly oxidative, highly lactated environment. This condition serves well as a metabolic definition of a "healing wound"[19] (Fig. 3–2).

The extent of vascular injury and inflammation are highly variable. However, even "insignificant" wounds contain areas of ischemia, where the healing cells exist in microscopic units, such as a few macrophages, a few fibroblasts, and perhaps no vessels. (For instance, patients have developed tetanus without displaying any sign of a wound.) These sites are slow to heal and vulnerable to infection.

Fibroblasts, endothelial cells, and inflammatory cells, the majority of wound cells, obtain most of their energy via aerobic glycolysis and thus survive easily, but function poorly in low PO_2 in wounds. As noted above, their important healing functions have a lower affinity for oxygen than the enzymes that ensure survival. For this reason, as PO_2 falls, wound healing fails well before the viability of normal tissue is in danger.

Although oxygen is essential to healing, wounds actually use rather little, less than one volume of oxygen per 100 mL of blood flow (assuming normal hemoglobin and perfusion).[6]

Wounds on the surface of the body, where vasoconstriction is a mechanism of thermal control and in those tissues whose vessels contract under "stress" (ie, are well supplied by sympathetic innervation), are particularly vulnerable to wound infection and uncertain healing. In practical terms, the sympathetic response is an enormously important item to wounds! As noted above, when perfusion falls, the fraction of delivered oxygen that is consumed increases, PO_2 in capillary blood falls, and healing and resistance to infection fall with it.[17,20]

Collagen must be deposited in this ischemic, relatively hypoxic environment. One of the challenges to healing, then, is to develop new vessels to support the added new tissues, ie, angiogenesis. New vessels need collagenous support. Indeed, they supply their own, but collagen can be deposited only in the presence of a considerable concentration of oxygen. Until these new vessels acquire blood flow, the necessary oxygen for collagen deposition must diffuse forward a considerable distance from the last free-flowing vessel. This requires a high arterial PO_2 so that diffusion can overcome the distance.

Wound PO_2 has been measured, and low PO_2 has been securely correlated to poor collagen deposition, easy infectability, and slow angiogenesis in human and animal wounds. These correlations have been supported by mechanistic findings in individual cells.

The PO_2 in the center of a dead space wound can be quite low.[2] Ten to 15 mm Hg has been measured. Without the "dead space," however, the PO_2 is higher by about 40 or 50 mm Hg (if the arterial PO_2 is normal), a figure one can accept as an estimate of "normal" at the wound edge. Administration of 100% oxygen at 1 ATA raises it to the region of 150 to 200 mm Hg. Oxygen at 2 ATA raises it to about 400 or above with a wide variation.[21] The PO_2 in a dead space itself may rise only to 90 or so during HBO depending on the size of the space.

A large variability in PO_2 and collagen deposition has been found by 7 to 10 days postoperatively in human surgical patients. Statistically most of the variability is due to vasoactivity and arterial PO_2. Most of the differences in collagen production are due to the variation in local PO_2. The simple fact is that when more oxygen is made available to healing tissue, more is used, and some of the added consumption contributes to accelerated healing. The amount of benefit one can get depends on the PO_2 levels reached.

In summary, decreased perfusion, increased diffusion distances, and a rising demand for oxygen in wounds due to inflammation all lead to local hypoxia, an oxidative environment, and local lactacidosis. Provision of oxygen to wounded tissue, where circulation is sufficient, raises tissue concentration (PO_2) in wounds and profoundly influences healing.

MECHANISMS

Immunity to Infection

The mechanism by which wounds resist bacterial infection is the most direct entry to the explanation of how oxygen works in wounds. Ischemic wounds are notoriously vulnerable to infection. This undoubtedly involves many mechanisms, but impaired bactericidal oxidant production by leukocytes appears to be the most important.[22]

Leukocytes migrate into wounds where they are "activated" by phagocytosis, among other things. When "activated" they adopt a number of functions. For one, they begin to consume oxygen in large quantities by converting it to oxidants that are inserted into the phagosomes where they kill engulfed bacteria by oxidizing their membranes.[23–25] The equation for the conversion is:

$$O_2 + glucose \rightarrow O_2^- + lactate + H^+$$

(The K_m for oxygen utilization is about 75 mm Hg)

The enzyme, the NADPH-linked oxidase, often called "phox" (*ph*agocytic *o*xydase) first converts oxygen to superoxide, in what is called the "*oxidative burst*." The term "burst" comes from the fact that oxygen consumption rises as much as 50-fold upon activation. About 98% of the oxygen consumed in this reaction is converted to oxidants. The superoxide is then converted to hydrogen peroxide and other oxidants, including peroxynitrite in other reactions (Fig. 3–3).

As noted above, the K_m of this oxygen is high (ie, is highly dependent on PO_2). That is, the oxygen concentration necessary to support superoxide formation at half the maximum rate, is high—about 75 mm Hg. The PO_2 at the wound edge is rarely above 50 mm Hg, if the subject is breathing air at one atmosphere. In surgical patients breathing air, therefore, this system operates at significantly less than half its potential. Reduced PO_2 markedly reduces bacterial killing.[22] Raising PO_2 from a reduced value repairs the loss and is capable of adding an increment, which may double the killing rate above that reached by wounds in patients breathing air. Many studies show that bacteria are cleared more rapidly from hyperoxic as opposed to hypoxic wounds and it is now agreed that assurance of adequate oxygen tension in wounds is an excellent means of preventing wound infections. It is approximately as powerful as specific antibiotics. Furthermore, the two are additive.[17,26–30]

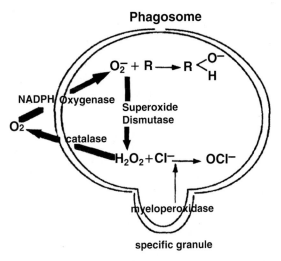

Fig. 3–3. When bacteria are phagocytosed, the NaDPH oxygenase is assembled in the phagosome membrane. Oxygen is converted to superoxide, which is injected into the phagosome. Various enzymes convert the superoxide to other bactericidal oxidants. Antioxidants in the granular membrane protect the cell. NADPH: nicotinamide adenine dinucleotide phosphate.

Au: Oxidase

The congenital absence of any of the several components of phox (as in chronic granulomatous disease of childhood) can produce a profound, usually fatal, susceptibility to the same organisms that infect wounds.[31] As oxygen tensions fall into the 20-mm Hg range, wounds approach this degree of vulnerability. It is now generally accepted that hypoxia of the magnitude seen clinically in human wounds, is a major source of vulnerability to infection. For example, ensuring an adequate PO_2 in wounds simply by maintaining body warmth, oxygen breathing, and blood volume support lowers postoperative wound infections by more than half![17,32] The effect is specific to the degree that wound PO_2 is elevated (which, on occasion, may require hyperbaric oxygen to achieve).

Nitric oxide, NO, is also bactericidal. It is formed from arginine and molecular oxygen by nitric oxide synthetase.

$$O_2 + arginine \rightarrow NO + citrulline$$

The rate of NO production is also proportional to local oxygen concentration. The K_m is uncertain and may be tissue specific, but, for most purposes, appears to be about 15 mm Hg.[33] This mechanism is separate from phox.

Studies in animals show that bacteria placed in wounds are cleared an order of magnitude faster when the subjects breathe oxygen; the added oxygen is transmitted to tissue. Human studies confirm this in terms of the incidence of postoperative wound infections. One must realize, however, that some ischemic tissue, including tissue that has healed (scarred) repeatedly, cannot be oxygenated by any means and must be debrided surgically and radically, back to bleeding tissue, before healing can be expected. This is particularly true of osteomyelitis in which oxygen therapy must be considered only part of a combined therapy with surgical debridement.

Collagen Synthesis and Infection

Oxygen concentration influences collagen synthesis, deposition, and cross-linking in at least three places in the synthetic pathway: gene transcription, post-translational modification, and extracellular cross-linking.[34–38]

In a mechanism that is still not fully understood, the combination of oxygen, lactate, and transition metals enhances intracellular oxidant production, which, in turn, stimulates collagen gene transcription, among many other stimuli.[39–41]

Although hypoxia is said to induce collagen gene transcription, the experimental conditions that were used in the experiments were actually hypoxia-followed-by-reoxygenation; a sequence that is a well established cause of oxidant production. The process is known as "oxidant stress" when excessive or as "oxidant signaling"

when in the physiologic range. The emerging view is that oxidant signaling enhances collagen gene transcription through several pathways, transforming growth factor beta (TGF-β) production and lactate production, for instance.[42]

As noted above, and contrary to conventional concepts, many biologic processes other than energy metabolism depend upon PO_2. Three oxygenases (enzymes that consume oxygen as a substrate) are critically important in collagen deposition. They are prolyl hydroxylase, lysyl hydroxylase, and lysyl oxidase.

The reason for the oxygen dependence of collagen secretion from the fibroblast is well understood. Proline, not hydroxyproline, is incorporated into in the procollagen peptides as they are synthesized. Later, in a post-translational step that occurs in the endoplasmic reticulum, prolyl hydroxylase inserts an oxygen atom into selected prolines, converting some of them to hydroxyprolines. The oxygen atom can be obtained *only from molecular oxygen*.[43] At this point, collagen peptides form their normal triple helical structure within the cell and can be exported into the extracellular space. Regardless of the rate of peptide synthesis, collagen is not released from cells, ie, deposited, until prolyl hydroxylase (and molecular oxygen) hydroxylates it. Since enzymatic reaction rates are hyperbolic with respect to the concentrations of their substrates (see Fig. 3–1), collagen deposition is 0 at $PO_2 = 0$, half-maximal at $PO_2 = 25$ (the K_m), and maximal only at above 200 mm Hg.[44] This is the entire physiologic range of PO_2 and beyond! These numbers may be tissue specific for some organs and/or cells.

Similarly, hydroxylated lysines, by the same type of mechanism (lysyl hydroxylase), assist extracellular cross-linking of collagen monomers into collagen fibrils. This step also requires oxygen and is analogous to proline hydroxylation. Its half-maximal rate also occurs at a PO_2 of approximately 25 mm Hg. If this step is incomplete, collagen fibers are weak.

Lastly, lysines in the collagen molecule are condensed by lysyl oxidase, yet another oxygen-requiring enzyme that assists in the extracellular polymerization of collagen. The K_m of this reaction is not well defined, but appears to be higher than 25 mm Hg. Thus, collagen cross-linking is probably even more susceptible to hypoxia than its deposition. If these steps are incomplete, collagen fibers are sparse and weak.

"Hypoxia" also stimulates the release of several growth factors and cytokines that induce collagen synthesis, particularly hypoxia-inducible factor (hif-1alpha), tumor-necrosis factor, transforming growth factor beta (TGF-β), interleukin-1(IL-1), and vascular endothelial growth factor (VEGF).[45] However, these functions appear to be duplicated, at least to some extent, by lactate and oxidant signaling.[46–48] On the other hand, hypoxia suppresses insulin-like growth factor-1 (IGF-1) synthesis between $PO_2 = 0$ and $PO_2 = 35$, as does a high lactate in the wound.[41] Paradoxically, IGF-1 deficiency is one of the few growth factors whose absence has been demonstrated to *suppress* collagen deposition in actual wounds.[49] The mechanism is unknown, but lack of IGF-1 probably contributes to the problems of hypoxia.

In summary, collagen deposition and both intra- and extracellular cross-linking are oxygen dependent. They are decelerated when perfusion and/or arterial PO_2 are below normal and accelerated when they are higher. As noted in the figure [as above in this section (Fig. 3–1)], this difference can be severalfold. The clinically important lesson is that collagen synthesis, cell replication, and oxidant production can be easily optimized by simple clinical means, such as warming to increase perfusion and breathing oxygen to increase arterial PO_2.

Collagen synthesis and deposition are also powerfully controlled by lactate. Adding enough lactate to animal wounds to raise concentration by only about 20% increases collagen deposition by 50%.[50] As noted above, lactate is generated by leukocytes. They are also *aerobically* glycolytic and contribute to the accumulation of lactate. This also comes about in two other ways. Smooth muscle cells and most cancer cells also generate lactate aerobically (that is, in the presence of oxygen). Last, lactate is also the by-product of anaerobic metabolism.[41]

Lactate also stimulates collagen gene transcription by stimulating its promoter and by activating prolyl hydroxylase, ie, collagen deposition. This appears to occur through a mechanism involving the pool of reduced nicotinamide adenine dinucleotide (NAD^+). The mechanism is complex. High lactate concentrations shift the equilibrium ratio of NAD^+/NADH in favor of NADH (reduced NAD) through the familiar action of lactate dehydrogenase that transfers hydrogens from accumulated lactate to NAD^+ with the production of NADH.[47]

The diminished NAD^+, in turn, has a vital consequence, namely, that its metabolites, particularly adenosine diphosphoribose (ADPR) production, are diminished. "ADPR" denotes the molecule that results when the "N" is removed from NAD^+.

The normal role of ADPR is important. It appears to suppress both collagen gene transcription in the nucleus and prolyl hydroxylase activity in the cytoplasm, thus (in the absence of lactate) inhibiting collagen synthesis and deposition when they are not "needed."[51] Injury, with its consequent accumulated lactate and lowered NAD^+, therefore, overcomes a repressive mechanism. Exposing fibroblasts to lactate, even in the presence of oxygen, reduces NAD^+ in favor of NADH and the net result is increased collagen deposition, which we know to be further accelerated by increased PO_2. Thus,

simultaneous elevation of lactate and PO_2 leads to increased collagen synthesis (and angiogenesis; see below).

All this runs contrary to classic thought. The standard questions that arise are: (1) shouldn't hyperoxia decrease lactate, and (2) isn't hypoxia necessary for lactate production? The demonstrated fact is that hyperoxygenation of wounded animals *does not* lower wound lactate levels.[19] Furthermore, addition of lactate, in the presence of oxygen, significantly enhances collagen production in fibroblasts in culture and/or wounds in animals.[52] Adding NAD^+ increases ADPR production and suppresses collagen production even in lactated and oxygenated cultured fibroblasts.

Angiogenesis

The logic of parsimony suggests that since macrophages, new blood vessels, and fibroblasts exist close together in wounds and act cooperatively (Fig. 3–2), the mechanisms of angiogenesis should be similar to those of collagen synthesis and deposition and should involve oxidants.[53] Angiogenesis is dependent upon collagen deposition (by endothelial cells) to give physical support to growing vessels.[54,55] In fact, the mechanisms of angiogenesis and collagen synthesis and deposition are strikingly similar.

It is well accepted that hypoxia leads to release of VEGF from many cell types.[56] It is not well known, but is nevertheless also true, that lactate stimulates VEGF release from macrophages, even in the presence of oxygen.[48] The mechanism currently appears to involve oxidant formation from oxygen, iron, and lactate.

This fact is particularly useful because the assumption that hypoxia is the single cause of VEGF release *in wounds* is incompatible with the fact that angiogenesis occurs best in well- or even hyperoxygenated wounds and is accelerated during hyperbaric oxygen therapy.[57,58] Hyperbaric oxygen exposure enhances angiogenesis in matrigel in implants in animal wounds.[59] Furthermore, *hypoxia truncates angiogenesis* both clinically and experimentally. There are several putative mechanisms for this: (1) hyperoxia enhances the endothelial response through oxidants and (2) small increases of peroxide, consistent with hyperoxia, also increase release of VEGF.[46] This argues for the central importance of lactate in healing, which fits the clinical facts. Both hypoxia and hyperoxia enhance VEGF release, which is lowest at normal tissue oxygen concentrations. Although a number of angiogenic substances are found in wound fluid, VEGF seems to be the most important.[60]

Of all the wound mechanisms, angiogenesis is by far the most important for take of skin grafts. Elevating oxygen tension, whether to normal or above normal, is the only angiogenic strategy that is known to be effective in ischemic tissue.

Epithelization

Although several animal studies have shown that epithelization is accelerated in the presence of oxygen, the mechanism is unknown.[61–63] Epithelial cells synthesize collagen just as endothelial cells do. By analogy with the above, it should be expected that oxygen and oxidants should be involved. However, both hyperbaric oxygen and topical oxygen have some difficulty reaching basal cells, largely, we think, because of the strong inflammatory reactions and the thick inflammatory exudates on the surface. Epithelial cells can extract oxygen directly from the ambient gas as well as from blood. No quantification is available. However, major differences in epithelization are observed in some patients during oxygen breathing. Epithelization has also been enhanced dramatically in some patients by *topical* application of oxygen![64,65]

Oxidants

This description of wound healing outlines an essential role for oxidants, which runs contrary to recent thinking that oxidant production is always damaging. Oxidant signaling, which requires only very low concentrations, is an established concept, but so is oxidant damage that occurs after very high or constant exposures.[46] There is a balance and wounds are well able to defend themselves against oxidant toxicity, being well protected by protein carboxylation and nitration, thiols, superoxide dismutase, catalase, and others. Wound fluid, for instance, destroys hydrogen peroxide almost instantly. Nevertheless, hydrogen peroxide is measurable in wounds at a few micromoles.[66] Since the antioxidant protection is excellent, this must mean that the throughput of oxidants is very high and that most is scavenged or consumed close to the point of production.

CHRONIC WOUNDS

Healing fails for many reasons and chronic (impeded) wounds result. For example, trauma, arteriosclerosis, venous insufficiency, diabetes, hypertension, arteritis, osteomyelitis, pressure necrosis, inflammatory disorders, and calciphylaxis are all potent inhibitors.

With some exceptions, chronic wounds are less well oxygenated than acute wounds. Most are on the lower extremity and are associated with arterial or venous insufficiency and/or excessive inflammation, all of which produce local hypoxia.

The healing potential of a lower extremity wound is directly related to its circulation. The circulation is currently best assessed by the transcutaneous PO_2 (TcPO₂) in its vicinity.[6,67] This measurement, however, must be carefully performed in order to isolate the physiologic and vasoactive variables. It must be done with the leg warmed under a cover of water vapor-impermeable substance and a blanket. The skin temperature must be within a degree or two of core temperature and should be recorded. The ideal method is to start with a well-hydrated, pain-free patient and then to obtain stability with the patient supine. A mask is used to add 100% oxygen. Once stability is again reached, the leg is raised 30 degrees. Stability is reached again, and the patient is measured sitting or standing. In this manner, artifact due to dehydration, pain, and cold are avoided and the effects of arterial and venous disease are isolated. A slight fall on elevation is normal; a large one is due to obstructive arterial disease. A rise above the supine value with standing is normal, but a large rise followed by a fall appears to be indicative of venous disease.

If the baseline TcPO₂ is over 30 mm Hg, especially if a plentiful response to oxygen occurs, the ulceration is not due to hypoxia. If it is less, hypoxia is a likely contributor. A PO_2 of 15 mm Hg or less without a rise due to oxygen spells a grave prognosis unless vascular surgery can be performed. Remember, though, that cold alone, even with normal arteries, can cause this level. A low PO_2 that responds to oxygen breathing suggests that hyperbaric oxygen will be helpful. Preferably, these values should be obtained after infection is controlled. *In other words, the capacity of oxygen to heal an ischemic wound is not estimated until the patient and wound are uninfected, well hydrated, free of pain, and warm.*

The degree of hypoxia in venous wounds has been debated, but the majority of evidence now supports the theory that chronic, repeated, intermittent ischemia and hypoxia followed by reperfusion and oxidant generation causes tissue death. The ischemia is caused by poor flow during prolonged standing. Reoxygenation occurs when raising the leg up toward heart level, restoring normal arterial/venous (A/V) pressure gradient and causing a transient period of reactive oxidant production. Prevention of stasis by pressure wrappings, the first treatment of choice, prevents the rise of venous pressure and accomplishes that same objective. Surgical interruption of venous perforators in or near the ulcer, thus preventing local ischemia/reperfusion, can be very helpful, but the healing time is still prolonged. After several recurrences of venous wounds, the skin and the local vasculature become scarred and atrophic. This raises a permanent obstacle to the transport of oxygen. Hyperbaric oxygen therapy is not usually a choice for venous ulcers unless they are hypoxic for other reasons as well. By far the most effective therapy for hypoxic wounds is revascularization, reduction of oxygen consuming inflammation and infection, warmth, and discontinuation of (vasoconstricting) tobacco use. All of these have the potential to raise the tissue oxygen concentration. If it is corrected, breathing oxygen can often be expected to raise wound PO_2 to recovery levels. Relatively few hyperbaric units observe all these conditions.

We are also persuaded that medical therapy is effective. Use of warmth in patients with active sympathetic nervous systems is usually helpful. In some cases, vasodilation with Clonidine® and/or calcium channel blockers, or possibly by ACE (angiotensin-converting enzyme) inhibitors is also helpful. One of the best uses of transcutaneous oximetry is in proving (or disproving) the efficacy of such therapies, since it is a system from which failure can be predicted in hours or days rather than waiting weeks in vain for an observable increase in healing. If TcPO$_2$ rises significantly as a result of treatment, the wound will almost invariably heal.

CLINICAL STRATEGIES

Correcting tissue hypoxia is more complex than simply breathing oxygen. Using wound oximeters, we have seen many surgical patients whose wound PO$_2$ is low and totally unaffected by breathing oxygen even though their vascular anatomy is normal and arterial PO$_2$ is significantly raised.[6] Yet, when given adequate fluid and warmed, their oximetry profile becomes normal. This emphasizes the importance of local perfusion. The most important causes of vasoconstriction are dehydration, blood volume loss, cold, pain, smoking, and fear. Expansion of blood volume and heat are more important than increasing red cell mass. The essential observation, however, is that for optimal results, all of these obstacles must be corrected *all at the same time* because any one is sufficient to cause maximal vasoconstriction. Consider what happens to your peripheral perfusion when you are relaxed, not smoking, well fed and happy, but cold! You have white fingers and toes.

For many years, warmth was been regarded as potentially harmful to chronic wounds. Furthermore, sympathetic innervation is supposed to be inoperative in diabetic legs. Nevertheless, warming often aids perfusion, as measured by transcutaneous PO$_2$. Furthermore, external warmth penetrates to the subcutaneous tissue and usually vasodilates and increases tissue PO$_2$.[16,68] We have not seen warmth lower it. A response to warmth predicts a therapeutic potential. Sympathetic overactivity is a frequent property of chronic wounds and preventing cold-mediated vasoconstriction is almost always beneficial.

Similarly, pain activates vasoconstriction. It is necessary to avoid the vicious cycle of pain/vasoconstriction/more pain, etc. Beta adrenergic blockade, diuretics, and smoking compound hypoxic problems and should be regulated. As nearly as anyone can tell, their harmful effects are due to limitation of oxygen supply. Many postoperative patients are blood volume depleted, in pain, cold, and beta blocked (perioperative beta blockade is commonly necessary). Correcting these vasoconstrictive stimuli, particularly cold and smoking, has led to significant decrements in postoperative wound infections,

up to 60% in the case of warming and oxygen during the operation and the immediate postoperative period. Wound PO$_2$ can also be elevated through the use of the alpha antagonist Clonidine in the patch dosage form, because blood volume changes and vasoconstriction occur very rapidly and the need for protection is constant. Many anesthesiologists like to use this strategy and this drug is excellent medication for short-term control of hypertension.[69]

In most cases, these strategies can be put into place arbitrarily. Some, particularly those involving chronic wounds, are best planned on the basis of transcutaneous oximetry, which should be available in all noninvasive vascular laboratories.[70]

HYPERBARIC OXYGEN

The most precise indication for hyperbaric therapy is a chronic wound in which periwound transcutaneous PO$_2$ is low and responds to oxygen breathing in a hyperbaric chamber with the ulcerated part warm and at heart level.

Hyperbaric oxygen treatment of chronic wounds has remained a controversial issue for many years, mainly because of our inability to effectively stratify chronic wounds and, therefore, predict responders. Transcutaneous oxygen measurement, while not perfect, has largely changed that situation. The authors themselves do not practice hyperbaric medicine but our experience, gained by referring patients, has been almost uniformly favorable when the above conditions are met. From all existing data, the beneficial effect on angiogenesis appears to be the most important of the several components that are affected by HBO inasmuch as prevention of major amputations in the long-term history of human ischemic diseases has now been documented.[71]

As experience with oximetry has expanded, the success rate of hyperbaric therapy has risen; indications have been clarified. Several prospective and blinded studies have recently been completed and, despite their relatively small size, the data seems quite clear that if the problem is ischemia (periwound hypoxia), and oxygen breathing raises periwound PO$_2$, hyperbaric oxygen can save limbs.[72,73] On the basis of the enzyme kinetics noted above, hyperbaric oxygen should bring little benefit to healing of normoxic wounds, and it does not.

One might also predict that hyperbaric oxygen would be of little benefit for chronic venous ulcers, since it adds little to the elevation of PO$_2$ that can be obtained by rest, elevation, and compression. This has been the general experience. The major exception would be in venous ulcers that have healed many times and are chronically scarred, thus setting up an oxygen diffusion block. It is well known that capillary density decreases with each subsequent healing.[74] In this case, a judgment would have to be made as to whether hyperbaric oxygen or radical debridement (or more likely both) is the best choice. Efficacy of the combination has not been tested.

One of the most fruitful applications has been in osteoradionecrosis. The published data is convincing. Several authors, including Marx, have noted a favorable influence on angiogenesis.[75–77]

The usual daily hyperbaric is usually only 90 minutes. How can such a short exposure have a significant effect? Although the current explanations may not be all-inclusive, they are helpful. First, tissue hyperoxia lasts about 2 hours to return to baseline after the 90-minute exposure is terminated.[21] Second, during the exposure, bacterial killing is increased. The effect of eliminating large numbers of bacteria probably has "downstream" significance, just as one would expect from a bolus of antibiotic. Third, angiogenesis, collagen synthesis, and epithelization are enhanced for 3–4 hours per treatment. The degree of infection becomes correspondingly less as treatment cycles add up. In fact, the very periodicity of hyperbaric administration may be partly responsible for its success. Cyclic therapy alternates the hypoxic drive to VEGF with the hyperoxic drive. Thus, alternation adds potential without incurring oxidant toxicity.

It is fascinating that hyperbaric and growth factor therapy for problem wounds have suffered from the same obstacles to clinical verification. In contrast, however, hyperbaric oxygen has been regarded with far more skepticism despite the fact that its rationale is more complete and its therapeutic capacities include problems that are beyond help by growth factors!

CONCLUSIONS

Hypoxia is the most common deficiency found in failed wounds and restoration of oxygen concentration in tissue allows wound cells to deposit collagen, to resist infection, to epithelize, and to develop new vasculature.

Although tissue hypoxia can stimulate the assembly of many mechanisms of healing, it frustrates each of them in the end. Lactate accumulation mimics hypoxia in most, if not all, wounds, and leaves the clinician in position to increase oxygen concentration (PO_2) in both acute and chronic ischemic wounds with benefits to almost all aspects of healing, as well as resistance to infection.

The following are important, practical rules for mitigating the hypoxia.

- PO_2 in wounds is profoundly influenced by the rate at which blood perfuses them. Perfusion is reduced by vasoconstriction, which is a response to low blood volume, pain, fear, smoking, cold, and vasoconstrictive drugs.
- Vasoconstriction can almost always be overcome using warmth, fluids, or medications, even in the hyperbaric chamber.

- Wound PO_2 also varies with arterial PO_2 and falls as the distance that oxygen has to diffuse to get to the healing wound cells increases.
- Surgical debridement, infection control, and hyperbaric oxygen are useful to overcome diffusion obstacles and excessive demand for oxygen due to inflammation.

Oxygen has a surprising diversity of effects in wounds. The rates of angiogenesis, collagen deposition, epithelization, and the ability of wounds to resist infection are all dependent on tissue oxygen concentration.

ACKNOWLEDGMENT

Supported by NIH NIGMS GM 27345-23.

REFERENCES

1. Sumpio BE. Foot ulcers. *N Engl J Med*. 2000;343(11):787–793.

2. Hunt TK, Dunphy JE. Effects of increasing oxygen supply to healing wounds. *Br J Surg*. 1969;56(9).

3. Barbul A. Postoperative wound infection. In: Cameron J, ed. *Current Surgical Therapy*, 4th ed. St. Louis: Mosby-Year Book; 1992:960–990.

4. Cousteau J, Cousteau JY, Alinat J. On the adaptation of man to underwater life in natural and synthetic compressed air. *C R Acad Sci Hebd. Seances Acad Sci D*. 1966;262(18):1962–1965.

5. Duff JH, Shibata HR, Vanschaik L, et al. Hyperbaric oxygen: A review of treatment in eighty-three patients. *Can Med Assoc J*. 1967;97(10):510–515.

6. Jonsson K, Jensen J, Goodson W, et al. Tissue oxygenation, anemia, and perfusion in relation to wound healing in surgical patients. *Ann Surg*. 1991;214:605–613.

7. Hunt TK, Zederfeldt B, Goldstick TK. Oxygen and healing. *Am J Surg*. 1969;118(4):521–525.

8. Hunt TK, Goodson WHI. Uncomplicated anemia does not influence wound healing. In: Tuma RF, White JV, Messner K, eds. *The role of hemodilution in optimal patient care*. Munich: Zukschwerdt Verlag; 1989:8.

9. Hunt T. The physiology of wound healing. *Ann Emerg Med*. 1988;17:1265–1269.

10. Hunt TK, Hopf H, Hussain Z. Physiology of wound healing. *Adv Skin Wound Care (Suppl. 2)*. 2000;13:6–11.

11. Silver IA. The measurement of oxygen tension in healing tissue. *Prog Resp Res*. 1969;3:124–135.

12. Gottrup F, Firmin R, Rabkin J, et al. Directly measured tissue oxygen tension and arterial oxygen tension assess tissue perfusion. *Crit Care Med*. 1987;15(11):1030–1036.

13. Myllyla R, Tuderman L, Kivirikko KI. Mechanism of the prolyl hydroxylase reaction. 2. Kinetic analysis of the reaction sequence. *Eur J Biochem*. 1977;80(2):349–357.

14. Hopf H, Viele M, Watson J, et al. Subcutaneous perfusion and oxygen during acute severe isovolemic hemodilution in healthy volunteers. *Arch Surg*. 2000; Dec. 135(12):1443–1449.

15. Hopf H, Swanson D, Hunt T. Moderate anemia does not decrease tissue oxygen in rabbits. *Wound Repair Regen*. 1993; 1(2):107.

16. Sheffield CW, Hopf HW, Sessler DI, et al. Thermoregulatory vasoconstriction decreases subcutaneous oxygen tension in anesthetized volunteers. *Anesthesiology.* 1992;77:A96.

17. Hunt TK, Hopf HW. Wound healing and wound infection. What surgeons and anesthesiologists can do. *Surg Clin North Am.* 1997;77(3):587–606.

18. Whitney JD. The influence of tissue oxygen and perfusion on wound healing. *Aacn Clin Issues Crit Care Nurs* 1990;1(3): 578–584.

19. Hunt TK, Conolly WB, Aronson SB, et al. Anaerobic metabolism and wound healing: An hypothesis for the initiation and cessation of collagen synthesis in wounds. *Am J Surg.* 1978; 135(3):328–332.

20. Hopf H, McKay W, West J, et al. Percutaneous lumbar sympathetic block increases tissue oxygen in *patients* with local tissue hypoxia in non-healing wounds. *Anesth Analg.* 1997;84:S305.

21. Rollins MD. Wound and subcutaneous tissue oxygen physiology. Doctoral thesis, University of California, San Francisco. 1999;111–130.

22. Allen D, Maguire J, Mahdavian M, et al. Wound hypoxia and acidosis limit neutrophil bacterial killing mechanisms. *Arch Surg.* 1997;132:991–996.

23. Babior BM. NADPH oxidase: An update. *Blood.* 1999;93(5): 1464–1476.

24. Gabig TG, Bearman SI, Babior BM. Effects of oxygen tension and pH on the respiratory burst of human neutrophils. *Blood.* 1979;53(6):1133–1139.

25. Babior BM. Oxygen-dependent microbial killing by phagocytes. *N Engl J Med.* 1978;198:659–668.

26. Knighton DR, Halliday B, Hunt TK. Oxygen as an antibiotic: The effect of inspired oxygen on infection. *Arch Surg.* 1984;119:199–204.

27. Knighton DR, Halliday B, Hunt TK. Oxygen as an antibiotic. A comparison of the effects of inspired oxygen concentration and antibiotic administration on in vivo bacterial clearance. *Arch Surg.* 1986;121(2):191–195.

28. Greif R, Akca O, Horn EP, et al. Supplemental perioperative oxygen to reduce the incidence of surgical-wound infection. Outcomes Research Group. *N Engl J Med.* 2000;342(3): 161–167.

29. Sessler DI, Akca O. Nonpharmacological prevention of surgical wound infections. *Clin Infect Dis.* 2002;35(11):1397–1404.

30. Jonsson K, Hunt TK, Mathes SJ. Oxygen as an isolated variable influences resistance to infection. *Ann Surg.* 1988;208: 783–787.

31. Babior B, Woodman R. Chronic granulomatous disease. *Semin Hematol.* 1990;27:247–259.

32. Kurz A, Sessler D, Lenhardt R, et al. Perioperative normothermia to reduce the incidence of surgical-wound infection and shorten hospitalization. *New Engl J Med.* 1996;334(19): 1209–1215.

33. Albina JE, Mastrofrancesco B, Vessella JA, et al. HIF-1 expression in healing wounds: HIF-1alpha induction in primary inflammatory cells by TNF-alpha. *Am J Physiol Cell Physiol.* 2001;281(6):C1971–1977.

34. Semenza GL. HIF-1, O(2), and the 3 PHDs: How animal cells signal hypoxia to the nucleus. *Cell.* 2001;107(1):1–3.

35. Semenza GL. HIF-1 and mechanisms of hypoxia sensing. *Curr Opin Cell Biol.* 2001;13(2):167–171.

36. Niinikoski J. Current concepts of the role of oxygen in wound healing. *Ann Chir Gynaecol.* 2001;90(Suppl 215):9–11.

37. Hunt TK, Pai MP. The effect of varying ambient oxygen tensions on wound metabolism and collagen synthesis. *Surg Gynecol Obstet.* 1972;135(4):561–567.

38. Eyre DR, Paz MA, Gallop PM. Cross-linking in collagen and elastin. *Annu Rev Biochem.* 1984;53:717–748.

39. Hussain MZ, Ghani AP, Hunt TK. Inhibition of prolyl hydroxylase by poly(ADP-ribose) and phosphoribosyl-AMP. Possible role of ADP-ribosylation in intracellular prolyl hydroxylase regulation. *J Biol Chem.* 1989;264:7850–7855.

40. Hussain MZ, Hunt TK, Bhatnagar RS. Metabolic regulation of prolyl hydroxylase activation. *Prog Clin Biol Res.* 1988;266: 229–236.

41. Trabold O, Wagner S, Wicke C, et al. Lactate regulates wound healing processes. *Wound Repair Regen.* 2003;11:504–509.

42. Kirkeby LT, Ghani QP, Enriquez B, et al. Stimulation of collagen synthesis in fibroblasts by hydrogen peroxide. *Mol Cell Biol.* 1995;6:44.

43. Kivirkko KI, L. R. Biosynthesis of collagen and its alterations in pathological states. *Med Biol.* 1976;54:159–186.

44. Hutton JJ, Tappel AL, Udenfriend S. Cofactor and substrate requirements of collagen proline hydroxylase. *Arch Biochem Biophys.* 1967;118:231–240.

45. Jiang BH, Semenza GL, Bauer C, et al. Hypoxia-inducible factor 1 levels vary exponentially over a physiologically relevant range of O_2 tension. *Am J Physiol.* 1996;271(4 Pt 1):C1172–1180.

46. Sen CK, Khanna S, Gordillo G, et al. Oxygen, oxidants, and antioxidants in wound healing: An emerging paradigm. *Ann NY Acad Sci.* 2002;957:239–249.

47. Zabel DD, Feng JJ, Scheuenstuhl H, et al. Lactate stimulation of macrophage-derived angiogenic activity is associated with inhibition of poly(ADP-ribose) synthesis. *Lab Invest.* 1996;74: 644–649.

48. Constant JS, Feng JJ, Zabel DD, et al. Lactate elicits vascular endothelial growth factor from macrophages: A possible alternative to hypoxia. *Wound Repair Regen.* 2000;8(5):353–360.

49. Wicke C, Halliday B, Allen D, et al. Effects of steroids and retinoids on wound healing. *Arch Surg.* 2000;135(11): 1265–1270.

50. Green H, Goldberg B. Collagen and cell protein synthesis by established mammalian fibroblast line. *Nature.* 1964;204:347.

51. Ghani QP, Hussain MZ, Zhang J, et al. Control of procollagen gene transcription and prolyl hydroxylase activity by poly[ADP-ribose]. In: Poirier E, Moreaer A, eds. *ADP-Ribosylation Reactions.* New York: Springer Verlag; 1992: 111–117.

52. Green H, Goldberg B, Todaro GJ. Differentiated cell types and the regulation of collagen synthesis. *Nature.* 1966; 212(62):631–633.

53. Cho M, Hunt TK, Hussain MZ. Hydrogen peroxide stimulates macrophage vascular endothelial growth factor release. *Am J Physiol Heart Circ Physiol.* 2001;280(5):H2357–H2363.

54. Haralabopoulos GC, Grant DS, Kleinman HK, et al. Inhibitors of basement membrane collagen synthesis prevent endothelial cell alignment in matrigel in vitro and angiogenesis *in vivo. Lab Invest.* 1994;71(4):575–582.

55. Missirlis E, Karakiulakis G, Maragoudakis ME. Angiogenesis is associated with collagenous protein synthesis and degradation in the chick chorioallantoic membrane. *Tissue Cell.* 1990; 22(4):419–426.

56. Ferrara N, Davis-Smyth T. The biology of vascular endothelial growth factor. *Endo Rev.* 1997;18:4–25.

57. Ketchum SA, 3rd, Thomas AN, Hall AD. Effect of hyperbaric oxygen on small first, second, and third degree burns. *Surg Forum.* 1967;18:65–67.

58. Sheikh AY, Gibson JJ, Rollins MD, et al. Effect of hyperoxia on vascular endothelial growth factor levels in a wound model. *Arch Surg.* 2000;135(11):1293–1297.

59. Gibson J, Angeles A, Hunt T. Increased oxygen tension potentiates angiogenesis. *Surg Forum.* 1997;87:696–699.

60. Nissen NN, Polverini PJ, Koch AE, et al. Vascular endothelial growth factor mediates angiogenic activity during the proliferative phase of wound healing. *Am J Pathol.* 1998;152(6):1445–1452.

61. Silver IA. Oxygen tension and epithelialization. In: Maibach HI, Rovee DT, eds. *Epidermal Wound Healing.* Chicago: Year Book Medical Publishers; 1972:291.

62. Winter GD. Oxygen and epidermal wound healing. *Adv Exp Med Biol.* 1977;94(673):673–678.

63. Kaufman T, Alexander JW, Nathan P, et al. The microclimate chamber: The effect of continuous topical administration of 96% oxygen and 75% relative humidity on the healing rate of experimental deep burns. *J Trauma.* 1983;23(9):806–815.

64. Kaufman T, Alexander JW, MacMillan BG. Topical oxygen and burn wound healing: A review. *Burns Incl Therm Inj.* 1983;9(3):169–173.

65. Edsberg LE, Brogan MS, Jaynes CD, et al. Topical hyperbaric oxygen and electrical stimulation: Exploring potential synergy. *Ostomy Wound Manage.* 2002;48(11):42–50.

66. Liu D, Liu J, Wen J. Elevation of hydrogen peroxide after spinal cord injury detected by using the Fenton reaction. *Free Radical Biol Med.* 1999;27(3-4):478–482.

67. Jorneskog G, Djavani K, Brismar K. Day-to-day variability of transcutaneous oxygen tension in patients with diabetes mellitus and peripheral arterial occlusive disease. *J Vasc Surg.* 2001; 34(2):277–282.

68. West J, Hopf H, Sessler D, et al. The effect of rapid postoperative rewarming on tissue oxygen. *Wound Repair Regen.* 1993; 1(2):93.

69. Hopf H, West J, Hunt T. Clonidine increases tissue oxygen in patients with local tissue hypoxia in non-healing wounds. *Wound Repair Regen.* 1996;4(1):A129.

70. Wütschert R, Bounameaux H. Determination of amputation level in ischemic limbs. Reappraisal of the measurement of TcPO$_2$. *Diabetes Care.* 1997;20(8):1315–1318.

71. Faglia E, Favales F, Aldeghi A, et al. Change in major amputation rate in a center dedicated to diabetic foot care during the 1980s: Prognostic determinants for major amputation. *J Diabetes Complications.* 1998;12(2):96–102.

72. Fife CE, Buyukcakir C, Otto GH, et al. The predictive value of transcutaneous oxygen tension measurement in diabetic lower extremity ulcers treated with hyperbaric oxygen therapy: A retrospective analysis of 1,144 patients. *Wound Repair Regen.* 2002;10(4):198–207.

73. Ratliff DA, Clyne CA, Chant AD, et al. Prediction of amputation wound healing: the role of transcutaneous PO$_2$ assessment. *Br J Surg.* 1984;71(3):219–222.

74. McEwen AW, Smith MB. Chronic venous ulcer. Hyperbaric oxygen treatment is a cost effective option. *BMJ.* 1997; 315(7101):188–189; author reply 189.

75. Feldmeier JJ, Hampson NB. A systematic review of the literature reporting the application of hyperbaric oxygen prevention and treatment of delayed radiation injuries: An evidence based approach. *Undersea Hyperb Med.* 2002;29(1):4–30.

76. Myers RA. Hyperbaric oxygen therapy for trauma: crush injury, compartment syndrome, and other acute traumatic peripheral ischemias. *Int Anaesth Clin.* 2000;38(1):139–151.

77. Marx RE, Johnson RP, Kline SN. Prevention of osteoradionecrosis: a randomized prospective clinical trial of hyperbaric oxygen versus penicillin. *J Am Dent Assoc.* 1985;111(1): 49–54.

4 Topical Oxygen Therapy as an Adjunctive Modality in Wound Healing

Francis Rossi, Eric S. Baskin, Shail N. Patel, and Adam J. Teichman

Introduction
History
Overview of Wound Healing
Topical Oxygen Therapy in Wound Healing
**Topical Oxygen Therapy Treatment Modalities
    and Mechanism**
    Burns
    Diabetic Foot Ulcers
    Pyodermagangrenosum
    Necrotizing Fasciitis

Equipment and Application Methods
    Patient Selection
    Equipment of Systematic versus Topical
        Oxygen Therapy
    Treatment Protocol
Summary
Case Study One
Case Study Two
Case Study Three
References

INTRODUCTION

Nonhealing wounds of various etiologies have reached epidemic proportions and have posed a constant challenge to the wound-care physician. Skin ulcerations may develop secondary to etiologies, such as arterial insufficiency, venous insufficiency, sickle cell anemia, diabetes mellitus, postsurgical infection, or traumatic injury, such as decubitus ulcerations or burns. Diabetes mellitus is most commonly associated with ulcerations and the complication of subsequent amputation.[1] Current studies reveal that the rate of lower-extremity amputation among diabetics is greater than forty times that of nondiabetics;[2] it is estimated that 25% of all diabetic hospital admissions are for pathologies associated with the diabetic foot.[1]

It is obvious why there are so many treatment therapies for wounds. Effective local wound care modalities designed to accelerate the wound-healing process are vital in today's medical environment. Systemic hyperbaric oxygen (systemic HBO) and, more recently, topical oxygen therapy are adjunctive wound-healing treatments many clinicians are employing in their wound-care protocol.

The purpose of this chapter is to familiarize the clinician with topical oxygen therapy as an adjunctive treatment in the wound-healing process of several etiologies. We will review the pathology of wound healing, the science behind hyperbaric medicine, both full-body and topical oxygen, products available for topical oxygen medicine, and review clinical case studies. It has been the authors' personal clinical experience that topical oxygen therapy is a worthy adjunctive therapy to the revitalization of indolent wounds. However, topical oxygen therapy is a controversial subject criticized by some as to its effectiveness.[3] There is a need for further objective and clinical research providing concrete confirmation of its clinical value and capabilities to the medical community.[4]

HISTORY

Bogaslav Fischer may be one of the earliest researchers of topical oxygen therapy. In the 1960s, Dr. Fischer was a neurologist at the New York University Medical Center in New York City. Prior to the popularity of hyperbaric medicine, Dr. Fischer's facility had a multiplace chamber. This unit was used for the standard treatment of divers with decompression sickness and patients with carbon monoxide poisoning. Dr. Fischer also used this modality in the treatment of multiple sclerosis and other neurological disorders. It was observed that patients afflicted by neurological diseases sustaining decubitus ulcers healed at an increased rate after receiving hyperbaric oxygen treatments. This observation eventually led to the development of a topical oxygen chamber designed specifically for wound care.

A working union was forged between Dr. Fischer and Mr. Phillip Loori of Jersey City, New Jersey in the mid 1970s. Dr. Fischer's early chamber exposed the wound to oxygen at a continuous pressure of 22 mm Hg. Mr. Loori and a team of engineers added the intermittent compression cycle to Dr. Fischer's original prototype, which allowed the unit to cycle up to 50 mm Hg each 35-second interval. This enhanced the clinical outcome with the Topox unit that is presently in use. Recently, there have been developments in topical oxygen therapy and other newly designed products are available to wound-care physicians.

Madalene Heng is a dermatologist and a noted researcher and author in the area of topical oxygen therapy. She has contributed several landmark studies, which have increased the understanding of the science behind topic oxygen therapy and its relationship to angiogenesis.

OVERVIEW OF WOUND HEALING

As we begin our discussion on topical oxygen therapy, one must first be fully versed in the pathophysiology of wound healing. This section will briefly review the traditional phases of wound healing and its classifications. The three stages of wound healing are the inflammatory, fibroproliferative, and the maturation phases.[5]

The inflammatory phase[5] encompasses approximately 10% of the healing process, also known as the substrate, or lag phase. This is due to the recruitment of proteins and healing factors to the wound at the time of insult. Initial vasoconstriction is proceeded by vasodilation and erythema, which lasts a total of 3 to 4 days. During this initial phase, neovascularization occurs.[5] Fibroblasts lay down collagen, which allows tensile strength to return to the damaged tissue. Superficially the epidermal epithelialization process occurs antagonistically with dermal inflammation. Cell mitosis continues throughout the healing process until contact inhibition occurs between epithelial cells, ultimately sealing the wound surface.

The fibroproliferative phase comprises approximately 20% of the healing process, which lasts from 3 to 21 days.[5] During this granulation phase of tissue healing, new collagen production and capillary buds continue to form until the wound contracts and epithelialization is complete. Fibroblasts are the primary cell

Table 4–1. Stages of Wound Healing

1. Inflamatory phase—10% Healing process, 3–4 days
2. Fibroproliferative phase—20% Healing process, 4–21 days
3. Maturation phase—70% Healing process, 21–360 days

type in the wound, as collagenation rapidly increases during this phase. After 14 days, the tensile strength of the wound approaches only 35% of the original strength of the local tissue. The main source of tensile strength in a surgical wound during this phase of wound healing is from the suture material inserted during primary closure.[5]

The maturation phase comprises approximately 70% of the healing process and lasts from approximately 3 weeks to 1-year postinsult.[5] During this phase, randomly arranged collagen fibers are debrided by enzymatic breakdown of macrophages.[5] New collagen fibers are produced and aligned in response to mechanical forces causing wound contraction to occur in a centripetal direction.

When wound healing is obstructed by systemic disease or other causes, the aforementioned phases are prolonged or inhibited (Table 4–1). During this time, the benefits of extrinsic modalities, including topical oxygen therapy can be beneficial to patient outcome.

TOPICAL OXYGEN THERAPY IN WOUND HEALING

Topical oxygen therapy, the application of oxygen at pressures greater than 1 atm at sea level (1 atm = 14.7 psi, 1 kg/cm^2, 101.3 kpa, 760 torr, or 760 mm Hg) is a form of therapy capable of providing favorable physiological, cellular, and biochemical effects that aid in revascularization of damaged tissue.[1] An increase in oxygen tension is achieved by raising the PO$_2$ in the circulating blood.[17] Oxygen serves as a fundamental healing element for chronic wounds in many ways. It is involved in collagen synthesis and plays a role in cross-linking, fibroblast enhancement, epithelialization, oxidative microbial killing, phagocytosis, and leukocyte function. Oxygen is also associated with angiogenesis, osteoclastic resorption, osteoblastic formation, and upregulation of platelet-derived growth factor receptor (PDGFR) in ribonucleic acid (RNA) activity. During topical oxygen therapy, oxygen is responsible for providing a gradient between the oxygen-deprived wound and surrounding soft tissues that encourages neovascularization.[3,6–8]

Topical oxygen therapy treatment is administered in two different ways: systemic and topical. Systemic topical oxygen therapy involves placing a patient in a chamber where pure oxygen is breathed at increased atmospheric

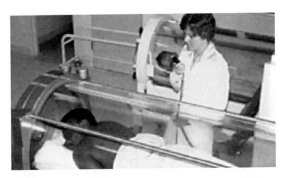

Fig. 4.1. Systemic full body hyperbaric oxygen chamber.

pressures (2–3 atm) once–twice daily for 10 to 60 treatments, depending on the condition. Blood (plasma) concentration of oxygen at sea level is 0.3 ml/dL.[9,10] When 100% oxygen is administered systemically at a hyperbaric pressure of 3 atm, the blood-oxygen concentration is approximately 6 mL/dL.[9,11] The oxygen courses through an individual's dermal capillaries to the vicinity of the ulcer. Subsequently, oxygen diffusion through the granulation tissue occurs at the base of the ischemic ulcer.[12] Systemic hyperbaric oxygen therapy is a useful therapy that can enhance wound healing, encourage granulation tissue formation, and expedite wound closure.[3,13,14] It can be life saving in acute conditions, such as carbon monoxide (CO) poisoning decompression syndrome, gas gangrene myonecrosis, and severe burns. (Fig. 4–1)[3,11,15]

Systemic hyperbaric oxygen therapy can pose risk to the patient, specifically to the central nervous system. Pulmonary toxicity, pulmonary edema, grand mal seizures, atelectasis, hemorrhage, and fibrosis are serious side effects that can be caused by systemic topical oxygen therapy. These risks have resulted in a set criterion for the institution of systemic oxygen therapy for chronic conditions.[6] The most common reported complication of full-body hyperbaric therapy is barotrauma of the ear. Other problems are round-window blow out, sinus squeeze, visual refractive changes, numb fingers, dental problems, and claustrophobia. Claustrophobia, in many instances, will require the administration of sedatives.[16]

The effect of topical oxygen therapy is to supplement oxygen to superficial tissue not sufficiently supplied from the systemic blood stream. The oxygen is applied directly to the open ulcer base, improving the oxygen content of the body fluids bathing the ischemic wound.[17] Studies show that during topical oxygen treatment, there is an increase in oxygen saturation of the plasma covering the ulcer and in it's superficial layer of granulation tissue, which, in turn, augments the healing process.[8] Topical oxygen delivery to the ischemic areas is separated by a thin layer of tissue fluid approximately 2 to 3 μm in thickness. Oxygen delivery to the healing tissue greatly depends on diffusion, and not on blood oxygen-carrying capacity.[19] Furthermore, uptake of oxygen at ulcer sites is also dependent on skin thickness and viability in ulcerations. Topical oxygen therapy requires lower pressures of 1.04 to 1.06 atm as opposed to 2 to 3 atm with systemic therapy to promote wound healing. Oxygen at pressures of up to 3 atm did not significantly elevate PO_2 within deeper layers; the vascular bed supplies these deeper layers. This may explain the usual lack of success in the healing of lower-extremity ulcers secondary to advanced arteriosclerosis. Note, that oxygen applied under ambient pressure has little penetrance of the epidermis.

Clinical research has been performed determining the efficacy of topical oxygen therapy with pressures of 22 to 50 mm Hg revealing that after 2 minutes of treatment termination the PO_2 returned to its original value.

Olejinczak described a two-phase wound healing process. The first phase is a cleansing and self-debriding period. This phase extends from 1 to 10 days, at which time the exudate disappears and the necrotic tissue sloughs off.[20,21] The wound demonstrates an appearance of fresh red granulation tissue on the surface with well-marked edges. The second phase is characterized by increased growth of granulation tissue filling the ulcer void. This occurs simultaneously with epithelial outgrowth.[20,21] Successful skin grafting of chronic ulcerations may follow the course of topical oxygen therapy.[19] When utilized, the therapeutic effects previously mentioned, aid in the overall healing prognosis.

Wound healing rates with topical oxygen therapy have been traditionally difficult to evaluate. Three randomized control trials have been performed in the past 10 years. Only one trial reported complete healing as an end point. Bouachour et al.[22] compared the efficacy of systemic topical oxygen therapy versus traditional therapies for acute crush injuries. The results demonstrated a 94.4% healing rate in systemic topical oxygen therapy-treated patients (100% O_2 at 2.5 atm) versus a 55.5% healing rate in patients receiving placebo (21% O_2 at 1.1 atm).[22,23] A limitation of this study is the fact that only acute wounds were investigated.

For example, necrotic and gangrenous wounds lacking adequate blood supply can develop further vascular damage from either reperfusion injury or oxygen toxicity, when exposed to oxygen at incorrect pressures. Heng et al.[24] demonstrated through a prospective randomized study, the efficacy of topical oxygen therapy at 1.004 to 1.013 atm in stimulating angiogensesis and healing of necrotic and gangrenous wounds. The results of the study support the theory that topical oxygen therapy decreases ulcer size and increases capillary density as compared to standard wound care (24). Oxygen levels of an ulcer must be greater than or equal to 40 mm Hg for wound fibroblasts to begin normal collagen production. Tissue oxygen tension is a major component in determining progress of wound healing.

Angiogenesis stimulation and regulation is crucial to the wound-healing cascade. The principle behind angiogenesis is similar to that of collagen synthesis and deposition. Lactate concentration and products of oxidation (NO, O_2^-, H_2O_2) activate macrophages to produce angiogenic substances that are chemoattractive.[24] As mentioned earlier, microbial killing capacity of neutrophil cells increase linearly with increased oxygen tension. Conversely, neutrophil cells also adhere to the cell walls of ischemic vessels and release unopposed free radicals and proteases causing reperfusion injury. Found in wounds lacking appropriate blood supply, these substances induce endothelial cell destruction, vasoconstriction, and tissue necrosis. This degenerative process increases the severity of the wound.[24,25] In oxygen-rich environments, angiogenesis is stimulated and leads to an increase in new vessel concentration. This is stimulated by many factors, Vascular endothelial growth factor (VEGF) being the most important factor in wound healing.[24] VEGF induces angiogenesis when exposed to oxidants and lactate. This growth factor is not inhibited by hyperoxia.

Patients with complicated wounds are often subjected to lengthy and costly stays in hospitals and extended-care facilities. The effects of long-term debilitation can dramatically deteriorate an individual's quality of life and mental health. Modalities such as topical and systemic HBO treatment may assist in stabilizing patients psychologically and physiologically by reducing the total recovery and healing time.

TOPICAL OXYGEN THERAPY TREATMENT MODALITIES AND MECHANISM

The two theorized mechanisms of systemic oxygen therapy administration provide increased oxygen diffusion throughout dermal capillaries that encompass the ulcer.[17] The first mechanism is by hyperoxia. This provides the biologic oxygen requirements to the wound, as previously discussed. The other mechanism is thought to be that nitric oxide (NO) production increases during systemic oxygen therapy.[3,7,8] Created when oxygen combines with L-arginine, NO activates guanylyl cyclase to cyclic adenylic acid (cyclic AMP). This is then thought to cause vasodilation, angiogenesis, and regulates wound matrix restoration.[3] Topical oxygen therapy involves enclosing the limb in an encased chamber with local application of oxygen, which poses minimal risk to the patient. The oxygen is applied directly to the base of the open ulcer. The treatment dissolves oxygen in tissue fluid and enhances the oxygen content of the intracellular fluid. This in turn directly saturates the ischemic cells inside the wound site. This process enhances endothelial cell proliferation, neovascularization, and epidermal cell migration in areas where previous ischemic changes have occurred.[26–29] This is an essential component in the wound-healing process because blood vessel concentration and oxygenation are increased.[17] Therefore, it is proposed that topical oxygen therapy may promote wound healing in areas of decreased blood vessel concentration and oxygenation potential.

The theorized mechanism of how topical oxygen therapy is administered bypasses the prolonged distances systemic oxygen takes to reach ischemic tissue. Studies have proved that the efficiency of oxygen diffusion is primarily dependent on delivery distance.[26] A thin layer of tissue fluid (approximately 2–3 μm in thickness) separates topical hyperbaric oxygen delivery into the ischemic areas (see Fig. 4–1). Conversely, with systemic administration of hyperbaric oxygen, the oxygen must diffuse over distances of 150 μm or more to reach ischemic tissues at the base of the ulcers (see Fig. 4–2). This explains why the topical delivery system requires lower pressures of 1.04–1.06 atm, rather than the systemic requirements of 2 to 3 atm.

With topical oxygen therapy delivery, only the wounded region is placed inside the chamber and oxygen is applied directly to the open ulcer base, which improves the oxygen content of the body fluids involved with the ischemic cells. The topical method has been shown to decrease the risk of systemic oxygen toxicity due to the avoidance of significant systemic oxygen absorption (see Fig. 4–3). The primary indication for topical oxygen therapy is an open wound. Systemic topical oxygen therapy has been utilized in multiple medical diseases; these conditions are outlined in Table 4–2.

Topical oxygen therapy is contraindicated and ineffective in patients with severe ischemia and wounds covered with a thick eschar. Acute thrombophlebitis/DVT (deep venous thrombosis) is also contraindicated because the device may exacerbate the condition (Table 4–3).

Systemic oxygen therapy is contraindicated in patients with development of or with acute pneumothorax and a

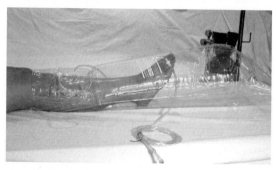

Fig. 4–2. O$_2$ boot.

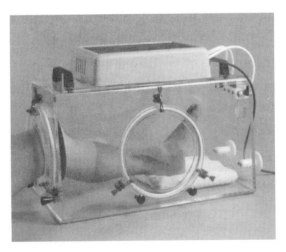

Fig. 4–3. Topical oxygen extremity chamber.

recurrent pulmonary leak at parietal or visceral pleura. A history of ear or sinus surgery is contraindicated, because there may be problems associated with rapid pressure changes. Patients undergoing chemotherapy may have reactions with the increased presence of oxygen. Systemic topical oxygen therapy may induce seizures in patients that have a prior history of the disorder. Claustrophobia is also a contraindication[3,11] (Table 4–4).

Table 4–2. Indications of Adjunctive Topical Oxygen Therapy[1]

Systemic Topical Oxygen Therapy	Topical Oxygen Therapy
Open wounds/diabetic foot ulcers	Diabetic foot ulcers
Air embolism	Burns
Gas embolism	Varicose ulcers
Decompression sickness	Pyodermagangrenosum
Carbon monoxide poisoning	Necrotizing fasciitis
Mild ischemic ulcers	
Clostridial gas gangrene myonecrosis	
Crush injury	
Compartment syndromes	
Osteoradionecrosis	
Compromise skin grafts and flaps	
Smoke inhalation	
Necrotizing fasciitis	

[1] In conjunction with all appropriate medical and surgical therapy as dictated by the standard of care.

Table 4–3. Contraindication of Adjunctive Topical Oxygen Therapy

Severe ischemia
Acute thrombophlebitis/ DVT
Wounds covered with eschar

Burns

Burn wounds have distinguishing characteristics and are very different from other types of lesions. Hunt et al.[27] observed that burns became edematous and hypoxic during the period of vascular impairment with little inflammatory change during the first few days. In one case, the reported tissue concentration (PO_2) level in the edematous tissue below the burn eschar was about one half the normal value.[27] During oxygenation of burn wounds, capillary budding appears throughout the formation of new granulation tissue. Burn wound healing has been shown to depend partly on maintaining tissue oxygen tension at or near the normal range of 0 to 20 mm Hg.[28,29]

Following a burn injury, persistent hypoxia, edema, and inflammation occurs within the wound. Topical oxygen therapy can aid in burn wound healing by increasing hydroxyproline levels and, collagen synthesis, as well as the preservation of adenosine triphosphate (ATP) in cell membranes. This action reduces excessive edema and inflammation normally observed in burn wounds.[28,29,30] This reduces the need for of surgical intervention and decreases healing time, which generates fewer complications.[28,29]

Diabetic Foot Ulcers

Throughout the course of this chapter, it has been discussed that topical oxygen therapy can improve the microvascular circulation by enhancing neovascularization of the wound.[12,17,18,26,31] This same theory is thought to improve the microvascualture in diabetic foot ulcers. The constraint in the treatment of ulcers is dependent on large vessel patency. Therefore, one must always evaluate the vascular status of the diabetic patient. Ankle–brachial indexes (ABI) may be utilized to evaluate the vascularity of diabetic patients. A low ABI may suggest the need for surgical intervention through

Table 4-4. Contraindications of Adjunctive Systemic Topical Oxygen Therapy

Acute pneumothorax
Recurrent pulmonary leak at parietal or visceral pleura
History of ear or sinus surgery
Chemotherapy
Seizure disorder

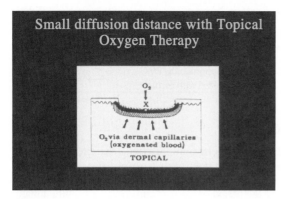

Fig. 4–4.

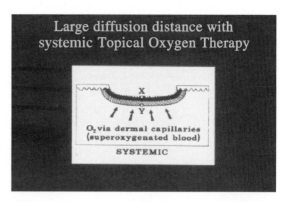

Fig. 4–5.

bypass grafting or angioplasty before topical oxygen therapy can be effective.[18,19,31] Oxygen toxicity plays a major role in diabetic ulcers as well. Glutathione levels are low in diabetic tissues, secondary to the abnormal carbohydrate metabolism ensued from inadequate insulin levels.[1,18] Topical oxygen therapy has been shown to increase the activity of glutathione peroxidase causing a decrease in glutathione levels in diabetic ulcers.[1] Andreoli et al.[1] found that a sufficient supply of reduced glutathione is essential to neutralize hydroperoxides and reactive oxygen species released by reperfusion of ischemic tissue.

Furthermore, diabetic microvascular involvement limits adequate delivery of antibiotics to tissue. The origins of this theory stem from decreased levels of prostacyclin secondary to endothelial cell damage and increased thromboxin levels released by platelets in injured diabetic tissue.[1] This imbalance has caused formation of platelet thrombi and associated disease.[1,5,12,18]

Christopher Attinger performed a study at Georgetown University on 12 patients with gangrenous achilles tendons, peripheral vascular disease, and transcutaneous peripheral O_2 (TcPO$_2$) levels of 11 to 17 mm Hg. Each patient received an average of 29.4 hours of topical oxygen therapy. TcPO$_2$ measurements rose to an average of 30 mm Hg. When each wound granulated, a skin graft was applied. All grafts went on to heal—10 out of 12 grafts remained stable during the 19-month follow-up course.[32]

The goal of diabetic ulcer treatment is the promotion of healthy granulation tissue and epithelialization. Adequate blood glucose control is required for optimum response to hyperbaric oxygen in the diabetic population.[1,18] Achieving optimum wound healing is multifactorial and not limited to appropriate local wound care alone. The limb salvage team must address all circumstances involved, such as vascular disease, necrotic tissue management, and adjunctive modalities, such as topical oxygen therapy.

Pyodermagangrenosum

This condition is usually associated with systemic disease such as inflammatory bowel disease, ulcerative colitis, Chron's disease, rheumatoid arthritis, active chronic hepatitis, paraproteinemias, and lymphomas.[18] Pyodermagangrenosum is a swiftly advancing pyogenic skin lesion, which eventually breaks down into an irregular confluent ulcer. An irregular base characterizes this disease with a blue hue parameter accompanied by severe pain.[17] Pyodermagangrenosum responds well to topical oxygen therapy without any definitive reason. The presumed theory is that areas of necrosis benefit from topical oxygen therapy because neovascularization, re-epithelialization, and collagen synthesis are stimulated in tissues with considerably low oxygen tension, in the 2 to 3 mm Hg range.[22]

Necrotizing Fasciitis

Necrotizing fasciitis is classically described as a rapidly progressing synergistic bacterial infection affecting full-thickness skin down to the fascia.[22,33] Necrotizing fasciitis leads to diffuse cutaneous gangrene and has a high mortality rate. Patients present clinically with advancing necrosis of epidermal and endothelial cells, compromising edema and hemorrhage.[17] This caused by the secretion of tumor necrosing factor-alpha (TNF-α) by activated macrophages, in the presence of lipopolysaccharides.[17,22] These lipopolysaccharides are present in the cell membranes of gram-negative bacteria aiding in the activation of TNF-α. TNF-α selectively damages the endothelial cells, via degranulation of neutrophils, from the release of superoxides. Subsequent vascular thrombosis and ischemic damage to infected tissues are the end result of this circumstance. After surgical debridement and antibiotic therapy, adjunctive topical oxygen therapy can be useful in long-term treatment of this condition. Topical oxygen therapy is particularly beneficial in these cases by its ability to increase superoxide dismutase in the tissues, combined with the induction of neovascularization.[34]

In a study performed by Ariseman et al., 29 patients with necrotizing fasciitis were treated with surgical débridement and antibiotics (controls) versus débridement, antibiotics, and topical oxygen therapy (treated). The study showed that the rate of mortality was 23% in the treated group compared with 66% in the control group.[22,33]

EQUIPMENT AND APPLICATION METHODS

Patient Selection

Patients with any stage III–IV ulcer/open wound with adequate vascular supply, as discussed above, qualifies for topical oxygen therapy.[25] Shallow ulcers, especially of neuropathic etiology, not grossly infected, will usually respond to conservative treatment. Patients' with compromised vascular status need to undergo thorough evaluation. Topical oxygen therapy treatment would be ineffective in patients without adequate arterial flow and should be referred for angiograms and revascularization work-up as needed.

Transcutaneous peripheral O_2 (TcPO$_2$) levels are recognized as a method for evaluation and selection for topical oxygen therapy.[4] Patients with TcPO$_2$ values greater than 40 mm Hg may heal without intervention.[3,4,22,33] If a patient's readings are less than 20 mm Hg, they will have a significantly decreased prognosis for healing. As more data and information becomes available, patient selection criteria will be more precise.

Equipment of Systemic versus Topical Oxygen Therapy

Administration of systemic topical oxygen therapy involves two different types of full-body chambers, including mono- and multiplaced systems.[26] The multiplace chamber accommodates two or more patients, where as the monoplace chamber can accommodate only one patient. These chambers tend to be expensive to maintain and difficult to sterilize, consequently causing cross-infection possibilities among patients using these chambers.[17]

The topical oxygen therapy equipment available at the time of publication of this volume is a rigid chamber constructed to fit and encompass a limb (see Fig. 4–2). These local chambers feature controlled-pressure sealing and automatic regulation control. In addition to nondisposable chambers, disposable one-piece chambers constructed to fit around the limb, made of polyethylene bags, are also available.[26]

TREATMENT PROTOCOL

First, culture the wound to determine if *Pseudomonas* is active within the wound. If present, wet approximately 1/2 of a dry sterile 4 × 4-cm-gauze pad with 1% acetic acid solution, and apply to the wound. This is performed to prevent growth of the organism. Next, remove all creams, ointments, and dressings prior to application of the unit, except in the presence of *Pseudomonas*. The wound is to be covered with moist environmental dressings after each treatment.

Topical oxygen therapy treatment schedules vary from 1 hour four times weekly to 90 minutes twice daily. It is the authors' preference that outpatients receive the therapy for 1 hour three to four times a week. In the inpatient or nursing home setting, patients can receive 60 to 90 minutes of treatment once or twice a day, depending on the condition of the wound and environmental circumstances.

Systemic topical oxygen therapy consists of 90 to 120 minutes at 2–2.5 atm, once or twice daily for 10–60 treatments.[17,22,33] Research performed on animal models has shown that a single treatment is superior to twice daily treatment, because the later stimulates excessive osteoclastic activity.[17]

SUMMARY

Topical hyperbaric oxygen may be utilized, under appropriate conditions, as an adjunctive treatment in the healing of dermal ulcerations. Advantages of topical hyperbaric oxygen include the convenience of receiving home treatment with minimal risk associated with this device.[22,33] In addition to low cost and lack of need for specialized equipment, topical oxygen therapy can provide the physician with another adjunctive tool in the armamentarium of treating complex wounds derived from multiple causative agents. Systemic oxygen therapy is a useful therapeutic adjunctive modality, which has been utilized in acute conditions, such as carbon monoxide poisoning, decompression syndromes, gas gangrene myonecrosis, and severe burns.[22,33] However, disadvantages of this treatment include the increase risk of systemic toxicity to the central nervous system and respiratory track.

The effects of topical oxygen therapy include improved collagen synthesis, angiogenesis, and as an aid to wound healing with its bactericidal and bacteriostatic properties.[1,12,18,35] The reduction of edema in traumatic injuries is another therapeutic effect of topical oxygen therapy. Control of relative hypoxia in traumatic tissue and stimulation of epithelial formation, provide further positive evidence for the use of topical oxygen therapy to heal chronic wounds.

Prior to the initiation of treatment program, the treating physician must obtain a full-patient physical exam and psychological evaluation. Positive outcomes involve patient compliance and physician competency.

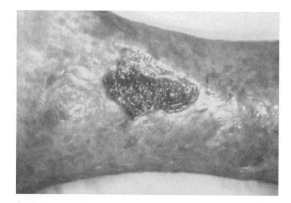

Fig. 4–6. Pre-topical oxygen therapy venous stasis ulcer of the left ankle.

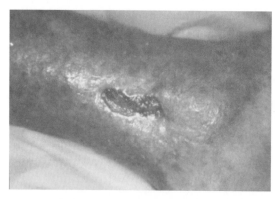

Fig. 4–7. Venous stasis ulcer after 21 hours of topical oxygen therapy.

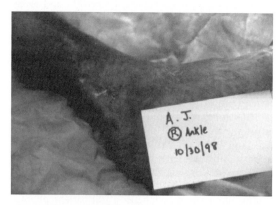

Fig. 4–8. Complete closure of the wound after 3 months of topical oxygen therapy.

Further research can aid in determining the future uses of this modality and its benefits to wound healing.

CASE STUDY ONE

Hispanic female, 78 years old, with a stasis ulcer left ankle with associated PVD. This ulcer had been non-healing for 6 years prior to our team being consulted. At the time of the consultation, she was being treated with collagen dressings. Pre-topical oxygen therapy TCPO$_2$ studies were taken and found to be 20 mm Hg. We did not change her wound care protocol, with the exception of the addition of topical oxygen therapy. After 21 hours of topical oxygen therapy therapy, her TCPO$_2$ rose to 50 mm Hg. We attained complete closure of the wound in 3 months (Figs. 4–6 to 4–7).

CASE STUDY TWO (Courtesy of Judy Horn PTCWS)

A severe diabetic ulcer of the right heel, which probed directly to bone status postdébridement. Patient

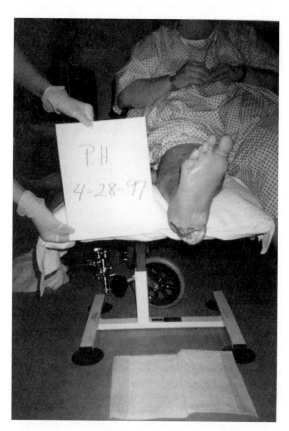

Fig. 4–9. Severe diabetic ulcer of the right heel, which probed directly to bone.

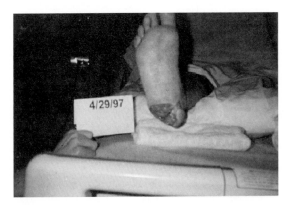

Fig. 4–10. Status post right heel debridement.

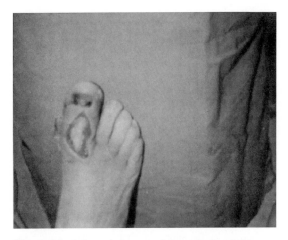

Fig. 4–12. Infected abscess of the right first MPJ.

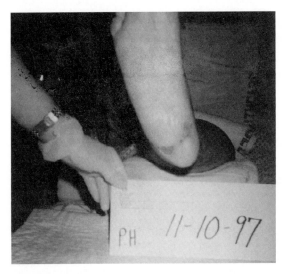

Fig. 4–11. Status post 6 months of BID topical oxygen therapy which closed the wound successfully.

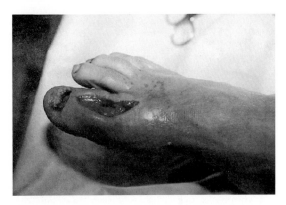

Fig. 4–13. Status post incision and drainage and debridement right first MPJ with 3 weeks topical oxygen therapy.

underwent two débridements while in hospital and 6 months of b.i.d. topical oxygen therapy, which closed the wound successfully (Figs. 4–9 to 4–11).

CASE STUDY THREE

Diabetic male, 64 years old, who presented with an infected abscess of the right first metatarsophalangeal joint (MPJ). The infection was incised, drained, and debrided. The patient was left with an ulcer down to the bone. Topical oxygen therapy was instituted along with antibiotic therapy and the patient was completely healed within a 6-week period (Figs. 4–12 to 4–14).

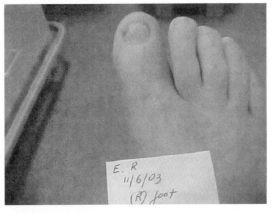

Fig. 4–14. Status post 6 weeks topical oxygen therapy along with antibiotic therapy.

REFERENCES

1. Andreoli SP, Mallett CP, Bergstein JM. Role of glutathione in protecting endothelial cells against hydrogen peroxide oxidant injury. *J Lab Clin Med.* 1986;108:190–198.

2. Allo MD., Lehman WL, et al. Human bite infections of the hand: Adjunct treatment with hyperbaric oxygen. *Infections Surg.* 1985;460–465.

3. Boykin JV. 5 Questions and answers about hyperbaric oxygen therapy. *Adv Skin Wound Care.* 2001;14:232–234.

4. Wattel F, Mathieu D, et al: Hyperbaric oxygen therapy in chronic vascular wound management. *Angiology.* 1990;41: 59–65.

5. Bowker JH, Pfeifer MA, *The diabetic foot,* 6th ed, Chap 19, St. Louis Missouri: Mosby, 2000;404–421.

6. Boykin JV: Hyperbaric oxygen therapy: A physiological approach to selected problem wound healing. *Wounds.* 1996; 8(6):183–198.

7. Boykin JV. The nitric oxide connection: Hyperbaric oxygen therapy, becaplermin, and diabetic ulcer management. *Adv Skin Wound Care.* 2000;13:169–174.

8. Buras JA, Stahl GL, et. al. Hyperbaric oxygen downregulates ICAM-1 expression induced by hypoxia and hypoglycemia: The role of NOS. *Am J Physiol Cell Physiol.* 2000; 278(2):C292–C302.

9. Lambertsen CJ, Kough RH, et al. Oxygen toxicity: Effects in man of oxygen inhalation at 1 and 3.5 atmospheres upon blood gas transport, cerebral circulation and cerebral metabolism. *J Appl Physiol.* 1953;5:471–86.

10. Boerema I, Meyne NG, Brummelkamp WK, et al. Life without blood: A study of the influence of high atmospheric pressure and hypothermia on dilution of the blood. *J Cardiovasc Surg.* 1960;1:122–146.

11. Tibbles PM, Edelsberg JS. Medical Progress: Hyperbaric-oxygen therapy. *N Engl J Med.* 1996;334:1642–1648.

12. Daniel IR, Pavot AP. et al. Topical oxygen therapy treatment of extensive leg and foot ulcers. *J Amer Podiatr Med Assoc.* 1985;75(4)196–199.

13. Sheffield PJ. Measuring tissue oxygen tension: A review. *Undersea Hyperb Med.* 1998;25:179–188.

14. Leslie CA, Sapico FL et al. Randomized controlled trial of topical hyperbaric oxygen for treatment of diabetic foot ulcers. *Diabetes Care.* 1998;11:111–115.

15. Wunderlich RP, Peters EJG, Lavery LA. Systemic hyperbaric oxygen therapy: Lower-extremity wound healing and the diabetic foot. *Diabetes Care.* 2000;23(10):1551–1555.

16. Kindwall EP. *Hyperbaric medicine practice.* Best Publishing Company, 1995;51–54.

17. Heng MCY. Topical hyperbaric therapy for problem skin wounds. *Dematol Surg Oncol.* 1993;19:784.

18. Heng MC, Harker J, et al. Enhanced healing and cost-effectiveness of low-pressure oxygen therapy in healing necrotic wounds: A feasibility study of technology transfer. *Ostomy Wound Manage.* 2000;46:52–61.

19. Diamond E, Forst MB, et al. The effects of hyperbaric oxygen on lower extremity ulcerations. *J Amer Podiatr Med Assoc.* 1982;72:4:180–185.

20. Olejniczak S, Zleiinski A, et al. Topical oxygen promotes healing of leg ulcers, *Med Times* 1976;104:12; 114–122.

21. Olejniczak S, Zleiinski A. Low hyperbaric therapy in the management of leg ulcers. *Mich Med* 1975;74:32: 707–712.

22. Kloth LC, McCulloch JM, Feeder JA. Use of hyperbaric oxygen in wound healing. *Wound healing: Alternatives in management,* Chap. 15, Philadelphia: F.A. Davis 2002:302–318.

23. Kloth LC, McCulloch JM, Feedar JA. Use of hyperbaric oxygen in wound healing. *Wound healing: Alternatives in management:* Chap. 17, Philadelphia: F.A. Davis 2002:405–413.

24. Heng MC, Harker J, et al. Angiogenesis in necrotic ulcers treated with hyberbaric oxygen. *Ostomy Wound Manage.* 2000;46:9;18–31.

25. Faglia E, Favales F. Adjunctive systemic hyperbaric oxygen therapy in treatment of severe prevalently ischemic diabetic foot ulcer. *Diabetes Care.* 1996;19:1338–1343.

26. Heng MCY, Pilgrim JP, and Beck FWJ. A simplified hyperbaric oxygen technique for leg ulcers. *Arch Dermatol.* 1984; 120:640.

27. Hunt TK, Zederfeldt B, Goldstick TK. Oxygen and healing. *J Surg.* 1962;118:521.

28. Kaufman T, Alexander JW, et al. Topical oxygen and burn wound healing: A review. Shriners Burn Institute, Cincinnati, Ohio.

29. Kaufman T, et al. Acceleration of wound healing and contraction of experimental deep burns by topical oxygen. *Surg. Forum* 1983;34:112.

30. Edsberg LE, Brogan MS, et al. Topical hyperbaric oxygen and electrical stimulation: Exploring potential synergy. *Ostomy/Wound Manage.* 2002;48:11:42–50.

31. Upson AV. Topical hyperbaric oxygen in the treatment of recalcitrant open wounds. *Clin Rep Phys Ther.* 1986;66:9; 1408–1412.

32. Attinger CE, Basile A, Delaney J. A simple solution for the partially gangrenous Achilles tendon: Split thickness skin graft. Presented at the Orthopedic Foot and Ankle Summer Meeting June 29, 1996.

33. Kernahan DA, Zing W, Kay WW. The effect of hyperbaric oxygen on the survival of experimental skin flaps. *Plast Reconstr Surg.* 1965;36:19.

34. Kalliainen LK, Gordillo GM, et al. Topical oxygen as an adjunct to wound healing: A clinical case series, *Pathophysiology.* 2003;9:81–87.

35. Schattner LZ. Topical hyperbaric oxygen an low energy laser therapy for chronic diabetic foot ulcers resistant to conventional treatment *Yale J Biol Ed.* 2001;74:2;95–100.

Negative-Pressure Wound Therapy (Vacuum-Assisted Closure)

Jeffrey A. Niezgoda and Barbara Schibly

Introduction to Vacuum-Assisted Closure
　History and Development
　Description
Mechanisms of Action
　Removal of Edema and Wound Exudate
　Reduction of Bacterial Load
　Angiogenesis
　Enhanced Cellular Proliferation
Literature Review
　Initial Studies
　VAC versus Traditional Wound Therapy
　Use of VAC in Complicated Wounds
　VAC and Skin Grafts

Indications for Vacuum-Assisted Closure
　Types of Wounds
　Contraindications and Precautions
Application Techniques
　Modifications and Technology
　　Improvements
Cost Analysis & Reimbursement Issues
Synergistic Wound Healing
　Oxygen and Wound Healing
　Hyperbaric Oxygen Therapy and VAC
The Future
References
Recommended Additional Reading

INTRODUCTION TO VACUUM-ASSISTED CLOSURE

History and Development

Vacuum-assisted closure, or VAC, is a noninvasive system that promotes wound closure through the application of topical, subatmospheric or "negative" pressure to the wound base. Developed at the Wake Forest University School of Medicine in Winston-Salem, North Carolina, VAC received FDA approval for commercial market distribution in 1995. Since then, vacuum-assisted closure has been used in the treatment of thousands of acute, subacute, and chronic nonhealing wounds in patients in the United States and throughout the world. This chapter discusses proposed mechanisms of action, indications, application techniques, and clinical outcomes, with a short discussion on the synergistic effect of VAC with other advanced wound-care technologies, such as hyperbaric oxygen therapy.

Description

The VAC system (Kinetic Concepts Inc, San Antonio, TX) consists of medical-grade open-cell polyurethane foam sponge, evacuation tubing, a fluid-collection canister, and a vacuum pump with adjustable settings. To apply the VAC system, the foam sponge is first cut to conform to the specific size and shape of the wound and is then placed into the wound cavity. The evacuation tube is either inserted into or attached to the foam sponge so that it exists parallel to the skin and the wound site. The sponge dressing is then covered with a thin adhesive film to create an airtight seal. This converts the previously open wound into a controlled closed system. After sealing the wound, the proximal end of the evacuation tube is attached to an effluent-collecting canister and the canister is connected to the adjustable vacuum pump (see Application Techniques.) Depending on the nature of the wound, the pump can deliver either continuous or intermittent subatmospheric pressures ranging from −50 to −200 mmHg. This negative pressure is transmitted equally through the open-cell foam sponge to all wound surfaces.

MECHANISM OF ACTION

The application of topical negative pressure has been shown to enhance wound healing by: (1) removing edema and chronic wound exudate, (2) reducing bacterial colonization, (3) enhancing the formation of new blood vessels, and (4) increasing cellular proliferation as the result of applied mechanical force. Although these actions are often discussed singularly, they are clearly interrelated and act synergistically.

Removal of Edema and Wound Exudate

Edema is a frequent characteristic of both acute and chronic wounds, which has a deleterious effect on wound healing because it compresses local microvasculature and decreases blood flow to injured tissues. As a consequence, delivery of oxygen and essential nutrients to the wound is impaired and wound exudate, which contains factors that inhibit the activity of fibroblasts, endothelial cells, and keratinocytes (tumor necrosis factor, proteases, etc.) cannot be effectively removed. Application of negative pressure to the wound site removes tissue edema, reduces interstitial pressure, and reopens local vasculature facilitating the delivery of oxygen and nutrients and the removal of wound exudate. Laser Doppler flow studies have shown significant increases in blood flow in wounds treated with negative pressure.

Reduction of Bacterial Load

In addition to containing factors that inhibit healing, wound exudate is an ideal medium for bacterial growth and the bacteriocidal action of neutrophils and macrophages is impaired in poorly perfused tissues due to low tissue oxygen tensions. By removing wound exudate and restoring blood flow, VAC therapy has been shown to significantly decrease wound bacterial counts after just 3 to 4 days of application. The occlusive dressing required for proper VAC function also helps prevent bacterial colonization of the wound site by providing an external shield while maintaining a moist environment conducive to wound healing.

Angiogenesis

Wounds that extend beneath the dermis of the skin undergo a proliferative phase of healing in which granulation tissue, consisting of newly formed blood vessels in a collagen matrix, fills in the wound cavity. As previously mentioned, chronic wound fluid contains substances that suppress the activity of cells responsible for the formation of collagen and new blood vessels (fibroblasts and endothelial cells). Withdrawal of this fluid from chronic or compromised wounds decreases the negative impact of these inhibitory factors and enhances the formation of granulation tissue. Mechanical distortion of cells within the wound bed caused by the application of negative pressure also increases the rate of angiogenesis (see below). Angiographic evaluation of patients treated with VAC therapy can demonstrate contrast enhancement in the tissues subjacent to the wound base. This finding suggests that neoangiogenesis is a result of negative pressure forces stimulating the wound base.

Enhanced Cellular Proliferation

The dynamic forces applied via VAC therapy result in enhanced cellular proliferation and increased angiogenesis. Cellular proliferation, in response to mechanical force, has long been recognized to occur in both bone and soft tissues. Distortion of cells by the application of mechanical force activates ionic channels within the cells and causes the release of biochemical mediators that stimulate cellular proliferation by increasing mitotic division. By applying negative force to the wound, VAC therapy pulls the wound edges closer together. This centrifugal tensile force, caused by the collapsing sponge within the wound, results in distortion of cells within the wound as well as the periwound tissue. VAC in the continuous mode causes a single release of chemical mediators, while the intermittent mode results in repetitive stressing of the cytoskeleton with multiple releases of proliferative chemical signals (mechanicochemical signaling). This is thought to explain the increase in granulation tissue formation observed when VAC is used in the intermittent mode.

LITERATURE REVIEW

Numerous studies have supported the use of VAC therapy in the management of a variety of acute, subacute, and chronic wounds, including wounds complicated by infection and the presence of exposed bone, tendon, and orthopedic hardware. VAC has also demonstrated utility in securing grafted tissue and healing graft donor sites.

Initial Studies

Working with a porcine wound healing model, Morykwas et al.[1] were first to demonstrate that negative pressure applied at 125 mm Hg increased blood flow fourfold, significantly reduced bacterial counts after 4 days, and improved muscle flap survival. Following this preliminary study, Morykwas and Argenta[2] examined the effects of VAC therapy on 300 patients with either chronic wounds (stage III and IV pressure ulcers and venous stasis ulcers open for a minimum of 1 week with no signs of healing), subacute wounds (wounds that had dehisced or had bone exposed for less than 7 days), and acute wounds (such as postsurgical wounds which had been open for less than 12 hours).

In the chronic wound group, 32% of pressure ulcers treated with VAC showed complete healing within 2 to 16 weeks, 46% showed more than 80% closure, and 15% showed 50 to 80% closure. All of the partially healed pressure ulcers in this group were improved significantly to allow for delayed primary closure or for closure by grafting. Venous stasis ulcers in this group formed granulation tissue after 4 to 6 days of VAC treatment. Of these wounds, 90% were suitable for skin grafting. Wounds in the subacute group responded more rapidly than chronic wounds. During the study period, 28% of the subacute wounds showed complete healing and the remaining 72% contracted to point where they could be closed with use of skin grafts or other methods. Patients in the acute wound group developed granulation tissue at an extremely rapid rate and healed even more quickly than the other two groups.

VAC versus Traditional Wound Therapy

In a controlled randomized prospective trial comparing healing rates of chronic wounds treated with VAC versus traditional wet to moist dressings, Joseph et al.[3] found that after 6 weeks of treatment, VAC-treated wounds showed a 78% reduction in wound volume compared to a 30% reduction volume in wounds treated with traditional dressings. Most notably, the average depth in VAC treated wounds was reduced by 66%, while the average depth of wet to moist-treated wounds was reduced by only 20%. Wounds treated with VAC, which did not achieve complete closure during the course of this study (chronic wounds of large volume may require 16 to 20 weeks for complete closure), developed a dense and viable layer of granulation tissue, whereas adequate granulation was rarely seen in the wet- to moist-treated wounds.

In a similar study, McCallon et al.[4] Compared the effect VAC therapy to treatment with saline-moistened gauze dressings in nonhealing diabetic foot ulcerations. Satisfactory healing of the ulcers occurred in an average of 22.8 days in the VAC-treated group compared to 42.8 days in the group treated with gauze dressings. During the period of observation, wound surface area decreased 28.4% in the VAC-treated group compared to only 9.5% in the gauze-treated group.

Use of VAC in Complicated Wounds

VAC therapy has been successfully used in the management of wounds complicated by exposed deep tissues, as well as underlying fracture. DeFranzo et al.[5] looked at the effect of VAC therapy on lower-extremity wounds overlying exposed tendon, bone and/or orthopedic hardware. He reported that these difficult wounds, when treated with VAC therapy, formed profuse granulation tissue covering both exposed deep tissues and hardware, and that 71 of the 75 wounds studied showed significant reduction in tissue edema and wound surface and were closed without complication.

Mullner et al.[6] conducted a prospective trial of VAC on 16 patients with infected soft tissue defects complicated by exposed bone and/or implants following rigid stabilization of lower leg fractures. Fourteen of the sixteen patients formed granulation tissue over the bone and hardware implants with a mean healing time of 16 days. Twelve of these wounds were then closed with split-thickness grafts. Two others healed by secondary intent. The two patients who did not respond to VAC therapy had active osteomyelitis underlying the wound. The authors concluded that VAC was an effective treatment for soft tissue defects complicated by exposed bone and/or hardware and a useful adjunctive treatment for wounds complicated by infection.

VAC and Skin Grafts

In addition to preparing wound beds for grafting, VAC has been successfully used as a method of securing skin grafts to difficult recipient beds. Unlike conventional bolsters, VAC prevents fluid collection beneath the graft and the contraction of the foam sponge in response to negative pressure ensures even contact between the entire wound bed and the transplanted skin regardless of wound bed irregularities. In addition, because the sponge is pliable, limited movement of the recipient surface can occur without compromising the graft. Schneider et al.[7] used VAC to secure over 100 grafts applied to various areas of body including feet, lower extremities, perineum, genitalia, trunk, hands, face and scalp. All but two of these grafts took completely. The two failures occurred in grossly contaminated, chronic wounds. No graft in this series was lost due to fluid accumulation beneath the graft and the VAC dressing was reportedly comfortable and allowed for early limited movement.

Molnar et al.[8] reported successful use of VAC to stabilize skin grafts immediately applied to exposed skull following removal of the outer table of bone in four patients with full-thickness scalp loss. Traditionally, this procedure requires two operations with a week or more in between to allow the inner table of bone to form granulation tissue before applying the graft. However, use of VAC for 3 to 4 days following one-step reconstruction resulted in 100% take of the grafts in each of these four cases.

Meara et al.[9] reported success using VAC in the treatment of nine degloving injuries requiring full-thickness grafts of the degloved skin. Seven of the nine grafts secured with VAC showed at least 95% take of the grafted skin even in areas where the skin was obviously traumatized or abraded. A full-thickness graft was also successfully applied in this series to a degloved area overlying an open medial malleolar fracture. Josty et al.[10] also reported successful use of the VAC to manage a degloving injury of the foot.

Re-epithelialization of graft donor sites has been shown to be enhanced by the use of VAC. Genecov et al.[11] measured the rate of healing in donor site wounds in a pig model and in humans and found that donor sites exposed to negative pressure healed at a much faster rate than sites treated with standard occlusive dressings. They concluded that VAC provided a simple and cost-effective method for treating donor graft sites.

INDICATIONS FOR VACUUM-ASSISTED CLOSURE

Types of Wounds

VAC is currently indicated for the treatment of acute and subacute wounds including dehisced incisions, split-thickness meshed skin grafts, muscle flaps, full-thickness burns, open sternal wounds, and infected wounds (following débridement), including cases of necrotizing fasciitis.

For chronic nonhealing wounds, VAC is indicated for the treatment of full-thickness wounds, including vascular wounds caused by arterial insufficiency or venous stasis, neuropathic wounds, and stage III and IV pressure ulcers. VAC has been successfully used on complicated wounds overlying exposed bone, tendon, and orthopedic hardware and in problematic anatomical areas including the perineum, hip, and sacrum. VAC therapy is especially useful in the management of any wound complicated by extensive tunneling and undermining.

Contraindications and Precautions

Relative contraindications for VAC include the presence of necrotic tissue in the wound bed, underlying untreated osteomyelitis and malignancy in or around the wound site. Fistulae opening to body cavities or organs are also currently listed as a contraindication to VAC therapy. However, VAC has been successfully used in select wounds complicated by fistulae and this complication may eventually be listed as a precaution. The authors have utilized VAC as an adjunctive technique in the management of several enterocutaneous fistulae. One particular success, a large abdominal wound complicated by the presence of several loops of exposed and fistulized small bowel, was closed by oversewing the fistula tracts and then grafting over the granulated bowel surfaces with split-thickness skin grafts following several weeks of VAC therapy. Current precautions include active bleeding at the wound site, difficult wound hemostasis, and anticoagulant use.

APPLICATION TECHNIQUES

VAC application is simple, easily learned, and associated with few reported complications. The VAC employs medical-grade polyurethane or polyvinyl alcohol sponge dressings that are fitted and cut with a scissors at the bedside to the appropriate size for each individual wound. The sponge is placed into the wound bed and then covered with an adhesive drape or tape to create an airtight seal. The sponge should completely fill the wound bed, especially in areas of tunneling or undermining. An evacuation tube is then placed within the sponge dressing by cutting a hole in the previously sealed sponge and inserting the tubing. Beveling the distal end of the fenestrated tube to be placed into the sponge is a useful technique. The dressing and the inserted tube are then resealed with additional tape and connected to a fluid collection canister contained within a portable computer-controlled vacuum machine. Once the pump is activated, assuming a good dressing seal has been established, a negative (subatmospheric) pressure at the wound surface interface will be created. The VAC pump provides a digital display, which guides the user through different options, such as continuous or intermittent negative pressure, and a range of negative pressure options (-50 to -200 mmHg). The dressing is changed every other day, typically on a Monday–Wednesday–Friday schedule in the outpatient setting.

Modifications and Technology Improvements

A portable and lightweight unit called the Mini-VAC is available for out patient use. This unit is typically reserved for use in wounds with minimal or limited drainage. Recent upgrades in VAC technology have been introduced with the release of the VAC–ATS (acute hospital version to replace the older first-generation VAC unit) and the VAC–Freedom (replaces the Mini-VAC). These newer units provide Therapeutic Regulated Accurate Care (TRAC) technology that optimizes delivery and control of the negative pressure with monitoring and feedback from the wound to the pump via special channels in the evacuation tubing. TRAC technology has also simplified application and connection of the distal end of the tubing to the sponge, with self-adhesive pads and an elbowed connection to the evacuation tubing. Modifications and specialized dressings are continually being introduced. A variety of sponge foam sizes and precut or perforated sponges are available. Specialized dressing kits for use on hand wounds, abdominal wounds, and large oversized wounds are also offered. Current industry research efforts are focused on utilization of the VAC sponge to potentially deliver antibiotics and a variety of topical agents to enhance the wound environment and further improve healing.

Positive patient outcomes are correlated to user knowledge and experience. Healthcare providers should become familiar with the equipment, as well as dressing application, removal, and monitoring.

COST ANALYSIS AND REIMBURSEMENT ISSUES

Wounds treated with VAC typically heal faster and require fewer dressing changes than those treated with traditional therapy resulting in shorter hospital stays, fewer office or home visits, less nursing care and fewer supplies. Not surprisingly, several studies have shown VAC to be cost effective when compared to standard therapies.

Philbeck et al.[12] reviewed records for 1032 home healthcare Medicare patients with stage III and IV trochanteric and trunk wounds treated with VAC after failing to respond to previous interventions. Healing rates and outcomes in this VAC-treated group were then compared to previously obtained outcome data for similar wounds treated with low air-loss surfaces and saline-soaked gauze therapy. They found that moist gauze-treated wounds took an average 247 days to heal at a cost of $23,465, whereas VAC-treated wounds healed in 97 days at a cost of $14,546.

In an independent analysis of the patient data used in the Philbeck study, the Weinberg Group looked specifically at wounds that were over 30 days old and had failed previous interventions ($n = 979$). The analysis showed that following VAC treatment, 77% of these wounds closed or were progressing toward closure. The Weinberg Group concluded that (1) VAC therapy would successfully heal more chronic wounds that would standard therapies, and (2) that VAC would cost $1,925 less per patient.

Argenta and Morkywas[2] assessed chronic wounds assigned to Diagnoses Related Group 263 (skin graft and/or debridement for skin ulcer or cellulitis) and found that use of VAC decreased overall treatment costs by 65%.

At our institution, we performed a retrospective review of 10 cases of large truncal wounds initially managed with VAC. Complete healing in this group was seen in 94 days. VAC therapy was used for an average of 63 days (range 34–118 days). VAC therapy was discontinued after wound bases were well granulated and all areas of tunneling and undermining had been eliminated. Patients were then managed with advanced topical wound granulating agents and dressing changes were continued on a Monday–Wednesday–Friday schedule. Cost data analysis was then performed, looking specifically at dressing supply and labor costs. The VAC group was then compared to estimate costs for managing these wounds using traditional wet-to-dry dressings on a very conservative schedule, twice daily. Assuming the same healing rate in both groups, VAC therapy was $1,160 less expensive than traditional wound care. An extrapolation cost analysis of our group using Philbeck's data (61% delayed healing with traditional wound care), found an impressive $11,634 cost saving for VAC therapy.

Costs for VAC equipment rental and dressing supplies will vary between institutions and geographic locations. Caregivers need to stay abreast of Medicare, state aid, and managed-care contracts regarding the reimbursement of VAC therapy, as they are continuously being reviewed and revised.

SYNERGISTIC WOUND HEALING

Multiple factors compromise wound healing. Advanced wound care technology is defined as a treatment that positively impacts the healing process by counteracting, eliminating or significantly decreasing at least two of these negative factors. VAC is an example of advance wound-care technology as it has been shown to increase blood flow to the wound, decrease bacterial colonization, edema, and wound exudate, as well as stimulate cellular proliferation via mechanical and chemical mechanisms. Other examples of advanced wound-care technologies include the Circulator Boot, Sonoca or the Ultrasound-Assisted Wound Treatment, Regenesis, and Hyperbaric Oxygen (HBO) therapy. All of these treatment modalities satisfy the definition of advanced wound-care technology as they all positively affect several impediments to wound healing. What started as an observation at our institution—enhanced healing rates in patients treated simultaneously with VAC and HBO therapy—has developed into a theory that we have named *synergistic wound healing*. The concept is that wound healing is hastened when two or more advanced technologies are utilized together and explains our clinical observations as well as our outcome data.

Oxygen and Wound Healing

The role of oxygen in wound healing is well known. Tissue hypoxia, defined as tissue oxygen tensions less than 30 mmHg, impairs wound healing, while correction of hypoxia with improved oxygen delivery has been shown to enhance all phases of the healing process.

Oxygen is essential to meet the metabolic demands of healing tissues and to prevent wound infection. Neutrophils and macrophages do not function efficiently in hypoxic environments, as they require oxygen tensions of at least 30 mmHg to kill bacteria. Oxygen itself has antibacterial properties that are lost when tissues become hypoxic. As a result, hypoxic wounds can quickly become infected. Infection and tissue hypoxia can lead to the loss of vascular membrane integrity, resulting in fluid extravasation and edema. Tissue edema can cause extrinsic compression of the microvasculature, further decreasing local blood flow, resulting in a downward cycle of increasing tissue hypoxia, additional injury, worsening infection, and further edema.

Oxygen is also necessary for proliferation of granulation tissue needed to fill in the wound cavity prior to epithelialization. Fibroblasts and endothelial cells are aerobic and require oxygen for replication, collagen synthesis, and maturation. The formation of new blood vessels (angiogenesis) in the wound bed is also an oxygen-dependent process. Finally, without adequate tissue oxygenation, epithelial migration cannot resurface the wound and wound closure will not be achieved.

Hyperbaric Oxygen Therapy and VAC

While tissue ischemia due to large vessel disease or atherosclerosis can often be corrected by endovascular intervention or revascularization procedure, tissues made hypoxic as the result of compromised flow through small vessels (arteriosclerosis) or due to injury to small vessels, such as those damaged by radiation or diabetes, cannot be surgically improved. However, tissues made hypoxic due to acute small vessel arterial insufficiency can frequently be oxygenated by increasing the oxygen-carrying capacity of the blood. When this occurs, the distance oxygen can diffuse from functioning capillaries increases and marginally viable tissue can be salvaged. Increasing the oxygen-carrying capacity of damaged or compromised arterial vessels can be accomplished by the use of hyperbaric oxygen therapy (HBOT). Breathing 100% oxygen at pressures greater than 1 ATA significantly increases the partial pressure of oxygen in the lungs, resulting in greatly increased plasma oxygen concentrations (at 3 ATA of pressure, breathing 100% oxygen will result in the dissolution of sufficient oxygen in the plasma to support life without presence of red blood cells), increased oxygen diffusion distances, and improved tissue oxygen tensions. To satisfy the definition of HBOT, the patient must inhale 100% oxygen, while entirely enclosed in a pressure vessel capable of generating pressures exceeding 1.4 ATA. Topical oxygen delivery devices do not deliver systemic/inhaled oxygen or exceed pressures of greater than 1.03 ATA and thus do not meet the criteria for hyperbaric oxygen. Typical HBOT sessions deliver 90 minutes of 100% oxygen at 2.4 ATA.

Hyperbaric oxygen has been shown to positively impact wound healing via multiple pathways. HBO therapy can stimulate angiogenesis, enhance cellular proliferation and functioning (neutrophils, fibroblasts, osteoclasts-blasts), augment epithelialization, up-regulate growth factor receptor sites, and decrease tissue edema. In addition, HBOT potentiates the activity of certain antibiotics and has direct antimicrobial effects. Since many of these positive effects are also achieved with VAC therapy, when HBOT is utilized in the management of a wound that is also being treated with VAC, the factors limiting healing are doubly impacted. This combined approach is synergistic and results in improved wound healing.

THE FUTURE

We have discussed the proposed mechanisms of action, indications, application techniques, current literature, and clinical outcomes of vacuum-assisted closure in the management of acute, subacute, and chronic nonhealing wounds. While much of the current literature is anecdotal and retrospective, there are currently several prospective and randomized clinical multicenter trials being conducted. Preliminary analysis of this data is favorable and supports the findings previously reported in the literature.

REFERENCES

1. Morykwas MJ, Argenta LC, Shelton-Brown EI, McGuirt W. Vacuum-assisted closure: A new method for wound control and treatment: Animal studies and basic foundation. *Ann Plast Surg.* 1997;38(6):553–562.

2. Argenta LC, Morykwas MJ. Vacuum-assisted closure: A new method for wound control and treatment: Clinical experience. *Ann Plast Surg.* 1997;38(6):563–577.

3. Joseph E, Hamori CA, Bergman S, Roaf E, Swann NF, Anastasi GW. A prospective randomized trial of vacuum-assisted closure versus standard therapy of chronic nonhealing wounds. *Wounds* 2000;12(3):60–67.

4. McCallon SK, Knoght CA, Valiulus, JP, Cunningham MW, McCulloch JM, Farinas LP. Vacuum-assisted closure versus saline moistened gauze in the healing of postoperative diabetic foot wounds. *Ostomy/Wound Manage.* 2000;46(8):28–34.

5. DeFranzo AJ, Argenta LC, Marks MW, Molnar JA, David LR, Webb LX, Ward WG, Teasdall RG. The use of a vacuum-assisted closure therapy for the treatment of lower-extremity wounds with exposed bone. *Plast Reconstruct Surg.* 2001;108: 1184–1191.

6. Mullner T, Mrkonjic L, Kwasny O, Vecsei V. The use of negative pressure to promote the healing of tissue defects: A clinical trial using the vacuum sealing technique. *Br J Plast Surg.* 1977;50: 194–199.

7. Schneider AM, Morykwas MJ, Argenta LC. A new and reliable method of securing skin grafts to the difficult recipient bed. *Plast Reconstruct Surg.* 1998;102(4):1195–1198.

8. Molnar JA, DeFranzo AJ, Marks MW. Single-stage approach to skin grafting the exposed skull. *Plast Reconstruct Surg.* 2000; 105(1):174–177.

9. Meara JG, Guo L, Smith JD, Pribaz JJ, Breuing KH, Orgill DP. Vacuum-assisted closure in the treatment of degloving injuries. *Ann Plast Surg.* 1999;42(6):589–594.

10. Josty IC, Ramaswamy R, Laing JHE. Vacuum-assisted closure: an alternative strategy in the management of degloving injuries of the foot. *Br J Plast Surg.* 2001;54:363–365.

11. Genecov DG, Schneider AM, Morykwas MJ, Parker D, White WL, Argenta LC. A controlled subatmospheric pressure dressing increases the rate of skin graft donor site reepithelialization. *Ann Plast Surg.* 1998;40(3):219–225.

12. Philbeck TE, Whittington KT, Millsap MH, Briones RB, Wight DG, Schroeder WJ. The clinical and cost effectiveness of externally applied negative pressure wound therapy in the treatment of wounds in home healthcare Medicare patients. *Ostomy/Wound Manage.* 1999;45(11):41–50.

13. Technology assessment of the VAC for in-home treatment of chronic wounds. Washington: The Weinberg group;1999.

RECOMMENDED ADDITIONAL READING

Fleischmann W, Becker U, Bischoff M, Hoekstra H. Vacuum sealing: indication, technique, and results. *Eur J Ortho Surg. Traumatol.* 1995;5:37–40.

Morykwas MJ, David LR, Schneider AM, Whang C, Jennings DA, Conty, C, Parker D, White WL, Argenta LC. Use of subatmospheric pressure to prevent progression of partial-thickness burns in a swine model. *J Burn Care Rehab.* 1999; 20:15–21.

Deva AK, Buckland GH, Fisher E, Liew SCC, Merten S, McGlynn M, Gianoutsos MP, Baldwin MAR, Lendvay PG. Topical negative pressure in wound management. *MJA* 2000;173: 128–131.

Zecha PJ, Reitz R, Hovius SER. Vacuum therapy as an intermediate phase in wound closure: A clinical experience. *Eur J Plast Surg.* 2000;23:174–177.

Sposato G, Molea G, DiCaprio G, Scioli M, La Rusca I, Ziccardi P. Ambulant vacuum-assisted closure of skin-graft dressig in the lower limbs using a portable mini-VAC device. *Br J Plast Surg.* 2001;54:235–237.

De Lange MY, Schasfoort RA, Obdeijn MC, Van der Werff JFA, Nicolai JPA. Vacuum-assisted closure: Indications and clinical experience. *Eur J Plast Surg.* 2000;23:178–182.

Scheufler O, Peek A, Kania NM Exner K. Problem-adapted application of vacuum occlusion dressings: Case report and clinical experience. *Eur J Plast Surg.* 2000;23:386–390.

Evans D, Land L. Topical negative pressure for treating chronic wounds: A systematic review. *Br J Plast Surg.* 2001;54: 238–242.

Deva AK, Sui C, Nettle WJS. Vacuum-assisted closure of a sacral pressure sore. *J Wound Care.* 1997;6(7):311–312.

Greer SE, Kasabian A, Galiano RD, Scott R, Longaker MT. The use of subatmospheric pressure during therapy to close lymphocutaneous fistulas of the groin. *Br J Plast Surg* 2000;53: 484–487.

Rosser CJ, Morykwas MJ, Argenta LC, Bare RL. A new technique to manage perineal wounds. *Infect Urol.* March–April 2000.

Tang, ATM, Ohri SK, Haw MP. Novel application of vacuum assisted closure technique to the treatment of sternotomy wound infection. *Eur J Cardio-thoracic Surg.* 2000;17:482– 484.

Hersh RE, Kaza AK, Long SM, Fiser SM, Drake DB, Tribble CG. A technique for the treatment of sternal infections using the vacuum assisted closure device. *Heart Surg Forum* 2001; 4(3): 211–215.

Hersh RE, Jack JM, Dahman MI, Morgan RF, Drake DB. The vacuum-assisted closure device as a bridge to sternal wound closure. Presented at the Southeastern Society of Plastic and Reconstructive Surgeons, Bermuda, June 4–8, 2000.

Obdeijn MC, de Lange MY, Lichtendahl DHE, de Boer WJ. Vacuum-assisted closure in the treatment of post-sternotomy mediastinitis. *Ann Thoracic Surg.* 1999;68:2358–2360.

Morykwas MJ Argenta LC. Nonsurgical modalities to enhance healing and care of soft tissue wounds. *J South Orthopedic Assoc.* 1997;6(4):279–288.

Greer SE, Duthi E, Cartolano B, Koehler K, Maydick-Youngberg D, Longaker MT. Techniques for applying subatmospheric pressure dressing to wounds in difficult regions of anatomy. *J Wound Ostomy Continence Nurs* 1999;26(5): 250–253.

Valenta AL. Using the vacuum dressing alternative for difficult wounds. *AJNR* April 1944;44–45.

Chua Patel CT, Kinsey GC, Koperski-Moen, KJ, Bungum LD. Vacuum assisted wound closure. *AJNR* 2000;100(12):45– 48.

Mcallon SK, Knight CA, Valiulus JP, Cunningham MW, McCulloch JM, Farinas LP. Vacuum assisted closure versus saline-moistened gauze in the healing of postoperative diabetic foot wounds. *Ostomy Wound Manager.* 2000;46(8):28–34.

Ballard K, Baxter H. Developments in wound care for difficult to manage wounds. Br J Nurs. 2000;9(7):405–412.

Mendez-Eastman S. Negative pressure wound therapy. *Plast Surg Nurs.* 1998;18(1):27–37.

Banwell PE. Topical negative pressure therapy in wound care. *J Wound Care.* 1999;8(2):79–84.

Alvarez AA, Maxwell GL, Rodriguez GC. Vacuum-assisted closure for cutaneous gastrointestinal fistula management. *Gynecol Oncol.* 2001;80:413–416.

6 Historical Aspects of Wound Healing

Bok Y. Lee and Marcelo C. DaSilva

Ancient and Primitive Medicine
Prehistoric Phases
Egyptian Medicine
Sumerian and Oriental Medicine
Greek Medicine
Greco-Roman Period (156 BC–AD 576)
Byzantine Period (AD 476–732)
Mohammedan and Jewish Period
  (733–1096)

Medieval Period (1096–1438)
The Renaissance (1453–1600)
Seventeenth Century: The Age of Individual
  Scientific Endeavor
Eighteenth Century: The Age of Theories
  and Systems
Nineteenth Century: The Beginning of Science
Modern Period
References

To primitive and modern alike, ceremonial is a shock-absorber, a mitigating diversion from the change become inevitable.

—Elsie Clews Parsons, 1914

There have been times when rigorous scholarship and academia in medicine led to great improvement in the quality of healing, and there have been times when medicine disappeared from its own history. Physicians are taught that only what is "relevant" counts and that they would practice medicine in ignorance of their past. But it is through knowledge of the history of our profession that physicians can understand the present and speculate on the future. The history of medicine is not just the history of physicians and their fields of specialization, nor is it just the history of how to treat diseases—it is a history of man's endeavors.

ANCIENT AND PRIMITIVE MEDICINE

Collective investigations of historians, ethnologists, archeologists, and sociologists reveal that phases of social anthropology converge to a single point: instincts of self-preservation and reproduction. Savage man, in his effort to cope with injury and hostile forces, created religious and ethical beliefs based on the necessity to survive. Civilized minds differ from the savage one in regard to evolution. Primitive minds lacked the ability to assign causes for phenomena. The convergence of all medical folklore is animism: the world crawls with invisible spirits that cause disease and death. As savage man advanced, knowledge was gained from experience; there followed herbal medicine, bone setting, and crude surgery as a means of livelihood for some individuals.[1] The history of wound care begins with man's first injury[2] and the art of healing is as old as humanity.[3] Surgery, however, has become a science of recent times.

Primitive surgery was rudimentary. Instruments included such items as a leaf-shaped flint or fish teeth. Primitive procedures included "blood letting," abscess emptying, scarifying tissues, trephining skulls, and performing circumcisions. Wounds were dressed with moss* or fresh leaves, ashes or natural balsams. The Chinese civilization utilized bread mold, "cupping," and moxisbution"† for the treatment of neurologic and

---

*Any of various green, usually small, nonvascular plants of the class Musci of the division Bryophta.
†Smoldering, soft wormwood leaves applied at acupuncture site.

muscle pain.[4] Signs of amputation have been found in prehistoric bones.

During the Bronze and Iron Ages, craftsmanship of metal improved. Surgical saws and files were plentiful from Egypt to Central Europe. Articulated surgical instruments, like scissors, appeared during the Gallo–Roman period.

Development of a rational, scientific concept of disease is essentially modern. Its origin is in the Greek Period, as written in the Hippocratic tract on *Ancient Medicine* (circa 430–420 BC): "... men came to learn by themselves how their own sufferings came about and cease, ... medicine has long had all its means at hand, and has discovered both a principle and a method, through which the discoveries made during a long period are many and excellent."

History suggests that permanent ignorance and superstition result from oppression of mankind by fanatical "leaders." Essential traits of folk and ancient medicine have been alike; in each case, an affair of attraction and spells, plant lore, and psychotherapy exists to reject the effects of supernatural agencies. When this pattern exists, there is no place for development of medicine. The primitive minds had natural standards and were worthy of consideration and scientific respect. "There is nothing men will not do, and there is nothing men have not done to recover their health and save their lives."[5]

PREHISTORIC PHASES

The prehistory of man begins with the origins of highly developed primates in the Oligocene epoch,[‡] the transformation of these in the Pliocene epoch,[§] and the extinction of the great mammals and dawn of Old Stone Age culture in the Pleistocene epoch (500,000 BC).[*] The question that arises about that period is, primarily, what was the relation of prehistoric man to medicine? It began with human and comparative anatomy; innumerable carvings, mural paintings, statuettes, and line engravings of man and animals. Found in caves of the Old Stone Age (Paleolithic[†] period, 150,000 to 35,000 BC), these works represented physiological and pathological findings. What were the primary reactions to agonizing wounds, fatal hemorrhage, terrifying diseases, suffocation, and

imminent death? From ancient medical German folklore we learn that the reaction was panic. Prehistoric trepining was performed by Neolithic[‡‡] man 10,000 years ago. Cauterization of skull wounds was a common Neolithic practice in northern France and evidence of it was found in a pre-Columbian skull from Peru. North American Indian remains of the pre-Columbian period reveal the results of inflammation of bone. Evidence of lesion of soft tissues in Neolithic man comes from the paleopathology of ancient Egypt.

EGYPTIAN MEDICINE

The oldest records of the history of medicine known are the medical papyri of ancient Egypt. Predating these are well-splinted fractures of the fifth dynasty (2750–2625 BC). The earliest known physician was Im-hotep of King Zoser's reign (third dynasty, 2980–2900 BC). A valuable medical papyrus (1600 BC) was found by Edwin Smith,[1,6] at Thebes in 1862, translated by J.H. Breasted. The Smith papyrus contains 48 cases of clinical surgery, examinations, semiology, diagnosis, prognosis, and treatment and a glossary of archaic terms. An important medical papyrus was obtained next. By Georg Ebers,[1,7] at Thebes in 1872 and translated by H. Joachim in 1890, which dates to about 1550 BC, the Ebers papyrus documented the first medical vocabulary, surgical methods, drug therapies, and techniques of splinting and bandaging of wounds.[3] The ancient Egyptians understood wound healing. They used honey, or *byt,* frequently, and described it as an aseptic, antiseptic, and antibiotic.[3,8] The Egyptians believed pus was helpful as long as it was not excessive and advocated draining suppuration from wounds.

SUMERIAN AND ORIENTAL MEDICINE

Sumerian tablets, which date to 2100 BC,[9] describe chronic wound care—washing, bandaging, plastering, and otherwise treating wounds. The Sumerians were skilled in mathematics and astronomy and created the decimal system of notations, weights, and measures. Medical practice in Babylon advanced in public esteem and was rewarded with adequate fees, which were carefully regulated by law.

GREEK MEDICINE

The chief of healing in Greek pantheon was Apollo, commonly called Alexikakos (the averter of ills), also known as *Paean,* as he treated and cured diseases with the

---

[‡]The geologic time and deposits of the epoch in the Tertiary period of the Cenozoic era that extended from the Eocene epoch to the Miocene epoch.
[§]The five epochs of the Tertiary period, are characterized by the appearance of distinctly modern animals.
[*]The earlier of the two epochs of the Quaternary period, characterized by the alternate appearance and recession of northern glaciation and the appearance of the progenitor of human beings.
[†]Designating the cultural period beginning with the earliest chipped stone tools, about 750,000 years ago, until the beginning of the Mesolithic age, about 15,000 years ago.

[‡‡]The cultural period beginning around 10,000 BC in the middle East and later elsewhere, characterized by the development of agriculture and making of polished stone implements.

root of the peony. Hence, the epithet "sons of Paean" was applied to physicians. Legend related that knowledge of medicine was communicated by Apollo and his sister Artemis to the centaur Chiron, son of Saturn. Chiron was entrusted with the rearing and education of the heroes Jason, Hercules, Achilles and, in particular Aesculapius, the son of Apollo by the nymph Coronis.[1] Among the legendary children of Aesculapius by his wife Epione were his daughters Hygieia and Panacea, who assisted in the temple rites and fed the sacred snakes.* Aesculapius is commonly represented with the sacred snake entwined around a rod, a miniature Omphalos, and a childish figure called Telesphorus, the god of convalescence.

The classical period (460–136 BC) of European medicine begins in the Age of Pericles, and its scientific developments center in the figure of Hippocrates (460–370 BC), who gave Greek medicine its scientific principles and its ethical ideals. He was a contemporary of Sophocles, Euripides, Aristophanes, Socrates, Plato, Herodotus, Thucydides, Phidias, and Polygnotus and lived when the Athenian democracy had reached its zenith. Not before or since have so many men of genius appeared within the same limits of space and time. The eminence of Hippocrates is threefold: (1) he dissociated medicine from theology and philosophy, (2) he crystallized the loose knowledge of medicine into a more systematic science, and (3) he gave physicians the highest moral inspiration. Hippocrates revolutionized the fundamentals of wound care by emphasizing the importance of light, stating that examination of a patient should be comfortable for the physician, and emphasized that the injured area should be compared to the corresponding uninjured area.

The formal writings on *Fractures, Dislocations, and Wounds of the Head* may be thought of as modern. Hippocrates argued, in *Wounds of the Head,* for decompressive trephining, even in contusions, and advised simple treatment for an open decompressed fracture. In *Wounds,* he infers that wounds should never be irrigated except with clean water or wine. He describes the dry state near the healthy, the wet to be diseased. He prescribes the aseptic advantages of extreme dryness and the avoidance of greasy dressings. This effort would bring the fresh edges of the wound to close apposition. Hippocrates recognized that "rest and immobilization are of capital importance." While describing symptoms of suppuration, he said" in such cases, medicated dressings, if applied at all, should be not upon the wound itself, but around it." If water was used for irrigation, it had to be pure or boiled. The hands and nails of the surgeon were to be clean. Hippocrates gave the first description of healing by first and second intention. He described the operating room environment as well

illuminated and discussed proper patient posture and the presence of capable assistants. About the surgeon's training he said, "War is the only proper school of the surgeon." Behind the phenomena of nature he hypothesized the existence of a tremendous power. Hippocrates founded the beside method of examining the patient, which is the distinct talent of all clinicians. His method of using the mind and senses as diagnostic instruments, his transparent honesty, his elevated concept of dignity of the physician's duty, and his respect for patients made him the "Father of Medicine."

After Hippocrates came Aristotle (384–322 BC) of Stagira. A pupil of Plato, Aristotle gave medicine the origins of botany, zoology, comparative anatomy, embryology, teratology, and physiology. He named the aorta and regarded the heart as the primary source of heat, sensation, and thought, a view upheld even in Harvey's writings. After the foundation of Alexandria (331 BC), Herophilus (335–280 BC), grandson of Aristotle, created the great school of anatomy at Alexandria, becoming known as the "Father of Scientific Anatomy." Herophilus made important advances in the study of the nervous system, including sensory and motor nerves. He wrote about wounds of the head, venous drainage of the skull, and the anatomic basis of wounds. Erasistratus (circa 310–250 BC) was an experimental physiologist who described the aorta and pulmonary valves, the chordae tendineae of the heart, and the capillary network of arteries and veins. In the third century BC, Alexandrine medicine was introduced in Mesopotamia and, in this way, Syria acquired some of Hippocrates' doctrine via Egypt.

GRECO–ROMAN PERIOD (156 BC–AD 576)

The northern half of the early Roman Empire was conquered by warriors. The southern half of Italy and Sicily were not occupied by northern invaders, but remained free as Magna Graecia from the sixth century BC to the tenth century AD. Magna Graecia introduced cultural influences that led to the School of Medicine of Salerno. After the destruction of Corinth (146 BC), Greek medicine migrated to Rome. The most eminent physicians came from the Schools of Pargamus, Ephesus, Tralles, and Miletus in Asia Minor. Greek medicine was respected in Rome through the personality, tact, and ability of Asclepiades of Bithynia (124 BC).

Roman medicine was almost entirely in Greek hands and produced names such as Aurelius Cornelius Celsus (25 BC–AD 50), who was also known as the "Latin Hippocrates." Celsus was not a physician, but he translated encyclopedia writings on medicine. He was ignored by Roman practitioners. His work went unrecognized until the Renaissance when *De re medicina* was one of

---

*The ancient Greeks, Egyptians, Cretans, and Hindus venerated the serpent as the companion of many gods.

the first medical books printed (1478). *De re medicina* consists of eight books. The first four described diseases treated by diet and regimen and the last four described those amenable to drugs and surgery. The third book contains a definition of insanity (*Insania*) and the first drawing of heart disease. The fourth book contains the four cardinal signs of inflammation: *rubor, tumor, calor,* and *dolar* (redness, swelling, heat, and pain). The fifth book classifies lists of drugs, pharmaceutical methods, and weights and measures. The sixth book describes disease of the skin and venereal disease. The seventh book is on surgery and describes the use of the ligature for bleeding vessels, management of cancer of the head, neck, and nose, hypertrophic scar, and proper dressing of wounds. Celsus said "the physician cannot apply the proper therapeutics without a correct diagnosis."[3]

Three Greek surgeons were contemporaries of Celsus: Heliodorus, Archigenes, and Antyllus. Heliodorus described the first ligation and torsion of blood vessels, surgery of hernias, and circular and flap amputations. Archigenes of Apamea used ligatures during surgical procedures. Antyllus treated aneurysms by applying two ligatures and cutting down between them, which became the method of treatment until John Hunter (1728–1793). This ancient period ends with a widely respected Greek physician, Galen of Pergamon (131–210). He founded experimental physiology and was the first experimental neurologist. He was a skilled practitioner and his theories dominated Western medicine for 1500 years.[3] He was the foremost contributor of experimental physiology prior to William Harvey (1578–1657) and treated wounded gladiators during mortal combats in Pergamon and Rome. During this period, he learned about human anatomy, the venous and arterial circulation, and wound healing. Galen wrote that, "The best physician has also to be a philosopher." His theory that suppuration is essential to the healing of wounds led to Arabic notions of healing by second intention. His concept of "*pus bonum et laudible*" was opposed by Mondeville, Paracelsus, and Paré, and lasted until Lister in 1881.[10]

BYZANTINE PERIOD (AD 476–732)

The Western Roman Empire lasted 500 years. The Eastern Empire lasted over 1,000 years (395–1453). The downfall of the Western Empire began when the Romans acquired a state where "wealth accumulates and men decay." Degeneration of mind and body, with consequent relaxation of morals, led to mysticism and respect for the supernatural. This paved the way for dogmatism and the mental inertia of the Middle Ages.

The demoralization, luxury, and sloth in the Eastern Empire became synonymous with the Byzantine Empire. Medical achievement was limited to the preservation of the language, culture, and literary texts of the Greeks. The habit of compilation established by Greek and Roman writers was expressed in four industrious compilers. Oribasius (325–403) wrote a treatis on medicine, *Euporista*, that was the most popular during the Dark Ages. Aetius of Amida, in the sixth century, described for the first time the ligation of the brachial artery above the sac for aneurysm, which evolved into the Hunterian method (1786).

MOHAMMEDAN AND JEWISH PERIOD (733–1096)

The Middle Ages were first influenced by Arabic authors, such as Rhazes (860–932), who described smallpox and measles. Haly ben Abbas, a Persian, was the author of *Almaleki*, containing an anatomical section that was the only source of knowledge at Salerno from 1070–1170. Ibn Sina or Avicenna (980–1037), "the Prince of Physicians," recommended wine as a wound dressing and was the first to describe the preparation and properties of sulfuric acid and alcohol.

During the second period of the Middle Ages, medicine greatly prospered during the Spanish dynasty (655–1236). Abulkasism, called Albucasis (1013–1106), was the author of a medico-surgical treatise called *Altasrif* (Collection), which contained three books. The first discussed the use of cautery; the second contained detailed descriptions of lithotripsy, amputations for gangrene, the treatment of wounds, and management of phlegmon and carbuncle; the third book dealt with fractures and dislocations.

Closely associated with Mohammedan medicine is the Jewish influence upon European medicine. During the Middle ages and long after, the destiny of the Jewish physicians in Europe was protected by monarchy and clergy. They were utilized as teachers in the Schools of Salerno and Montepellier because of their scientific knowledge. The prohibition of Jewish physicians by Popes Paul IV (1555–1559) and Pius V (1566–1772) was lifted by Pope Gregory XIII in 1584. It was not, however, until the beginning of the modern industrial movement that Jewish physicians had access to the universities.

MEDIEVAL PERIOD (1096–1438)

The Middle Ages are described as a period of conflict between feudalism and ecclesiasticism, or Church and State. The School of Salerno was the first independent medical school. It aroused the healing art from 500 years of stagnation. Salerno was known by Romans as the ideal health resort. Its medical teachings produced surgeons like Roger (Ruggiero Frugardi) of Palermo and Roland (Rolando Capelluti) of Parma. Roger studied many important areas in medicine, one being the healing of wounds by second intention. The medical school of Salerno was abolished by Napoleon in November 1881.

The authority on surgery in the 14th and 15th centuries was Guy de Chauliac (1300–1368). He introduced medical education at Toulouse, Montpellier, and Paris and taught a special course in anatomy at Bologna, becoming the most erudite surgeon of his time. He believed in resecting cancer at an early state with a knife. Guy de Chauliac wrote *Wounds and Fractures* in 1363, which included instructions on bandaging, suturing, compresses, drains, and the treatment of keloids.[3] Despite his knowledge and clinical experience, he was known as a reactionary in wound healing. He stated that, "The healing of a wound must be accomplished by the surgeon's interference: salves, plasters and other interventions."

Another pupil of the School of Montepellier was Arnold de Villanova (1235–1311) of Spain, who described suture materials and their differences. He wrote, in relation to wound healing, "in large wounds one should use sutures and silk thread should be tied at short distances . . . a collection of pus is best dissolved by incision and cleaning out the purulent material, to put off the opening of an abscess brings many dangers with it . . . where veins and arteries are notably large, incision and deep cautery should be avoided.

During the Middle Ages, the Crusades awakened nationhood, an idea of citizens against barons. In the struggle between collectivism and individualism, intellectual independence was ostracized if it did not agree with Church or State. Popes and kings supported advances in medicine by building universities and hospitals and by encouraging individuals. This, however, was done by suppression of experimental science. Until the Renaissance, there was neither induction nor experimentation.

THE RENAISSANCE (1453–1600)

Humanistic revival of classical art, architecture, literature, and science originated in Italy in the 14th through the 16th centuries and, later, spread throughout Europe. Known as the Renaissance, it marked the transition from medieval to modern times. Many factors led to the defeat of individualism by authority inflicted upon mankind, gunpowder being the most important. The use of gunpowder and bullets during the Renaissance eventually led to the end of feudalism. It changed the role of surgeons into an active and aggressive one. Resurgence of Greek culture was brought into Italy by the Byzantine scholars after the fall of Constantinople (Istanbul) in 1453. This Renaissance revival reached its peak with the medical leaders of the 16th century. These leaders were Parcelsus, Versalius, and Paré.

Philippus Aureolus Theophrastus Bombastus von Hohenheim, or simply Paracelsus (1493–1541), was the forerunner of chemical pharmacology and therapeutics. His coarseness of fiber often hindered his ability to think "straight and see clear." The son of a physician, he had a peculiar "disaffection" for those who disagreed with his views and writings. He was one of the few who advanced medicine by debating about it. He traveled all over Europe, collecting information from regional folklore. Practically the only asepsist between Mondeville and Lister, he taught that nature heals wounds. As a theorist, Paracelsus believed in the descent of living organisms from primordial ooze, anticipating Darwin's observation that "the strong wore down and prey upon the weak." Andreas Vesalius (1514–1564), was a commanding figure in European medicine after Galen and before Harvey. He introduced anatomy as a living science. He taught students to dissect and inspect the partis *in situ* and wrote *De Fabrica Humani Corporis* in 1543. He was the first to diagnose and describe aneurysm of the abdominal and thoracic aorta (1551). Disregarded by his old teacher, Sylvius, and persecuted by his colleagues, Vesalius burned his manuscripts and left Padua to work as a court physician to Emperor Charles V.[1]

Abroise Paré (1510–1590), a barber's apprentice, worked as a dresser at Hotel Dieu in Paris. He became an army surgeon in 1537 and was the only "Protestant" to be spared (by royal mandate) at St. Bartholomew. Paré's contribution to medicine related to the treatment of gunshot wounds: "diseases not curable by iron are curable by fire." During the Battle of Villaine, Paré's supply of boiling oil was depleted and he applied milder treatments to amputation wounds. He practiced with meticulous cleanliness and epitomized these words: "I make the wound, God heals it," ending dogma of laudable pus.

SEVENTEENTH CENTURY: THE AGE OF INDIVIDUAL SCIENTIFIC ENDEAVOR

In the 17th century, medicine produced physicians such as William Harvey (1578–1657), who graduated from Padua. Not since Vesalius had a body of work by one writer so influenced modern medicine. Harvey reviewed theories of blood in motion, showed their inadequacy, and proceeded to prove that the heart acts as a muscular force pump in propelling blood continuously and in a cycle. For Harvey, the primary necessity underlying all his actions was personal observation. He wrote to Riolan: " . . . by my observations and experiments, and not to demonstrate by causes and probable principles, but to confirm it by sense and experience, as by a powerful authority, according to the rule of the anatomists.[11]" He published *De Motu Cordis* in 1628.

The introduction of the microscope was made in the last half of the 17th century by Anton van Leeuwenhoek (1632–1723), a Dutch naturalist, who devoted his private life to studying natural history. He had 247 microscopes and observed small particles in ordinary pond water, calling them "animalcules." Leeuwenhoek was the first to describe spermatozoa, red blood cells, sarcolemma, and microorganisms in the teeth. He also accurately described the morphology of bacterial chains and clumps. He demonstrated capillary anastomosis between the arteries and veins, which Malpighi observed in 1660, completing Harvey's demonstration. The greatest microscopist was Marcello Malpighi (1628–1694), the founder of histology and profession of anatomy at Bologna and Pisa. He discovered the rete mucosum, or Malpighian layer of skin, and demonstrated pulmonary capillary anastomosis between arteries and veins and capillaries (1600). Prior to Harvey, respiration was regarded as a means of refrigeration and not combustion. Malpighi demonstrated that blood changes from venous to arterial in the lungs, but did not correlate how or why humans breathe. Robert Boyle (1627–1691) demonstrated that necessity of air for life and combustion through experiments involving flames and animals. In 1665, Robert Hooke (1635–1703), in his treatise *Micrographia*, described microscopic units that made up cork, naming these units "cells." In 1667, he proved that by attaching a bellow to the trachea of a dog with an open thorax, life could be maintained by artificial means. Antoine-Laurent Lavoisier (1743–1794) discovered oxygen as the true element in the interchange of gases in the lungs. Lavoisier demonstrated that respiration is the analog of combustion, the chemical products of carbon dioxide and water.

EIGHTEENTH CENTURY: THE AGE OF THEORIES AND SYSTEMS

John Hunter (1728–1793), a Scottish surgeon, came to London in 1748 and was taken in by his brother, William Hunter (1718–1783), who was also a surgeon. During the expedition of Belleisle (1761), John Hunter acquired a unique knowledge of gunshot wounds. He was the first to classify healing by *primary and secondary intention* and to describe granulation tissue in healing wounds. As a surgical pathologist, he described shock, phlebitis, pyemia, and intussusception and studied inflammation, gunshot wounds, and surgical treatment related to the vascular system. In 1790, he first introduced artificial feeding via a flexible tube passed into the stomach. He described inflammation as not a disease by a nonspecific response that has a "salutary" effect on its host. John Hunter recognized the possibility of tissue acceptance for transplants.[3] He referred to a female calf, the nonidentical twin of a male, which matured into a sterile cow lacking immunogenicity. This antedated the works of Carrel, Guthrie, and Sir Peter Brian Medawar on tissue transplantation and acquired immunologic

tolerance, respectively. Hunter's position in science is based on the fact that he was the founder of experimental and surgical pathology as well as comparative physiology and anatomy.

NINETEENTH CENTURY: THE BEGINNING OF SCIENCE

Great industrial and social–democratic movements of man followed the political revolutions in America and France and intensified feelings for intellectual and moral liberty. The publication of works such as Hemholtz's *Conservation of Energy* (1847) and Darwin's *Origin of Species* (1859) led to true advancements in medicine. Physics, chemistry, and biology were finally studied as objective laboratory sciences. Prior to 1850 and afterward, advancements in medicine primarily came from France, as Germany was recovering from the Thirty Years War. Virchow published *Cellular Pathology*, which described new forms of disease.

Theodor Schwann (1810–1882), born near Duseldorf, described the constitution of tissues: "The elementary parts of all tissues are formed of cells in an analogous, though very diversified, manner . . . " His cell theory was published 1839. He discovered the sheath of neurons that bears his name. Schwann proved the necessity of air for development in the embryo and also addressed spontaneous generation. In 1836, he proved that putrefication was produced by living organisms. Following research by Schleiden and Schwann, cells became the primary subject of investigation. Virchow (1858) published works on continuity of cellular development and its importance in pathology. The cell became known as the structural and physiological unit in all living organisms. Anatomic studies became more progressive and more histological. The "seats and causes" of disease were regarded as cellular elements of the body. Jacob Henle (1809–1885), a German pathologist, is recognized as the identifier of epithelial tissues of the body (1836–1837). He maintained that a physician's duty was to prevent and cure disease and believed disease to be a deviation from normal physiologic processes. He published *Allgemeine Anatomie* in 1841, a book on microscopic histology.

The rise of modern medicine includes a German pathologist, Rodolf Virchow (1821–1902), the founder of cellular pathology. Virchow graduated in Berlin in 1843. He was the first to observe leukocytosis. Virchow described the "body as a cell-state in which every cell is a citizen," and, in 1856, created the doctrine of embolism. He articulated the cell theory in 1858: "Every animal appears as a sum of vital units, each of which bears in itself the complete characteristics of life." A pupil of Virchow, Julius Cohnheim (1839–1884) made microscopic observations of initial vasodilatation and changes in blood flow and subsequent edema caused by increased permeability. He demonstrated, in opposition to Virchow, that an essential feature of inflammation included passage of white blood cells through walls of capillaries and that pus and pus cells are formed away from the blood. Diapedesis was described by Addison; however, Cohnheim's investigations traced the migration of stained leukocytes.

Advances in scientific medicine during the second half of the 19th century were characterized by the introduction of the biological or theory of evolution by Charles Robert Darwin (1809–1882). Darwin graduated from Cambridge and worked for 20 years prior to publishing *On the Origin of Species by Means of Natural Selection* (1859). Darwin's work in biology introduced cellular pathology, bacteriology, and parasitology, which had been previously referred to as the germ theory. Louis Pasteur (1822–1895) graduated in chemistry in 1847 from the École normale in Paris. His work included writings on molecular asymmetry (1848), fermentation (1857), spontaneous generation (1862), preventive vaccinations (1880), and discovery of the anaerobic and aerobic characteristics of bacteria. In November 1877, Robert Koch (1843–1910), after working with bacillus anthrax, published methods of fixing and drying bacterial films. He used coverslips for staining and photographing, as well as identification and comparison. Joseph Lister (1827–1912), an English surgeon, graduated from the University of London in 1852, becoming house surgeon and professor at the University of Glasgow. Lister, interested in the high mortality from surgical infections, which included his own 45% mortality rate for amputations, was attracted by Pasteur's work and experimented with zinc chloride and sulfites. He stumbled by "chance" upon carbolic acid, which was used to disinfect sewage in Carlisle. In 1867, he published the results of 2 years' work *On the Antiseptic Principle in the Practice of Surgery*. In 1874, Lister sent Pasteur a letter acknowledging his work in relation to antiseptic surgery.

Born in Saint Julien (Rhone), Claude Bernard (1813–1878), a physiologist from France, is regarded as a founder of experimental medicine, that is, the artificial production of disease by chemical and physical manipulation. His achievements include the discovery of effects of vasodilator and vasoconstrictor nerves on circulation.

The theory of evolution, combined with the cell theory, provided the intellectual framework that developed biology into an experimental science. It branched into biochemistry and genetics. In 1865, Austrian monk Gregor Mendel described the basic rules of heredity, but it was not until 1900 that his theory was widely accepted. Fredrich Miescher, in 1871, isolated what may have been DNA from the nuclei of dead white blood cells. Elie Metchnikoff (1845–1916), a Russian biologist, demonstrated how amoeboid cells in connective tissues and blood engulf solid particles and bacteria, destroying them by phagocytosis. He called them "phagocytes" and related their function as scavengers. He described inflammation as the effect of phagocytosis to the site of injury by chemotaxis. He upheld the theory of immunity as phagocytosis.

MODERN PERIOD

Ancient surgeons were able to care for wounds and hemorrhage by cleansing and bandaging. Paul Ehrlich's (1854–1915) lock-and-key theory of antigen–antibody recognition was instrumental in furthering the understanding of immunochemical principles of wound healing. Sir Thomas Lewis established that chemical substances, locally induced by injury, mediated the vascular changes in inflammation. In 1897, Eduard Buchner demonstrated that chemical transformation could be performed by cell extracts.

By 1900, 16 of the 20 standard amino acids that form proteins had been identified. That same year, Emil Fischer proposed the correct mechanism for formation of chemical links in protein: peptide bonds between adjacent amino acids. In 1935, threonine was the last amino acid discovered.

In 1928, while studying staphylococcus variants, Sir Alexander Fleming (1881–1955) observed that a mold contained in one of his cultures caused the bacteria in its vicinity to undergo lysis. The mold belonged to the genus *Penicillium notatum* and was named penicillin. Fleming's career was devoted to investigating human defenses that control bacterial infection.[12] Alexis Carrel's (1873–1944) and C. C. Guthrie's work on the effects of exudation on fibroblast proliferation found in an inflammatory site suggested that humoral substances present within the inflammatory environment stimulated tissue repair. Their studies led to research in growth factors, cytokines, substrates, hormones, cell-to-cell communication, and the effects of inflammation on cell function and replication.

Sir Peter Medawar, in 1944, devised three characteristics of immune system responsiveness: recognition of nonself, memory, and specificity. He examined the histology of rejection and suggested that the mononuclear cell (lymphocyte) had an important role in allograft destruction.[13] Studies by Paul Ehrlich led to immunoassays. Names in molecular biology include Michael Tswett and his analytical methods and Martin Synge's partition chromatography. In 1953, Frederick Sanger reported the complete amino acid sequence of human insulin.[14, 15] Myles Partridge separated pure amino acids using column chromatography and others contributed to the identification, isolation, and sequencing of proteins. In 1951, Linus Pauling suggested the helical arrangement for certain parts of protein chains.

The modern era of molecular cell biology, concerned with how genes govern cell activity, began in 1953 when James D. Watson and Francis H. C. Crick postulated the double-helical structure of deoxyribonucleic acid (DNA).[16] In 1961, Francois Jacob and Jacques Monod suggested that protein products of certain genes regulate activity of other genes. Soon after, proof that messenger ribonucleic acid (mRNA) carries information from DNA to protein-synthesizing machinery, discovery of the genetic code, and discovery that proteins are translated by transfer RNA (tRNA) and ribosomes were reported.[17] Technical advances in molecular biology in the 1970s were greatest in analysis and manipulation of DNA. Enzymes that are able to cut DNA were discovered. These enzymatic scalpels are called restriction endonucleases and their discovery accounts for DNA cloning and sequencing. Throughout the years, the cell has become an organism in which the controlled and integrated actions of genes produce specific sets of proteins that build characteristic structures and carry out specialized enzymatic activities, preserving the species and perpetuating the process of life. Man's concept of the cell has come a long way from its original characterization as a simple unit of living matter.

ACKNOWLEDGMENT

This article was reproduced with permission from B. Y. Lee and B. Herz. *Surgical Management of Cutaneous Ulcers and Pressure Sores,* published by Hodder Arnold, 1998.

REFERENCES

1. Garrison FH. *An Introduction to the History of Medicine,* 4th ed. Philadelphia: Saunders; 1929.

2. Wideman DM, Rovee DT, Alvarez OM. Wound dressings: Design and use. In: Cohen IK, Diegelmann RF, Lindblad WJ, eds. *Wound Healing; Biochemical and Clinical Aspects*; Philadelphia: Saunders; 1992:562–580.

3. Brown H. Wound healing research through the ages. In Cohen IK, Diegelmann RF, Lindblad WJ, eds. *Wound Healing; Biochemical and Clinical Aspects*; Philadelphia: Saunders; 1992: 5–18.

4. Weingarten MS. Obstacles to wound healing, *Wounds* 1993: 5(5):238–244.

5. Holmes OW. *Medical Essays*; Boston, MA; 1883.

6. Breasted JH. *The Edwin Smith Surgical Papyrus*. Chicago: University of Chicago Press; 1930.

7. Ebbell B. *The Papyrus Ebers. The Greatest Egyptian Medical Document*; London: Oxford University Press; 1937.

8. Majno G. *The Healing Hand: Man and Wound in the Ancient World*; Cambridge, MA: Harvard University Press; 1975.

9. Caldwell MD. Topical wound therapy—An historical perspective. *J Trauma* 1990; 30(S12):S116–S122.

10. Lister J. An address on the treatment of wounds. *Lancet* 1881; 863:90.

11. Whitteridge G. *William Harvey and the Circulation of the Blood*. New York: Neale Watson Academic Publications; 1971.

12. Gilman AG, Rall TW, Nies AS, Taylor P. *Goodman and Gilman's The Pharmacological Basis of Therapeutics*; 8th ed. New York and Oxford: Pergamon Press; 1990:1065.

13. Amos DB, and Sanfilippo F. The immunology of transplants antigens. In Sabiston DC, Jr, ed. *The Biological Basis of Modern Surgical Practice*; 14th ed. Philadelphia: Saunders; 1991: 346.

14. Brown H, Sanger F, and Kitai R. The Structure of pig and sheep insulins, *Biochem J.* 1955:60:556–565.

15. Sanger F. Sequences, sequences, and sequences, *Ann Rev Biochem.* 1988:57:1–28.

16. Watson JD, Crick FHC. Molecular structure of nucleic acids. A structure for deoxyribose nucleic acid. *Nature* 1953:171: 737–738.

17. Darnell J, Lodish H, Baltimore D. *Molecular Cell Biology*; 2nd ed. New York: Scientific American Books; 1990:1–15.

Electrical Stimulation in Wound Repair

Joseph McCulloch

Overview of Medical Electricity
The Rationale for use of Electrical Stimulation in Wound Healing
  Endogenous Bioelectric System
Therapeutic Currents
  Direct Current
  Pulsed Current
Research Evidence

  Circulatory Effects of ES
  Effects of ES on Wound Tensile Strength
Clinical Evidence Supporting ES in Wound Healing
Clinical Application of ES
  Precautions
Summary
References

A variety of physical modalities have been used clinically in an effort to facilitate wound healing. These include ultraviolet radiation,[1] ultrasound,[2] hydrotherapy,[3] and electrical stimulation (ES). Of all the physical agents, the greatest amount of evidence from clinical trials supports the use of electrical stimulation. This is particularly true for the treatment of chronic stage III and IV pressure ulcers.[4–7]

The success of ES in clinical trials resulted in the Agency for Health Care Policy and Research recommending that a course of ES treatment be considered for stage II, III, and IV pressure ulcers that did not respond to conventional therapies. This recommendation was published in the Clinical Practice Guideline *Treatment of Pressure Ulcers.*[8] In addition, in 2002, the Centers for Medicare and Medicaid Services (previously known as the Health Care Financing Administration) issued a national coverage policy stating that "For services performed on or after April 1, 2003, Medicare will cover electrical stimulation for the treatment of wounds only for chronic stage III or stage IV pressure ulcers, arterial ulcers, diabetic ulcers and venous stasis ulcers."[9]

OVERVIEW OF MEDICAL ELECTRICITY

Anyone reading the clinical research literature on ES is often confused by the broad variety in terminology that exists. It is helpful in understanding the science, therefore, to provide a brief description of some of the terms that might be encountered. The following terminology comes from a monograph entitled *Electotherapeutic Terminology in Physical Therapy* produced by the Section on Clinical Electrophysiology of the American Physical Therapy Association.[10]

Charge (Q)—a fundamental property of matter. Matter can be either positively or negatively charged or be electrically neutral. An electrically neutral substance can gain electrons and become negatively charged or lose electrons and become positively charged. Charge is measured in units called Coulombs. One Coulomb contains 6.28×10^{18} electrons. When electrical stimulation is used in wound care, charge is delivered in the microcoulomb range.

Charge Density—a measure of electrical charge per unit of cross-sectional area of the electrode. In wound care, this is again in the microcoulomb range and would be represented by $\mu C/cm^2$. Charge density is inversely related to electrode size. Therefore, current density would be less when a larger electrode is used.

Voltage (V)—the driving or electromotive force capable of moving electrons or ions through a conductor (in this case wound tissue) between two or more electrodes applied to the body. The voltage between two points is determined by the separation of the charges between the points. This means that one region has an excess of electrons as compared to the other. The regions, therefore, are "polarized" with respect to each other (one is negative and the other positive). *Current (I)*—the rate of flow of charged particles (electrons or ions) past a specific point, in a specific direction. Current is measured in amperes (A) and is defined mathematically by the formula

$$I = C/t$$

where *I* equals amperes, *C* equals Coulombs, and *t* equals time in seconds. In electrical stimulation for wound care, we attempt to mimic the bioelectric currents typically seen in tissues, which is in the milliampere (mA) range.

Resistance (R)—measured in ohms (Ω), resistance is the property of a conductor that opposes the flow of electrons. In wound care, the skin offers a greater resistance to current than does the open wound.

Anode—the positively charged pole of an electrical circuit.

Cathode—the negatively charged pole of an electrical circuit.

THE RATIONALE FOR USE OF ELECTRICAL STIMULATION IN WOUND HEALING

The rationale for the use of ES in wound healing stems from the fact that an endogenous bioelectric system exists within the human body that enhances the healing of bone fractures and soft-tissue wounds.[11] When problems ensue that result in failure of this system, therapeutic levels of ES may be delivered to the wounded tissue from an external source in an attempt to mimic the body's natural bioelectric currents.

Endogenous Bioelectric System

It is not news that endogenous electrical currents exist in the body. These include such things as the transmembrane voltages found in cell membranes and action potentials and electrical impulses that travel along peripheral nerves. What may not be as well known, however, is the existence of measurable currents in skin, wounds, and the cells that facilitate wound repair.

It has been known since 1945 that endogenous bioelectric circuits exist in humans, other mammals, and amphibians and that these circuits can facilitate wound healing.[12–17] Electropositive voltages have been recorded from the dermis of superficial wounds and electronegative

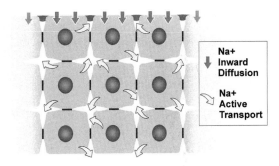

Figure 7–1. Sodium transport through the epithelium (modified from Vanable[17]).

voltages have been detected from the intact skin.[12,14,15] As described by Vanable,[17] these transepithelial potentials (TEPs) result from sodium (Na^+) diffusing from the outside of epidermal cells to the inside via channels in the apical membrane of the skin's mucosal surface. As sodium ions enter the outer cells of the epithelium, they migrate along a steep electrochemical gradient. As the ions enter a cell, they can then diffuse to other cells in the epithelium. This creates about a 50 mV potential across the epithelium. The process is represented graphically in Fig. 7–1.

TEPs of human skin have been measured and reported by Foulds and Barker.[16] They detected voltage ranging from 10 to 60 mV, depending on the region being measured. The average voltage for all of the skin sites measured was - 24 mV (Fig. 7–2) This negative outer charge is attributed, to a great degree, to the diffusion of sodium from the surface to the interior epithelial cells.

Skin Battery Potentials

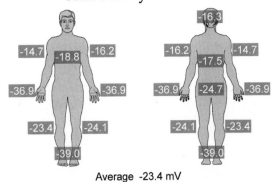

Average -23.4 mV

Figure 7–2. Average human skin battery potentials (modified from Foulds and Barken[15]).

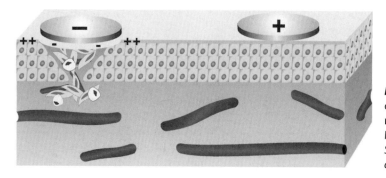

Figure 7-3. Migration of positively charged ions (neutrophils and epidermal cells) toward the cathode. (From McCulloch, JM. *Therapeutic Modalities Stimulate Wound Management, Biomechanics* April 2004, p. 67, with permission).

When a break occurs in the skin, the homeostatic mechanism just described becomes altered. The TEP provides the stimulus for measurable current to move outward because of the low resistance provided by the loss of skin. This effectively produces a short circuit of the skin battery. Jaffee and Vanable[18] found that the skin immediately bordering the wound developed a steep, lateral voltage gradient that fell from 140 mV/mm at the wound edge to 0 mV/mm just 3 mm laterally.[18] This gradient is felt to be a stimulus to repair. Interesting is the fact that when a scab is allowed to develop, the lateral voltage gradient is eliminated.[15] On the other hand, in experimental wounds that were covered with an occlusive dressing that prevented desiccation, a measurable postwounding current of injury of 29.6 ± 8.6 mV was noted.[19]

With knowledge that a skin battery potential exists, it was logical to question whether the potential could be affected by outside forces, in particular, electrical stimulation. Research has demonstrated that when appropriate levels of electricity are delivered to a wound, positively charged ions in the tissues (Na^+, K^+, H^+) and cells, such as fibroblasts and activated neurtophils, migrate toward the negative electrode (cathode) (see Fig. 7–3). Conversely, negatively charged ions (Cl^-, HCO_3^-, P^-) and cells, such as epidermal, macrophages and neutrophils, migrate toward the positive electrode (anode) (see Fig. 7–4). This process, termed galvanotaxis, is summarized in Table 7–1 and provides the foundation for the use of ES in wound healing. While most of these studies report *in vitro* data, a few have involved work on humans and animals.

Eberhardt and colleagues[20] examined the cell composition of wound exudate in 10 wounds treated with ES for 30 minutes. They noted that 69% of the cells counted after 6 hours of ES were neutrophils. This compared to 45% for the control wounds. The authors attributed this 24% difference to ES. Mertz and associates[21] evaluated epidermal migration in pig wounds following ES. They utilized a monophasic pulsed-current (described later in this chapter) for 30 minutes twice daily for 7 days. Macroscopic examination of the epidermis revealed that wounds treated with negative polarity on day 0 followed by positive polarity on days 1 through 7 demonstrated a 20% improvement in epithelialization compared to those receiving treatment with with positive or negative polarity alone. Another finding of interest was that when the polarity was alternated daily between positive and negative there was a 45% inhibition in epithelialization. This suggests that cellular migration is somewhat dependent on endogenous bioelectric signals.

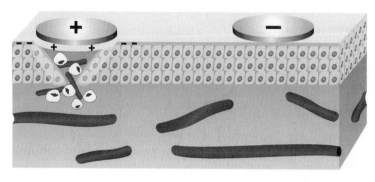

Figure 7-4. Migration of negatively charged ions (activated neutrophils and fibroblasts) toward the anode. (From McCulloch, JM. *Therapeutic Modalities Stimulate Wound Management, Biomechanics.* April 2004, p. 67, with permission.

Table 7–1. Galvanotaxis in wound healing

Cells and polarity	Biological effects	Citations
Macrophage (−)	Phagocytosis and autolysis	Orida and Feldman[50] Fukushima et al.[51] Eberhardt et al.[20]
Neutrophil (−) Activated neutrophil (+)	Phagocytosis and autolysis	Monguio[52]
Epidermal (−)	Epithelialization	Cooper and Schliwa[53] Mertz et al.[21]
Fibroblast (+)	Fibroplasia	Bourguignon et al.[45]
Myofibroblast (+)	Contraction	Stromberg[54]

THERAPEUTIC CURRENTS

Before discussing further studies on the effects of ES on various wound-related events, it is appropriate to first explain the types of electrical currents available clinically and why particular forms of ES are commonly used in wound healing. Electrical currents are broken down into two major categories: direct current (DC) and alternating current (AC). An additional category, labeled "pulsed" currents, has been adopted for clinical use. This is not a third type of current but instead describes how other currents are "packaged" and delivered to the patient to achieve a desired therapeutic result. In addition, all of the currents under discussion can be classified further by waveform phases, symmetry, and resultant net charge delivered to the patient. Figure 7–5 provides a breakdown of the different currents and their associated characteristics.

Direct Current

Direct current (DC) (Fig. 7–6) is defined as the continuous, unidirectional flow of charged particles for at least 1 second.[10] Since DC is continuous and has no pulses, there is no associated waveform. When DC is delivered through an electrolytic solution, the current causes migration of charged ions of sodium (Na^+) and chloride (Cl^-). Na^+ migrates toward the cathode (negative pole) and reacts with water to form NaOH (sodium hydroxide). Cl^-, on the other hand, migrates toward the anode (positive pole) and reacts with water to form HCl (hydrochloric acid). Prolonged delivery of DC to an individual can, therefore, produce caustic products in the superficial layers of the skin by the creation of alkaline or acidic pH changes. This was used in earlier days of ES to produce, respectively, softening and hardening of tissues and was termed *medical galvanism.* Such changes in the skin are not desirable in wound care. Therefore, if DC is to be used, clinicians typically decrease current intensity to less than 1.0 mA and generally to the microamperage (μA) range.

Pulsed Current

Pulsed current (PC) is defined as the brief, unidirectional or bidirectional flow of charged particles separated by a brief period of no flow.[10] The period of no flow is typically

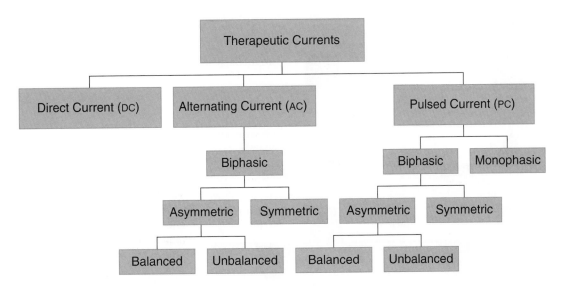

Figure 7–5. Therapeutic currents and their waveform characteristics.

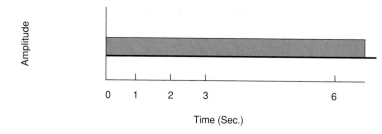

Figure 7–6. Graphic representation of direct current (DC) (from Kloth, LC and McCulloch, JM, eds. *Wound Healing Alternatives in Management*, 3rd ed, Philadelphia: F. A. Davis 2002, p 279, with permission).

of longer duration, thereby isolating each pulse as a specific electrical event. PC can vary widely and is generally described by its waveform, amplitude, duration, and frequency.

The term waveform refers to the visual configuration of current or voltage in relation to amplitude. Waveforms can be either monophasic (a single phase) or biphasic (two opposing phases) and can vary in shape. Some of the more common shapes are sine, square, triangular, and spike (Fig. 7–7) A phase begins with the initiation of a current or voltage and is represented graphically by the initial departure of the signal from the isoelectric baseline. The phase ends when the tracing returns to the baseline. In a monophasic pulse, there is a very short duration of stimulation (typically well less than 1 second). The benefit of such a stimulation is that galvanotaxis can occur without the caustic chemical build up associated with longer phase durations.

Various monophasic waveforms have been described in the wound-healing literature. These include rectangular waveforms[22, 23] and the classic twin-peaked waveform generated by high-voltage pulsed current machines (HVPC)

(Fig. 7–7).[5, 24] HVPC units deliver signals that are very short in duration (2–20 μseconds) with high peak currents but low total currents. These currents have also been erroneously named high-voltage galvanic currents implying that the signals are DC in nature. However, there have been no significant pH changes noted in the skin with the use of HVPC.

Biphasic pulsatile currents also provide for a brief duration of ionic movement. The difference from monophasic currents, however, is that the direction of flow is constantly changing. Current flows in one direction for a fraction of a second then reverses and travels in the opposite direction. In some cases the reversal is instanteous, while in others there is a short millisecond delay before reversal occurs. As demonstrated in Fig. 7–6 b and c, biphasic waveforms can be symmetrical or asymmetrical. In a symmetric biphasic waveform, all of the variables such as amplitude, duration, and shape of the wave above and below the baseline are identical. In an asymmetric biphasic waveform, one or more of the variables are different for each phase. Biphasic waves can also be balanced or

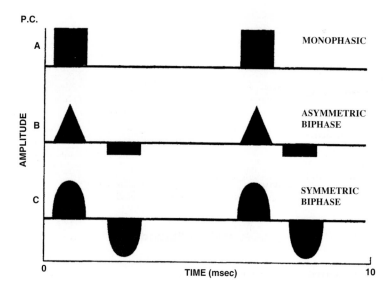

Figure 7–7. Graphic representations of pulsed current (PC) showing (A) monophasic PC, (B) asymmetric biphasic PC, and (C) symmetric biphasic PC (From Kloth, LC and McCulloch: *Wound Healing: Alternatives in Management* 3rd ed. Philadelphia, FA Davis, 2002, p 280, with permission).

unbalanced, which refers to whether there is a net difference in charge. Unbalanced waveforms produce a net charge different from zero.

RESEARCH EVIDENCE

As stated at the outset, there is an abundance of support from laboratory and clinical studies for use of ES in wound care. In addition to the galvanotaxic cellular effects previously mentioned, there is evidence that ES inhibits bacterial growth, improves blood flow, reduces edema, stimulates fibroplasia, improves wound tensile strength, and speeds healing in chronic wounds.

Antibacterial Effects of ES

Wounds that remain unhealed for any significant period of time will inevitably become colonized with bacterial organisms. Exactly what role this plays in continued nonhealing remains unclear, but minimizing bacterial colonization is thought to be advantageous.[25] ES has been demonstrated in several in vitro trials to be effective in inhibiting and killing bacteria. Rowley and associates examined the effects of ES on both Escherichia coli B[26] and Pseudomonas aeruginoga.[27] In the first study, cathodal stimulation in the microamperage (<1.0 μA) and milliamperage (>1.0 mA) range were shown to be effective in killing Escherichia coli. Similar effects were noted in the second study that involved treatment of Pseudomonas-infected rabbit skin wounds with cathodal DC at an intensity of 1000 μA. It is likely that these findings are related to the pH changes noted to occur with DC stimulation.

Guffey and Asmussen[28] decided to see if HVPC could also produce the bactericidal properties seen with DC. They compared milliamperage HVPC with milliamperage DC and demonstrated that after two 30-minute trials, neither anodal or cathodal HVPC applied at amplitudes between 50 and 800 mA had any inhibitory effect on Staphylococcus aureus. However, anodal and cathodal DC stimulation at 1, 5, and 10 mA did inhibit growth.

Several studies, however, have demonstrated HVPC to be effective in inhibiting bacterial growth. Szuminsky and colleagues[29] observed bactericidal effects from both the cathode and anode when 500 V of current was delivered into culture medium containing four species of bacteria. Kincaid and Lavoie[30] likewise found that growth of several microorganisms was inhibited at the anode and cathode with HVPC stimulation at 250 V for 2 hours.

In summary, cathodal stimulation with microamperage DC (nonnoxious) has been demonstrated to be most effective in killing bacteria in vitro. HVPC, while effective, must be delivered for several hours and, if used in humans, the intensity of stimulation would be such that significant sensory and motor effects would be observed.

Circulatory Effects of ES

When evaluating the effect of ES on circulation, several mechanisms of action must be considered. These include release of various vasoactive substances in the vascular system, the action of these substances on the nervous system, and effects of muscle contraction on intramuscular blood flow.

Kaada[31] examined several of these factors. In one study, he treated 10 patients with leg ulcers with transcutaneous electrical nerve stimulation (TENS). The stimulation consisted of monophasic pulsed current at an intensity of 15 to 30 mA for 30 to 45 minutes 3 times per day. Treatment (cathode) electrodes were applied to the web space of the ipsilateral hand. The anode was placed over the distal ulna of the ipsilateral wrist. He reported that all of the ulcers, some of which had received treatment for years, healed completely. He proposed that remote stimulation of muscles in the hand was responsible for this finding and suggested several modes of action. The first mode was activation of a central serotonergic link that prevented sympathetic vasoconstriction. Second, it was hypothesized that there was a release of vasoactive polypeptide into the plasma. A final possible mechanism was activation of a segmental axon reflex that caused vasodilation. The first mechanism is supported by other findings that serotonin inhibitors block the vasodilation response.[32, 33]

Several animal studies have evaluated the effect of exogenous muscle stimulation on blood flow. ES of skeletal muscle at low frequencies (2–20 pulses per second) at intensities greater than 10% of maximum voluntary contraction has been demonstrated to increase local intramuscular blood flow.[34,35] These findings were supported in human studies by Currier and associates[36] who used 2500 Hz AC stimulation to produce isometric contractions in calf muscles. Using Doppler flowmetry on the popliteal artery, they demonstrated increased flow in the stimulated leg during the first minute and for a period of poststimulation. Similar results were obtained by Tracy and colleagues[37] who noted increased flow in the femoral artery following pulsed contractions of the quadriceps at frequencies of 10, 20, and 50 pulses per second.

It is an accepted fact that edema can complicate healing and compromise tissue perfusion. ES has been shown to be effective in reducing lower-extremity edema by stimulating muscle contraction, thereby assisting the calf muscle pump in facilitating venous and lymphatic return.[38,39] ES has also been used successfully in preventing postsurgical deep venous thrombosis (DVTs) by improving venous blood flow.[40,41]

Effects of ES on Wound Tensile Strength

For a wound to be successfully healed, it must not only be re-epithelialized but must also demonstrate adequate tensile strength to assure tissue integrity. Several studies have evaluated what role ES might play in facilitating fibroplasia and increasing the tensile strength of the wound scar.

Assimacopoulos[42] evaluated the effects of ES on rate of healing and scar tensile strength in rabbit wounds treated with microcurrent DC stimulation. Treated wounds not only healed 25% faster than those of the controls, but their scars were noted to have more dense connective tissue and parallel arrangement of collagen fibers.

Carey and Lepley[43] also observed an increase in wound tensile strength following microcurrent (200–300 μA) stimulation with DC. Cathodal-treated wounds had double the tensile strength of anodal-treated wounds in four cases. In the fifth case, the cathodal-treated wound was 50% stronger than the anodal-treated wound.

While low-intensity stimulation with DC has resulted in an increase in tensile strength, evidence from studies with HVPC is not as clear. While Brown and associates[44] found that HVPC-treated wounds in rabbits attained closure statistically faster than controls, there was no difference in wound tensile strength between the two groups. Bourguignon and colleagues,[45] however, did note in an *in vitro* study of HVPC and human fibroblasts, that protein stimulation and DNA synthesis occurred in response to ES. Maximal effects occurred at 50–75 V at a frequency of 100 Hz. It was interesting to note that intensities greater than 250 V were inhibitory to both protein synthesis and DNA. This demonstrates an important factor in ES. More is not necessarily better.

CLINICAL EVIDENCE SUPPORTING ES IN WOUND HEALING

While some of the evidence presented to this point has been derived from human trials, the preponderance has addressed *in vitro* and animal studies. A large body of evidence exists in the form of case reports, controlled, and randomized controlled clinical trials to support ES as a valuable adjunctive treatment for chronic, recalcitrant wounds.

As Kloth[46] notes, in clinical trials, wound treatments are frequently compared with the so-called "standard of care" for a particular wound (pressure, venous, diabetic). This implies that the only thing different in how a subject is treated is the additional experimental variable under study, in this case ES. When significant findings are noted in ES clinical trials, it is important to note that in the time period the subject is not receiving ES, they are receiving standard care. This is often up to 23 hours per day. It should be evident, therefore, that in cases where ES-treated wounds were demonstrated to heal at a faster rate than controls that ES should be seriously considered as an effective adjunct to management.

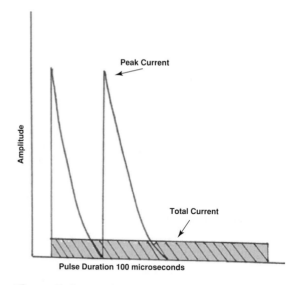

Figure 7–8. Graphic representation of high-voltage pulsed current (HVPC) wave form demonstrating high peak current with low average current.

While a variety of currents have been evaluated in the clinical management of chronic wounds, most of the present-day evidence supports use of HVPC (Fig. 7–8). Kloth and colleagues [5] performed some of the initial work with this form of current in the treatment of pressure ulcers. In a controlled study, 16 patients with stage IV ulcers were randomly assigned to either a standard treatment or experimental group. Subjects in the experimental group received 45 minutes of HVPC 5 days per week. Standard care was provided for the remainder of the time. Control subjects received 45 minutes of sham therapy, which consisted of electrode application, but no current being delivered. This likewise was followed by standard care. Patients in the experimental group healed completely in a mean of 7.3 weeks. Control patient wound size increased a mean of 29% during this same time.

Griffin and colleagues[47] performed a similar study on 17 patients with spinal cord injury who had stage II, III, and IV pressure ulcers. All subjects were treated daily with standard of care. In addition, experimental subjects received 60 minutes of cathodal HVPC on 20 consecutive days. Measurements of ulcer size were taken before and after treatment on days 5, 10, 15, and 20. On each of these days, ulcers in the HVPC group had significantly greater wound area reductions than those in the sham group.

Drawing on the successes seen with ES in the management of pressure ulcers, several researchers have begun to evaluate the effectiveness of this modality in treatment of neuropathic ulcers in persons with diabetes. Peters and associates[48] conducted a randomized, double-blind, placebo-controlled pilot trial utilizing HVPC. The ES was delivered 8 hours per night through a microprocessor-controlled unit to one-half of the forty subjects enrolled. The control subjects received sham therapy. Five patients withdrew (2 experimental, 3 placebo) due to severe infections. Patients were followed for 12 weeks or until the wound healed, whichever came first. The authors reported full healing of 65% of the ES-treated wound compared to 35% of the control wounds. The findings were statistically significant.

Lundeberg and colleagues[49] also looked at ES in wound healing of neuropathic ulcers. The stimulator used, however, delivered a pulsed biphasic signal at an intensity of current strong enough to evoke a strong paresthesia. This differs substantially from the monophasic, mild tingling paresthesia signals delivered with HVPC units. The authors randomly assigned 64 subjects to treatment or placebo groups (ES or sham) and treatment was delivered for 20 minutes twice daily for 12 weeks. A comparison was made of percentages of healed ulcer area and number of healed ulcers at 2, 4, 6, 8, and 12 weeks. Significant differences existed in healed ulcers area and number of healed ulcers at 12 weeks for ES-treated ulcers compared to the control group.

CLINICAL APPLICATION OF ES

As stated earlier, most of the current day evidence supports the use of HVPC in the treatment of chronic wounds. Such devices allow clinicians to select an electrode polarity that is galvanotaxic to the particular cells needed at any point in the wound-healing continuum, but, in addition, does not produce the electrochemical side effects so problematic with other types of stimulation.

If it is determined that ES is appropriate as an adjunctive treatment for a chronic wound, the following guidelines of application should be followed:

1. The clinician should first débride as much necrotic tissue, particularly eschar, as possible from the wound. Such tissue provides a resistance to electricity and can result in current being unevenly distributed in the tissue.

2. Following débridement, irrigate the wound with normal saline.

3. Loosely fill the wound cavity with saline-moistened gauze or one of the commercially available conductive hydrogel dressings. The wound should not be firmly packed.

4. Place a treatment electrode over the moistened gauze. This electrode can be purchased commercially or can be made simply by shaping a piece of aluminum foil to the proper size. Electrodes should be smaller than the surface area of the gauze to prevent them from making direct contact with the surrounding skin.

5. A reference electrode is placed some distance away from the wound. In general, current penetration is proportional to the distance between the electrodes. The further apart the electrodes, the deeper the penetration.

6. Connect the electrodes to the HVPC stimulator being sure to select the proper polarity for the treatment electrode based upon the type of cell you wish to attract to the wound. Remember that opposite charges attract. (Refer to Table 7–1 and Fig. 7–3 and 7–4.) If commercial electrodes are used, connecting pins and leads will be provided. If an electrode is made with aluminum foil, an alligator clip attachment with a pin adaptor (purchased from any electronics store) should be used. The alligator clip is connected to the foil with care being taken to avoid the clip coming in contact with the skin.

7. Secure electrodes in place with elastic wraps or devices supplied by the equipment manufacturer.

8. Set the HVPC device to a frequency of 100 pulses per second. Turn on the device and increase the intensity until the patient reports a mild tingling paresthesia. This is typically between 75 and 100 V.

9. Treatments are generally given 1 hour per day.

Precautions

Anytime electrical current is being used, precautions should be taken to prevent electrochemical burns. As previously stated, the likelihood of this occurring is greatly reduced with the use of HVPC. Should the clinician decide that DC stimulation is desired, the patient should be monitored closely and checked frequently. This is particularly important in patients with altered sensation.

Care should also be taken to assure that electrodes are appropriately moistened and positioned. The failure to adequately moisten electrodes can result in a nonuniform distribution of the current. This is also the situation that can occur if an electrode comes in contact with the skin. This produces an area of high current density and a burn can result.

Keeping these factors in mind, ES can be a safe and effective modality and few contraindications exist to its use. Treatment around any area of suspected basal or squamous cell carcinoma should be avoided as ES may cause an increase in mitogenic activity. In addition, ES is generally contraindicated over the pericardium, carotid sinus, phrenic nerve, parasympathetic nerves and ganglia, and the larynx or in proximity to a cardiac pacemaker.[46] In the past, ES has been noted to be contraindicated in the presence of osteomyelitis since it might promote the premature closure of an infected site. There has been little evidence to support this and ES may be beneficial in helping to treat infection through cathodal stimulation in conjunction with antibiotic therapy.

SUMMARY

Electrical stimulation, as an adjunct to the treatment of chronic wounds, has been well supported in the literature. While much of the earlier research focused on the use of direct current, more evidence has surfaced in recent years of the benefits of high-voltage pulsed current as an effective and safe modality when combined with standard wound care.

REFERENCES

1. Nussbaum E. Comparison of ultrasound/ultraviolet-C and laser for treatment of pressure ulcers in patients with spinal cord injury. *Phys Ther.* 1994;74:812.

2. Dyson M, Pond J, Warwick J, et al. The stimulation of tissue regeneration by means of ultrasound. *Clin Sci.* 1995;35.

3. Loehne H. Wound debridement and irrigation. In: Kloth L, McCulloch J, eds. *Wound Healing Alternatives in Management.* 3rd ed. Philadelphia: FA Davis; 2002:568.

4. Wolcott L, Wheeler P, Hardwick H, et al. Acclerated healing of skin ulcers by electrotherapy. *South Med J.* 1969;62:795–801.

5. Kloth L, Feedar J. Acceleration of wound healing with high voltage, monophasic, pulsed current. *Phys Ther.* 1988;68: 503–508.

6. Wood J, Evens P, Schallreuter K, et al. Treatment of decubitus ulcers: A new approach. *J Invest Dermatol.* 1992;98:4.

7. Akers T, Gabrielson A. The effect of high voltage galvanic stimulation on the rate of healing of decubitus ulcers. *Biomed Sci Instrum* 1984;20:99–100.

8. Bergstrom N, et al. US Department of Health and Human Services. Public Health Service, Agency for Health Care Policy and Research. Clinical Practice Guidelines No. 15. *AHCPR Publication No.* 95-0652; 1994.

9. Government Report. Coverage and billing requirement for electrical stimulation for the treatment of wounds. Bethesda: Department of Health and Human Services, Centers for Medicare and Medicaid Services; 2002:1-4.

10. Committee ES. Electrotherapeutic terminology in physical therapy. Alexandria, VA: American Physical Therapy Association, Section on Clinical Electrophysiology; 2000:1–60.

11. Kloth L, McCulloch J. Promotion of wound healing with electrical stimulation. *Adv Wound Care.* 1996;9:42–45.

12. Cunliffe-Barnes T. Healing rate of human skin determined by measurements of electrical potential of experimental abrasions: Study of treatment with petrolatum and with petrolatum containing yeast and liver abstracts. *Am J Surg.* 1945; 69:82.

13. Borgens R, Jr., Vanable JW, Jr., Jaffe LF. Bioelectricity and regeneration: Initiation of regeneration by minute currents. *J Exp Zool.* 1977;200:403.

14. Illingsworth C, Barker A. Measurement of electrical currents emerging during the regeneration of amputated finger tips in children. *Clin Phys Physiol Meas.* 1980;1:87.

15. Barker A. The glabrous epidermis of cavies contains a powerful battery. *Am J Physiol Regul Integr Comp Physiol.* 1982;11.

16. Foulds I, Barker A. Human skin battery potentials and their possible role in wound healing. *Br J Dermatol.* 1983;109: 515.

17. Vanable JJ. Integumentary potentials and wound healing. In: Borgans R, et al., eds. *Electric Fields in Vertebrate Repair.* New York: Alan R. Liss; 1989:183.

18. Jaffee L, Vanable JJ. Electric fields and wound healing. *Clin Dermatol.* 1984;2:34.

19. Cheng K. Confirmation of the electrical potential induced by occlusive dressing. *Eighth Annual Symposium on Advanced Wound Care.* San Diego, CA: Health Management Publications; 1995.

20. Eberhardt A, Szczypiorski P, Korytowski G. Effect of transcutaneous electrostimulation on the cell composition of skin exudate. *Acta Physiol Polonica.* 1986;37:41.

21. Mertz P. Electrical stimulation: Acceleration of soft tissue repair by varying the polarity. *Wounds.* 1993;5:153.

22. Weiss D, Eaglstein W, Falanga V. Exogenous electric current can reduce the formation of hypertrophic scars. *J Dermatol Surg Oncol.* 1989;15:1272.

23. Feedar J, Kloth L, Gentzkowl G. Chronic dermal ulcer healing enhanced with monophasic pulsed electrical stimulation. *Phys Ther.* 1991;71:639.

24. Fitzgerald G, Newsome D. Treatment of a large infected thoracic spine wound using high voltage pulsed monophasic current. *Phys Ther.* 1993;73:355.

25. Kirsner R. Wound Bed Preparation. *Ostomy Wound Manage.* 2003;49:2.

26. Rowley B. Electrical current effects on E coli growth rates. *Proc Soc Exp Biol Med.* 1972;139:929.

27. Rowley B, McKenna J, Chase G. The influence of electrical current on an infecting microorganism in wounds. *Ann NY Acad Sci.* 1974;238:543.

28. Guffey J, Asmussen M. *In vitro* bactericidal effects of high voltage pulsed current versus direct current against *Staphylococcus aureus. J Clin Electrophysiol.* 1989;1:5.

29. Szuminsky N, Albers A, Unger P. Effect of narrow, pulsed high voltages on bacterial viability. *Phys Ther.* 1994;74:660.

30. Kincaid C, Lavoie K. Inhibition of bacterial growth *in vitro* following stimulation with high voltage, monophasic pulsed current. *Phys Ther.* 1989;69:651.

31. Kaada B. Vasodilation induced by transcutaneous nerve stimulation in peripheral ischemia (Raynaud's phenomenon and diabetic polyneuropathy). *Eur Heart J.* 1982;3:303.

32. Kaada B, Eielson O. In search of the mediators of skin vasodilation induced by transcutaneous nerve stimulation: I. Failure to block the response by antagonists of endogenous vasodilators. *Gen Pharmacol.* 1983;4:623.

33. Kaada B, Eielson O. In search of the mediators of skin vasodilation induced by transcutaneous nerve stimulation: II. Serotonin implicated. *Gen Pharmacol.* 1983;14:635.

34. Wakim K. Influence of frequency of muscle stimulation on circulatin in the stimulated extremity. *Arch Phys Med Rehabil.* 1953;34:291.

35. Mohr R, Akers T, Wessman H. Effect of high voltage stimulation on blood flow in the rat hind limb. *Phys Ther.* 1987;67:526.

36. Currier D, Petrilli C, Threlkeld A. Effect of graded electrical stimulation on blood flow to healthy muscle. *Phys Ther.* 1986;66:937.

37. Tracy J, Currier DP, Threlkeld A. Comparison of selected pulse frequencies from two different electrical stimulators on blood flow in health subjects. *Phys Ther.* 1988;68:1526.

38. Miller B, Gruben K, Morgan B. Circulatory responses to voluntary and electrically induced muscle contractions in humans. *Phys Ther.* 2000;50:53.

39. Heath M, Gibbs S. High voltage pulsed galvanic stimulation effects of frequency of current on blood flow in the human calf muscle. *Clin Sci.* 1992;82:607.

40. Nicolaides A, Kakkar W, Field E. Optimal electrical stimulus for prevention of deep vein thrombosis. *Br Med J.* 1972;3:756.

41. Lindstrom B, Korsan-Bengtsen K, Jonsson O. Electrically induced short-lasting tetanus of the calf muscle for prevention of deep vein thrombosis. *Br J Surg.* 1982;69:203.

42. Assimacopoulos D. Wound healing promotion by the use of negative electric current. *Am Surg.* 1968;34:423.

43. Carey L, Lepley D. Effect of continuous direct electric current on healing. *Surg Forum.* 1962;13:33.

44. Brown M, McDonnell M, Menton D. Electrical stimulation effects on cutaneous wound healing in rabbits. A follow-up study. *Phys Ther.* 1988;68:955.

45. Bourguignon C, Bourguignon L, et al. Electrical stimulation of protein and DNA synthesis in human fibroblasts. *FASEB J.* 1987;1:398.

46. Kloth L. Electrical Stimulation for Wound Healing. In: Kloth L, McCulloch J, eds. *Wound Healing Alternatives in Management.* 3rd ed. Philadelphia: FA Davis; 2002:296.

47. Griffin J, Tooms R, Mendius R. Efficacy of high voltage pulsed current for healing of pressure ulcers in patients with spinal cord injury. *Phys Ther.* 1991;71:433.

48. Peters E, Lavery L, Armstrong D. Electric stimulation as an adjunct to heal diabetic foot ulces: A randomized clinical trial. *Arch Phys Med Rehabil.* 2001;82:721–725.

49. Lundeberg T, Eriksson S, Malm M. Electrical nerve stimulation improves healing of diabetic ulcers. *Ann Plastic Surg.* 1992; 29:328–331.

50. Orida N, Feldman J. Directional protrusive pseudopodial activity and motility in macrophages induced by extra-cellular electric fields. *Cell Motil.* 1982;2:243.

51. Fukushima K. Studies of galvanotaxis of leukocytes. *Med J Osaka Univ.* 1953;4:195.

52. Monguio J. Uber die polar wirkung des galvanischen stromes auf leukozyten. *Z Biol.* 1933;93:553.

53. Cooper M, Schliwa M. Electrical and ionic controls of tissue cell locomotion in DC electrical fields. *J Cell Physiol.* 1985; 103:363.

54. Stromberg B. Effects of electrical currents on wound contraction. *Ann Plast Surg.* 1988;21:121.

8

Antioxidant Effects of Ultra-Low Microcurrents in Wound Healing

Bok Y. Lee, Alfred J. Koonin, Keith Wendell, and John Hillard

Introduction
Oxidation and the Formation of Free Radicals
Antioxidants and Their Effects on Free Radicals
Mitochondria and Their Role in Free-Radical Damage
The Electron and Its Role in Electric Currents

Ultra-Low-Level Microcurrents as Antioxidants
  Methods
  Results
Summary
References

INTRODUCTION

Otto Van Guericke, who rotated a ball of solidified sulfur to create static electricity in 1672, invented the first electric instrument made by man. Amber was the first material used to generate electricity, which could be generated by rubbing it with the hands. Static electricity machines were the first instruments and, with the machine age by the 18th century, were powerful enough to destroy superficial tissue and be used for cauterization. Ultraviolet ray machines invented by Strong in 1897 were still in use in 1937.

Direct current grew rapidly with the invention of the battery. The electric cell pile allowed the generation of higher voltages than the usual 2 V by connecting them in series. This reaction then provided a convenient and readily available source of direct current. Salandier is credited as the first to apply direct current to acupuncture needles; later, moist conductive pads were introduced. Galvanic is another word used to describe direct current therapy. Today's galvanic instruments are a direct descendant of this early invention, practically without change.

With the discovery of alternating current by Tesla and the invention of the Vacuum Tube by Edison, and improved by DeForrest, tubes were universally used. House mains were used to eliminate the nuisance of recharging or replacing batteries for the energy-gobbling appetites of the vacuum tubes.

The limitation of tubes, as far as frequencies were concerned, was primarily due to the matching trans-

formers, which, although they did well in the audible human range of 20 to 20,000 cycles per second, did not produce frequencies below 10 Hertz because the output could not be coupled easily to the patient. With the advent of the rediscovery of solid-state technology, the transistor was capable of bridging the gap.

Frequency, which is the rate of occurrence of repetition, is used in physical therapy to describe the number of cycles per second of the output wave. Since electrical waves travel at approximately 186,000 miles or so per second, the length of each wave is calculated by dividing the repetitions per second into the known speed. In honor of Hertz, a German scientist who discovered and measured radio waves, "Hertz" (abbreviated Hz) are cycles per second. Clinical research has shown that the frequencies in the ultra-low frequency range of 0.1 and 0.3 Hz, seem to have longer lasting effects, although relief is not as rapid as in higher frequencies of 10 to 100 Hz.

The initials AC mean alternating current. Most physical therapy equipment use electrical waves that are alternating positive then negative in each half cycle to complete one complete wave. Whereas direct current (DC) flows in one direction only, AC flows in alternating directions depending on whether it is the negative or positive phase. The upper half is considered the positive cycle, while the lower portion is the negative cycle.

Radio waves overlap into frequencies in the audible range, starting as low as 5000 Hz. Above 1000 Hz, we do not find physical therapy using any frequencies until 2,000,000 Hz (2 megahertz, MHz), where interferential frequencies of 2000 to 4000 Hz are not considered as therapeutic since only the lower 0 to 200 Hz have been used for therapy. Ultrasound instruments use this to vibrate their sound heads. The resulting output is mechanical, but not electrical, so that a nonelectrical conductive substance can be employed.

The next higher frequency is the short-wave diathermy at 27 MHz. These were originally equipped with large insulated rubber pads. However, it is still possible to burn the patient. It is thus, wise to wrap the patient in several layers of heavy towels for additional insulation. Currently most units employ an isolating drum inductor to reduce this hazard. Outputs from these units are usually 300–500 W, so care is advised on their application. The cords leading to these pads are usually cut to match the wavelength and are "hot" with radio frequency (RF). They also should be carefully routed to avoid painful RF burns. A safer form of diathermy is the microwave or radar type. At frequencies of 2450 MHz, the wavelength is so short that a reflector-type antenna can be used to direct the energy to the desired area. Most units have outputs of 100 W and depend upon increased circulation rather than heating. Higher frequencies include the heat lamps, infrared, and colors of the visible light ranges. Medical laser, x rays, and cosmic rays complete the high end of the spectrum.

The healing effects of electricity have always been poorly understood. However, with the advent of subatomic particle physics and the electron theory of electrical current, explanations of electricity acting as an antioxidant have become more likely.

In order to understand how electrical currents can function as an antioxidant, the formation and effects of free radicals and their interaction with antioxidants needs to be understood.

OXIDATION AND THE FORMATION OF FREE RADICALS

We know that the atom is made up of protons, neutrons, and electrons. An inert oxygen molecule (Fig. 8–1) is stable because the outer shells contain 8 electrons arranged in 4 pairs. When molecules with weak bonds split, they can leave atoms with unpaired electrons—which is what free radicals are. This produces an atom or molecule seeking an electron to make up a stable pair. Molecular oxygen is one of the most important substances on earth. Oxygen comprises 21% of the atmosphere, 89% of seawater by weight, and at least 47% of the earth's crust.

In the 1840s, Michael Faraday discovered that oxygen is attracted to a magnet, but it took until 1925 to discover the reason. Why oxygen is magnetic was clarified by Robert Millikan using at that time the recently developed quantum theory. His analysis showed that molecular oxygen has two unpaired electrons in its

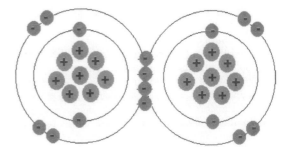

Figure 8-1. An inert oxygen molecule which is stable because the outer shells contain 8 electrons arranged in 4 pairs.

lowest energy state (Fig. 8–2). The existence of unpaired valence electrons in a stable molecule is very rare in nature and confers high chemical reactivity, which is why oxygen is unique.

The chemical reactions leading to this reactive state are either oxidation or reduction. Oxidation is a loss of electrons; reduction is a gain of electrons. These reactions always occur in pairs, that is, when one molecule is oxidized, another is reduced. Highly reactive molecules can oxidize molecules that were previously stable, leading to unstable molecules, such as free radicals.

A free radical is a chemical species with an unpaired electron that can be neutral, positively, or negatively charged. Although a few stable free radicals are known, most are highly reactive. In free-radical chain reactions, the radical product of one reaction becomes the starting material for another, propagating free-radical damage.

The three steps in free-radical chain reactions are initiation, propagation, and termination. In the initiation phase, free radicals are formed from molecules that readily give up their electrons. An example of this is hydrogen peroxide. In the propagation phase, the chain carrying the radicals are alternately consumed and produced. In the termination phase, the free radicals are

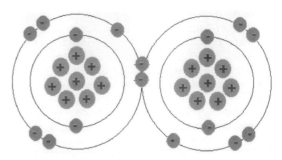

Figure 8-2. Molecular oxygen has 2 unpaired electrons in its lowest energy state.

destroyed. Thus, without termination by an agent, such as an antioxidant, a single free radical can damage numerous molecules.

There are four common oxygen metabolites in biologic systems that are free radicals; superoxide anion ($O_2^{-\bullet}$), hydrogen peroxide (H_2O_2), hydroxyl radicals ($OH^\bullet$), and singlet oxygen ($^1O_2$). The ($\bullet$) represents the unpaired electron. These free radicals can be generated via a number of mechanisms including normal physiologic processes and those resulting from external factors. For example, singlet oxygen is generated by photosensitization reactions wherein a molecule absorbs light of a given wavelength exciting the molecule. This excited molecule transfers the increased energy to a molecule of oxygen-producing singlet oxygen, which can then attack other cell components. The quantum theory of atomic and molecular structure is required to explain the unique properties of molecular oxygen. Suffice it to say that in the ground state, the valence electrons of oxygen spin parallel to each other. When these electrons are elevated into a higher energy orbital, the spins are inverted to create an antiparallel pair, thus creating a singlet oxygen. There are two kinds, Σ and Δ, the former being of higher energy. The primary function of carotenoids is to scavenge free radicals, particularly singlet oxygen produced in this manner.

A certain amount of oxidative function is necessary for proper health. For example, oxidative processes are used by the immune system to kill microorganisms. Sometimes, however, the level of toxic reactive oxygen intermediates overcomes the antioxidative defenses of the host, resulting in excessive free radicals. This state is called *oxidative stress*. These free radicals can induce local injury by reacting with lipids, proteins, and nucleic acids. The interaction of free radicals with cellular lipids leads to membrane damage and the generation of lipid peroxide by-products.

ANTIOXIDANTS AND THEIR EFFECTS ON FREE RADICALS

Antioxidants are chemicals that have the ability to donate electrons without becoming free radicals themselves. Cells contain a number of antioxidants that have various roles in protecting against free-radical reactions. The major water-soluble antioxidant metabolites are glutathione (GSH) and vitamin C (Fig. 8–3), which reside primarily in the cytoplasm and the mitochondria.

Glutathione (Fig. 8–4), is a tripeptide composed of glutamic acid, cysteine, and glycine convalently joined end-to-end. Glutathione peroxidase is an enzyme that catalyzes the reaction between GSH and hydrogen peroxide, leading to water and oxidized glutathione (GSSH) that is stable.

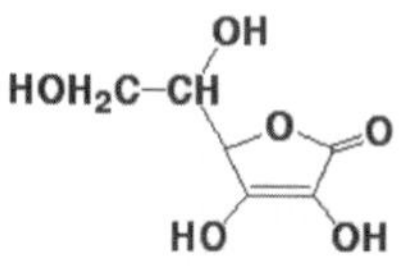

Figure 8-3. The major water soluble antioxidant metabolites are glutathione (GSH) and vitamin C which are primarily in cytoplasm and mitochondria.

Vitamin E and the carotenoids are the main lipid-soluble antioxidants (Fig. 8–5). Vitamin E is the major fat-soluble antioxidant in the cell membrane. Its role is to break the chain of lipid peroxidation. Despite the actions of antioxidant nutrients, some oxidative damage will occur and accumulation of this damage throughout life is believed to be a major factor in aging and disease.

MITOCHONDRIA AND THEIR ROLE IN FREE-RADICAL DAMAGE

The cell is a complex structure. The mitochondrion is the powerhouse of the cell and is where free radicals can do most of their damage.

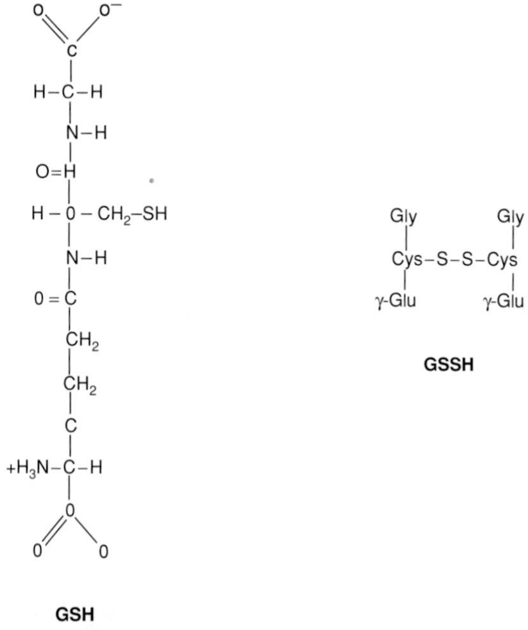

Figure 8-4. Glutathione (GSH) is a tripeptide made up of glutamic acid, cysteine and glycine covalently joined end to end. Glutathione peroxidase is an enzyme that catalyzes the reaction between (GSH) and hydrogen peroxide leading to water and oxidized glutathione (GSSH) that is stable.

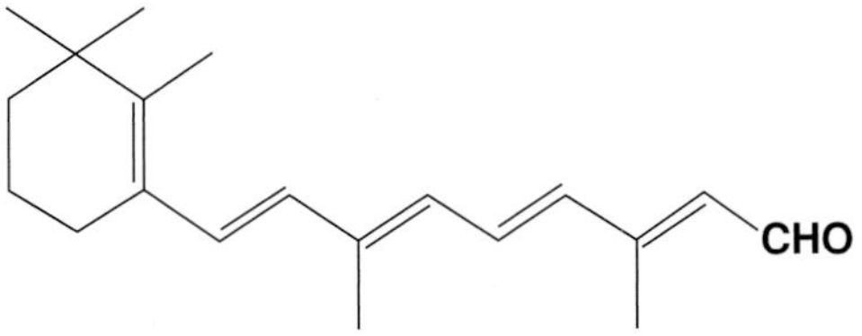

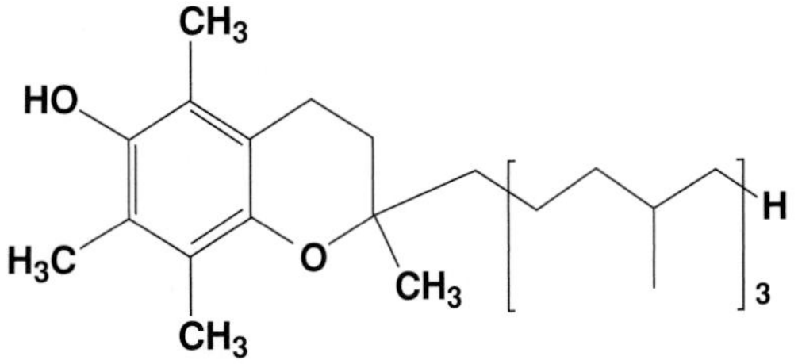

Vitamin A

α-tocopherol (Vitamin E)

Figure 8-5. Vitamin E and the carotenoids are the main lipid soluble antioxidants.

Mitochondria have an outer and inner membrane (Fig. 8–6). The inner membrane is arranged in folds called the cristae mitochondriales. Strands of mitochondrial DNA and ribosomes are located in the matrix.

The food we eat is oxidized to produce high-energy electrons that are converted to stored energy. This energy is stored in high-energy phosphate bonds in the form of adenosine triphosphate (ATP). The metabolic process goes through the Emden–Meyerhof (glycolysis) pathway ending in the Kreb's or citric acid cycle. The electron transfer chain is on the cristae, where ATP is produced under the influence of ATP synthase in the form of elementary particles on the cristae, which explains how the mitochondria run at the ATP pump. This is an aerobic process. In the absence of oxygen, 1 molecule of glucose will yield 4 molecules of ATP. In the presence of oxygen, the Krebs cycle produces 24 to 28 molecules of ATP from 1 molecule of glucose; 4 molecules are produced from glycolysis. This entire oxidation process taking place in the mitochondria is what makes it more susceptible to the formation and effects of free radicals (Fig. 8–7).

THE ELECTRON AND ITS ROLE IN ELECTRIC CURRENTS

The oxidative process takes place at a subatomic level with the electron being the main player. Electrons are the smallest of the charged subatomic particles. They fall into a group called *Leptons*. Electrons have a mass of (m_e) of 9.1095×10^{-31} kg (0.51100 MeV/c^2) and charge of -4.8032×10^{-10} esu (1.6022×10^{-19}C), this being the lowest charge detectable.

The electrostatic unit or esu, is the unit of electrical charge. When two equal electric charges 1 cm apart,

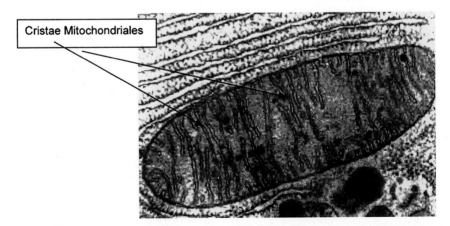

Cristae Mitochondriales

Figure 8-6. Mitochondria have an outer and inner membrane. The inner membrane is arranged in folds called the cristae mitochondriales. The matrix contains strands of mitochondrial DNA and ribosomes.

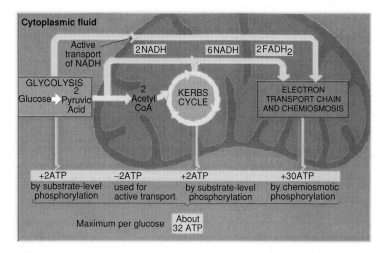

Figure 8-7. The metabolic process goes through the glycolysis pathway to end in the Kreb's or citric acid cycle. This process is aerobic producing 24–28 molecules of ATP from on glucose molecule going through the Kreb's cycle plus the 4 molecules from glycolysis.

exert a force of 1 dyne on each other, each charge is 1 esu in magnitude.

By knowing the charge of an electron, we can see that 1 esu is equivalent to two billion (2×10^9) electrons. Another unit of charge commonly used is the Coulomb (C). One Coulomb is a unit equivalent to three billion (3×10^9) esu or six billion (6×10^{18}) electrons. One ampere (Amp or A) is one Coulomb per second. Therefore, a current flow of 1 Amp is equivalent to the flow of 6×10^{18} electrons per second.

For an electric current to flow, it needs a pathway called a conductor. Certain materials, such as metals, are better conductors than others, based on the ability of a good conductor to propagate the flow of electrons. Copper is an excellent conductor because it contains a single electron in its outer shell (Fig. 8–8).

The ease of flow of an electrical current depends not only on the conductive material, but also on the size of the current and the width of the pathway. For instance, a current of a constant size, will pass more readily down a wire of wide diameter than it will down a wire of narrow diameter, since the narrower wire has a higher resistance.

The same will apply if the diameter of the wire is constant but the size of the current varies. A smaller current will pass more readily than a large one. Voltage is also required to propagate the current. Voltage is a measure of the electrical potential. Simply stated, voltage is a measure of the electrical pressure trying to force the propagation of current flow. If the resistance increases due to either a decrease in the diameter of the conductor or an increase in the size of the electrical charge, the effect will be an increase in the conversion of energy to heat. Applied to the human body this heat can be damaging.

ULTRA-LOW-LEVEL MICROCURRENTS AS ANTIOXIDANTS

Ultra-low-level microcurrents are those below the milliamp range (Table 8–1).

To see if these ultra-low currents could work as an antioxidant, we chose the chronic skin wound model. The reason for this was that most of these lesions are found in debilitated patients with poor immune systems, who

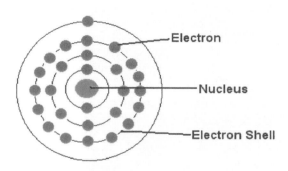

Copper Atom

Figure 8-8. Copper is an excellent conductor due to the single electron in its outer shell.

Table 8–1. Ultra-low-level microcurrents

milliAmpere (mA) = 10^{-3} A
microAmpere (μA) = 10^{-6} A
nanoAmpere (nA) = 10^{-9} A
picoAmpere (pA) = 10^{-12} A
femtoAmpere (fA) = 10^{-15} A
attoAmpere (aA) = 10^{-18} A

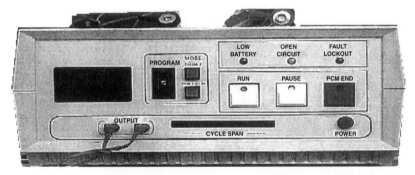

Figure 8-9. The device used in wound healing experiment that produced a current range of 3 mA down to 100 nA.

probably have a high concentration of free radicals. Further, the wounds themselves are generally necrotic and infected, with poor healing potential and a high concentration of free radicals in the local area. The idea was to isolate the injured area as part of the circuit and thereby infuse a steady stream of electrons through the area with as little resistance as possible. The resistance would be reduced using a low-level current and by increasing the diameter of the conductor. The frequency of the current would also have to be low in order to prevent the electrons from traveling in short bursts. A low frequency would allow the electrons to move in a steady stream.

Method

A device* (Fig. 8–9) was used that produced a current range of 3 mA down to 100 nA. The frequency used produced a cycle lasting approximately 23 minutes and was designed to switch the direction of current flow half way through the cycle. The device runs on a rechargeable battery producing a square-wave bipolar current with a voltage ranging between 5 up to a maximum of 40 V. The voltage range will vary proportionately with the resistance in tissues. The device will not function if the range goes beyond 40 V.

The electrodes are applied (Fig. 8–10) in two layers using tap water as a conducting medium. Water is a very poor conductor of electricity, but the minerals in tap water are sufficient to carry the current into the tissues. Also wraps cover a large surface area thus reducing resistance and allowing an optimum number of electrons to flow freely into the tissues.

Patients were treated for approximately 3.5 hours per day, 5 days a week, until the lesion had healed. A

12-week maximum was allowed for healing to take place. All patients were inpatients and were on wound care treatments for at least 3 months, prior to this study, with no observable improvements in their condition.

The 25 patients treated had lesions present for an average of 18.5 months. The etiology of the lesions varied (Table 8–2).

For approximately 23 minutes per day, the subjects were wrapped, above and below the wound, with spongy bandages, soaked in water. Conductive silicone electrodes were then wrapped over these and attached to the device with stud clips (Fig. 8–10). For the first cycle (23 minutes), the device was set at a current output of 3 mA. For the subsequent eight cycles of treatment (approximately 3 hours), the device was set at an output of 400 nA. Twenty-five chronic wounds were treated, which were present for a period ranging from 3 to 60 months. These wounds did not respond to standard therapy. Ages of the patients in the study varied from 20 to 85 years old. Twenty-three of the lesions were stage III or IV.

Results

Of the lesions, 92% were stages III or IV. The age of the lesions varied from 6 to 60 months, with an average of 18.5 months. Healing of the lesions, occurred in 100% in an average of 48 hours of treatment, (ie, an average of 16 days). Some of the results are summarized as follows:

Patient #5 (Fig. 8–11*A*), was a 74-year-old male with diabetes, congestive cardiac failure, and chronic obstructive pulmonary disease. This chronic stage IV ulcer of his right heel had been present for 3 years. He had been in the hospital for 6 months during which time he had specialized care to the ulcer with no noticeable improvement. The only change to his regular treatment and dressing regimen was the addition of the electrical therapy, as described. After ten treatments over a 2-week

*The G4 Ultra-Low Current Device supplied by EPRT Technologies, Inc (formally Electroregenesis, Inc.) PO Box 278, Pacific Palisades, California 90272.

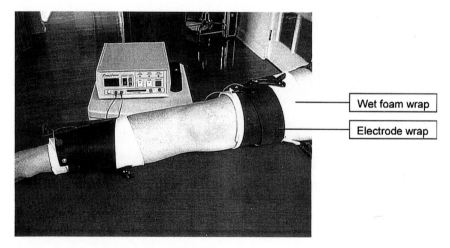

Figure 8-10. Application of electrode wraps.

period, there was complete healing of the wound (Fig. 8–11*B*).

Patient #12 (Fig. 8–12*A*) was a 22-year-old male paraplegic with stage IV decubitus ulcer of his left heel present for over 1 year. The standard wound care over a 5-month period produced no change in the ulcer. After 26 treatments over 6 weeks with the ultralow current electrical device, there was complete healing of the lesion (Fig. 8–12*B*).

Patient #17 (Fig. 8–13*A*) which was a 53-year-old paraplegic with stage III ulcer of the right knee, present for over 9 months. He had been under his present wound care regime for 3 months with no improvement. After 3 treatments with the ultralow current electrical device, the lesion completely healed (Fig. 8–13*B*).

Of the 25 chronic wounds treated, 8 were patients under 50 years of age, 7 were between 50 and 70 years old, and 10 were over 70. Rate of wound closure was measured by the reduction of size in square centimeters

Table 8–2. Etiology of chronic wounds

AIDS
Arterial insufficiency
Cerebrovascular accident
Chronic obstructive pulmonary disease
Chronic renal failure
Congestive cardiac failure
Spinal cord injury
Traumatic brain injury
Venous stasis

per day. The rate of closure was then averaged according to the three groups described above, (ie., under 50 years of age, between 50 and 70, and over 70). Comparison was also made between the length of time the lesion was present and the length of time of treatment.

Two of the wounds were rated as stage II, while the rest were stage III or IV. The average rates of healing (Fig. 8–14) for the three age groups were (in cm^2/day) 20–50 years of age, 0.74; 50 to 70 years of age, 0.73; and >70 years of age, 0.73. It was also found that the length of time that treatment was necessary for complete healing was directly proportional to the time of duration of the lesion (Fig. 8–15).

Although no surgical débridement was performed, all the necrotic tissue appeared to reabsorb spontaneously and be replaced with healthy granulation and/or skin.

SUMMARY

In conclusion, 25 chronic skin ulcers present for an average of 18.5 months, which did not respond to standard conservative treatment in a hospital setting, were treated with the ultralow current, ultralow frequency device. Of the 25 ulcers, 100% showed response to the treatment; 100% healed in a maximum time of 7 weeks. Average time of healing was 48 hours of treatment over 16 days. Surgical debridement was unnecessary as the necrotic tissue appeared to disappear spontaneously. The ages of the patients ranged between 20 and 85 years of age, divided into three groups: 20 to 50, 50 to 70, and greater than 70 years of age. The rate of healing was measured in square centimeters per day. The length of time of

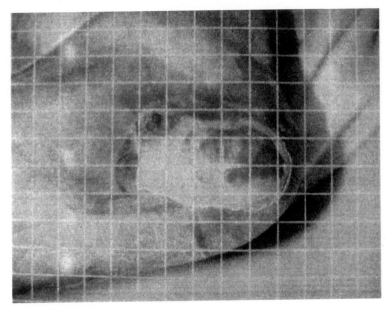

A

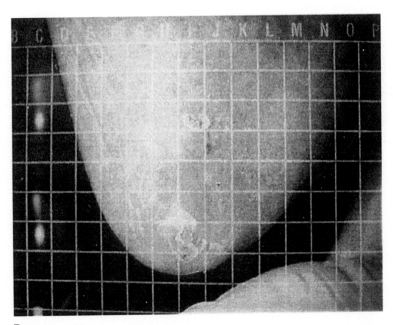

B

Figure 8-11A. Patient was 74 year old male with diabetes, CHF and COPD. Chronic stage IV ulcer of right heel present for 3 years. ***B.*** After 10 treatments with ultra-low current electrical device over a 2 week period there was complete healing of the wound.

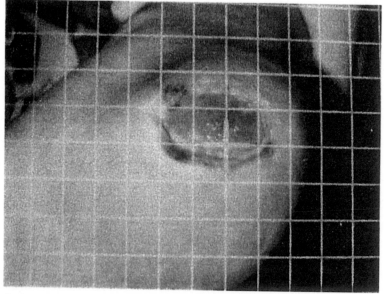

A

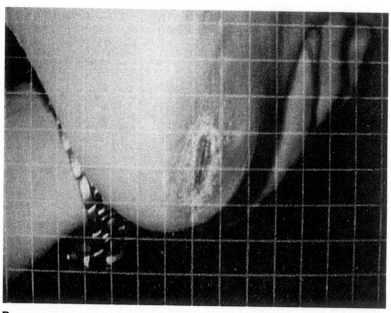

B

Figure 8-12A. Patient was 22 year old male paraplegic with stage IV ulcer of left heel present for over 1 year. ***B.*** Following 26 treatments over 6 weeks with ultra-low current electrical device, there was complete healing of lesion.

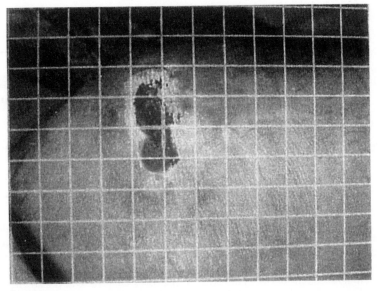

A

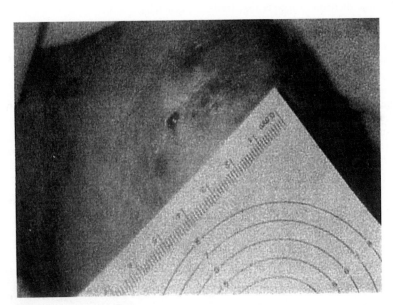

B

Figure 8-13A. Patient was 53 year old paraplegic with stage III ulcer of right knee present for over 9 months. **B.** Following 3 treatments with the ultra-low current electrical device, the lesion was completely healed.

Healing Rate Related to Age

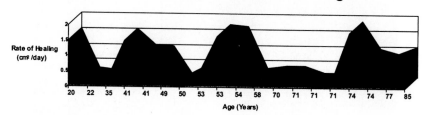

Figure 8-14. Average rates of healing for the 3 age groups.

treatment was also compared to the duration of the lesion (Fig. 8–15).

Many studies have shown that the rate of wound healing of an individual is directly proportional to their age. From this study it can be seen that treating chronic skin ulcers with the ultralow current device eliminates the age factor by equalizing the healing rate at all ages (Fig. 8–14). The only limiting factor in healing time with this method seems to be the duration of the lesion (Fig. 8–15). This study, therefore, suggests that treatment with the ultra-low current device eliminates the restrictions that aging brings to the healing process.

It is also known that the lower the frequency of an electrical device, the more permanent the effects of the device. This observation was borne out of this study. To date, none of the healed lesions has shown any sign of recurrence after a period ranging from 6 to 18 months.

From what we know about the effects of free radicals and the mechanism of antioxidants in neutralizing them, we can see a remarkable similarity in the action of the ultralow currents used in this study. The steady flow of electrons in a relatively low concentration appears to act exactly as one would expect from any antioxidant. The fact that these electrons are focused on a small region of the body may explain why healing changes appeared so rapidly. The actual regeneration of the tissue coupled with the absence of the age factor in healing and the concomitant improvement noticed in the patients' general condition all point to a highly potent antioxidant effect on the local tissues as well as generally.

Further studies need to be carried out, such as skin biopsies, tensile strength, tissue oxygenation and more accurate assessment of the patients' general condition. A larger double-blind placebo study is currently being established to cover these and other parameters.

Current studies show evidence that a low-concentration steady stream electron flow produced in the manner described acts as a highly potent antioxidant that can be focused to any area of the body and opens a door to studying this type of technology in many disease processes that are initiated by free radicals.

Completely Healed Lesions

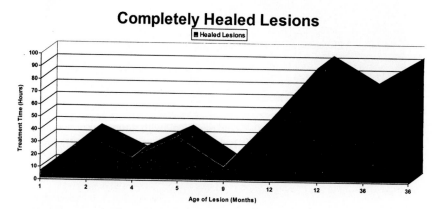

Figure 8-15. Length of time of treatment necessary for complete healing was directly proportional to the time of duration of lesions.

REFERENCES

Adams AK, Wermuth EO, McBride PE. Antioxidant vitamins and the prevention of coronary heart disease. *Am Fam Physician.* 1999;60:895–904.

Auer BL, Auer D, Rodgers AL. Relative hexoxaluria, crystalluria and hematuria after megadose ingestion of vitamin C. *Eur J Clin Invest.* 1998;28:695–700.

Azzi A, Boscoboinik D, Clement S. Vitamin E mediated response of smooth muscle cell to oxidant stress. *Diabetes Res Clin Pract.* 1999;45:191–198.

Bates CJ, Walmsley CM, Prentice A, Finch S. Does vitamin C reduce blood pressure? Results of a large study of people aged 65 or older. *J Hypertens.* 1998;16:925–932.

Bendich A. Beta-carotene and the immune response. *Proc Nutr Soc.* 1991;50:263–274.

Bielory L, Gandhi R. Asthma and vitamin C. *Ann Allergy.* 1994;73:89–96.

Block G. Vitamin C and cancer prevention: The epidemiologic evidence. *Am J Clin Nutr.* 1991;53:270S–282S.

Blumberg JB, Couris RR, Bernardi VW. The rationale for vitamin E supplementation. *Pharmacist.* 1998;23:111–119.

Brown KM, Morrice PC, Duthie GG. Erythrocyte vitamin E and plasma ascorbate concentrations in relation to erythrocyte peroxidation in smokers and nonsmokers: Dose response to vitamin E supplementation. *Am J Clin Nutr.* 1997;65:496–502.

Brown L, Rimm EB, Seddon JM, et al. A prospective study of carotenoid intake and risk of cataract extraction in US men. *Am J Clin Nutr.* 1999;70:517–524.

Bulger EM, Helton WS. Nutrient antioxidants in gastrointestinal disease. *Gastroenterol Clin North Am.* 1998;27:403–419.

Bucca C, Rolla G, Farina JC. Effect of vitamin C on transient increase of bronchial responsiveness in conditions affecting the airways. *Ann NY Acad Sci.* 1992;669:175–186.

Calabrese V, Scapagnini G, Catalano C, Dinotta F, Geraci, D, Morganti, P. Biochemical studies of a natural antioxidant isolated from rosemary and its application in cosmetic dermatology. *Int J Tissue React.* 2000;22(1):5–13.

Calabrese V, Randazzo SD, Morganti PG, Rizza V. An *ex vivo* biochemical model to study the antioxidant clinical properties of cosmetic products in human antiaging skin care. *Drugs Exp Clin Res.* 1999;25(1):43–49.

Cheeseman KH, Holley AE, Kelly FJ, et al. Biokinetics in humans or RRR-alpha-tocopherol: The free phenol, acetate ester, and succinate ester forms of vitamin E. *Free Radic Biol Med.* 1995;19:591–598.

Christen S, Woodall A, Shigenaga MK, et al. Gamma-tocopherol traps mutagenic electrophiles such as NOx and complements alpha-tocopherol physiologic implications. *Proc Natl Acad Sci U.S.A.* 1997;94:3217–3222.

Christen WG, Jr. Antioxidants and eye disease. *Am J Med.* 1994;97:14S–17S.

Clinton SK. Lycopene: Chemistry, biology and implications for human health and disease. *Nutr Rev.* 1998;56:35–51.

Cohen HA, Neuman I, Nahum H. Blocking effect of vitamin C in exercise-induced asthma. *Arch Pediatr Adolesc Med.* 1997;151:367–370.

Cook JD, Watson SS, Simpson KM, et al. The effect of high ascorbic acid supplementation on body iron stores. *Blood.* 1984;64:72–76.

Combs GF, Jr, Gray WP. Chemopreventive agents: Selenium. *Pharmacol Ther.* 1998;79:179–192.

Corrigan JJ. Jr, Marcis FI. Coagulopathy associated with vitamin E ingestion. *J Am Med Assoc.* 1974;230:1300–1301.

Curhan GC, Willett WC, Speizer FE, Stampfer, MJ. Intake of vitamin B6 and C and the risk of kidney stones in women. *J Am Soc Nephrol.* 1999;10:840–845.

Daviglus ML, Orencia AJ, Dyer AR, et al. Dietary vitamin C, beta-carotene and 30 year risk of stroke: Results from the Western Electric Study. *Neuroepidemiology.* 1997;16:69–77.

Delcourt C, Cristol JP, Tessier F, et al. Age related macular degeneration and antioxidant status in the POLA Study. *Arch Ophthalmol.* 1999;117:1384–1390.

de la Fuente M, Ferrandez MD, Murgos MS, et al. Immune function in aged women is improved by ingestion of vitamins C and E. *Can J Physiol Pharmacol.* 1998;76:373–380.

Douglas RM, Chalker EB, Treacy B. Vitamin C for preventing and treating the common cold. *Cochrane Database Syst Rev.* 2000;2:CD000980.

Du Nouy PL. Cicatrization of wounds III. The relation between the age of the patient, the area of the wound and the index of cicatrization. *J Exper Med.* 1916.

Flatt A, Pearce N, Thomson CD, et al. Reduced selenium in asthmatic subjects in New Zealand. *Thorax.* 1990;45:95–99.

Forastiere F, Pistelli R, Sestini P, et al. Consumption of fresh fruit rich in vitamin C and wheezing symptoms in children. *Thorax.* 2000;55:283–288.

Gardner SE, Franz RA, Schmidt FL. Effects of electrical stimulation on chronic wound healing: A meta-analysis. *Wound Repair Regener.* 1999;7(6):495–503.

Gerster H. The potential role of lycopene for human health. *J Am Coll Nutr.* 1997;16:109–126.

Gey KF, Stahelin HB, Eichholzer M. Poor plasma status of carotene and vitamin C is associated with higher mortality from ischemia heart disease and stroke. Basel Prospective Study. *Clin Invest.* 1993;71:3–6.

Giovannucci E, Ascherio A, Rimm EB, et al. Intake of carotenoids and retinol in relation to risk of prostate cancer. *J Natl Cancer Inst.* 1995;87:1767–1776.

Goodman DS, Goodman DS. Vitamin A and retinoids in health and disease. *N Engl J Med.* 1984;310:1023–1031.

Greenberg ER, Baron JA, Stukel TA, et al. A clinical trial of beta carotene to prevent basal-cell and squamous-cell cancers of the skin. The Skin Cancer Prevention Study Group. *N Engl J Med.* 1990;323:789–795.

Hemilia H. Vitamin C and common cold incidence: A review of studies with subjects under heavy physical stress. *Int J Sports Med.* 1996;17:379–383.

Hennekens CH, Buring JE, Manson JE, et al. Lack of effect of long-term supplementation with beta-carotene on the incidence of malignant neoplasms and cardiovascular disease. *N Engl J Med.* 1996;334:1145–1149.

Institute of Medicine. *Dietary Reference Intakes for Vitamin C, Vitamin E, Selenium, and Carotenoids.* Washington DC: National Academy Press; 2000.

Jacques PF, Chylack LT, Jr. Epidemiologic evidence of a role for the antioxidant vitamins and carotenoids in cataract prevention. *Am J Clin Nutr.* 1991;53:352S–355S.

Johnston CS, Thompson LL. Vitamin C status of an outpatient population. *J Am Coll Nutr.* 1998;141:366–370.

Kalayci O, Besler T, Kiline K, et al. Serum levels of antioxidant vitamins (alpha tocopherol, beta carotene, and ascorbic acid) in children with bronchial asthma. *Turk J Pediatr.* 2000;42: 17–21.

Kappus H, Diplock AT. Tolerance and safety of vitamin E: A toxicological position report. *Free Radic Biol Med.* 1992; 13:55–74.

Karakucuk S, Ertugrul Mirza G, Faruk Ekinciler O, et al. Selenium concentrations in serum, lens, and aqueous humour of patients with senile cataract *Acta Ophthalmol Scand.* 1995; 73:329–332.

Kelloff GJ, Crowell JA, Steele VE, et al. Progress in cancer chemoprevention: Development of diet-derived chemopreventive agents. *J Nutr.* 2000;130:467S–471S.

Kim JM, White RH. Effect of vitamin E on the anticoagulant response to warfarin. *Am J Cardiol.* 1996;77:545–546.

Kloth LC, McCulloch JM. Promotion of wound healing with electrical stimulation. *Advanced Wound Care.* 1996:9(5):42–45.

Knekt P, Heliovaara M, Rissanen A, et al. Serum antioxidant vitamins and risk of cancer. *BMJ.* 1992;305:1392–1394.

Knekt P, Heliovaara M, Aho K, et al. Serum selenium, serum alpha-tocopherol and the risk of rheumatoid arthritis. *Epidemiology.* 2000;11:402–405.

Kohlmeier L, Kark JD, Gomez-Garcia E, et al. Lycopene and myocardial infection risk in the EURAMIC study. *Am J Epidemiol.* 1997;146:618–626.

Lee IM. Antioxidant vitamins in the prevention of cancer. *Proc Assoc Am Physicians.* 1999;111:10–15, Accepted for publication.

Levine M, Dhariwal KR, Welch RW, et al. Determination of optimal vitamin C requirements in humans. *Am J Clin Nutr.* 1995;62:1347S–1356S.

Levine M, Conry-Cantilena C, Wang Y, et al. Vitamin C pharmacokinetics in healthy volunteers: Evidence for a recommended dietary allowance. *Proc Natl Acad Sci U.S.A.* 1996;93: 3704–3709.

Levine M, Ramsey SC, Daruwala R, et al. Criteria and recommendations for vitamin C intake. *JAMA.* 1999;281:1415–1423.

Loria CM, Klag MJ, Caulfield LE, Whelton PK. Vitamin C status and mortality in U.S. adults. *Am J Clin Nutr.* 2000;72: 139–145.

Loudon GM. *Organic chemistry.* Menlo Park, CA: Benjamin/ Cummings; 1988.

Maress-Perlman JA, Brady WE, Klein BE, et al. Diet and nuclear lens opacities. *Am J Epidemiol.* 1995;141:322–334.

Meyers DG, Maloley PA, Weeks D. Safety of antioxidant vitamins. *Arch Intern Med.* 1996;156:925–935.

Meydani SN, Meydani M, Blumberg JB, et al. Vitamin E supplementation and *in vivo* immune response in healthy elderly subjects. *JAMA.* 1997;277:1380–1386.

Micozzi MS, Brown ED, Edwards BK, et al. Plasma carotenoid response to chronic intake of selected foods and beta-carotene supplements in men. *Am J Clin Nutr.* 1992;55:1120–1125.

Monteleone CA, Sherman AR. Nutrition and asthma. *Arch Intern Med.* 1997;157:23–34.

Ness AR, Khaw KT, Bingham S, Day, NE. Vitamin C status and blood pressure. *J Hypertens.* 1996;14:503–508.

Padayatty SJ, Levine M. Vitamin C and myocardial infarction: The heart of the matter. *Am J Clin Nutr.* 2000;71:1027–1028.

Paiva SAR, Russel RM. Beta-carotene and other carotenoids as antioxidants. *J Am Coll Nutr.* 1999;18:426–433.

Pallast EB, Schouten EG, de Waart FG, et al. Effect of 50- and 100-mg vitamin E supplements on cellular immune function in noninstitutionalized elderly persons. *Am J Clin Nutr.* 1999; 69:1273–1281.

Pandey DK, Shekelle R, Selwyn BJ, et al. Dietary vitamin C and beta-carotene and risk of death in middle-aged men. The Western Electric Study. *Am J Epidemiol.* 1995;142: 1269–1278.

Paolisso G, Esposito R, D' Alessio MA, Barbieri M. Primary and secondary prevention of atherosclerosis: Is there a role for antioxidants? *Diabetes Metab.* 1999;25:298–306.

Peters, EM, Goetzsche JM, Grobbelaar B, Noakes TD. Vitamin C supplementation reduces the incidence posttrace symptoms of upper-respiratory-tract infection in ultramarathon runners. *Am J Clin Nutr.* 1993;57:170–174.

Psathakis D, Wedemeyer N, Oevermann E, et al. Blood selenium and glutathione peroxidase status in patients with colorectal cancer. *Dis Colon Rectum.* 1998;41:328–335.

Reavley N. *The new encyclopedia of vitamins, minerals, supplements & herbs.* New York, NY: M. Evans; 1998.

Richard MJ, Roussel AM. Micronutrients and aging: Intakes and requirements. *Proc Nutr Soc.* 1999;58:573–578.

Rimm EB. Antioxidants for vascular disease. *Med Clin North Am.* 2000;84:239–249.

Ruiz RF, Martin PG, Lopez MC, et al. Plasma levels of vitamins A and E and the risk of acute myocardial infarct. *Rev Clin Esp.* 1997;197:411–416.

Russo MW, Murray SC, Wurzelmann JI, et al. Plasma selenium levels and the risk of colorectal adenomas. *Nutr Cancer.* 1997; 28:125–129.

Sahyoun NR, Jacques PF, Russell RM. Carotenoids, vitamin C and E and mortality in an elderly population. *Am J Epidemiol.* 1996;144:501–511.

Seddon JM, Christen WG, Manson JE, et al. The use of vitamin supplements and the risk of cataract among U.S. male physicians. *Am J Public Health.* 1994;84:788–792.

Seifter E, Mendecki J, Holtzman S, et al. Role of vitamin A and beta-carotene in radiation protection: Relation to antioxidant properties. *Pharmacol Ther.* 1988;39:357–365.

Semba RD. Vitamin A, immunity and infection. *Clin Infect Dis.* 1994;19:489–499.

Sheffet A, Cytryn AS, Louria DB. Applying electric and electromagnetic energy as adjuvant treatment for pressure ulcers: A clinical review. *Ostomy Wound Manage.* 2000;46(2):28–33, 36–40,42–44.

Simon JA, Hudes ES, Browner WS. Serum ascorbic acid in cardiovascular disease prevalence in U.S. adults. *Epidemiology.* 1998;9:316–321.

Singh RB, Ghosh S, Niaz MA, et al. Dietary intake, plasma levels of antioxidant vitamins and oxidative stress in relation to coronary artery disease in elderly subjects. *Am J Cardiol.* 1995; 76:1233–1238.

Sun Y. Free radicals, antioxidant enzymes and carcinogenesis. *Free Radic Biol Med.* 1990;8:583–599.

Tavani A, Negri E, D' Avanzo B, La Vecchia C. Beta-carotene intake and risk of nonfatal acute myocardial infarction in women. *Eur J Epidemiol.* 1997;13:631–637.

Troisi, RJ, Willett WC, Weiss ST, et al. A prospective study of diet and adultonset asthma. *Am J Respir Crit Care Med.* 1995; 151:1401–1408.

Tsao CS, Salimi SL. Effect of large intake of ascorbic acid on urinary and plasma oxalic acid levels. *Int J Vitam Nutr Res.* 1984; 54:245–249.

Urivetzky M, Dessaris D, Smith AD. Ascorbic acid overdosing: A risk factor for calcium oxalate nephrolithiasis. *J Urol.* 1992; 147:1215–1218.

van den Brandt PA, Goldbohm, RA, van't Veer P, et al. A prospective cohort study on selenium status and the risk of lung cancer. *Cancer Res.* 1993;53:4860–4865.

Vitoux D, Chappuis P, Arnaud J, et al. Selenium, glutathione peroxidase, peroxides, and platelet functions. *Ann Biol Clin (Paris).* 1996;54:181–187.

Watkins ML, Erickson JD, Thun MJ, et al. Multivitamin use and mortality in a large prospective study. *Am J Epidemiol.* 2000;152:149–162.

Weijl NI, Cleton FJ, Osanto S. Free radicals and antioxidants in chemotherapy-induced toxicity. *Cancer Treat Rev.* 1997;23: 209–240.

Winkler BS, Boulton ME, Gottsch JD, Sternberg P. Oxidative damage and age-related macular degeneration. *Mole Vis.* 1999; 5:32.

Yang G, Zhou R. Further observations on the human maximum safe dietary selenium intake in a seleniferous area of China. *J Trace Elem Electrolytes Health Dis.* 1994;8:159–165.

Yang GQ, Wang SZ, Zhou RH, Sun SZ. Endemic selenium intoxication of humans in China. *Am J Clin Nutr.* 1983;37: 872–881.

Yang GQ, Xia YM. Studies on human dietary requirements and safe range of dietary intakes of selenium in China and their application in the prevention of related endemic diseases. *Biomed Environ Sci.* 1995;8:187–201.

Yu BP. Aging and oxidative stress: Modulation by dietary restriction. *Free Radic Biol Med.* 1996;21(5):651–668.

Zheng W, Sellers TA, Doyle TJ, et al. Retinol, antioxidant vitamins, and cancers of the upper digestive tract in a prospective cohort study of postmenopausal women. *Am J Epidemiol.* 1995; 142:955–960.

Lymphedema and Wound Healing: A Case for Codependence

John M. Macdonald,

Introduction
The Hidden Epidemic
Lymphedema and Edema
Lymphedema and Wound Healing
  Clinical Observations

Lymphedema Therapy and the Open Wound
Summary
References

INTRODUCTION

The relationship between lymphedema, lymph stasis, and wound healing has received little attention. When this connection is discussed, it is almost always in relation to venous ulcers. This chapter will assert that lymphatic pathology is a principle inhibitory factor for proper healing in the great majority of chronic wounds, regardless of etiology. With the emergence of the discipline of "Wound Care," specialized centers have become commonplace world wide. Understanding the science of lymphology as it relates to wound healing is critical to the clinical excellence of these centers. Programs for wound care and lymphedema should be integrated. Current evidence based support defining the relationship will be presented. The principles of compression therapy for wound related lymphedema will be discussed.

Historically, medical progress often begins with a chance observation that leads to exciting, new therapies. This has been especially true for the developing science of wound care. The principles of moist wound healing, débridement, and wound protection were first observed in clinics and then taught by anecdotal presentations of observations and results. In time, these principles become evidence-based as clinicians and basic scientists test and define their observations. Once precepts are tested in practice, broader applications are developed, along with a tendency to promote therapy that is more esoteric and, more expensive. The clinician sometimes

assumes that "bioengineered/new" is better when, in fact, a "better mouse trap" has not been developed. Not surprisingly, therefore, when a "new" therapy is based on an obvious, but often disregarded, physical finding, acceptance comes slowly. Ignaz Semmelweiss merely asked obstetricians to wash their hands in the 1840s. The rest is history.

Current textbooks and review articles are uniform in listing the local and systemic factors that inhibit wound healing. Didactic lists include foreign body, elevated matrix metalloprotease, oxygen deficiency, and the like. Lymph stasis or lymphedema, if mentioned at all, receives little or no discussion. The important differentiation between edema and lymphedema is found in the lymphedema literature and rarely in current wound care literature. This chapter will assert that an understanding of lymphedema as it relates to wound healing is essential for proper therapy.

THE HIDDEN EPIDEMIC

Lymphedema is a chronic, incurable condition (localized lymphedema secondary to trauma and chromic wounds may be the exception), characterized by an abnormal collection of fluid (lymph) as a result of an anatomical alteration of the lymphatic system. Estimates state that worldwide, one person in 30 is afflicted with some form of lymphedema. This figure does not include the millions suffering from chronic venous disease.[1] Until the past decade, the medical community, particularly in North America, has ignored the majority of these patients.

Lymphedema is differentiated into "primary lymphedema" and "secondary lymphedema." Primary lymphedema, the result of a congenital malfunction of the lymph system accounts for 10% of all lymphedema patients. The symptoms of primary lymphedema may not present until the second or third decade of life. Secondary lymphedema can be caused by many factors. The most recognizable are associated with lymphadenectomy, radiation, venous disease, and postsurgical complications. Lymphedema secondary to joint replacement and venous harvesting comprises an ever-growing problem. The most common cause of lymphedema is filariasis, a disorder caused by infection with larvae that is transmitted to humans by mosquito and infects more than 90 million people worldwide (see Table 9–1).

Many therapies have been tried in the past with little success, such as surgery (debulking and lymphovenous anastomosis), diuretics, and pneumatic pumps.[2] Because of the chronicity of symptoms, therapy has been very difficult and is, in a sense, palliative. Pharmacological treatment with benzopyrones (coumarin) has shown promise but because of serious side effects has not been approved for use in the United States.[3]

Comprehensive decongestive physiotherapy (CDP) is the gold standard throughout the world for the treatment of lymphedema. This therapy consists of manual lymph drainage (MLD), compression bandaging, related exercise, patient education in prevention, and self-care, and is widely accepted because of the contributions of the Foeldi[4] and the Casley-Smith.[5] Until recently, CDP was relatively unknown in North America. The pioneering work of Lerner[6] and Boris[7] introduced CDP to America in the late 1980s. The therapy is now eliciting the notice of the medical profession because of the excellent results achieved. As will be discussed, the treatment of lymphedema related to chronic wounds is derived from CDP principles used to treat nonwound-related lymphedema.

Table 9–1. Causes of lymphedema

Primary	Secondary
Birth	Surgery
Praecox-adolescent	Infection
Tarda-Age 35+	Trauma
	Chronic wound
	Tumor
	Radiation
	Venous disease
	Neurological
	Filariasis

LYMPHEDEMA AND EDEMA

In order to understand the pathophysiology of lymphedema as it relates to treatment, clinicians must differentiate edema from lymphedema. This is especially important in addressing the relationship of lymphedema and wound healing.

Traditionally, edema/edematous is used to describe any limb or organ that becomes swollen. In fact, two classifications of edema—"high-protein edema" and "low-protein edema"—should be used. The arbitrary dividing line of protein in concentration in edema fluid 1 g/dl (ie, 1 g %). Most of the excess fluid is present because of the colloidal osmotic pressure of the excess protein. Lymphedema is "high-protein edema." Edema, in contrast to lymphedema, is primarily water. The lymphedema associated with acute and chronic wounds is sometimes called "post-traumatic lymphedema." Table 9–2 lists the etiology of edema. Acute trauma is usually followed by a transudative "low-protein edema." If the lymphatic collecting anatomy is damaged (ie, in an open wound), true lymphedema rapidly develops. Unless the lymphedema is pre-existing, collectors proximal and distal to the lesion are normal.[8]

LYMPHEDEMA AND WOUND HEALING

To appreciate the relationship of lymphedema to wound healing, clinicians should review their understanding of chronic venous insufficiency and venous ulceration. Chronic venous insufficiency leads to venous hypertension, which results in a high filtration pressure and causes increased fluid to appear in the tissues (ie, increased lymphatic waterload). When the lymphatic transport capacity is exceeded by the water load, a state of low-protein edema occurs because of this dynamic failure. Constant

Table 9–2. Etiology of edema

Passive Hyperemia
Chronic venous insufficiency
Circulatory
Congestive heart failure
Pregnancy
Inactivity

Hypoproteinemia
Malnutrition
Malabsorption
Renal disease

Active Hyperemia
Inflammation
Allergy

lymphatic hypertension causes infiltration of lymph into the perilymphatic tissues resulting in fibrosclerosis and lymphangitis. Protein permeability increases and lymphatic damage follows. Subsequently, lymphedema/lymph stasis (high-protein edema) becomes the underlying pathology that contributes to the formation of venous ulcers.

Venous ulcers often exhibit many of the characteristics of the nonvenous chronic wound: normal arterial blood supply, colonized bacterial contamination, and healthy granulation tissue. With compression and control of the lymphedema, in addition to conventional wound care, these wounds will, in the majority of cases, heal. Given the exact same parameters in nonvenous, acute, and chronic wounds throughout the body, controlling the lymphedema will result in enhanced wound healing.[9] In the author's clinic, in excess of 80% of patients with lower extremity, nonvenous chronic wounds have demonstrated generalized limb or periwound lymphedema (data accumulated April–November 2000). The degree varied from trace to four plus pitting. These findings were present with multiple types of wounds (ie, ischemic, diabetic, and traumatic). Many of these patients had no prior history of lymphedema. Eliminating the lymphedema improves healing. In many instances, the enhanced rate of healing has been dramatic.

Surprisingly, although lymphedema control in the therapy of venous ulcers is widely accepted, the same principle applied to nonvenous ulcers has required a leap of faith. A search of the wound literature up until 2001 provides some explanation. A recent, preliminary search using the phrase "wound healing + lymphedema" resulted in one match.[10] This relationship is almost always discussed within the context of venous disease.

Clinical Observations

How do clinical observations translate into evidence-based conclusions at the clinical and basic science level? Many years of research will be required to define exactly how lymphedema inhibits wound healing. In fact, currently, considerable information/observations support this assumption.

The most obvious effect from lymphedema is swelling. This can result in abnormal function at both the tissue and cellular level. Distance between tissue channels can affect metabolic exchange, causing a shift toward anaerobic metabolism. Because cells are more widely separated, the exchange of gases between plasma membranes is likely to be affected. In chronic venous insufficiency, the removal of lymphedema results in a significant increase in transcutaneous oxygen tension.[11]

Alteration in tissues produced by simple injections of protein are almost identical with those of subacute and chronic lymphedema.[12] Mani states, "The chronic effects of edema on the viso-elastic properties of connective tissue are unknown. It is reasonable to assume that pools of edema will squash, squeeze, stretch, or affect the crimping and orientation of dermal collagen bundles."[13]

Open wounds studied by the injection of dye have demonstrated significant reduction in lymphatic channel regeneration as compared to arterial and venous angiogenesis.[14] Trauma increases lymphatic flow, and outflow obstruction with accumulation of the waste products generated in the wound healing process is a likely factor in wound healing.[15]

Tissues surrounding acute and chronic wounds are characterized by collections of third-space or interstitial fluid. This collection of fluid mechanically compromises the microvascular and lymphatic system, thereby increasing capillary and venous afterload. Consequently, the delivery of oxygen and nutrients and the discharge of inhibitory factors and toxins is affected.[16,17]

Removing excess chronic wound fluid is thought to remove inhibitory factors present in the fluid. Studies have shown that fluids removed from chronic wounds suppress the proliferation of keratinocytes, fibroblasts, and vascular endothelial cells *in vitro*.[18,19]

Argenta and Morykwas, in their investigations related to vacuum-assisted closure of wounds, have provided invaluable insight into the consequences of lymphedema. The technique removes chronic edema leading to increased blood flow and enhanced formation of granulation tissue.[20]

LYMPHEDEMA THERAPY AND THE OPEN WOUND

Compression is the cornerstone therapy for lymphedema that complicates the acute and chronic wound. While MLD can be used under certain circumstances (eg, reconstructive plastic surgery, extremity decompression proximal to compression bandaging), using MLD in proximity to the wound is neither time-, nor cost-efficient. After the wound is healed, CDP may be indicated if persistent swelling is a problem. Limb elevation, when practical, is obviously helpful. Using diuretics is rarely indicated as primary therapy and, in fact, can impair fluid mobilization by extracting water from the lymph. Diuretics are useful in treating limb swelling when a significant degree of edema superimposed on the underlying lymphedema is evident, as in chronic congestive failure. The use of pneumatic pumps for the treatment of lymphedema with or without an open wound is controversial and must be used with strict patient supervision.[21]

A variety of compression wraps are used in the treatment of lymphedema (see Table 9–3). Multiple combinations of bandages are available and their application

Table 9–3. Compression wraps used in wound care

Unna boot
Short-stretch bandage
Long-stretch bandage
Cotton padding
Self-adherent crepe dressing
Multiple combination dressings

is dictated by patient presentation. The degree of swelling, diabetes, neuropathy, arterial insufficiency, and chronic congestive heart failure must be considered. Local skin conditions, wound characteristics, and patient mobility influence the choice. In applying compression, frequently reassessing the condition of the limb and creatively matching the dressing to the patient's diagnosis is critical. When compression is applied improperly, even limbs with normal circulation may be harmed.

The mechanics of "resting pressure" and "working pressure" need to be understood. Short-stretch bandages have a high working pressure and a low resting pressure. In the relaxed limb, these bandages provide a comfortable degree of support, but the total pressure increases significantly when the muscles contract against fixed resistance. This results in an effective, intermittent massage that forces interstitial fluid into normal functioning lymphatic collectors. Thus, when properly applied, the compression wrap becomes a dynamic part of the wound dressing.

The impact of external limb compression on vascular dynamics is a concern. Properly applied bandages, even in the compromised limb, can be effective. An important technical point in the bandage technique is to use (in selected patients) a layer of cotton/gauze padding as the primary wrap to separate the short-stretch bandage from the skin. This affords a measure of protection from the resting pressure. In addition, limbs with a smaller circumference and bone protuberance (eg, anterior tibial ridge) should be protected with foam padding. In most patients, with normal arterial perfusion and sensation, a reasonable margin of error in applying compression is present. In these patients, most of the commonly used methods are safe when bandages are applied with regard to the patients comfort and the clinical observation of capillary return.

In patients with insensate or ischemic limbs, special precautions are required. Studies are now in progress to define the hemodynamics that clinically appear to permit such application. The report of Mayrovitz and Larson[22] demonstrating increased leg pulsatile flow effected by compression bandaging, may have special significance. In areas of the body that do not permit bandage compression (eg, the trunk, head, and buttocks),

vacuum-assisted closure is a logical alternative to compression bandaging.

SUMMARY

Despite numerous bioengineering product refinements, good wound care is driven by adherence to the fundamentals: modifying systemic and local factors, where possible, and, controlling infection and wound protection. Proper wound healing is also dependent upon identifying wound-related lymphedema/lymph stasis and the mobilization of the fluid. With increased awareness will come research verification and precise safety guidelines for compression. The case for the codependence of wound healing and lymphedema will be obvious.

REFERENCES

1. Casley-Smith JR. Frequency of lymphedema. In: Casley-Smith JR, ed. *Modern Treatment for Lymphedema*. 5th ed. Adelaide, Australia: The Lymphedema Association of Australia; 1997: 81–84.

2. Casley-Smith JR. Surgery and microsurgery for lymphedema. In: Casley-Smith JR, ed. *Modern Treatment for Lymphedema*. 5th ed. Adelaide, Australia: The Lymphedema Association of Australia; 1997:294–295.

3. Casley-Smith JR. There are many benzo-pyrones for lymphedema. *Lymphology*. 1997;30–38.

4. Foeldi E, Foeldi M, Weissleder H. Conservative treatment of lymphedema of the limbs. *Angiology*. 1985;86:171–180.

5. Casley-Smith JR. Complex physical therapy: The first 200 Australian limbs. *Austr J Dermatol*. 1992;33:61–68.

6. Ko D, Lerner R, Klos G, Cosimi A. Effective treatment of lymphedema of the extremities. *Arch Surg*. 1998; 133:452–458.

7. Boris M, Weindorf S, Lasinski B, et al. Lymphedema reduction by non-invasive complex lymphedema therapy. *Oncology*. 1994;8:95–106.

8. Casley-Smith JR. Pathology of oedema—causes of oedemas. In Casley-Smith JR, ed. *Modern Treatment for Lymphedema*. 5th ed. Adelaide, Australia: The Lymphedema Association of Australia; 1997:41–46.

9. Weissleder H, Schuchhardt C, eds. *Lymphedema—Diagnoses and Therapy*. 2nd ed. Bonn, Germany; Kagaer Kommunication; 1997:29–33.

10. Mallon EC, Ryan T. Lymphedema and wound healing. *Clin Dermatol*. 1994;12:89–93.

11. Kolari PJ, Pekanmaki K, Pohjola RT. Transcutaneous oxygen tension in patients with posttraumatic ulcers: Treatment with intermittent pneumatic compression. *Cardiovasc Res*. 1988; 22:138–141.

12. Gaffney RM, Casley-Smith JR. Excess protein as a cause of chronic Inflammation and lymphedema: biochemical estimations. *J Pathol*. 1981:133;243–272.

13. Mani R, Ross JN. The study of tissue structure in the wound environment in chronic wound healing. In: mani R, Falanga V, Shearman CP, Sandeman D, eds. *Clinical Measurement and Basic Science*. Philadelphia: Saunders;1999:139.

14. Eilska O, Eliskova M. Secondary healing wounds and their lymphatics. *Europ J Lymphol.* 2000;8(31):64.

15. Szczesny G, Olszewski WL. Lymphatic and venous changes in posttraumatic edema of lower limbs. *Europ J Lymphol.* 2000; 8(31):60.

16. Reuler JB, Cooney TG. The pressure sore pathophysiology and principles of management. *Ann Intern Med.* 1981;94: 661–665.

17. Witkowski JA, Parish LC. Histopathology of the decubitus ulcer. *J Am Acad Dermatol.* 1982;6:1014–1021.

18. Falanga V. Growth factors and chronic wounds: The need to understand the microenvironment. *J Dermatol.* 1992;19: 667–672.

19. Bucalo B, Eaglstein WH, Falanga V. Inhibition of cell proliferation by chronic wound fluid. *Wound Repair Regen.* 1993;1: 181–186.

20. Argenta L, Morykwas M. Vacuum-assisted closure: A new method for wound control and treatment; clinical experience. *Ann Plast Surg.* 1997;38:563–576.

21. Boris M, Weindorf S, Lasinski B. The risk of genital edema after external pump compression for lower limb lymphedema. *Lymphology.* 1998;31:15–20.

22. Mayrovitz H, Larson P. Effects of compression bandaging on leg pulsatile blood flow. *Clin Physiol.* 1997;17: 105–117.

Role of Matrix Macromolecules in the Etiology and Treatment of Chronic Ulcers

Seth L. Schor, Ana M. Schor, Robert P. Keatch, and Jill Belch

Introduction
The Acute Wound-Healing Cascade
  Cell and Tissue-Level Events
  Cell Activation: A Critical First Step
Cytokines and Matrix Macromolecules:
  Interdependent Mediators of Cell Activation
  Matrix Modulation of Cell Behavior: A
    Spectrum of Mechanisms
  The Reciprocity of Cytokine and Matrix
    Signaling

Matrikines: Protease-Generated Fragments
  of Matrix Macromolecules Displaying
  "Cytokine-Like" Bioactivities
MSF: A Genetically Truncated Isoform
  of Fibronectin
Etiology of Impaired Wound Healing:
  A Question of Critical Balance
Future Prospects
Summary
References

INTRODUCTION

Tissue response to injury is driven by the sequential activation of different cell populations. Although cytokines have long been recognized to play a key role in mediating these events, the extracellular matrix (ECM) has, until relatively recently, been considered to play a passive role in wound healing, essentially confined to providing a physical scaffold for cell attachment and migration. This rather limited view of matrix functionality is no longer tenable. Indeed, the past decade has witnessed a profound change in perspective, with the ECM now acknowledged to complement cytokines in orchestrating the ordered progression of acute wound healing. In view of the important clinical implications of this paradigm shift, the objective of this chapter is to highlight emerging opportunities for utilizing ECM bioactivity in developing improved patient management strategies. Toward this end, we shall (1) outline the key events of the acute wound-healing cascade, (2) identify the diverse mechanisms whereby ECM constituents contribute to the control of wound healing, (3) introduce MSF, a recently cloned matrix-dependent modulator of wound healing, (4) indicate the convergent mechanisms responsible for

the etiology of impaired wound healing associated with diverse pathologies, and (5) speculate how the potent bioactivities of MSF and an appropriate ECM may be utilized to develop more efficacious therapeutic strategies.

THE ACUTE WOUND-HEALING CASCADE

Cell and Tissue-Level Events

Acute wound healing proceeds through a series of overlapping stages involving (1) the formation of a blood clot and fibrin-based provisional matrix, (2) the ingress of neutrophils and monocytes into the wound site, (3) epithelial cell migration and coverage of the wound, (4) the outgrowth of new blood vessels from pre-existing ones (a process referred to as *angiogenesis*) and their comigration with fibroblasts into the wound site to produce granulation tissue, (5) matrix degradation and redeposition by granulation tissue fibroblasts and vascular cells, and (6) the gradual transformation of granulation tissue into a relatively acellular mature scar consisting predominantly of Type I collagen bundles.[1–3] This cascade of events involves the spatial and temporal coordination of key cell and tissue-level events, including cell migration, angiogenesis, and matrix remodeling.

Cell migration in wound healing is initiated and coordinated by soluble *mitogenic* factors (such as cytokines) and matrix macromolecules.[4] The migratory response of cells to soluble factors may be resolved into two distinct components: *chemokinesis*, defined as the stimulation of random cell migration in response to an isotropic concentration of soluble mitogenic factor, and *chemotaxis*, defined as the stimulation of directional cell migration by a spatial concentration gradient of mitogenic factor. The ECM may also influence cell migration as a consequence of *haptotaxis*, defined as directional-cell migration along a concentration gradient of a solid-phase matrix macromolecule. Directional-cell migration (both chemotaxis and haptotaxis) is a particularly important feature of wound healing, contributing to re-epithelialization, angiogenesis, and the ingress of both leukocytes and stromal cells into the wound.

The initiation, directionality, and appropriate cessation of angiogenesis are central to the progression of an effective wound healing response.[5,6] Angiogenesis is a complex process involving a number of distinct stages, including (1) the activation of vascular endothelial cells and pericytes, and their migration through the vessel basement membrane into the perivascular three-dimensional macromolecular martrix, (2) the formation of sprouts by these cells and their directional migration into the wound site, and (3) the morphogenetic interaction of the sprouting cells, culminating in the formation of a patent new vessel in functional continuity with the parental one.

Changes in the ECM begin with the formation of the provisional matrix and continue throughout the remainder of the wound-healing response as a consequence of controlled matrix degradation (predominantly by members of the matrix metalloproteinase family) and the deposition of newly synthesized matrix constituents.[7,8] The neomatrices produced by progressive remodeling processes provide the structural scaffold for cell adhesion and migration, and furnish key regulatory cues controlling the ordered progression of wound healing. Exploring the various mechanisms, whereby the ECM contributes to the control of wound healing, constitutes the central theme of this chapter.

Cell-Activation: A Critical First Step

The initiation of wound healing is marked by the *activation* of relevant cell populations. In spite of its common usage, the term "cell activation" remains a difficult to define phenomenon, variously used to describe the changes in cell morphology, migratory behavior, proliferation, adhesive characteristics and gene expression that accompany wound healing, as well as other tissue responses to stress. All of the major cell types involved in the wound-healing response (ie, inflammatory cells,

keratinocytes, fibroblasts, and vascular endothelial cells) undergo an activation process, which is collectively required for the commencement of a sustained wound-healing response. In this context, stromal cell activation has been reported to be a particularly critical requirement for granulation tissue formation and keratinocyte migration.[9] The complementary process of *cell deactivation* (ie, a return to the resting phenotype), commonly in concert with the apoptosis (ie, programmed cell death) of residual activated cells, marks the end of the wound-healing response. As cell activation is of such central importance to wound healing, it is not surprising that a considerable amount of effort continues to be devoted to defining the precise alterations in gene expression by which it may be defined more precisely.[10,11]

Cytokines and other soluble regulatory molecules have long been recognized to induce cell activation by receptor-mediated signaling. Platelet derived growth factor (PDGF) and transforming growth factor beta-1 (TGF-β1) are released from activated platelets at the beginning of the wound-healing response and are considered to provide the initial cell activation stimuli. The cytokine profile at the wound site is subsequently augmented by the release of other cytokines by infiltrating neutrophils and activated macrophages. The wound milieu continues to be modified as a consequence of the arrival of activated keratinocytes, fibroblasts, and vascular endothelial cells, which release a new wave of cytokines. Cytokines may accordingly be considered to be both inducers (mediators) of cell activation and markers of the activated phenotype. In addition to their role in cell activation, cytokine gradients also contribute to the ordered progression of wound healing by promoting chemotaxis and angiogenesis.[12,13]

Alterations in cell–matrix interactions have recently been recognized to be a key feature of the activation process. For example, changes in the expression of members of the integrin family of matrix receptors, cell adhesion molecules, matrix macromolecules, matrix metalloproteinases, and tissue inhibitors of matrix metalloproteinases have consistently been reported to be molecular markers of activation.[10,11] As is the case with cytokines, these molecules function as both mediators and molecular markers of cell activation.

CYTOKINES AND MATRIX MACROMOLECULES: INTERDEPENDENT MEDIATORS OF CELL ACTIVATION

Matrix Modulation of Cell Behavior: A Spectrum of Mechanisms

The composition and physical organization of the ECM exert a profound effect upon cell behavior during various physiological and pathological processes, including embryonic development[14] and wound healing.[15,16] These functions of the ECM are mediated by a number of mechanisms involving receptor-mediated signaling and mechanochemical signal transduction, all of which ultimately culminate in the induction or modulation of intracellular signaling pathways (Table 10–1).

A considerable amount is known regarding receptor-mediated signaling of cytokines. In general, this involves: (1) cytokine ligation by specific cell-surface receptors, (2) the phosphorylation and dephosphorylation of molecular constituents of diverse intracellular signaling pathways, and (3) resultant changes in the pattern of gene expression and/or functional state of the cytoskeleton. Downstream mediators of cytokine bioactivity include other cytokines, as well as a chemically diverse spectrum of soluble effectors.[17,18] Common matrix macromolecules (including collagen, fibronectin, fibrin, and hyaluronan) have also been reported to elicit signal-transduction cascades as a consequence of their ligation by cell-surface receptors.[19] This receptor-mediated signaling is elicited by the ligation of specific amino acid motifs within the matrix macromolecule by members of the integrin family of cell-surface receptors.[20,21] For example, the RGD tripeptide motif, first identified as mediating cell adhesion to fibronectin, is also present in a number of other matrix macromolecules

and is a ligand for integrin $\alpha5\beta1$ (the "classical" fibronectin receptor), as well as other integrins, including $\alpha3\beta1$, $\alpha v\beta1$, $\alpha v\beta3$, and $\alpha v\beta6$. Additional cell-adhesion motifs have subsequently been identified in fibronectin and other matrix macromolecules. It should be noted that (1) the same bioactive amino acid motif may be present within several matrix macromolecules, (2) a given matrix constituent may contain a number of different adhesion motifs, and (3) the same amino acid motif may be a ligand for several integrin receptors. This level of diversity and redundancy affords the cell with a complex input of signals. Even fibrinogen, a soluble macromolecular constituent of plasma previously thought to contribute to wound healing solely by its plasmin-catalyzed conversion into the insoluble fibrin mesh of the provisional matrix, is now recognized to elicit a receptor-mediated signal-transduction cascade.[22] These matrix-induced signal cascades converge with their well-characterized cytokine-induced counterparts, thereby generating a multitier circuitry of regulatory pathways.[23,24]

In addition to receptor-mediated signal-transduction pathways, the solid-phase nature of the ECM allows it to provide a number of topologic cues. For example, vascular endothelial cells persistently adopt a resting ("cobblestone") monolayer when cultured *on the surface* of a native Type I collagen gel in the absence of exogenous angiogenic factors. The addition of angiogenic factors to these cultures induces the formation of a network of activated (sprouting) cells underneath the cobblestone monolayer. In this newly encountered three-dimensional environment, the sprouting cells form complex tubular structures and migrate into the underlying three-dimensional matrix. Significantly, resting endothelial cells spontaneously adopt a sprouting phenotype when they are directly plated *within* a three-dimensional collagen gel in the absence of exogenous angiogenic factors, thereby suggesting that in this culture environment the endothelial cells produce endogenous angiogenic factors.[25–27] These two cell culture environments only differ in terms of the topology of endothelial cell contact with the collagenous matrix: (ie, in the "on gel") culture protocol endothelial contact with the collagen substratum is confined to their basal surface, whereas in the "in gel" protocol cell contact with the collagen matrix is uniform along the entire plasma membrane. The observed induction of an activated cell phenotype in response to this topologic cue (ie, shift from two- to a three-dimensional matrix environment) is consistent with the postulated role of the geometry and tension of cell–matrix interactions in defining cytoskeletal organization, with its ultimate impact on gene expression.[28,29] Extrapolating to the *in vivo* situation, these results suggest that the movement of endothelial cells during angiogenesis from their

Table 10–1 Diverse mechanisms whereby the ECM may modulate cell behavior[1]

Biochemical composition
  Receptor-mediated signaling
  Re-expression of onco-fetal isoforms

Cytokine presentation

Physicochemical
  Mechanochemical signaling
  Geometry of cell interaction
  Micro- and nanoscale topographical features

Degradation products
  Matrikines/ matricryptins

Generation of truncated bioactive isomers
  MSF

Working in concert, these various mechanisms determine the bioinductive properties of the extracellular matrix, including its ability to function in a permissive or nonpermissive fashion with respect to the support of cytokine signaling.

two-dimensional luminal position into the three-dimensional stromal compartment may be sufficient *in itself* to induce changes in gene expression. According to this view (1) angiogenic factors produced by non-endothelial cells may principally function to induce the initial stages of endothelial cell activation (including their migration into the perivascular stroma) and provide a chemotactic stimulus for the directed migration of the sprouts into the wound site, whereas (2) angiogenic factors endogenously produced by the sprouting endothelial cells may be principally responsible for mediating the morphogenetic cell–cell interactions required for neovessel maturation.

Nanoscale and microscale topologic features of the substratum influence the anchorage, orientation, and directed migration (contact guidance) of cells *in vitro*.[30] The pattern of gene expression is modulated by physical forces transmitted (via cell-surface receptors) from the ECM to the cytoskeleton in a manner that has been postulated to affect chromatin organization and gene expression.[31,32] The imposition of both static and dynamic mechanical loading on cells at the wound site (as a consequence of wound contracture and tissue movement) also affects gene expression and has been implicated in fibroblast activation to a myofibroblast phenotype.[33,34]

The Reciprocity of Cytokine and Matrix Signaling

Cytokines and matrix macromolecules are pleiotrophic effectors, each capable of influencing several aspects of cell behavior. This inherent complexity is further enhanced by the fact that the bioactivities attributed to a particular cytokine or matrix molecule are not invariant, but critically dependent upon the tissue "context" of the target cell population.[35] For example, members of the TGF-β family of cytokines may variously stimulate, inhibit, or have no effect on the migration of target dermal fibroblasts, depending on the nature of the macromolecular substratum.[36,37] The consequence of this matrix dependence is that the same cytokine may have quite different effects upon a target cell population at different stages of wound healing in response to ongoing matrix remodeling. Indeed, it is now clear that all aspects of the wound-healing response, including cell migration and angiogenesis, are regulated by the dynamic and reciprocal interplay of cytokines and matrix macromolecules.[6,35,38–40]

Cytokines and matrix macromolecules affect each other's bioactivities by a number of mechanisms (Table 10–1). As indicated above, this interdependence may reflect *cross talk* between their respective intracellular signal-transduction pathways whereby the net effect upon cell behavior reflects the strength of a signal at critical convergent points. The reverse *inside-out* signaling

results in either the affinity of a cytokine receptor at the cell surface being modified by matrix-mediated signal-transduction pathways, or the reciprocal modification of matrix receptor affinity by cytokine signaling.[40] Cytokines affect the synthesis of matrix macromolecules, including regulating the balance between "fetal" and "adult" isoforms,[10,41,42] thereby altering the matrix milieu and its consequent signaling capacity. Indeed, the precise spectrum of matrix macromolecules induced by transcription factors (such as *ets*) is strictly context dependent, being responsive to the cytokine and matrix profile in the microenvironment.[43] Biological activities ascribed to a particular cytokine may be mediated by the induced matrix constituent;[35] conversely, cell–matrix interactions may exert a reciprocal effect upon the expression of cytokines and their cell-surface receptors. Finally, the correct presentation of certain cytokines to their cell-surface receptors is dependent upon their prior binding to matrix macromolecules.[44]

An important biologic concept to have emerged in the past decade is that wound healing and its constituent processes (chemotaxis and angiogenesis) are regulated by the *critical balance* of stimulators and inhibitors, rather than the *absolute concentration* of any one effector.[39,45,46] Stimulators and inhibitors of these key wound-healing events include cytokines and matrix macromolecules.[39,47–49] This insight has significant implications for our understanding of the pathogenesis of chronic nonhealing ulcers, as well as the development of more clinically efficacious means of treating these pathologies.

Matrikines: Protease-Generated Fragments of Matrix Macromolecules Displaying "Cytokine-Like" Bioactivities

As indicated above, the matrix scaffold to which cells are attached can modulate cell behavior by a number of mechanisms involving receptor-mediated cell signaling, topological cues, and mechanochemical signal transduction. It is now apparent that matrix macromolecules may also affect cell behavior by a distinct mechanism involving their degradation into bioactive soluble fragments. In this situation, matrix metalloproteinases (as well as other matrix-degrading enzymes) degrade constituents of the ECM into soluble fragments, which express a broad spectrum of neobioactivities not manifest by the full-length molecule. These bioactive matrix fragments have variously been referred to as *matrikines,*[50] in recognition of their matrix origin and cytokine-like neobioactivity, and *matricryptins,*[51] in recognition of their matrix origin and functional crypticity in the full-length matrix molecule. Matrikines (the term employed in this chapter) are now recognized to play a crucial role in a number of important biologic processes.[52]

Fibronectin is an ubiquitously distributed ECM molecule. It is a source of diverse matrikines and is accordingly well suited to serve as a prototype for matrix signaling by this mechanism. Fibronectin is a modular glycoprotein consisting of a number of protease-resistant "functional domains" named on the basis of their specific binding affinities for other matrix macromolecules and members of the integrin family of matrix receptors. Starting at the N-terminus, these functional domains include (Fig. 10–1): *Hep1/Fib1* (N-terminal low-affinity binding to heparin and fibrin), *Gel-BD* (binding to gelatin/collagen), *Cell-BD* (RGD-mediated binding to cell-surface integrins), *Hep2* (high-affinity heparin binding), and *Fib2* (C-terminal fibrin-binding site). The functional domains are, in turn, built from "structural homology modules",[53] of which there are three (designated Types I, II, and III). The considerably smaller amino acid-adhesion motifs provide the minimal peptide unit required for ligation by integrin receptors. The RGD recognition sequence (located within the tenth Type III module) was the first such amino acid motif demonstrated to mediate cell adhesion.[54] Subsequent studies have identified other bioactive amino acid motifs in fibronectin (including LDV, REDV, and IGD), which promote the adhesion and migration of various target cell types.[55–59] Alternative splicing at three locations within human fibronectin pre-messenger ribonucleic acid (mRNA) results in the expression of approximately 20 distinct isoforms characterized by the inclusion or deletion of two particular Type III modules (designated EDA and EDB) and various segments of IIICS.[60,61] Certain of these isoforms (eg, those retaining the EDA and/or EDB) are referred to as "oncofetal" on the basis of their enhanced expression during fetal development and in various pathologies, including cancer and wound healing.[62] All of these isoforms have molecular masses in the region of 250 kDa and are, therefore, considered to be "full length."

The protease-resistance of fibronectin functional domains ensures that they are consistently generated by limited proteolysis of matrix fibronectin, both *in vitro* and *in vivo*.[63] In addition to expressing the specific binding affinities they mediate when part of the full-length molecule, the liberated functional domains function as matrikines in that they also express a number of neoactivities that are cryptic within full-length fibronectin: ie, (1) the inhibition of Schwann cell proliferation[64] and the stimulation of adipocyte differentiation[65] by the N-terminal fibrin/heparin-binding domain, (2) the potent stimulation fibroblast migration by the gelatin-binding domain,[66] (3) the stimulation of monocyte migration[67] and induction of protease gene expression[68] by the cell-binding domain, and (4) an RGDS-independent stimulation of cell migration[69] by the C-terminal fibrin-binding domain. Various lines of

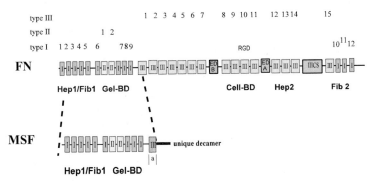

Fig. 10–1. The modular structure of fibronectin and MSF.
FN. Fibronectin consists of the following functional domains: *Hep1/Fib1* (N-terminal low-affinity binding to heparin and fibrin), *Gel-BD* (binding to gelatin/collagen), *Cell-BD,* (RGD-mediated binding to cell-surface integrins), *Hep2* (high-affinity heparin binding), and *Fib2* (C-terminal fibrin-binding site). Each functional domain is composed of three possible homology modules: types I, II and III. The RGD integrin recognition motif is located in the tenth type III module.
MSF. Predicted amino acid sequence of MSF is identical to that of fibronectin up to and including the peptide module coded by exon III-1a. MSF terminates in a 10 amino acid sequence (VSIPPRNLGY) not present in any previously identified fibronectin isoform. Bioactive IGD motifs are present in the seventh and ninth type I modules.

evidence indicate that the expression of such neoactivities results from the release of steric hindrance operative in the full-length native molecule. In this regard, Fukai and collaborators[70] demonstrated that fibronectin isolated from plasma by conventional purification protocols (involving exposure to high concentrations of urea, a potent denaturing agent) mediated an RGDS-dependent stimulation of cell migration, whereas fibronectin isolated by a gentler ion-exchange chromatography protocol did not. Fibronectin isolated by ion-exchange chromatography could be induced to display mitogenic activity by subsequent exposure to urea. Hydrodynamic and light-scattering data confirmed that exposure of nondenatured fibronectin to urea induced significant conformational changes in the molecule, which correlated with the enabling of RGDS-dependent migration-stimulating activity. In contrast, the cryptic biological activities of the N-terminal Fib-1 domain (induction of adipocyte differentiation) and C-terminal Fib-2 domain (RGDS-independent stimulation of migration) were not expressed by denatured fibronectin and required a more extensive alteration in conformation induced by proteolytic cleavage.[70] Cryptic sites within fibronectin may also be exposed by the stretching of fibronectin ECM fibrils in response to cell-imposed mechanical loading.[71]

In the context of the present discussion, the mitogenic activity cryptic within the gelatin-binding domain of fibronectin[66] is of particular relevance as it is extremely potent (with a half-maximal activity manifest in the femtomolar concentration range) and strictly matrix dependent (ie, stimulates the migration of target fibroblasts adherent to a *native*, but not *denatured*, type I collagen substratum). This potent mitogenic activity is mediated by two IGD amino acid motifs present within the seventh and ninth type I structural modules via signaling through integrin $\alpha v\beta 3$ and is competitively inhibited by cell-binding domain signaling through integrin $\alpha 5\beta 1$.[59,66] These findings have a number of implications for the role of the gelatin-binding domain (as well as other fibronectin-derived matrikines) in wound healing: namely, these matrix derivatives may exert effects on target cells at concentrations previously regarded as too low to be biologically relevant and their bioactivity may be modulated during wound healing as a consequence of ongoing matrix remodelling, as well as the generation of other proteolytically generated matrix fragments.

Potent matrikines are also generated by the degradation of other matrix/serum glycoproteins including collagen Type IV and Type XVIII[72,73], laminin,[74,75] plasminogen,[76] and fibrinogen.[77] The neobioactivities expressed by these matrikines may be expected to affect wound healing by virtue of their modulation (both stimulation and inhibition) of angiogenesis,[72,73,76,78,79] as well as other critical processes.

Matrikines may, in addition, be generated by the degradation of nonproteinaceous matrix constituents, such as hyaluronan, a widely distributed matrix glycosaminoglycan. Oligosaccharide degradation products of hyaluronan have been shown to be potent stimulators of angiogenesis.[80] These hyaluronan fragments exert this effect by binding to their receptors (CD44 and RHAMM) on target endothelial cells[81] and signaling through the MAP kinase signal-transduction pathway.[82]

MSF: A GENETICALLY TRUNCATED ISOFORM OF FIBRONECTIN

We have recently cloned *migration stimulating factor* (MSF), a novel cell-activation molecule which is transiently up-regulated during wound healing and exhibits a number of potent bioactivities of particular relevance to different stages of the wound-healing process.[83] Sequence analysis of MSF cDNA indicates that it is identical to the 5′ end of fibronectin, with the addition of a novel 175 nt 3′-tail consisting of a 30 nt coding sequence, followed by a 3′ untranslated region containing five inframe stop codons and a cleavage/polyadenylation signal. Chromosome mapping and sequencing of genomic DNA indicate that MSF is derived from the fibronectin gene and that its unique 175 nt 3′-tail is generated by retention of the intron separating fibronectin exons III-1a and III-1b and its cleavage and polyadenylation during subsequent mRNA maturation. The deduced MSF protein consists of (1) the intact 70-kDa N-terminus of fibronectin (containing the entire Fib1/Hep1 and Gel-BD regions and the first portion of module III-I), and (2) a unique 10 amino acid C-terminus (VSIPPRNLGY), as coded by the first 30 nt of the retained intron (Fig. 10–1). MSF is the first truncated isoform of human fibronectin to be identified.

Recombinantly expressed human MSF stimulates fibroblast migration and hyaluronan synthesis with a bell-shaped dose-response identical to that of the gelatin-binding domain of fibronectin (Gel-BD), with half-maximal activity achieved in the femtomolar concentration range (Fig. 10–2). These potent bioactivities of MSF are efficiently inhibited by TGF-β1.[84] The migration of other cell types, including epithelial and vascular endothelial cells, is also stimulated by MSF. Recent observations also indicated that both MSF and Gel-BD are potent angiogenic factors, both *in vitro* and in various *in vivo* assays (AM Schor, manuscripts in preparation). Significantly, MSF bioactivity is completely abolished by a function neutralizing anti-Gel-BD monoclonal antibody, but unaffected by antibodies raised against the N-terminal Fib1/Hep1 domain or the unique MSF C-terminal decapeptide. The IGD amino acid motif is a highly conserved feature of the fibronectin type I structural module[53] and is present at two locations (I-7 and I-9) within the gelatin-binding domain

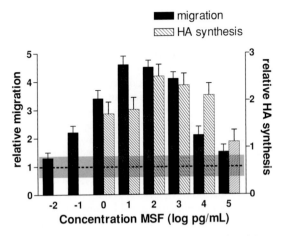

Fig. 10–2. The effect of MSF on target skin fibroblasts. Dose-response of adult skin fibroblasts to MSF in terms of its stimulation of cell migration and hyaluronan synthesis. Assay details as previously described.[37,59]

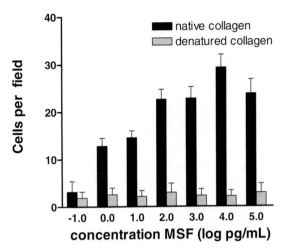

Fig. 10–3. The matrix dependence of fibroblast mitogenic response to MSF. Dose response of adult skin fibroblasts to MSF as ascertained in the transmembrane migration assay using filters coated with native or denatured type I collagen. Assay details as previously described.[59]

of MSF (Fig. 10–1). Small synthetic peptides containing the IGD motif express all of the bioactivities of MSF.[59] Recent *in vitro* mutagenesis studies confirm that MSF bioactivity is mediated by these IGD motifs.[83] All of the bioactivities manifest by MSF and Gel-BD are cryptic within full-length fibronectin.

The mitogenic response of target cells to MSF is strictly matrix dependent. In the case of fibroblasts, enhanced migration is apparent by cells adherent to *native*, but not *denatured*, type I collagen (Fig. 10–3), whereas target endothelial cells are responsive on both substrata. Endothelial cells also responded to MSF when adherent to matrices of cellular fibronectin, plasma fibronectin, and type IV collagen, but were nonresponsive when adherent to matrices of thrombospondin-1 and full-length hyaluronan.

Initial observations using an MSF-specific bioassay revealed the presence of detectable quantities of MSF in wound fluids collected from healing surgical wounds.[85] Subsequent immunohistochemical studies have utilized MSF-specific antibodies (raised against its unique C-terminal decapeptide) to document its pattern of expression in acute human wound healing. For this purpose, an initial 3-mm full-thickness punch biopsy was taken from healthy volunteers at day 0, thereby providing a sample of normal skin in addition to producing the wound. A second 6-mm punch biopsy, this encompassing the healing wound and a rim of perilesional skin, was taken from the 24 recruited volunteers at different times thereafter. MSF staining was first apparent at day 3 and was confined to the migrating edge of epithelial cells (AM Schor, manuscript in preparation). The intensity

of epithelial staining was significantly increased at days 7 and 14; stromal cell staining was also apparent at these times. In the majority of specimens, staining declined to negligible levels by day 21. There was a significant increase in vascularity at days 7 and 14. These results provide the first direct experimental evidence that MSF is transiently expressed by keratinocytes, fibroblasts, and vascular endothelial cells during the acute wound healing response in healthy controls. Our data further indicate that there is a clear temporal sequence of cell activation, with keratinocytes at the migrating edge of the wound being the first to show evidence of MSF expression. Pilot data further suggest that MSF is not present in detectable quantities in chronic leg ulcers or histologically normal perilesional skin at presentation (Fig. 10–4A,B) and re-expressed by ulcer fibroblasts and endothelial cells, and (to a lesser extent) by the advancing epithelial sheet, when healing is initiated in responsive patients by compressive dressing (Fig. 10–4C).

It should be noted that MSF and Gel-BD are functionally equivalent, but produced by distinct mechanisms, presumably under independent control: (ie, Gel-BD) is a matrikine produced by the proteolytic degradation of matrix fibronectin, whereas MSF is a truncated isoform of fibronectin generated by alternative splicing of the fibronectin gene transcript. This functional convergence provides tissue cells with two independent mechanisms of locally generating equivalent neobioactivities, one by degradation of the extracellular matrix (Gel-BD)

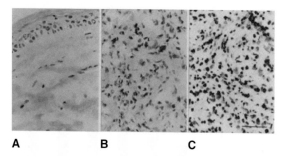

Fig. 10–4. MSF expression in a venous stasis ulcer at presentation and following the induction of wound healing. Little or no staining with anti-MSF monoclonal antibody in perilesional skin (**A**) and ulcer at presentation (**B**). High levels of MSF expression in healing ulcer 7 weeks after application of pressure bandage (**C**). Specimens kindly provided by Professors C McCollum and M Ferguson, University of Manchester.

and the other by control of fibronectin gene transcription (MSF). The capacity of producing MSF by a genetic mechanism affords the cell with a means of selectively producing a functional equivalent to Gel-BD without the necessity of generating a mixture of proteinase-generated matrikines expressing a complex array of (sometimes competing) neobioactivities. As previously discussed in the context of Gel-BD neobioactivity, the matrix-dependence of MSF provides a "tissue-level" means of modulating its effect on target cells in pathologies characterized by matrix remodeling: ie, temporal changes in matrix composition may progressively render adherent cells responsive or nonresponsive to MSF.

Finally, it should be noted that fibronectin functionality has been reported to be critically modulated by its self-association into fibrillar aggregates of "super fibronectin".[86] Cells display enhanced adhesion to super fibronectin, with a reciprocal decrease in migratory activity. Significantly, super fibronectin formation is mediated by an amino sequence coded by exons III-1a and III-1b. The truncation of MSF translation at exon III-1a and the consequent absence of the super fibronectin signal may support its function as a physiological counterpoise to the migration-inhibiting activity of super fibronectin.

ETIOLOGY OF IMPAIRED WOUND HEALING: A QUESTION OF CRITICAL BALANCE

Perturbations in cell activation contribute to the etiology of many apparently disparate pathological conditions, including aberrant wound healing and cancer.[87,88] As discussed above, the initiation of cell activation during wound healing is controlled by a finely tuned balance between stimulatory and inhibitory signals and it, therefore, follows that a disruption in this balance may result in pathological sequellae. The matrix may contribute to this balance by a number of mechanisms (Table 10–1) which are subject to temporal variation during wound healing as a consequence of matrix remodeling, as well as changes in the expression of matrix receptors in relevant cell populations. In this context, it should be noted that overexpression of matrix metalloproteinases has commonly been reported to be a feature of chronic ulceration.[89,90] Indeed, dermal fibroblasts isolated from normal skin of patients with diabetes display elevated levels of MMP-2 and -3 production, thereby suggesting that this perturbation may precede (and possibly contribute to) ulcer development.[91] Overexpression of MMPs may interfere with the initiation and/or maintenance of an efficacious wound-healing cascade by degrading the matrix sufficiently to impair its ability to function as a biosignaling scaffold, as well as result in the production in a broad spectrum of matrikines eliciting a net balance of negative signaling.

Impaired local perfusion is a principal etiological factor in ulcer development.[92] Critical deficiencies in vascular perfusion may occur at different sites within the vascular tree. For example, atherosclerotic arterial disease affects approximately 20% of men over 70 years of age, often leading to the development of peripheral ulcers and gangrene. Venous disease is more common, with venous ulcers affecting approximately 2.5% of the population. Blood flow through capillaries can be impeded as a result of vessel spasm (eg, Raynaud's Syndrome) and vasculitic occlusion. Microvessel obstruction is also a common complication of diabetes mellitus, often encountered in association with large vessel disease. As discussed above, the maintenance of a normal wound healing response is dependent upon the generation of new blood vessels. The induction of angiogenesis, both in terms of the generation of collateral vessels in the perilesional tissue and the provision of a new microvascular bed at the wound site, is, therefore, a rational clinical objective and may provide an efficacious means of improving the management of patients with chronic ulceration. As discussed in the following section, the development of the next generation of patient management strategies should take into account our growing understanding of the role played by the matrix in controlling stromal cell activation and angiogenesis.

FUTURE PROSPECTS

Wound healing in the early gestation fetus is a regenerative process characterized by a minimum of scar formation.[93] Several lines of evidence indicate that this desirous outcome is not dependent upon the unique character of the intrauterine environment, but is an inherent property of fetal skin, especially its constituent fibroblast population.[94,95] Fetal skin fibroblasts differ from their adult counterparts by a number of potentially relevant phenotypic characteristics.[96] The challenge is to identify those particular characteristics which are responsible for the regenerative nature of fetal wound healing and devise means whereby these may be effectively deployed in the adult to "kick-start" the healing of chronic ulcers. MSF would appear to be a key candidate on the basis of its constitutive expression by fetal fibroblasts and potent bioactivities, including the stimulation of cell migration, hyaluronan biosynthesis, and angiogenesis. The oral mucosa is a "privileged" site in the adult in that it retains a fetal-like mode of regenerative wound healing; it is, therefore, of interest that gingival fibroblasts are unusual in that they continue to express a fetal-like phenotype with respect to their persistent production of MSF in the adult.[97]

Fetal skin fibroblasts differ from adult cells in terms of their elevated basal level of migration and hyaluronan synthesis.[98,99] Initial data with function neutralizing anti-MSF antibodies have confirmed that these two phenotypic characteristics of fetal fibroblasts are mediated by MSF. Fetal skin has a significantly higher content of hyaluronan compared to adult skin[100] and fetal wound healing differs from its adult counterpart in terms of the magnitude and persistence of the accompanying elevation in hyaluronan content.[101,102] The experimental depletion of hyaluronan in healing fetal wounds (by the application of *Streptomyces* hyaluronate lyase) results in the acquisition of a more adult-like mode of healing.[103] Conversely, the application of either hyaluronan gel or (more recently) ester cross-linked sheets have been reported to promote the healing of different chronic wounds, including diabetic foot ulcers.[104] The *in situ* induction of hyaluronan synthesis by topically applied MSF may prove more clinically efficacious than applied hyaluronan as a consequence of the physiological deposition pattern (perhaps in combination with specific binding proteins) of the former.

As discussed in preceding sections, the induction of angiogenesis is a critical event in acute wound healing and is required for the induction of a healing response in chronic ulcers.[5] It is, therefore, not surprising that a considerable amount of interest is currently devoted to the identification of novel and clinically efficacious pro- and antiangiogenic agents.[105] Proangiogenic agents will most probably need to be administered locally, as patients with chronic ulcers (due to a local insufficiency in vascular perfusion) may suffer from excessive angiogenesis at other sites, eg, retinopathy in

patients with diabetes.[106] Angiogenic factors (such as MSF and its mimetics) may be applied to a wound site by different means. The pharmacological approach simply involves application of the active compound in an inert delivery vehicle. Application of wound-healing cytokines (either singly or in combination) has resulted in limited clinical success.[107,108] Other workers have explored the use of locally administered matrikines as part of a clinical management strategy aimed at evoking a regenerative response.[21] Although useful in certain applications, it is our contention that the clinical efficacy of this approach may be compromised as a consequence of the existence of a suboptimal macromolecular matrix in the recipient wound site. To address this issue, a complementary "tissue-engineering" approach involves the implantation of matrices, which can provide a permissive scaffold for soluble regulatory molecules produced by the host cells.[109–111] Although some clinical success has been obtained using this approach, it is commonly observed that the lack of sufficient infiltration of the graft by host blood vessels results in its nonintegration and poor clinical outcome.[112] In order to circumvent this problem, a number of investigators have explored the possibility of incorporating a soluble bioactive (angiogenic) factor in combination with a bioengineered matrix scaffold.[113] Our work makes it clear that great attention should be given to the choice of matrix scaffold, which must be (among other criteria) permissive for the particular soluble bioactive employed. Data suggesting the potential clinical utility of MSF incorporated into a native type I collagenous matrix have been obtained in an animal model. This matrix is derived from dermis and is composed of densely packed collagen bundles, and, as indicated in Fig. 10–5A does not support the significant ingrowth of fibroblasts and capillaries, even after 28 days following subcutaneous implantation in rats. In contrast, the prior incorporation of MSF into the matrix resulted in a marked stimulation of fibroblast and capillary ingress (Fig. 10–5B). A complementary approach might involve manipulating the tissue matrix by the application of agents that modify matrix deposition and/or degradation.[114]

SUMMARY

Normal wound healing proceeds through a series of stages orchestrated by the critical balance of stimulatory and inhibitory factors. The interdependent signaling of cytokines and the ECM provide such stimulatory and inhibitory cues and collectively establish the dynamic tissue context of wound healing. It is now recognized that the ECM may modulate wound healing by a number of mechanisms, including (1) receptor-mediated cell signaling and cross talk with cytokine-induced

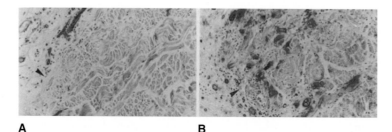

A   **B**

Fig. 10–5. Effects of MSF on angiogenesis and fibroblast migration into collagenous matrices subcutaneously implanted in rat. ***A***. *Control implant.* Blood vessels and fibroblasts principally confined to the host tissue surrounding the implanted matrix. ***B***. *MSF impregnated implant.* Significantly higher numbers of infiltrating blood vessels and fibroblasts in the matrix. All tissues fixed and paraffin-embedded 28 days after implantation. Arrowhead marks the edge of the implant. Blood vessels stained brown with biotinylated Griffonia (Bandeiraea) Simplicifolia Lectin I. Specimens kindly provided by Dr R Oliver, University of Dundee.

pathways, (2) the re-expression of bioactive oncofetal isoforms, such as EDA and EDB fibronectins, (3) cytokine presentation, (4) the liberation of matrikines by local proteolysis, (5) micro- and nanoscale topological features and geometry of interaction with the plasma membrane, and (6) mechanochemical signal transduction resulting from the imposition of matrix-mediated mechanical loading. The bioinductive activity of the ECM, including its capacity to support/modulate the action of soluble factors (such as MSF) on target cells is determined by the net input of these diverse signaling mechanisms. Impaired wound healing may result from perturbations in the critical balance of stimulatory factors, inhibitory factors, and the inductive/modulatory activity of the extracellular matrix. It follows that the therapeutic manipulation of ECM signaling may provide a novel and clinically efficacious target. Our initial data suggest that MSF plays a hitherto unrecognized role in acute wound healing and may afford a novel means of improving the management of patients with recalcitrant nonhealing wounds.

ACKNOWLEDGMENTS

Author's data included in this chapter were obtained in studies funded by: The Dystrophic Epidermolysis Bullosa Research Association (DEBRA), Sir Jules Thorn Charitable Trust, Scottish Office Department of Health, Tenovus Scotland, Joint Diabetes UK and Research Into Ageing Studentship, National Institutes of Health, USA (NIH grant number: 1 RO1 DK9144-01), The Royal Society, The Roche Organ Transplantation Research Foundation (ROTRF, 378986359), Tayside Area Oncology Fund, and the Anonymous Charitable Trust.

REFERENCES

1. Clark RAF. Wound repair: Overview and general considerations. In: Clark RAF, ed. *The Molecular and Cellular Biology of Wound Repair.* 2nd ed. Plenum Press: New York; 1996: 3–50.

2. Martin P. Wound healing: Aiming for perfect skin regeneration. *Science.* 1997;276:75–81.

3. Steed DL. Wound-healing trajectories. *Surg Clin. North Am.* 2003;83:547–555.

4. Manes S, Mira E, Gomez-Mouton C, et al. Cells on the move: A dialogue between polarization and motility. *IUBMB Life.* 2000;49:89–96.

5. Tonnesen MG, Feng X, Clark RA: Angiogenesis and wound healing. *J Invest Dermatol Symp Proc.* 2000;5:40–46.

6. Li Zhang YP, Kirsner RS. Angiogenesis and wound repair: Angiogenic growth factors and the extracellular matrix. *Microsc Res Tech.* 2003;60:107–114.

7. Ravanti L, Kahari VM. Matrix metalloproteinases in wound repair (review). *Int J Mol Med.* 2000;6:391–407.

8. Armstrong DG, Jude EB. The role of matrix metalloproteinases in wound healing. *J Am Podiatr Med Assoc.* 2002;92:12–18.

9. McClain SA, Simon M, Jones E, et al. Mesenchymal activation is the rate-limiting step of granulation tissue induction. *Am J Pathol.* 1996;149:1257–1270.

10. Wang JF, Olson ME, Ball DK, et al. Recombinant connective tissue growth factor modulates porcine skin fibroblast gene expression. *Wound Repair Regen.* 2003;11:220–229.

11. Wary KK, Thakker GD, Humtsoe JO, et al. Analysis of VEGF-responsive genes involved in the activation of endothelial cells. *Mol Cancer.* 2003;2:25–37.

12. Moulin V. Growth factors in skin wound healing. *Eur J Cell Biol.* 1995;68:1–7.

13. Gillitzer R, Goebeler M. Chemokines in cutaneous wound healing. *J Leukoc Biol.* 2001;69:513–521.

14. Lonai P. Epithelial mesenchymal interactions, the ECM and limb development. *J Anat.* 2003;202:43–50.

15. Chiquet-Ehrismann R, Chiquet M. Tenascins: Regulation and putative functions during pathological stress. *J Pathol.* 2003;200:488–499.

16. Haider AS, Grabarek J, Eng B, et al. *In vitro* model of "wound healing" analyzed by laser scanning cytometry: Accelerated healing of epithelial cell monolayers in the presence of hyaluronate. *Cytometry.* 2003;53A:1–8.

17. Condeelis J. The biochemistry of animal cell crawling. In: Soll DR, Wessels, eds. *Motion Analysis of Living Cells.* New York: Wiley-Liss; 1998:85–100.

18. Schwentker A, Vodovotz Y, Weller R et al. Nitric oxide and wound repair: role of cytokines. *Nitric Oxide.* 2002;7:1–10.

19. Clark RA, Brugge JS. Integrins and signal transduction pathways: the road taken. *Science.* 1995;268:233–239.

20. Yamada KM. Adhesive recognition sequences. *J Biol Chem.* 1991;266:12809–12812.

21. Meiners S, Mercado ML. Functional peptide sequences derived from extracellular matrix glycoproteins and their receptors: Strategies to improve neuronal regeneration. *Mol. Neurobiol.* 2003;27:177–196.

22. Pereira M, Simpson-Haidaris PJ. Fibrinogen modulates gene expression in wounded fibroblasts. *Ann NY Acad Sci.* 2001; 936:438–443.

23. Damsky CH, Ilic D. Integrin signaling: Its where the action is. *Curr Opin Cell Biol.* 2002;14:594–602.

24. Hynes RO. Integrins: Bidirectional, allosteric signaling machines. *Cell.* 2002;110:673–687.

25. Schor AM, Schor SL, Allen TD. The effects of culture conditions on the proliferation and morphology of bovine aortic endothelial cells in vitro: Reversible expression of the sprouting cell phenotype. *J Cell Sci.* 1983;62:267–285.

26. Canfield AE, Boot-Handford RP, Schor AM. Thrombospondin gene expression by endothelial cells in culture is modulated by cell proliferation, cell shape and the substratum. *Biochem J.* 1990; 268:225–230.

27. Schor AM, Ellis I, Schor SL: Collagen gel assay for angiogenesis. Induction of endothelial cell sprouting. In: Murray JC. ed. *Methods in molecular medicine, vol 46: angiogenesis protocols.* Totowa, NJ: Humana Press; 2001;145–162.

28. Ingber D. Tensegrity: The architectural basis of cellular mechanotransduction. *Annu Rev Physiol.* 1997;59:575–599.

29. Cukierman E, Pankov R, Yamada KM. Cell interactions in three-dimensional matrices. *Curr Opin Cell Biol.* 2002;14: 633–639.

30. Curtis A, Wilkinson G. Topographical control of cells. *Biomaterials.* 1997;18:1573–1583.

31. Curtis A, Wilkinson O. Reaction of cells to topography. *J Biomater Sci Polymer Ed.* 1998;9:1313–1329.

32. Geiger B, Bershadsky A, Pankov R, et al. Transmembrane cross talk between the extracellular matrix–cytoskeleton cross talk. *Natl. Rev. Mol. Cell Biol.* 2001;2:793–805.

33. Chiquet M. Regulation of extracellular matrix gene expression by mechanical stress. *Matrix Biol.* 1999;18:417–426.

34. Gabbiani G. The myofibroblast in wound healing and fibro-contractive disease. *J Pathol.* 2003; 200:500–503.

35. Schor SL. Cytokine control of cell motility: Modulation and mediation by the extracellular matrix. *Prog Growth Factor Res.* 1994;5:223–248.

36. Ellis I, Schor SL. The interdependent modulation of hyaluronan synthesis by TGFβ-1 and extracellular matrix: Conse-quences for the control of cell migration. *Growth Factors.* 1995; 12:211–222.

37. Ellis IR, Banyard J, Schor SL. Motogenic and biosynthetic response of adult skin fibroblasts to TGFβ isoforms (-1, -2, and -3) determined by "tissue response unit": Role of cell density and substratum. *Cell Biol Int.* 1999;23:593–602.

38. Sutton AM, Canfield AE, Schor SL et al. The response of endothelial cells to TGF-β1 is dependent upon cell shape, proliferative state, and the nature of the substratum. *J Cell Sci.* 1991;99:777–787.

39. Canfield AE, Schor AM. Evidence that tenascin and thrombospondin-1 modulate sprouting of endothelial cells. *J Cell Sci.* 1995;108:797–809.

40. Smyth SS, Petterson C. Tiny dancers: The integrin-growth factor nexus in angiogenic signaling. *J Cell Biol.* 2002; 158:17–21.

41. Borsi L, Castellani P, Risso AM, et al. Transforming growth factor beta regulates the splicing pattern of fibronectin messenger RNA precursor. *FEBS Lett.* 1990;261:175–178.

42. Zhao Y, Young SL. TGF-beta regulates expression of tenascin alternative splicing isoforms in fetal rat lung. *Am J Physiol.* 1995;268:L173–L180.

43. Trojanowska M. Ets factors and regulation of extracellular matrix. *Oncogene.* 2000;19:6464–6471.

44. Bottaro DP. The role of extracellular matrix heparan sulfate glycosaminoglycan in the activation of growth factor signaling pathways. *Ann NY Acad Sci.* 2002;961:158.

45. Iruela-Arispe ML, Dvorak HF. Angiogenesis: A dynamic balance of stimulators and inhibitors. *Thromb Haemost.* 1997;78: 672–677.

46. Phillips SJ. Physiology of wound healing and surgical wound care. *ASAIO J.* 2000;46:S2–S5.

47. Steffensen B, Hakkinen L, Larjava H. Proteolytic events of wound healing: Coordinated interactions among matrix metalloproteinases (MMPs), integrins and extracellular matrix macromolecules. *Crit Rev Oral Biol Med.* 2001;12:373–398.

48. Motegi K, Harada K, Pazouki S, et al. Evidence of a bi-phasic effect of thrombospondin-1 on angiogenesis. *Histochem J.* 2002;34:411–421.

49. Dasu MR, Barrow RE, Spies M, et al. Matrix metalloproteinase expression in cytokine stimulated human dermal fibroblasts. *Burns.* 2003;29:527–531.

50. Schor SL, Schor AM. Tumour–stroma interactions. Phenotypic and genetic alterations in mammary stroma: Implications for tumour progression. *Breast Cancer Res* 2001;3:373–379.

51. Davis GE, Bayless KJ, Davis MJ, et al: Regulation of tissue injury responses by the exposure of matricryptic sites within extracellular matrix molecules. *Am J Pathol.* 2000;156:1489–1498.

52. Schenk S, Quaranta V. Tales from the crypt[ic] sites of the extracellular matrix. *Trends Cell Biol.* 2003;13:366–375.

53. Hynes, R. *Fibronectins.* New York: Springer-Verlag; 1990.

54. Pierschbacher MD, Ruoslahti E. Cell attachment activity of fibronectin can be duplicated by small synthetic fragments of the molecule. *Nature.* 1984;309:30–33.

55. McCarthy JB, Chelberg MK, Mickelson DJ, et al. Localization and chemical synthesis of fibronectin peptides with melanoma adhesion and heparin binding activities. *Biochemistry.* 1988;27:1380–1388.

56. Humphries MJ. The molecular basis and specificity of integrin-ligand interaction. *J Cell Sci.* 1990;97:585–592.

57. Mould AP, Humphries MJ. Identification of a novel recognition sequence for the integrin α4β1 in the COOH-terminal heparin binding domain of fibronectin. *EMBO J.* 1991;10, 4089–4095.

58. Woods A, McCarthy JB, Furcht LT, et al. A synthetic peptide from the COOH-terminal heparin-binding domain of fibronectin promotes focal adhesion formation. *Mol Biol Cell.* 1993;4:605–613.

59. Schor SL, Ellis I, Banyard J, et al. Motogenic activity of the IGD amino acid motif. *J Cell Sci.* 1999;112:3879–3888.

60. French-Constant C: Alternative splicing of fibronectin: Many different proteins but few different functions. *Exp Cell Res.* 1995;221:261–271.

61. Kornblihtt AR, Pesce CG, Alonso CR, et al. The fibronectin gene as a model for splicing and transcription studies. *FASEB J.* 1996;10:248–257.

62. French-Constant C, Van De Water L, Dvorak HF. Reappearance of an embryonic pattern of fibronectin splicing during wound healing in the adult rat. *J Cell Biol.* 1989;109:903–914.

63. Wysocki AB, Grinnell F. Fibronectin profiles in normal and chronic wound fluid. *Lab Invest.* 1990;63:825–831.

64. Muir D, Manthorpe M. Stromelysin generates a fibronectin fragment that inhibits Schwann cell proliferation. *J Cell Biol.* 1992;116:177–185.

65. Fukai F, Iso T, Sekiguchi K, et al. An amino-terminal fibronectin fragment stimulates the differentiation of ST-13 preadipocytes. *Biochemistry.* 1993;32:5746–5751.

66. Schor SL, Ellis I, Dolman C, et al. Substratum-dependent stimulation of fibroblast migration by the gelatin-binding domain of fibronectin. *J Cell Sci.* 1996;109:2581–2590.

67. Clark RAF, Wikner NE, Doherty DE, et al. Cryptic chemotactic activity of fibronectin for human monocytes resides in the 120-kDa fibroblastic cell-binding fragment. *J Biol Chem.* 1988;263:12115–12123.

68. Tremble PM, Damsky CH, Werb Z. Fibronectin fragments, but not intact fibronectin, signalling through the fibronectin receptor induce metalloproteinase gene expression in fibroblasts. *Matrix Suppl.* 1992;1:212–214.

69. Fukai F, Suzuki H, Suzuki K, et al. Rat plasma fibronectin contains two distinct chemotactic domains for fibroblastic cells. *J Biol Chem.* 1991;246:8807–8813.

70. Fukai F, Ohtaki M, Fugii N, et al. Release of biological activities from quiescent fibronectin by a conformational change and limited proteolysis by matrix metalloproteinases. *Biochemistry.* 1995;34. 11453–11459.

71. Ohashi T, Kiehart DP, Erickson HP. Dynamics and elasticity of the fibronectin matrix in living cell culture visualized by fibronectin-green fluorescent protein. *Proc Natl Acad Sci U S A.* 1999;96:2153–2158.

72. Hangai M, Kitaya N, Xu J, et al. Matrix metalloproteinase-9-dependent exposure of cryptic migratory control site in collagen is required before retinal angiogenesis. *Am J Pathol.* 2002;161:1429–1437.

73. Colorado PC, Torre A, Kamphaus G, et al. Anti-angiogenic cues from vascular basement membrane collagen. *Cancer Res.* 2000;60:2520–2526.

74. Khan KM, Falcone DJ. Selective activation of MAPK9erkl/2) by laminin-1 peptide alphal 1 :ser(2091)-Arg(2108 regulates

75. Khan KM, Laurie GW, McCaffrey TA, et al. Exposure of cryptic domains in the alpha 1-chain of laminin-1 by elastase stimulates macrophages urokinase and matrix metalloproteinase-9 expression. *J Biol Chem.* 2002;277:13778–13786.

76. O'Reilly MS, Holmgren L, Shing Y, et al. Angiostatin: A novel angiogenesis inhibitor that mediates the supression of metastasis by a Lewis lung carcinoma. *Cell.* 1994;79:315–328.

77. Lishko VR, Kudryk B, Yakubenko VP. Regulated unmasking of the cryptic binding site for integrin alpha M beta 2 in the gamma C-domain of fibrinogen. *Biochemistry.* 2002;41: 12942–12951.

78. D'Amore PA. Tales of the cryptic: Unveiling more angiogenesis inhibitors. *Trends Mol. Med.* 2002;8:313–315.

79. Pirie-Shepard SR. Regulation of angiogenesis by the hemostatic system. *Front Biosci.* 2003;8:286–293.

80. Lees VC, Fan TP, West DC. Angiogenesis in a delayed revascularization model is accelerated by angiogenic oligosaccharides of hyaluronan. *Lab Invest.* 1995;73:259–266.

81. Savani RC, Cao G, Pooler PM, et al. Differential involvement of the hyaluronan (HA) receptors CD44 and receptor of HA-mediated motility in endothelial cell function and angiogenesis. *J Biol Chem.* 2001;276:36770–36778.

82. Slevin M, Kumar S, Gaffney J. Angiogenic oligosaccharides of hyaluronan induce multiple signaling pathways affecting vascular endothelial cell mitogenic and wound healing responses. *J Biol Chem.* 2002;277:41046–41059.

83. Schor SL, Ellis IR, Jones SJ, et al. Migration Stimulating Factor (MSF): A genetically-truncated onco-fetal fibronectin isoform expressed by carcinoma and tumor-associated stromal cells. *Cancer Res.* 2004; 63: 8827–8836.

84. Ellis I, Grey AM, Schor AM, Schor SL. Antagonistic effects of transforming growth factor beta and MSF on fibroblast migration and hyaluronic acid synthesis: Possible implications for wound healing. *J Cell Sci.* 1992;102:447–456.

85. Picardo M, McGurk M, Schor SL. Identification of migration stimulating factor in wound fluid. *Exp Mol Pathol.* 1992;57: 8–21.

86. Morla A, Zhang Z, Ruoslahti E. Superfibronectin is a functionally distinct form of fibronectin. *Nature.* 1994; 367:193–196.

87. Satyanarayana K, Shoskes DA. A molecular injury-response model for the understanding of chronic disease. *Mol Med.* 1997;3:331–334.

88. Tuan T-L, Nichter LS. The molecular basis of keloid and hyptrophic scar formation. *Mol Med.* 1998;4:19–24.

89. Fray MJ, Dickinson RP, Huggins JP. A potent, selective inhibitor of matrix metalloproteinase-3 for the topical treatment of chronic dermal ulcers. *J Med Chem.* 2003;46:3514–3525.

90. Lohmann R, Ambrosch A, Schultz G, et al. Expression of matrix-metalloproteinases and their inhibitors in the wounds of diabetic and non-diabetic patients. *Diabetologia.* 2002;45: 1011–1016.

91. Wall SJ, Sampson MJ, Levell N, et al. Elevated matrix metalloproteinase-2 and -3 production from human diabetic dermal fibroblasts. *Br J Dermatol.* 2003;149:13–16.

92. Buhler-Singer S, Hiller D, Albrecht HP, et al. Disturbances of cutaneous microcirculation in patients with diabetic legs:

macrophage degradative phenotype. *J Biol Chem.* 2000;275: 4492–4498.

Additional parameters for a new therapeutic concept? *Acta Dermatol Venereol.* 1994;74:250–256.

93. McCallion RL, Ferguson MWJ. Fetal wound healing and the development of antiscarring therapies for adult wound healing. In: Clark RAF. ed. *The Molecular and Cellular Biology of Wound Repair.* 2nd ed. New York: Plenum Press; 1996: 561–600.

94. Ferguson MWJ, Howarth GF. Marsupial models of scarless fetal wound healing. In Adzick NS, Longaker MT. eds. *Fetal Wound Healing.* New York: Elsevier Scientific; 1992: 95–124.

95. Lorenz HP, Longaker MT, Whitby DJ, et al. Scarless fetal skin repair is intrinsic to the fetal fibroblast. *Surg Forum.* 1992; 43:696–697.

96. Schor SL, Ellis I, Banyard J, et al. Fetal-like phenotypic characteristics of gingival fibroblasts: Potential relevance to wound healing. *Oral Dis.* 1996;2:155–166.

97. Irwin CR, Picardo M, Ellis I, et al. Inter- and intra-site heterogeneity in the expression of fetal-like phenotypic characteristics by gingival fibroblasts: Potential significance for wound healing. *J Cell Sci.* 1994;107:1333–1346.

98. Schor SL, Schor AM, Rushton G, et al. Adult, fetal and transformed fibroblasts display different migratory phenotypes on collagen gels: Evidence for an isoformic transition during fetal development. *J Cell Sci.* 1985;73:221–234.

99. Chen J, Grant ME, Schor AM, et al. Differences between adult and foetal fibroblasts in the regulation of hyaluronate synthesis: Correlation with migratory activity. *J Cell Sci.* 1989;94:577–589.

100. West DC, Shaw DM, Lorenz P, et al. Fibrotic healing of adult and late gestation fetal wounds correlates with increased hyaluronidase activity and removal of hyaluronan. *Int J Biochem Cell Biol.* 1997;29:201–210.

101. Krummel TM, Nelson JM, Diegelmann RF, et al. Fetal response to injury in the rabbit. *J Pediatr Surg.* 1987;22:640–644.

102. Longaker MT, Chiu ES, Adzick NS, et al. Studies in fetal wound healing: V. A prolonged expression of hyaluronic acid characterizes fetal wound healing. *Ann Surg.* 1991;213: 292–296.

103. Mast BA, Haynes JH, Krummel TM, et al. *In vivo* degradation of fetal wound hyaluronic acid results in increased fibroplasia, collagen deposition and neovascularization. *Plast Recontr Surg.* 1992;89:503–509.

104. Ballard K, Cantor AJ. Treating recalcitrant diabetic wounds with hyaluronic acid: a review of patients. *Ostomy Wound Manage.* 2003;49:37–49.

105. Mazitschek R, Baumhof P, Giannis A. Peptidomimetics and angiogenesis. *Mini Rev Med Chem.* 2002;2:491–506.

106. Martin A, Komada MR, Sane DC. Abnormal angiogenesis in diabetes mellitus. *Med Res Rev.* 2003, 23:117–145.

107. Kunimoto BT. Growth factors in wound healing: The next great innovation. *Ostomy Wound Manage.* 1999;45:56–64.

108. Bennett SP, Griffiths GD, Schor SL, et al. The use of growth factors in the treatment of chronic diabetic foot ulcers. *Br J Surg.* 2003;90:133–146.

109. Clark RA. Fibrin and wound healing. *Ann NY Acad Sci.* 2001;936:355–367.

110. Badylak SF. The extracellular matrix as a scaffold for tissue reconstruction. *Semin. Cell Develop Biol.* 2002;13:377–383.

111. Tonello C, Zavan B, Cortivo R, et al. *In vitro* reconstruction of human dermal equivalent enriched with endothelial cells. *Biomaterials.* 2003;24:1205–1211.

112. Cassell OC, Hofer SO, Morrison WA, et al. Vascularization of tissue-engineered grafts: The regulation of angiogenesis in reconstructive surgery and disease states. *Br J Plastic Surg.* 2002;55:603–610.

113. Bottaro DP, Liebmann-Vinson A, Heidaran MA. Molecular signaling in bioengineered tissue microenvironments. *Ann NY Acad Sci.* 2002;961:143–153.

114. Fray MJ, Dickinson RP, Huggins JP. A potent, selective inhibitor of matrix metalloproteinase-3 for the topical treatment of chronic dermal ulcers. *J Med Chem.* 2003;46: 3514–3525.

11 Management of Acute Wounds

Zahid B. M. Niazi and Justin Sacks

Historical Background
Wound Characteristics
Wound Management
General Principles
Dressings
  Types of Dressing
Suture Material, Tapes, and Glues
  Sutures

Staples
Tapes
Tissue Adhesives
Specific Wounds Requiring Special Attention
Hyperbaric Oxygen Therapy
Specific Procedures for Wound Closure
  Types of Flaps
References

Acute wound management should incorporate the basics, which consists of knowing the mechanism of injury, stabilizing the patient, provision of tetanus coverage, and then débriding and irrigating wounds prior to attempting wound closure. All wounds, whether accidental or iatrogenic, ie, surgical, need to be brought into bacterial balance prior to closure either primarily or by delayed primary, secondary, or tertiary intention. Numerous reconstructive options can be used including skin grafts, local or free flaps for wounds with tissue deficit or those requiring coverage of important underlying structures. Dressings play an important role in wound management as these can provide a moist environment with an appropriate pH, as exemplified by hydrocolloid dressings, or a closed system, as exemplified by a vacuum-assisted closure (VAC) dressing.

HISTORICAL BACKGROUND

The history of medicine correlates closely with the history of wound management. Ritualistic teachings passed from one generation to the next are historically the first evidence of formalized wound care. The "three healing gestures" described around 2200 BC on an ancient clay tablet discuss washing the wound, applying plasters, which were considered wound-healing remedies, and bandaging the wound.[1] Ancient physicians of Egypt, Greece, India, and Europe practiced methods of wound care that gave particular importance to foreign body removal, cleansing of the wound, approximating skin edges, and protecting the

wound with clean bandages. The apposition of wounds in the early and middle ages was with flax, hemp, fascia, hair, linen strips, pig's bristles, reeds, grasses, and even the mouth parts of pincher ants.

The use of gunpowder and its associated sequelae, blast wounds, accelerated the pace of acute wound management. In the 1300s and for the next several hundred years, open wounds were treated more aggressively than previously described. The physician took a more active role than just cleanliness and the application of clean dressings. Gunpowder was felt to be a poison and treating the wound with oils, cautery, and scalding water was thought to be the appropriate way to drive out the "poison."

Ambroise Paré, a French army surgeon, helped usher in the modern era of acute wound care in the 16th century. During his first campaign at the battle of Villaine, he treated gunshot wounds in the standard fashion with hot oils. At one point he ran out of oil and dressed the soldiers wounds with a mixture of egg yolk, oil of roses, and turpentine. He observed the soldier's wounds treated with hot oils were swollen and painful. Wounds treated more conservatively were found to heal rapidly and without associated complications. Paré described this new treatment and vowed "never so cruelly to burn poor wounded men."[2]

As evidenced in other areas of medicine, the major wars of the 19th and 20th century have contributed to wound care. The violent mechanism of injury assaulted the human body in ways never before experienced in the history of mankind. It was not until the aseptic techniques, as advocated by Lister, that infection rates decreased and surgical wound care became more popular and successful.

With the advent of the scientific methodology and advances in molecular biology, the cellular changes that occur during wound healing have become clear. This knowledge has helped to advance the management of the acute wound. Concurrent to this advancement in basic science, there have also been advances in products used to repair wounds. In the early 1900s, natural organic protein products including silk, cotton, and catgut became available. Polyester and Nylon were the first synthetic materials available in the 1940s. In the 20th century, major advances, included the introduction of antibiotics, which began with the discovery of penicillin by Ian Fleming in 1929. This augmented the physician's arsenal in dealing with acute wounds.

However, the most significant advances during the 20th century for the management of acute wounds has been the availability of healthy and reliable wound coverage options. Reconstruction of the simple acute wounds may be carried out with skin grafts and or local flaps, but the more complex wounds require more complex local or distant flaps. The evolution of muscle and musculocutanoeus flaps, fascia, and fasciocutaneous flaps, based on axial blood supplies, have augmented the management of the acute wound, while microvascular tissue transplantation has paved the way for an unparalleled advance in acute wound management.

WOUND CHARACTERISTICS

The definition of an acute wound is the traumatic loss of normal structure and function as a result of a noxious insult to recently uninjured tissue. The ability of the living creatures to heal an acute wound is fundamental to its survival. In the human body, this has been studied closely. Three phases of wound healing are recognized. These can be classified on both the macroscopic and the microscopic level and are the inflammatory, proliferative, and remodeling phases. These are well documented; we will touch upon some of the more pertinent points briefly.

From a surgeon's perspective, knowledge of the anatomy and physiology of skin forms the basis of management protocols. Skin is a bilaminate structure generally 1.2 mm in thickness with a range of 0.5 to 6 mm. It is the largest organ in the body with its main function being protection. It protects against injury, regulates fluid loss or gain, monitors and controls temperature, provides immunologic surveillance, and controls invasion of microorganisms. Dermis is 20 to 30 times thicker than the epidermis and contains nervous, vascular, lymphatic, and support structures for the epidermis. The fibrous component of the dermis provides the durable matrix and is composed of collagen with type I being the most common. Type III collagen is found in higher concentrations in fetal development and early stages of wound healing. The nonfibrous or noncollagenous portion is mainly composed of glycosaminoglycans and their proteoglycans. Collagen synthesis peaks at 7 days postinjury. This is coincident with a rapid increase in tensile strength. The healing wound achieves the greatest mass at 3 weeks and then gradually remodels itself over the next 6 to 12 months. The wound will achieve only 15 to 20% of its ultimate strength by 3 weeks and only 60% by 3 to 4 months. It continues to regain strength slowly until 18 to 24 months.

Immediately after injury, the wound edges retract, thus increasing the size of the defect. This retraction occurs as the normal skin tension pulls along the lines of minimal tension. Wounds perpendicular to the normal skin tension lines place the wound under greater tension and thus may result in larger scars. Over the next few days the wound size shrinks as the edges move toward the center. This phenomenon is called *wound contraction* and is independent of presence of collagen or epithelialization. It is a normal physiologic process that is different from contracture, which results from scar shortening. Contracture becomes more apparent whenever the normal healing process is prolonged and can result in formation of hypertrophic scars. It is important to realize that an optimal inflammatory phase and decreased wound tension will help in producing a thinner, more aesthetic scar. The magnitude of static skin tension is directly related to ultimate scar width. Uneven, jagged wounds have greater surface area than linear lacerations. Therefore, skin tension is distributed over a greater area and is less per unit of tissue. Meticulous reapproximation of tissues results in a reasonable scar.

Karl Langer, a German anatomist, described the existence of natural skin tension lines from his observations in the 18th century. The clinical implications of his work is a recommendation to place incisions in the direction of Langer's lines or natural skin creases. Skin forces produced by muscular contraction and flexion/extension influence healing and scar size. These dynamic forces are greater where skin elasticity is necessary for function. Lacerations parallel to skin folds, lines of expression, and joints do not impair function and usually form excellent scars. The reverse is true for wounds that traverse the Langer's or joint lines where as these scars are more prone to dehiscence or hypertrophic formation.

Delayed wound healing results from interference in the normal pattern of wound healing. This can occur during coagulation, inflammation, collagen synthesis, the immune response, epithelializaton, and scar contraction with remodeling.[3] Local or systemic attributes of the organism can interfere with the healing process at any of these components of the wound-healing process. Local factors include ischemia, infection, foreign bodies, radiation, and trauma. Systemic factors affecting wound healing include age, alcoholism, diabetes, hepatic dysfunction, nutritional deficiencies, and uremia. These local and systemic factors all can interfere with wound healing. The key to management of the acute wound is to treat these factors in conjunction with the acute wound.

A patient with peripheral vascular disease or in an immunocompromised state may heal poorly. Other specific risk factors for wound morbidity are: delay in treatment of the acute injury; a crushing mechanism; deep penetrating wounds; high-velocity missiles; and contamination with saliva, feces, soil or other foreign bodies. Bacteria disrupt the normal healing process. They interfere with the inflammatory phase and collagen deposition. In addition, they interfere with epithelialization and wound contraction. Bacterial loads greater than 100,000 organisms per gram of tissue retard the wound-healing process.[4] Every effort must be made to reduce the bacterial count of a wound. This will include strict debridement of all devitalized tissue and foreign material. Anything that can act as a nidus for infection, must be removed in an appropriate manner.

As early as 3 hours after acute trauma, bacteria can proliferate to a level to cause infection. Lacerations produced by fine cutting instruments resist infection better than those due to crush. Reduction of blood flow to wound edges may increase infective concentration 100-fold. High-velocity missile injuries can produce damage far beyond their tract. Wounds contaminated by foreign material have high infection rate despite adequate therapeutic measures. Saliva and feces have a concentration of bacteria approximately double that needed to produce infection. The presence of soil in the wound raises the infective potential of bacteria.

Epithelialization is a mechanism whereby cells migrate across the wound to seal it. Cells in the basal cell layer in the wound edge show mitosis within hours of injury. The presence of eschar or other debris impedes this process. This can be reinitiated by proper cleansing and debridement of the wound. Furthermore, a clean wound if kept moist and protected will show epithelialization proceeding at a maximum rate. In a surgically repaired laceration, epithelialization bridges the defect within 24–48 hours. The new tissue proceeds to thicken and grow downward, beginning to resemble the layered structural characteristics of an uninjured epidermis within 5 days. Simultaneously, keratin formation loosens the overlying scab.

WOUND MANAGEMENT

An acute wound is considered a compromise in the inherent structure of the skin and subcutaneous tissues. When evaluating an acute open wound, the basic principles of

medical management should be followed. This includes stabilizing the patient, providing tetanus coverage and completing a detailed history and physical examination. An important component of wound management is to identify the mechanism of injury. This sets the foundation for the next few steps that will be undertaken, including immediate wound debridement and irrigation. Prophylactic antibiotic coverage may be needed depending on the type of the wound, the depth of the injury, the surface area involved, the deeper structures affected and, in some patients, the associated physiologic response of the body to the wound and the wounding agent. Systemic effects of the wound may require other medical management in an acute setting necessitating intensive care monitoring. All wounds whether accidental or iatrogenic need to be brought into bacterial balance prior to closure either by primary, delayed primary, secondary or tertiary intention.

A clinical diagnosis of structures damaged can be confirmed by exploring the wound in a sterile environment under local or general anesthesia. The wound is debrided of necrotic tissue, contaminated tissue, and foreign bodies are removed. Hematomas are evacuated and hemostasis secured. If tissues need to be revascularized, there is only a narrow window of opportunity to do so and the patient should be transferred in a stable condition to centers capable of providing appropriate care. A simple wound extending to the dermis or subcutaneous tissue can be closed primarily. A wound with damaged and exposed fascia, muscle or bone might require repair of structures and local or distant flaps to help close the acute wound. In some patients, further studies, such as angiography might need to be obtained to evaluate the vascularity of the wound, if wound coverage requires transfer of a free flap. Patients with burn wounds requiring hospitalization also need specialized care and these patients should be started on an appropriate resuscitation regimen, stabilized, and then transferred.

In certain cases, open wounds may need to be temporized, if the patient is either not stable or requires sequential procedures by the plastic surgical or other teams. These temporizing measures can take the form of nonadherent fabrics, absorptive normal saline and gauze dressings, occlusive biologic and nonbiologic dressings, and additional creams and ointment dressings.[5] Mechanical devices have also been developed to perform the function of standard dressings for the acute wound that is unable to be closed primarily. The VAC (vacuum-assisted closure device by KCI) has been developed for this need. It consists of a piece of foam covered by an occlusive dressing connected to a suction pump. This device has shown to increase local blood flow, decrease edema, reduce bacterial proliferation, and augment granulation tissue formation in wounds.[6]

Digital and extremity wounds require specific evaluation. Finger lacerations rarely gape. To examine these wounds properly, the digit and extremity are placed through a full range of active and passive movement. This enables identification of injured structures, specifically tendons and muscles, which may have been in a different state of tension and are located at a more proximal or distal location than the skin laceration. Wounds may need to be extended to properly identify all damaged structures and for their repair.

Some foreign bodies may not be visible on plain x-ray films. These include organic substances like wood and also glass less than 1 mm in thickness. These patients may need further investigation and a thorough examination, under tourniquet, if the wounds are located on extremities. Failure to perform these investigations under hemostatic conditions can cause undue harm to adjacent tissue.

GENERAL PRINCIPLES

Accidents resulting in lacerations are one of the most common reasons for a person to visit an emergency room (ER). There are 11 million ER visits per annum in the United States secondary to traumatic lacerations.[7] The enormity of the number of these injuries creates a need for the health care provider to have a protocol that will simplify the management of these acute wounds.

The wound characteristics dictate the type of repair or reconstruction needed to attain a healed wound. Wounds are classified as simple and complex. Simple wounds, consist of those with a cutaneous laceration but have no tissue deficit. These are usually cleaned and repaired in the ER by coaptation of the skin layers. Some simple wounds that involve a larger body surface area or those in a child may require surgery under general anesthesia. Complex wounds are those that either fail attempts at closure or the nature of the defect/injury is such that it requires more than simple debridement and reconstruction.

Lacerations are common skin wounds and can be handled by following the basic principles. In most instances, supporting the dermis with a resorbable suture that provides wound support for at least an 8 to 10-week period, produces the most aesthetically pleasing scar. Dead space must be obliterated to decrease the risk of hematoma or seroma formation. The epidermal sutures can then be placed without tension and can be removed early to prevent railroad-track suture.

Crush injuries are the result of intense, focal pressure placed on hard and soft tissue structures. Natural disasters, structural collapse, falls, high-speed motor vehicle accidents, and the unfortunate sequelae of war are some examples of crushing trauma that the tissues of the human body are exposed to.

In the ER or upon initial evaluation it is often difficult to assess viability of tissue structures. One way is to observe the wound in a temporal manner. Another way is to give the patient intravenous fluoroscein. This substance is helpful in predicting the survival of compromised tissue. Based on this information, it is required to acknowledge that these wounds may require a "second-look" procedure prior to definitive wound closure or coverage. This is not unreasonable if the goal is to preserve as much native tissue as possible in the acute wound while not compromising wound healing.

Abrasions are superficial injuries through varied levels of the dermis. These wounds need to be scrubbed thoroughly to remove all foreign bodies. This will prevent traumatic tattoo formation.

Most nonmilitary wounds can be closed primarily. This is based on the understanding that these injuries occur from low-velocity trauma. The zone of injury is not as extensive as those compared to the so-called military injuries, since the force of the injury is not as tremendous. The wound is washed with an antimicrobial solution. The pulse lavage is a tool that is helpful not only in delivering large amounts of irrigation but also delivers it at high pressures to an acute wound. Local or general anesthesia is used to accurately probe the wound in order to determine the extent of injury. The wound is sharply débrided of its nonvascularized tissue and all foreign bodies are removed.

Military wounds are considered a different entity. These are wounds caused by high-velocity weapons and devices. The standard management of acute wound care should be adhered to. However, these wounds often require reexplorations 24 to 48 hours after initial injury and temporizing procedures are performed in instances where the patient must first be medically stabilized. Once the patient is stable, reconstructive options can be evaluated. Either the patient can be closed primarily or there will be a need for more complicated reconstruction of the tissues. In these type of high-velocity injuries, delayed closure should always be considered first.

All wounds contain some level of bacterial innoculum. The role of débridement and lavage decreases this innoculum and allows effective primary closure. If a tissue deficit is present then keeping the bacterial count low with dressings is an important intermediate step prior to wound coverage with skin grafts, local, or distant flaps. Successful adherence of biologic dressings, such as cadaver or xenograft, indicate acceptable bacterial count and infers that one can proceed with formal reconstruction using autologous tissue.

Wound infection occurs when the number of pathogenic organisms in the wound exceeds the ability of the wound to control them. In most species, this level is 100,000 bacterial organisms per gram of tissue. When the levels of bacteria are higher than this level, the wound healing process is inhibited. Débridement is the most effective and important way of decreasing the bacterial load of wound. Devitalized tissue is removed along with infected tissue. Frequent dressing changes, is another form of conservative débridement that is beneficial for improved wound care.

Systemic antibiotics are of little use if necrotic tissue persists in the wound. There is no proven benefit in wound healing to administer systemic antibiotics prior to wound closure. In addition there is inadequate penetration of the antibiotics into granulating beds. In general, the goal of acute wound care is for wounds to be closed primarily. However, there are instances where this is not possible. The acute wound may be allowed to contract and heal secondarily under specific circumstances.

When considering wound-management options, if all tissues are present, than primary closure is performed usually within the first 24 hours. Delayed primary closure is defined as closure around 4–5 days. In other situations, the acute wound is allowed to heal secondarily with the development of granulation tissue and subsequent epithelialzation. There are particular instances where there is an absence of soft tissue in order to close an acute wound. In such instances, advancement closure or local tissue rearrangement by advancement or transposition flaps can be performed. The areas where the flaps are mobilized from may need coverage. These defects are called secondary defects and they may require other flaps or skin grafts. Tissues imported from a distance to provide coverage can include pedicled or free flaps. The imported tissues may be cutaneous, fascial, muscle, combination, or deeper structure flaps, including bones, tendons, and nerves.

Other principles to keep in mind include the following. Wounds with high static and dynamic tension that require meticulous closure cannot be closed with staples or tape. Wound edges should be everted if using a stapling device for wound closure. When deep sutures are placed, this reduces tension to the skin but no sutures are to be placed in adipose tissue. Use sutures in the dermal layer if using cyanoacrylate glue for skin apposition in those wounds that require more than simple or single-layer closure. A careful surgical technique includes avoiding blind clamping of a wound edge or deep structures, as this is likely to cause irreparable damage. While suturing wounds, the suture needle should enter perpendicular to skin for even-depth wounds and even-sized bites of the wound edges should be taken. Wounds with uneven edges require a shallow bite of the higher edge and a deeper bite of the lower edge (higher high and lower low) for good coaptation. It is well documented that even 5% povidone iodine solution is toxic to polymorphonuclear neutrophil leukocytes whereas a 1% solution is safe and effective with little or no toxicity. Preoperative hair removal by razor is shown to increase chances of wound infection by three to nine times. Evidence suggests that 0.9% normal saline solution may be as effective when used with high-pressure syringe irrigation (7–8 pounds per square inch or psi) when compared with commercial irrigation techniques (50–70 psi). In general, pressures greater than 7 psi significantly decrease the number of bacteria. A 30-cc syringe with an 18-gauge needle or angiocatheter can yield adequate pressures for wound irrigation.

DRESSINGS

Dressings create a microenvironment that affects the biology of healing. The optimum wound climate must not interfere with the activity of fibroblasts and macrophages. The production of granulation tissue and migration of epithelial cells must be optimized.

Several factors need to be considered. Certain dressings prevent evaporation of water and keep tissues moist. A drying wound produces a thick hardened scab that impedes the process of epithelialization. Excess fluid can cause maceration and may become potential for infection. Gaseous permeability is essential as epithelialization increases in the presence of oxygen. The dressings should be impermeable to bacteria and other particulate matter. Newly developed tissues should not be traumatized by the dressings or during change of dressings. Thus, the ideal dressing should be nonadherent, permeable to water vapor, but not to bacteria, and should absorb some fluid, but it will not dessicate the wound.

Vapor-permeable membranes improve healing and decrease patient discomfort. Wounds covered with vapor-permeable dressings fill with granulation tissue before re-epithelializing. This is a unique phenomenon specific to moist wound healing (factor in fluid increases rate of fibroblast production).

Types of Dressings

There are innumerable dressings on the market; we will discuss only a few of the ones more commonly used.

1. The traditional wet to dry dressings have a place in débriding infected and or necrotic wounds.

2. Nonadherent dressings like telfa or Vaseline-impregnated dressings are excellent for protecting skin grafts and newly laid epithelium, decreasing the amount of pain that the patient undergoes during dressing changes.

3. Cotton balls soaked with mineral oil dressings are excellent for molding and compressing wounds and grafts. These dressings are hygroscopic and do not become caked with blood. Thus, they are easier to

remove, with less chances of damage to the new graft and are relatively less painful for the patient during dressing changes.

4. Calcium alginate dressings have been developed from seaweed. They have been shown to promote development of granulation tissue and are also used as dressings over dermal wounds, including split-thickness skin graft (STSG) donor sites. In the latter instance, the dressings can be kept in place until the wound heals.

5. Biobrane is a synthetic dressing developed for cutaneous dermal injuries including second-degree skin burns and STSG donor sites. These dressings can be kept in place until the wound heals.

6. Hydrocolloid dressings provide a closed wound, which promotes healing and protects the neoepithelium. These may require changing every 3 to 5 days.

7. Negative-pressure closed-system dressings, like the VAC, were developed by Morykwas et al.[6] and have revolutionized the conservative management of a wound. These dressings have been noted to have beneficial effects in wound-edge blood flow and proliferation of granulation tissue, while maintaining a closed-wound environment. The excess secretions from the wound are removed without soiling the patients' clothes or the bed. It significantly decreases the nursing time involved in changing dressings, as they may not need to be changed for 2 to 5 days. It is comfortable for the patient and, in some instances like sternal wounds, it can significantly decrease the patient's pain as it stabilizes the wound.

8. Opsite or Tegaderm dressings are semipermeable occlusive dressings that provide a closed wound. These dressings also do not need to be changed until the wound heals, unless they develop a leak or excess fluid develops beneath the dressing. Thus, an ideal dressing helps protect wounds, immobilize the area, evenly compress the wound site, absorbs secretions, and is aesthetically acceptable.

SUTURE MATERIAL, TAPES, AND GLUES

Sutures

An ideal suture is inert to metabolism, resistant to infection, has great tensile strength, does not tear tissue, is easy to work with, and available in cutting and noncutting needles. Suture material can be classified according to its absorbability. In general, those materials that maintain their tensile strength more than 60 days are considered nonabsorbable, while those that absorb in less than 60 days are called absorbable. The second classification relies on the source and nature of the material. Biologic substances like catgut, collagen, silk, linen, and cotton produce the greatest tissue reaction and, in general, have the lowest tensile strength but they usually have good knot security. Synthetic substances like Polyester (Dacron), Polyamide (Nylon), Polypropylene (Prolene), Polyglycolide and Polylactide Polymers (Dexon, Vicryl), Polydiaxonon (PDS), and steel have more tensile strength and less tissue reaction. These sutures tend to be more difficult to handle and have less knot security.

Staples

Staples are useful in rapidly closing wounds, but attention has to be given to evert the wound edges to get good coaptation. These also do not have a tissue reaction, but, if not applied correctly or if all the wound is being supported by the staples alone, then they can result in wound dehiscence in the early phase of healing or poor scars in the latter phase of healing.

Tapes

Steristrips or tapes are useful for coapting wounds or supporting closed wounds. These cannot be used for hairy areas and the area of application has to be maintained dry. These closures have the highest dehiscence rate as they have one of the lowest tensile strength.

Tissue Adhesives

The common medical tissue adhesives in use are the 2-octylcyanoacrylates. These came to the American market in 1988, but have been in common use in Europe and Canada for a couple of decades. If tissue adhesive is used on the skin, then topical antibacterial or other moisturizers cannot be used. If a wound is deep then the deeper layers have to be supported with sutures before coapting the skin with the tissue adhesive to decrease the incidence of dehiscence and poor scarring. For the superficial wounds, it is a useful technique as local anesthetic may not be needed, which makes the ER visits a little less unpleasant for children.

SPECIFIC WOUNDS REQUIRING SPECIAL ATTENTION

The management of human and animal bites, require special attention due to the polymicrobial nature of the innoculum. These wounds may present as avulsions, lacerations, punctures, or scratches. Although these wounds may look innocuous they often can lead to infection with the potential for even greater morbidity. Animal bites are generally polymicrobial and contain both aerobic and anaerobic flora. The majority of organisms, recovered from the wound are usually from the mouth of the offending agent and not from the patient's own skin flora. *Pasteurella multocida* is generally found in animal bites. *Staphylococcus aureus* and α-hemolytic streptococci are the most common organisms isolated in the wound resulting from a human bite. *Eikenella corrodens* is a predominant aerobe found in the human bite wound.

The symptoms found after a bite depend on the animal species inflicting the injury.[8] Venomous animals can cause severe systemic symptoms, such as shock, whereas human and dog bites do not cause immediate symptoms. However, because of the direct introduction of oral and skin flora into the wound the infection, if it occurs, can proceed rapidly. Vigilance is paramount here. A proper history must be obtained and, if indicated, the local health department must be notified. The wound and related structures must be evaluated. Range of motion of extremities, if involved, must be assessed and documented. Both aerobic and anaerobic wound culture should be obtained. Wounds that are contaminated with soil, fungal, and mycobacterial cultures should be evaluated. Animal and human bite wounds can generate significant force and this must be considered. A radiograph should be performed to search for occult fractures.

All bite wounds should be irrigated, explored, and débrided of devascularized tissue and closed if appropriate. The critical maneuver is to reduce the high level of the inoculum from either the human or animal bite. Bites of the hand are at increased risk for deeper infections because sharp teeth can penetrate into tendon sheaths. Primary closure should be delayed. Tendon or nerve repair should also be delayed until the wound is considered clean and not capable of causing infection.

Bites to the face require meticulous management. These wounds either human or animal should be appropriately treated with irrigation and débridement. The wound should then be loosely approximated with strict surveillance. Facial wounds should be considered for primary closure to minimize a poor cosmetic result. However, they are at higher risk for infection and should be followed appropriately.

Other bite wounds in other regions of the body can be left open and clinically observed for 24 to 48 hours. Delayed primary closure is appropriate here as long as it is done in an appropriate fashion. All patients should be placed on antibiotics. The wound culture results are usually polymicrobial and should be treated with a broad-spectrum antibiotic. A 1 to 2 week course is appropriate for infections limited to soft tissue. For infections involving the joints or bones, a 3-week therapy is required.

Bite wounds, human or animal, can lead to potentially very serious complications. These wounds must be diagnosed in a timely fashion and treated correctly in order to maximize the healing process. A few specific situations are discussed. Cat bites result in 10 to 40% infection of all wounds. The organisms involved are *Staphylococcus*, *Streptococcus*, and *Pasteurella multocida*. The antibiotic of choice is augmentin. Dog bites result in 6 to 16% infection of wounds and are treated in a similar fashion. The common hand bite wounds are with *Eikinella corrodens* and *Bacteroides*. The treatment of choice is oral augmentin for early infection; intravenous antibiotics (ampicillin and sulbactam) is used for later infections. Intraoral lacerations result in 6 to 12% infection, but this rate is doubled in through and through lacerations as compared to simple mucosal lacerations. Foot puncture wounds result in 15% infection of all wounds. In these cases, *Pseudomonas* is the usual organism causing osteomyelitis (nearly 90%).

HYPERBARIC OXYGEN THERAPY

Hyperbaric oxygen therapy implies that oxygen is being delivered under pressure and this modality of treatment is specific for certain resistant wounds, including necrotizing fasciitis and osteomyelitis.

SPECIFIC PROCEDURES FOR WOUND CLOSURE

A proper analysis of the wound needs to be performed, with overall consideration given for the medical status of the patient. An acute wound closure begins by first assessing the defect, which can be the result of burn, infection, trauma, tumor ablation or any combination of these situations. The vascular status of the wound must be established. In addition, the acute wound must be evaluated for its bacterial and fungal status.

The reconstructive ladder is a template, which can help guide the physician. However, this is only a linear template. All wounds are different. The key is to always address the idea of form and function when reconstructing a wound. If these ideas are taken into account then an optimal result will follow. Direct primary closure is the first rung on the ladder. This is the simplest technique and should always be the first option. If wound tension precludes primary closure, then a skin graft can be considered next. This option is viable if the wound bed contains the vascular status to support a skin graft. However, a skin graft cannot supply coverage over an area lacking adequate vascularity, paratenon or over bone lacking periosteum. A skin graft also does not take in the presence of infection.

In situations where skin grafts are not a viable option, than the acute wound will require a more complex closure. Local flaps based on a random pattern or axial blood supply may be used, assuming that local tissue destruction has not precluded their use. The zone of injury must be adequately assessed for the safe use of local flaps. More complex approaches using distant flaps from local regional body areas can also be used based on an axial blood supply.

Microvascular tissue transplantation represents the most complex portion of the reconstructive ladder. This portion of the management requires the greatest investment of time and patience from the reconstructive surgeon. For some wounds, microvascular transplantation can represent the initial reconstructive option, even though it is considered the most complex. Such a decision is based on a careful analysis of the acute wound and knowing what the best option would be in certain situations.

Skin grafts can be transferred from one part of the body to another. They are of two types: split-thickness (STSG) and full-thickness skin grafts (FTSG). It is an autograft and the skin has no blood supply of its own. Imbibition takes place during the first 24 to 48 hours to nourish the graft. This is until inosculation takes place, which gives the skin graft a new blood supply.

STSG consist of epidermis and variable levels of dermis. The skin graft is usually harvested using a dermatome. A majority of the donor sites heal by epithelialization with dressings in 7 to 14 days unless the donor sites become infected and convert to a full-thickness tissue loss. In such instances, the donor sites become wounds requiring further reconstruction. Great care must be taken in the maintenance of skin graft donor sites. They can usually be covered with a semiocclusive or an occlusive dressing. The dressing might require frequent changing or drainage, if serous fluid collects below the bandage or the bandage is soaked through. Certain dressings can typically be left intact and not changed until the underlying donor site has re-epithelialized.

A STSG will have more secondary contraction than a FTSG. This is based on the ingrowths of the myofibroblasts. When STSG are placed in certain wounds, it is imperative to visualize how that graft will appear or undergo contraction and if it will cause significant morbidity later. For example, in a full-thickness tissue loss over a joint surface of the hand, a thicker skin graft would be more appropriate for closure. This would prevent joint contracture, which can be usually seen with thinner skin grafts.

A FTSG consists of the epidermis and full thickness of the dermis. There is no subcutaneous adipose tissue included. Potential donor sites for a FTSG are limited, secondary to the fact that no epithelial cells remain following harvest and these sites cannot heal by themselves. These defects must be closed primarily compared to the STSG, which can be allowed to re-epithelialize on its own. A FTSG in the head and neck area provides a good color match if harvested from the head and neck area. These grafts maintain their size and have less secondary contraction as compared to a STSG.

The next level of acute wound coverage is based on local flaps. Initially the subdermal plexus was thought to be the blood supply to the skin. Recent research has shown that the true blood supply to the skin is based on axial blood supply and perforator vessels from the vessels. However, flaps based on the subdermal plexus as the presumed blood supply are still used significantly in the coverage of an acute wound. The tenet that must be adhered too, however, is that the local flap must be out of the zone of injury. Viable tissue must be able to be transported into an acute wound for closure to become successful and the bacterial status of the wound to be appropriate.

Types of Flaps

The types of flaps available for wound coverage will be discussed briefly as detailed descriptions are beyond the scope of this chapter. Local flaps include advancement, rotation, transposition, and interpolation. An advancement flap is a type of local flap in which the skin and subcutaneous tissue undergo stretching in order to move in a straight line to fill the defect. A variant of the advancement flap includes the single pedicle advancement flap that is rectangular or square and is simply advanced into the wound defect. Burow's triangles can be removed at the base to increase the advancement. A V–Y advancement flap is created, by making a V-shaped incision adjacent to the wound defect, basing the blood supply on the subcutaneous tissue. The V-shaped flap is advanced and the incision is then closed in the form of a Y.

Rotation, transposition, and interpolation flaps have in common a pivot point and an arc of rotation through which the local flap is transferred. A rotation flap is a semicircular piece of skin and subcutaneous tissue that rotates into the primary defect, but the design incorporates coverage of the secondary defect. A transposition flap can be of different shapes and sizes, but the traditional description by Duformental was of a rhomboid-shaped flap of skin and subcutaneous tissue that is transposed around a pivot point into the primary defect. The secondary defect is covered by advancement flap closure in most instances or by a skin graft. Other examples of transposition flaps are, a Z-plasty, rhomboid flap, and fasciocutaneous flaps. The techniques described are different from an interpolation, as the defect and the flap edge are in contact prior to transfer. An interpolation flap is comprised of a skin and subcutaneous tissue flap that is rotated around a pivot point into a defect that contains normal tissue between the donor site and the defect. These flaps are a variant of island flaps.

Distant flaps are those that are created a considerable distance from the wound defect and can be transferred in a variety of ways. In a direct transfer, the flap is designed and raised, its vascularity is confirmed, and the flap is then transferred by bringing the wounded site close to the flap-bearing area or vice versa. The flap is then inset into the defect. Vessels from the wound bed grow into the insetted portion of the flap. This process is usually complete after 2 to 3 weeks. Examples of such a flap include the cross-leg flap for lower-extremity defects, the forehead flap for facial defects, and the groin flap for upper-extremity defects. After the flap develops a local attachment and blood supply the flap is then divided from its origin and the insetting of the flap is completed. Indirect transfer of distant flaps is rarely used. Examples of this include the Crane principle, where regions of the body are used as an intermediary prior to final soft-tissue coverage.

Soft-tissue flaps can be transferred for wound coverage based on a random blood supply, which includes the subdermal plexus. These flaps can also be transferred based on named arteries. Using these named arteries, flaps of tissue involving bone, muscle, fascia, and cartilage can be incorporated into the development of a flap that will help facilitate the complex closure of an acute wound. These flaps are called composite tissue flaps and contain multiple types of tissue.

The axial-pattern flap lends itself to specific vascular territories. These mapped-out vascular territories, which include skin and subcutaneous tissue, can be raised based on the named axial pedicle. Examples of such flaps are the latissimus dorsi myocutaneous flap, which can be elevated and raised based on the thoracodorsal vessels. This myocutaneous pedicle flap can be used to cover wound defects in the head and neck, in the thorax, upper extremity, and the abdomen. This flap can also be used for breast reconstruction. In addition, this flap can be transferred as a functional muscle for defects of the biceps, triceps or pectoralis major muscle.

Other examples include the pectoralis major muscle or myocutaneous flap, and fascial or fasciocutaneous flaps. These flaps are not delayed and the blood supply is never severed. These flaps can be transferred over significant distances based on the length of the supplying vascular pedicle. By releasing muscle from areas of insertion and origin, the three-dimensional potential of the axial pedicle flap is greatly increased in the coverage of acute wounds. These flaps bring stable coverage to acute wounds. A new blood supply is recruited, which is invaluable in augmenting the circulatory status of a compromised wound.

Microvascular composite tissue transplantation is based on the premise that a known vascular pedicle with its associated flap tissue can be transferred to a known recipient vessel in the proximity of the acute wound.

The anastamosis of the blood supply is performed using an operating microscope or surgical loupes. The same axial pedicle composite flaps, which formerly were restricted by the length of the arc of rotation of their vessels, can now be set free of these limitations. Using microvascular technology, anastamosis of vessel lumens ranging from 0.5 to 2.5 mm or more can be safely accomplished.

Free-flap transfer allows the surgeon to take tissue from any part of the body and transfer it safely to the acute wound. The only limitations are the suitability of the wound bed and the skill of the surgeon. Microvascular composite tissue transplantation allows the donor tissue to be reconstructed into a myriad of three-dimensional constructs to fill the acute wound defect. This is a grand leap from the surgical community of even the late last century and will continue to augment the beneficial results of acute wound repair and reconstruction.

In the reconstruction of an acute wound, some basic concepts need to be adhered to. The defect of the donor site is called a secondary defect and this should not result in another acute open wound with no potential to heal or result in loss of function. The harvesting of bone, muscle, adipose tissue, and skin form an area will create a defect in itself. The donor site should have the potential to heal with dressings or be reconstructed in the same operation. This is *paramount*. An appropriate soft and hard tissue must be chosen to reconstruct the resultant secondary defect. Finally, the form and function of the individual patient must always be considered when evaluating an acute wound and reconstructing it with appropriate care and consideration, the management of an acute wound will be successful with minimal morbidity.

REFERENCES

1. Yardley PA. *A Brief History of Wound Healing.* Oxford: Clinical Communications; 1998.

2. Paré A. *Cinq Livres de Chirurgie.* Paris; 1572.

3. Steed DL. Wound-healing trajectories. *Surg Clinics Am.* 2003; 83(3):547.

4. Robson MC, Stenberg BD, Higgins JP. Wound healing alterations caused by infection. *Clin Plast Surg.* 1990;17(3): 485–492.

5. Lionelli GT, Lawrence WT. Wound dressings. *Surg Clinics N Am.* 2003;83(3):617.

6. Morykwas MJ, Argenta LC, Shelton-Brown EI, McGuirt W. Vacuum-assisted closure: A new method for wound control and treatment: Animal studies and basic foundation. *Ann Plast Surg.* 1997;38(6):553–562.

7. McCabe C. Trauma: An annotated bibliography of the literature—2001. *Am J Emerg Med.* 2002;20(4):352–366.

8. Brook I. Microbiology and management of human and animal bite wound infections. *Prim Care Clin Office Pract.* 2003; 30(1):25.

Noninvasive Evalution of the Cutaneous Circulation

Bok Y. Lee and Lee E. Ostrander

Introduction
Anatomy of the Microcirculation
Physiology of Capillary Perfusion
Neural Control of Cutaneous Blood Flow
Noninvasive Assessment of Cutaneous
   Circulation
Cutaneous Perfusion
   Xenon-133 Washout
   Laser Doppler
   Fluorometry

Perfusion Pressure
Holstein's Isotope Techniques
Skin Perfusion Pressure Using Laser Doppler
Cutaneous Pressure Photoplethysmography
Oximetry
Transcutaneous Oxygen Tension
Subcutaneous Oxygen Tension
Near-Infrared Reflectance Oximetry
Other Methods
References

INTRODUCTION

The body's microcirculation, or system of capillaries, is responsible for the delivery of nourishment and the removal of waste products. Assessment of the cutaneous circulation can provide insight as to the cause and management of many pathologic conditions, particularly diseases affecting the peripheral vascular system. In this chapter, we present a brief review of the anatomy and physiology of the microcirculation and a review of methods available for the noninvasive assessment of circulation.

ANATOMY OF THE MICROCIRCULATION

In human skin, there is a dense system of capillary loops in the papillae of the corium that empties into a sub-capillary venous plexus that contains a major fraction of the cutaneous blood volume. The microvascular bed is a subunit of the circulatory system and is less than 100 μm in diameter. The microvascular bed (Fig. 12–1) begins with the terminal arteriole, with vessel walls com-

posed of an inner layer of epithelium, an internal elastic lamina, and a surrounding sheath of at least two continuous layers of vascular smooth muscle cells. Arterioles, which arise from the terminal arteries, have a single continuous layer of vascular smooth muscle. Next are the metarterioles, with a single discontinuous layer of vascular smooth muscle cells. The metarterioles often have a band of vascular smooth muscle cells at the origin—the precapillary sphincter. The capillaries arise from the metarteroiles and consist of a single layer of endothelial cells and a basement of membrane surrounded by a fine, reinforcing network of reticular collagen fibers. The capillaries are classified as being either arterial or venous, depending on whether they are closer to the metarterioles (arterial capillaries) or the draining collecting venules (venous capillaries).

The walls of the capillaries function as a selectively permeable membrane. Endothelial cells that form a single layer range from 0.1 to 3 μm in thickness (Fig. 12–2). Between the cells is an intercellular space of about 100 Å in width. Almost all spaces have a constricted area about 40 Å wide. Within the cells are many small vesicles that continually join with the inner and outer cell membranes, contributing to the transport of materials across capillary walls.

Note: Chapter 12 was reproduced with permission fom B.Y. Lee and B. Herz, *Surgical Management of Cutaneous Ulcers and Pressure Sores,* published by Hodder Amold, 1998.

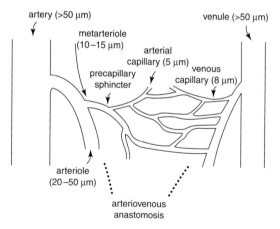

Fig. 12–1. Diagrammatic representation of a microcirculatory unit. Reproduced with permission from B.Y. Lee and B. Herz, *Surgical Management of Cutaneous Ulcers and Pressure Sores;* published by Hodder Arnold, 1998.

In the microcirculation, sympathetic vasoconstrictor innervation usually extends only as far as the arterioles but, in some instances, may be found in the metarterioles. Metarterioles, in general, as well as precapillary sphincters, are under local control, being influenced by tissue waste products, oxygen deprivation, or other factors. These vessels usually show a rhythmic vasomotion of alternating vasodilation and vasoconstriction. Arteriole changes in vessel caliber are more irregular. Venules, in general, receive few sympathetic vasoconstrictor nerves.

In terms of function, the microvascular bed can be divided into (1) resistance vessels—arterioles, metarterioles, and precapillary sphincters—which together control organ blood flow; (2) exchange vessels—the capillaries; and (3) reservoir vessels—venules and veins.

PHYSIOLOGY OF CAPILLARY PERFUSION

Perfusion and function of the capillaries are regulated and affected by a number of factors. Vasoconstriction or vasodi-

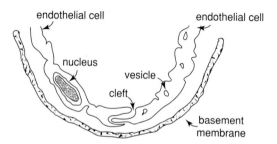

Fig. 12–2. Diagrammatic representation with electron microscopy of a cross section through a capillary. Reproduced with permission from B.Y. Lee and B. Herz, *Surgical Management of Cutaneous Ulcers and Pressure Sores;* published by Hodder Arnold, 1998.

lation alters the diameter of the arterioles and, therefore, influences the amount of blood flow that enters the capillaries. Vasoconstriction and vasodilation are regulated by both sympathetic and parasympathetic fibers and catecholamines, such as epinephrine and norepinephrine. In addition, pharmacologic agents (eg, alpha stimulators, beta blockers) will affect arteriolar diameter. In many tissues, arteriovenous shunts may open to cause a complete bypass of the capillary bed. Increases in cardiac output elevate arterial blood pressure and increase capillary blood flow. Elevation in arterial blood pressure caused by arteriolar constriction, however, decreases capillary blood flow. The presence of precapillary sphincters also influences the amount of blood reaching the capillaries and it is possible that capillaries may open and close because of the intrinsic contractibility of capillary endothelial cells. Such capillary constriction and dilation are independent of action by the arterioles. Essential components appear to be anoxia and histamine production. A capillary is closed from 60 to 95% of the time; therefore, as few as 5% of all capillaries are open at any one time, although the open 5% are constantly being changed. Thus, all capillaries are perfused, in turn.

Blood viscosity is an important factor in capillary blood flow. Viscosity is influenced by plasma protein concentration and hematocrit, among other factors, such as capillary size. Capillaries vary in size from 4 to 10 μm in diameter and are thus frequently much smaller than red blood cells, which average 7 μm in diameter. Red blood cells are required to deform themselves to pass through a capillary and are, therefore, a factor in blood viscosity. Blood viscosity decreases as capillary size diminishes, promoting capillary blood flow. However, this is a limited phenomenon, because at a critical diameter, capillary blood flow dramatically decreases as blood viscosity sharply increases, possibly because of the sticking of red blood cells in the capillaries. The deformability of red blood cells can be adversely affected by bacterial endotoxins, swelling of the cells by fluid absorption, and low pH.

An important factor in the noninvasive evaluation of the cutaneous circulation is tissue pressure. Severe increases in tissue pressure can virtually shut off capillary flow. Total tissue pressure is typically close to atmospheric. External pressure increases interstitial fluid pressure, which, at about 12 mm Hg, increases capillary arteriolar pressure, leading to filtration of fluid from the capillaries, edema, and autolysis. Unrelieved pressure is a primary cause of pressure sore formation.

The permeability of the capillary membrane can be expressed as the amount of water per minute that is forced through the membrane at a given pressure. Most exchange between blood and extracellular fluid takes place through the clefts between the cells of the capillary wall because of the presence of a hydrophobic layer of lipoprotein in the cell wall.

The plasma volume and the volume of the interstitial space are controlled by factors at the capillary level: plasma oncotic pressure, hydrostatic pressure, oncotic pressure of the interstitial fluid, and hydrostatic pressure of the interstitial space. Plasma oncotic pressure develops because of the restricted passage of large molecules such as proteins. Albumin makes up 51% of the plasma proteins. Because of its high concentration and relatively low molecular weight, it is primarily responsible for determining the oncotic pressure. Other plasma proteins include globulin (17%), fibrinogen (4%), and other miscellaneous proteins (28%). The plasma oncotic pressure is approximately 25 mm Hg. The capillary hydrostatic pressure ranges from 32 mm Hg at the arterial capillaries to about 15 mm Hg at the venous capillaries. The mid-capillary hydrostatic pressure is about 25 mm Hg. The interstitial fluid oncotic pressure is assumed to be very small. The tissue hydrostatic pressure is similarly difficult to measure, but is about 1.8 mm Hg.

NEURAL CONTROL OF CUTANEOUS BLOOD FLOW

Determinants of cutaneous blood flow include the direct, local, and reflex effects of central and peripheral heating. Cutaneous resistance vessels are significantly regulated by the sympathetic nervous system. One factor regulating the cutaneous vascular resistance is the frequency of the impulses over sympathetic nerve fibers that are tonically vasoconstrictive. At normal room temperature, the cutaneous resistance vessels demonstrate basal tone (vascular resistance independent of innervation). In contrast, cutaneous arteriovenous anastomoses possess little basal tone and are regulated by a tonic neural discharge. The elimination of this tonic neural discharge produces a maximum passive dilation. In the thigh and calf of a cool subject, a weak vasoconstrictor tone is maintained; active vasodilation, however, takes over when the subject is heated.

The heating or cooling of cutaneous areas induces vasomotor changes in the skin that are partly due to the return of heated or cooled blood to central areas (eg, the hypothalamus) that may mediate vasomotor responses. In humans, central thermoreceptors are quite sensitive; for example, a 0.15°C increase in oral temperature reflexly dilates the hand.

Baroreceptors also exert an influence over the cutaneous resistance vessels. Carotid sinus hypertension causes a reflex vasodilation. Baroreceptors also play a role in the intense cutaneous vasoconstriction that accompanies severe hemorrhage.

At the beginning of exercise, veins and the cutaneous resistance vessels constrict, but then relax as the central body temperature rises. The extent of the increase in skin blood flow during exercise is a result of the competing drives for vasoconstriction caused by the exercise and vasodilation caused by the generation of heat by the exercising muscles.

The primary response of the cutaneous circulation to an elevation in skin temperature is a four-to fivefold increase in flow. This response is under direct control, as this increase in flow occurs even with denervation. If one cools the whole body, cutaneous vasoconstrictor tone increase, depressing the local effects of heating. Thus, for example, local heating of the hand with lower body temperature produces a lesser increase in the skin blood flow than the same heat intensity applied at a normal body temperature. The vasodilation of heated skin paradoxically adds heat to the body as heat is gained when the surface to deep body temperature gradient is reversed. The high skin flow, however, does remove heat from the underlying skin, preventing burning. As mentioned, cold constricts cutaneous blood vessels, and the response to local cold is greater in a cold person than in a warm one. At about 15°C in a cold subject, hand blood flow is minimized. If, however, the local temperature is brought to below 10°C, the intense vasoconstriction of the fingers or toes is interrupted by the "hunting reaction" (periods of vasodilation). Induced vasodilation is free of sympathetic control but does seem to rely on a somatic nerve supply, probably through an axon reflex, where nerve impulses from a sensory ending pass to an effector organ along the divisions of a nerve fiber without passing through a nerve cell.

Cutaneous vasomotor tone can also be affected by a single stroking of the skin with a finger or other blunt object. A "white reaction" appears caused by blood being mechanically forced from the venous plexi. A more forceful mechanical stimulation causes "triple response." A red line appears initially, due to dilation, followed by a flare, probably due to an axon reflex. With strong enough stimulation, a wheal develops secondary to increased permeability of the capillaries, leading to the loss of fluid and protein.

The veins of the skin have a rich sympathetic innervation and are more responsive to sympathetic stimulation than resistance vessels, although this difference is associated with a difference in structure. Veins, however, are similar to the resistance vessels in that they are under vasoconstrictor control. Local skin cooling decreases venous compliance; healing has minimal direct effect. With a cool body temperature, the cutaneous veins constrict proportionately to the severity of the exercise.

NONINVASIVE ASSESSMENT OF CUTANEOUS CIRCULATION

Skin survival can be adversely affected by a variety of pathological conditions that diminish cutaneous circulation and interfere with tissue maintenance and healing.[1-3]

The skin is one of the few directly visible organs of the body. The first line of circulatory assessment is, therefore, to observe the appearance of the skin, the temperature of the skin, and the presence of blanching and of intraoperative wound bleeding. These can be combined with hands-on examination, including palpation and pulse findings.[4,5] The data may differentiate the circulatory status, particularly in patients with difficult healing. Examples of these problem cases are seen with diabetics and peripheral vascular disease. The cutaneous tissues also can offer an element of undesired surprise. The failure of the circulation in cutaneous tissue can be silent; the loss or impending loss may not be visibly apparent until hours or even days after the damage has occurred. For these reasons, more sophisticated and quantitative methods deserve consideration in order to monitor and assess the circulation in the cutaneous tissue where risk of tissue loss exists. The methodologies employ a variety of physical principles for their success, including the use of optical methods,[6] radioisotope indicators, and electrochemical sensing.

CUTANEOUS PERFUSION

Circulatory assessment can be made by noninvasive measurement of blood perfusion within the skin. Several methods are described here.

Xenon-133 Washout

The use of xenon-133 by Moore and others[7-9] has provided excellent results, but has not received widespread clinical acceptance. The technique of xenon-133 washout requires the injection of a radioactive substance into the body. As described by Malone et al.[9] in the selection of amputation level, patients are placed supine and allowed to equilibrate for 15 minutes at a room temperature of 22 to 27°C. The xenon-133, dissolved in saline (0.05 mL; 100–500 μc), is injected intradermally in two parallel injections, 2 cm apart, medial and lateral to a point indicated by the surgeon. The needle is kept in place for about 10 seconds and a slight pressure is applied over the injection site for about 5 seconds. The activity of the xenon-133 is monitored for 10 minutes. A computer generates the time-activity curves for the disappearance of the xenon. The cutaneous blood flow is calculated using the Kety–Schmidt treatment of the Fick flow equation:

$$\frac{\text{Skin blood flow (mL)}}{100 \text{ g of tissue per minute}} = \frac{10\alpha K}{P}$$

where K is the slope constant of xenon-133, α is the blood–skin coefficient for xenon-133, and P is the specific gravity of skin. Using this technique, local skin blood flow

in the range of 0.6 to 2.2 mL per 100 g of tissue per minute has been found to be indicative of good healing.

Laser Doppler

Another method for perfusion measurement employs Doppler frequency shifts of laser light. The laser Doppler method continues to be a subject of further research study and the instrumentation is commercially available. An advantage of this technique is that readings are rapidly obtained. Laser Doppler is sensitive to blood flow velocity in capillaries, but may not always be as specific as fluorometry to blood flow changes.[10] Laser Doppler can produce artifacts, in which zero blood flow may result in a nonzero reading because of random movements of blood cells.

In a variant of the laser Doppler method, heat is applied to the skin in the area of the laser Doppler sensing element. With this version of the Doppler system, the accuracy in predicting the healing outcome for ischemic wounds has been reported to be similar to that for transcutaneous oxygen measurement.[11] Another study reported that laser Doppler velocimetry, in combination with measurement of platelet-derived growth factor (PDGF), served as a prognostic indicator for the healing of ulcers and ischemic lesions of the lower limb.[12]

Fluorometry

Fluorometry is a method that contributes to the direct observation of blood circulation in the tissues. Measurement requires the introduction of fluorescein dye into the vasculature, which is then distributed by the circulation of the blood. An ultraviolet light source illuminates the skin and excites the dye in the vessels lying beneath the surface of the skin. The dye fluoresces, thereupon emitting a yellow–green light that can be observed visually. The assessment of circulation is limited by several factors, such as skin coloration, timing of dye injection and observation, and the limitations of the eye in observing graduations of light intensity. Therefore, instrumented and quantitative versions of the fluorometric method have been investigated.

Quantitative measurement of the fluorescence has been reported by Silverman and colleagues for assessing skin flap survival, skin viability prior to amputation, and intestinal viability.[13-18] The perfusion fluorometer quantifies the tissue fluorescence. A light source in the blue wavelengths of 450 to 500 nm is transmitted via a fiber optic cable to illuminate a selected tissue site. The transmitted light excites the fluorescein within the tissue in an area of approximately 2.5 cm² beneath the tip of the probe. The fluorescein emits light in the range of 520 to 550 nm, a portion of which is directed via fiber optics back to the fluorometer. The returning light travels to a photomultiplier tube and electronics, which produces a direct and quantitative readout of dye fluorescence.

Fluorometry is not a continuous reading. In most subjects, the dye is tolerated well, but a few subjects will show a reaction. A reported 0.6% incidence of anaphylactoid reactions[19,20] can be seen with bolus fluorescein injection.

Perfusion Pressure

Another set of techniques for assessing cutaneous circulation makes use of the pressure with which the blood enters the tissues. The basic measurement concept is an application of pressure to the skin surface to balance the driving pressure of the blood. Instrumentation is then applied to identify the minimum pressure at which perfusion of the tissue ceases or the maximum pressure at which perfusion is reestablished. The perfusion may be monitored in this test by any of several methods, including radioisotope clearance, laser Doppler, and photoplethysmography. Of these various methods, one study reported that the most accurate measurement used radioisotope clearance, and that laser Doppler was the simplest to use. Low agreement with the other methods was observed for the photoplethysmographic method.[21] The quality of results will depend upon the technique used and the quality of the particular instrumentation employed.

Holstein's Isotope Techniques

Holstein used the degree of external pressure required to halt isotope washout.[22–25] As with the xenon-133 washout method previously described, this technique is somewhat time consuming and requires injection of a radioactive substance. Holstein et al. dissolved $[^{133}I^-]$ antipyrine (4-$[^{133}I^-]$-iodoantipyrine) in sterile water and histamine diphosphate and injected the combination intradermally (0.1 mL). The gamma emission was measured for 3 to 5 minutes. External pressure was then increased to give a stepwise decrease in the washout rate. Pressure increments of 20 to 40 mm Hg were observed for 3 minutes, followed by 5-mm Hg increases, which were observed for 5 minutes at each level. The "flow cessation external pressure" is estimated as a pressure 3 mm Hg above the last pressure that allowed detection of a minimal washout. Using this technique, Holstein et al[23] found the skin perfusion pressure in normal subject to be approximately 10 mm Hg lower than systemic mean arterial blood pressure. In the assessment of wound healing in below-knee amputation, Holstein et al.[25] reported a skin perfusion pressure > 30 mm Hg to yield the highest postoperative success and a perfusion pressure < 20 mm Hg to yield poor results.

Skin Perfusion Pressure Using Laser Doppler

Another recent variation on measurement of skin perfusion pressure replaces the radioactive indicator of perfusion with measurements of perfusion using the laser Doppler flowmeter.[26] The laser Doppler system measures perfusion at a lesser depth than does the isotope, but the laser Doppler system is much simpler to apply, no radioactive materials are used, and measurements can be done more rapidly. Studies with this system suggest that prediction of wound healing following amputation is practicable. The measurement method was applied to assess the outcome for 53 amputations ranging from major amputations to toe amputations. A pressure of 30 mm Hg or better showed a prediction of healing of 90%; a value of less than 30 mm Hg had a healing failure of 75%.

Cutaneous Pressure Photoplethysmography

Cutaneous pressure photoplethysmography has also been reported as advantageous in measuring cutaneous perfusion pressure for determining amputation level and predicting the results of revascularization.[27–29] Cutaneous pressure photoplethysmography does not directly rely on the shape of the arterial pulse of the main trunk arteries because the critical pressure readings occur where waveforms begin or cease, independent of wave shape.

One study evaluated 25 patients and 9 normal subjects with this technique. Of the 25 patients, 10 were postoperative amputees (follow-up of 3 ± 3 years) studied to determine the cutaneous perfusion pressure required to maintain a healed stump. Five of the patients were candidates for bypass surgery (disabling claudication), and the remaining 10 patients were prospective amputees (gangrene). Bypass patients were followed up for 3 ± 1 month and postoperative amputees for 4 ± 3 months.

The cutaneous pressure photoplethysmograph senses blood flow in the skin at various skin-bearing pressures with the use of a hand-held probe. The photoplethysmograph probe contains a small light source and a photosensitive cell that responds to light reflected from the cutaneous vascular bed. A recorder prints out a permanent waveform (Fig. 12–3). A pressure sensor within the probe is calibrated using a known loading force on the surface of the probe and the skin-bearing pressure is directly shown on a digital display in millimeters of mercury. The probe is placed at the desired site and a waveform obtained. The waveform is obliterated with the manual application of gradually increasing pressure (Fig. 12–4). When the pressure is gradually released, the pressure reading at the point when the photoplethysmographic waveform returns, is recorded as the cutaneous pressure.

In the retrospective study of amputees, cutaneous pressure photoplethysmographic measurements were made above the knee and at the stump. For the prospective patients (amputees and bypass patients) and the normal subjects, measurements were made at four locations: the chest, 10 cm proximal to the knee joint, at midcalf, and over the dorsum of the foot.

Anterior   Posterior

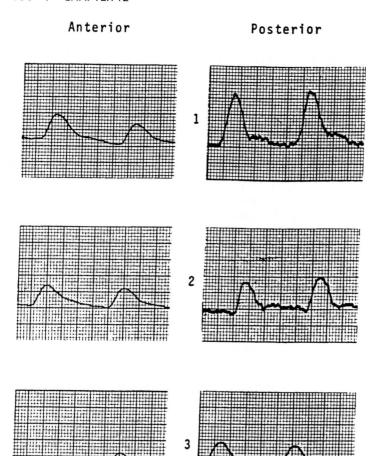

Fig. 12–3. The photoplethysmographic waveform is printed and becomes a permanent part of the patient's record. Reproduced with permission from B.Y. Lee and B. Herz, *Surgical Management of Cutaneous Ulcers and Pressure Sores;* published by Hodder Arnold, 1998.

The cutaneous pressures obtained are shown in Table 12–1. In normal subjects, a dorsum of foot: chest index greater than 1.0 was obtained. In the five patients with disabling claudication, an index of > 0.50 was obtained preoperatively. Postoperatively, an increase in the index to > 0.80 was accompanied by excellent clinical improvement. Nine of the prospective amputees had below-knee or more distal amputations: six had primary healing and three required revision. One patient with an above-knee amputation healed primarily. In the seven healed patients, the preoperative indices were > 0.90 above knee, > 0.70 at midcalf, and < 0.35 at the dorsum of the foot. In the four patients with below-knee amputation, the dorsum of the foot index was < 0.25 and was > 0.60 at the level of amputation. At the level of amputation the cutaneous pressure was 78.0 ± 30.1 mm Hg in healed patients preoperative, which increased to 90.0 ± 4.0 mm Hg postoperatively. In contrast, three patients without primary healing had a cutaneous pressure of 40.7 ± 8.1 mm Hg at the level of amputation and 27.3 ± 17.5 mm Hg over the dorsum of the foot preoperatively. Postoperatively, no improvement was seen (mean change: −1.0 ± 1.4 mm Hg). In two patients with healed distal amputation (one Syme's and one digital amputation), preoperative dorsum of the foot cutaneous pressure was 57.0 ± 7.1 mm Hg, which increased to 65.0 ± 29.6 mm Hg postoperatively. In the ten retrospective amputees (all below-knee), above knee cutaneous pressure was 122 ± 46.3 mm Hg and midcalf pressure was 91.2 ± 30.1 mm Hg, which was very similar to the cutaneous pressure at the stump of the prospective amputees.

Oximetry

Another way to assess cutaneous circulation is to measure the oxygen present within the cutaneous layers.

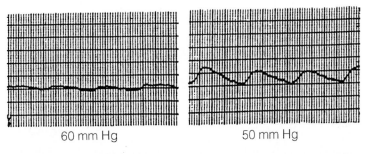

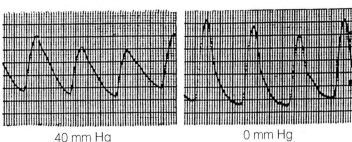

Fig. 12–4. With the application of pressure the cutaneous pressure photo-plethysmograph waveform is obliterated; the pressure at which the waveform returns with gradual release of pressure is the cutaneous pressure. Reproduced with permission from B.Y. Lee and B. Herz, *Surgical Management of Cutaneous Ulcers and Pressure Sores;* published by Hodder Arnold, 1998.

If circulation is poor in the presence of normal tissue metabolic loading, or if the delivered oxygen levels are low, the oxygen levels of the blood within the tissue will be low.

TRANSCUTANEOUS OXYGEN TENSION

The measurement of transcutaneous oxygen tension has long been an integral part of neonatal medicine and more recently has been applied to evaluating the cutaneous circulation in adults.[30–33] Transcutaneous oxygen measurements ($TcPO_2$) reflect changes in tissue perfusion and metabolic status. The technique is relatively simple and noninvasive, involving the application of a small sensing unit to the surface of the skin. The electrode within the sensor contains a heating unit that evaluates the skin temperature, causing localized hyperemia. Oxygen within the blood diffuses through the skin and

Table 12–1. Cutaneous pressure photoplethysmographic measurements in predicting outcome of amputation or revascularization*

Subjects	Cutaneous Perfusion Pressure (mm Hg)			
	Chest	**Above Knee**	**Midcalf**	**Dorsum of Foot**
Normal (n = 9)	144.8 ± 35.0	146.0 ± 35.4	149.9 ± 38.6	150.9 ± 41.0
Claudication (n = 5)				
Preop	140.2 ± 30.4	130.3 ± 51.0	110.3 ± 48.1	73.4 ± 26.2
Postop	121.3 ± 64.0	111.0 ± 30.9	116.0 ± 39.1	98.0 ± 56.1
Prospective amputees[1] (healed, preop) (n = 7)	119.6 ± 19.4	108.9 ± 21.8	89.7 ± 32.8	41.1 ± 19.9
Prospective amputees[2] (nonhealed) (n = 3)	—	—	40.7 ± 8.1 (postop)	27.3 ± 17.5 (preop)
Retrospective amputees (n = 10)	—	122.0 ± 46.3	91.2 ± 30.1	—

[1]One patient had above-knee amputation.
[2]Midcalf pressure at level of amputation.
*Source: Katsamouris et al.[32]
Reproduced with permission from B.Y. Lee and B. Herz, *Surgical Management of Cutaneous Ulcers and Pressure Sores;* published by Hodder Arnold, 1998.

is sensed by an oxygen-sensing electrode. In 49 patients, Katsamouris et al.[32] demonstrated that in successful revascularization procedures $TcPO_2$ increases significantly, whereas it remains unchanged or decreases in the presence of poor results (Table 12–2). In a further study of 10 patients monitored intraoperatively, $TcPO_2$ increases of 4 to 50 mm Hg immediately following re-establishment of blood flow were associated with good results. Cina et al.[31] have also found $TcPO_2$ to successfully identify the presence of vascular disease and distinguish among different levels of severity (Table 12–3). Using $TcPO_2$ measurements, Rhodes and Cogran[33] have found, following otherwise successful revascularization, that nonhealing foot ulcers that remain are "islands of ischemia" caused by microangiopathy, scarring, or a discontinuity of pedal artery flow. Franzeck et al.[30] have additionally reported $TcPO_2$ measurements of 36.5 ± 17.5 mm Hg to be predictive of primary healing of an amputation, whereas failed amputations had $TcPO_2$ measurements in the range of 0 to 3 mm Hg.

The transcutaneous measurement is predominantly a measurement of arterialized blood reaching the skin and does not necessarily reflect venous status. Roszinski and Schmeller[34] found that in chronic venous insufficiency, the $TcPO_2$ measurements did not correlate with tissue intracutaneous measurements determined with needle probes and concluded that skin damage in patients with chronic venous insufficiency is not necessarily associated with hypoxia.

SUBCUTANEOUS OXYGEN TENSION

Rather than measuring oxygen through the skin, a catheter containing an oxygen sensor can be inserted into the skin layers. The sensor can be an oxygen-sensing polarographic electrode or one of the more recent devices, such as an oxygen-sensing fluorescence-quenching optode.[35] Because this method is invasive, its primary use has been as a research tool. In clinical studies of this method, it has been described as a reliable indicator of blood loss and peripheral perfusion.[36]

NEAR-INFRARED REFLECTANCE OXIMETRY

The illumination of tissues for medical purposes goes back as far as 1912, with a light torch applied to illuminate soft tissue (diaphanography) to visualize lesions within the breast.[37] Today's successful use of pulse oximetry followed from these early origins. However, pulse oximetry has been used primarily for transmission of light through tissue thickness, where pulsatile changes of blood within tissue can be monitored.

In the early use of reflectance spectrography, the surface of the skin was flooded with light and instrumentation was used to quantitatively measure the light returning.[38,39] However, reflectance methods using light flooding do not measure as deeply as methods using point light sources. The results of experimental studies and modeling have shown that the depth to which photons travel can be related to parameters of surface reflectance, and to the optical properties of the biological medium. Measurements of oxygen in deeper layers of cutaneous tissue now appear possible using methods known, respectively, as time- and space-resolved reflectance spectroscopy.

The time-resolved method is also described as photon time-of-flight measurement.[40] This method selectively examines the distribution of photon travel times between a point of photon incidence on the skin surface

Table 12–2. Transcutaneous oxygen tension measurements over the dorsum of the foot pre- and postoperatively (7 days postoperatively)[1,*]

	Transcutaneous Oxygen Tension (mm Hg)					
	Good Results			**Poor Results**		
Diagnosis	**Preop**	**Postop**	**N**	**Preop**	**Postop**	**N**
Claudication	46 ± 8	60 ± 10^2	14	41 ± 5	41 ± 2^4	3
Rest pain	15 ± 10	53 ± 13^2	15	25 ± 7	22 ± 8^4	4
Impending gangrene	5 ± 3	45 ± 11^3	3	6 ± 1	8 ± 7^4	2
Ischemic ulcer	21 ± 19	52 ± 13^2	6	43 ± 24	24 ± 3^4	2

[1] $p < .001$.
[2] $p > .05$.
[3] $p < .03$.
[4] $p < .03$.

*Source: Katsamouris et al.[32]

Table 12–3. Transcutaneous oxygen tension measurements in distinguishing severity of peripheral vascular disease*

Subjects	Transcutaneous Oxygen Tension (mm Hg)		
	Chest	**Calf**	**Foot**
Normal[1]	65 ± 6	64 ± 8^3	64 ± 8^4
($n = 10$)			
Claudication	64 ± 15	52 ± 10	46 ± 10^4
($n = 26$)			
Rest pain	65 ± 8	40 ± 10^2	17 ± 9^4
($n = 19$)			
Impending gangrene	60 ± 9	26 ± 17	5 ± 2
($n = 10$)			

[1] Normal subjects > 45 years of age; $TcPO_2$ inversely correlated ($p < .005$). The difference between younger and older than 45 years was significant ($p < .01$).
[2] $p < .015$ (p value between adjacent values vertically).
[3] $p < .003$ (p value between adjacent values vertically).
[4] $p < .001$ (p value between adjacent values vertically).
*Source: Cina et al.[31]

Reproduced with permission from B.Y. Lee and B. Herz, *Surgical Management of Cutaneous Ulcers and Pressure Sores;* published by Hodder Arnold, 1998.

and another point at which is placed a photon-capturing detector. Space-resolved methods look instead at the averaged intensity of returned light generally distributed over multiple distances from light source to detector.

Because oxygenation of the blood is wavelength dependent, the application of two or more light wavelengths (usually red and infrared) in combination with reflectance of up to a few centimeters can be used to measure oxygenation via light reflectance at a depth within biologic tissue. The method is also sensitive to other chromophores such as carboxyhemoglobin and methemoglobin. However, additional light wavelengths may assist in reducing the effect of these artifacts on oxygen measurement.[41]

Other Methods

Nuclear magnetic resonance principles upon which magnetic resonance imaging is based also provides a means for tracking perfusion.[42] Because capillary perfusion follows a tortuous path and the linear velocity is low, phasing techniques suitable for large vessels are not applicable. However, tracking of a bolus of injected contrast material is possible.

Included in the category of other methods is the evaluation of wound healing through wound histology. If the circulation is impaired, one would expect that the cutaneous wound healing would be impaired. The test consists of applying a Simplate II bleeding-time device to create standardized wounds within the skin. The authors[43] have concluded that this method allows evaluation of tissue repair performance with relative safety, even for patients with peripheral vascular disease and diabetes mellitus.

REFERENCES

1. Silver IA, Cellular microenvironment in healing and nonhealing wounds. In: Hunt TK, Heppenstall RB, Pines E, Rovee D, eds. *Soft and Hard Tissue Repair.* New York: Praeger, 1984: Chap. 4.

2. Knighton DR, Oredsson S, Banda M, Hunt, TK, Regulation of repair: Hypoxic control of macrophage mediated angiogenesis. In: Hunt, Heppenstall, Pines, Rovee, eds. *Soft and Hard Tissue Repair.* New York: Praeger; 1984: Chap. 3.

3. Kerrigan CL, Daniel RK. Skin flap failure: Pathophysiology. *Plast Reconstr Surg.* 1983;72:76.

4. Romano RL, Burgess EM. Level selection in lower extremity amputations. *Clin Orthop.* 1971;74:177.

5. Lee BY, Trainor FS, Kavner D, Crisologo JA, Shaw W, Madden JL. Assessment of the healing potentials of ulcers of the skin by photoplethysmography. *Surg Gynecol Obstet.* 1972;148:232.

6. Lubbers DW. Optical sensors for clinical monitoring. *Acta Anaesthesiol Scand Suppl.* 1995;104:37–54.

7. Moore WR. Determination of amputation level: Measurement of skin blood flow with xenon 133. *Arch Surg.* 1973;107:798.

8. Moore WS, Henry RE, Malone JM, Daly MJ, Patton D, Childers SJ. Prospective use of xenon Xe133 clearance for amputation level selection. *Arch Surg.* 1981;116:86.

9. Malone J, Leal JM, Moore WS, et al. The "gold standard" for amputation level selection, Xenon 133 clearance. *J Surg Res.* 1981;30:449.

10. Liu AJ, Cummings CW, Trachy RE, Venous outflow obstruction in myocutaneous flaps: Changes in microcirculation detected by the perfusion fluorometer and laser Doppler. *Otolaryngol Head Neck Surg.* 1986;94:165.

11. Padberg FT, Jr, Black TL, Hart LC, Franco CD. Comparison of heated probe laser Doppler and transcutaneous oxygen measurements for predicting outcome of ischemic wounds. *J Cardiovasc Surg.* 1992;33:715–722.

12. Martins R, Rao S. Laser Doppler velocimetry and platelet-derived growth factor as prognostic indicators for the healing of ulcers and ischaemic lesions of the lower limb. *Cardiovasc Surg.* 1995;3:285–290.

13. Ostrander LE, Lee BY, Silverman DA, Groskopf RA. Constant infusion fluorometry to predict flap survival. *Decubitus.* 1988; 2:40.

14. Sloan GM, Sasaki GH. Noninvasive monitoring of tissue viability. *Clin Plast Surg.* 1985;12:185.

15. Silverman DG, Rubin SM, Reilly CA, Brousseau DA, Norton DJ, Wolf GL. Fluorometric prediction of successful amputation level in the ischemic limb. *J Rehabil Res Develop.* 1985; 23–28.

16. Silverman DG, Rubin SM, Reilly CA, Brousseau DA, Norton KJ, Bartley E, Neufeld GR. Fluorometric quantification of low dose fluorescein delivery to predict amputation site healing. *Surgery.* 1987;101:335.

17. Silverman DG, Cedrone FA, Hurford WE, Bering TG, LaRossa DD. Monitoring tissue elimination of fluorescein with the perfusion fluorometer: A new method to assess capillary blood flow. *Surgery.* 1981;90:409.

18. Weisman RA, Pransky SM, Silverman DA, Lyons KM, Denneny JC, III, Vidas MD, Kimmelman CP. Clinical assessment of flap perfusion by fiberoptic fluorometry. *Ann Otol Rhinol Laryngol.* 1985;94:226.

19. LaPiana EF, Penner R. Anaphylactoid reaction to intravenously administered fluorescein. *Arch Opthal.* 1968;79:161.

20. Stein, MR, Parker CW. Reactions following intravenous fluorescein. *Am J Opthal.* 1971;72:861.

21. Malvezzi L, Castronuovo JJ, Jr, Swayne LC, Cone D, Trivino JZ. The correlation between three methods of skin perfusion pressure measurement: Radionuclide washout, laser Doppler flow, and photoplethysmography. *J Vasc Surg.* 1992;15:823.

22. Holstein P, Lassen NA. Radio-isotope-clearance technique for measurement of distal blood pressure in skin and muscles. *Scand J Clin Lab Invest Suppl.* 1973;128:143.

23. Holstein P, Lund P, Larsen B, Shoemacker T. Skin perfusion pressure measured as the external pressure required to stop isotope washout: Methodological considerations and normal values on the legs. *Scand J Clin Lab Invest.* 1977;37:649.

24. Holstein P, Doney H, Lassen NA. Wound healing in above-knee amputations in relation to skin perfusion pressure. *Acta Orthop Scand.* 1979;50:59.

25. Holstein P, Sager P, Lassen NA. Wound healing in below knee amputations in relation to skin perfusion pressure. *Acta Orthop Scand.* 1979;50:49.

26. Andera HM, James K, Castronuovo JJ, Jr, Byrne M, Deshmukh R, Lohr J. Prediction of amputation wound healing with skin perfusion pressure. *J Vasc Surg.* 1995;21:823–829.

27. Lee BY, McCann WJ, Trainor FS, Thoden WR, Kavner D. Noninvasive assessment of wound healing potentials and determination of amputation level. *Contemp Surg.* 1980;17:20.

28. Lee BY, Thoden WR, Madden JL, McCann WJ. Cutaneous pressure photoplethysmography: A new technique for noninvasive evaluation of peripheral arterial occlusive disease. *Contemp Surg* 1984;25:39–43.

29. Lee BY, Ostrander LE, Thoden WR, Madden JL. Use of cutaneous pressure photoplethysmography in managing peripheral vascular disease. *Contemp Surg.* 1987;30:58.

30. Franzeck UK, Talke P, Bernstein EF, Fronek A, Goldbranson FL. Transcutaneous PO_2 measurements in peripheral arterial occlusive disease. In: Messmer K, ed. *Microcirculation and Ischemic Vascular Diseases: Advances in Diagnosis and Therapy.* Chicago: Abbott Laboratories; 1981:160.

31. Cina C, Katsamouris A, Megerman J, Brewster DC, Straghorn EC, Robinson, JG, Abbott WJM. Utility of transcutaneous oxygen tension measurements in peripheral vascular disease. *Int Cardiovasc Soc.* 1983 (abstr.).

32. Katsamouris AN, Cina C, Robinson J, Megerman J, Straghorn EC, Brewster DC, Abbott WJM. Intra-and postoperative assessment of revascularization procedures utilizing a transcutaneous PO_2 electrode. *Surg Forum.* 1983;34:461.

33. Rhodes GR, Cogan F. "Island of ischemia": Transcutaneous PO_2 (PO_{2tc}) documentation of pedal malperfusion following lower limb revascularization. *7th Annu Surg Symp.* 1983;81 (Abstr.).

34. Roszinski S, Schmeller W. Differences between intracutaneous and transcutaneous skin oxygen tension in chronic venous insufficiency. *J Cardiovasc Surg.* 1995;36:407–413.

35. Hopf HW, Hunt TK. Comparison of Clark electrode and optode for measurement of tissue oxygen tension. *Oxygen Transport Tissue.* 1994;345:841–847.

36. Powell CC, Schultz SC, Burris DG, Drucker WR, Malcolm DS. Subcutaneous oxygen tension: A useful adjunct in assessment of perfusion status. *Crit Care Med.* 1995;23:867–873.

37. Cutler M. Transillumination as an aid to diagnosis of breast lesions. *Surg Gynecol Obstet.* 1929;48:721.

38. Afromonwitz MA, Callis, JB, Hemibach DM, DeSoto LAA, Norton MK. Multispectral imaging of burn wounds: A new clinical instrument for evaluating burn depth. *IEEE Trans Biomed Eng.* 1988;35:842.

39. Jones BM, Sandes R, Greenlagh RM. Monitoring skin flaps by colour measurements. *Br J Plast Surg.* 1983;36:88.

40. Chance B, Nioka S, Kent J, McCully K, Fountain M, Greenfeld R, Holtom G. Time resolved spectroscopy of hemoglobin and myoglobin in resting and ischemic muscle. *Analyt Biochem.* 1988;174:69.

41. Findlay GH. Carbon monoxide poisoning: Optics and histology of skin and blood. *Br J Dermatol.* 1988;119:45.

42. Altobelli SA, Caporihan A, Fukushima E, Majors PD. Liquid flow velocity determination by NMR imaging. *IEEE Eng Med Biol Soc 11th Annu Conf.* 1989: 50.

43. Olerud JE, Odland GF, Burgess EM, Wyss CR, Fisher LD, Matsen EA. A model for the study of wounds in normal elderly adults with peripheral vascular disease or diabetes mellitus. *J Surg Res.* 1995;59:349–360.

13 Pathophysiology of Diabetic Foot Lesions and Their Treatment with the Circulator Boot

Richard S. Dillon

Lower-Extremity Amputations
  Lower-Extremity Amputations (LEA) in Diabetics and Nondiabetics
  Lower-Extremity Amputations (LEA) Associated with Diabetes
Intermittent Claudication and Ischemic Disease
  Claudication and Its Prognosis
  Treatment of Claudication
  Estrogen Replacement Therapy a Risk Factor?
Diabetic Neuropathy
  Incidence and Diagnosis
  Hyperglycemia and Glycosylation in Neuropathy
  Neuropathy and Nerve Compression Syndromes
  Vascular Aspects of Diffuse Diabetic Neuropathy
  Cholinergic Neuropathy
  Vascular Aspects of Acute Painful Diabetic Neuritis
Reactive Hyperemia and Vascular Dysfunction
  Reactive Hyperemia (Post-Tourniquet) and Use of Pneumatic Boots
  Other Stimuli and Reactive Hyperemia
Effects of Smoking and Buerger's Disease
  Risks of Smoking and Vascular Disease
  Pathophysiological Effects of Smoking
  Buerger's Disease or Thromboangiitis Obliterans (TAO)
Diffuse Vascular Disease and Operative Risk Assessment
Infected Wounds

  Risk Factors in the Elderly
  Recognition of Infection
  Tissue Damage from Infection
  Osteomyelitis
  Problems with Antibiotic Therapy
  Morbidity of Foot Infections
  Antibiotics and Surgery for Foot Infections
  Sepsis and Septic Shock
  Circulator Boot and Local Antibiotic Therapy of Soft-Tissue Infections and Osteomyelitis
Cholesterol Emboli and Trash Feet
Vascular Hormones and Clotting Factors
  Relationship to *in vitro* Studies
  Collecting Blood Samples
  Hypercoagulability States
  Fibrinolysis and Fibrinolytic/ Anticoagulation Therapies
  Prostacyclin (PGI)
  Nitric Oxide
  VEGFs (Vascular Endothelial Growth Factors)
  Erythrocyte Sedimentation Rate and C-Reactive Protein ... Guides of Healing
Hyperinsulinemia and Insulin Resistance
  Weight Gain and Hyperinsulinemia
The Circulator Boot and Its Differences from Other Boots
  History of Vascular Boots and Effects on Vascular Tests
  Circulator Boot Versus ECP Devices
  Circulator Boot Therapy for PVD Versus Invasive Procedures

Cardiosynchronous External Compression Boots and the Heart

Method of Treatment and How the Boot Works

Effect of Booting on Hemodynamic Variables

How Does the Boot Work?

Patient Data

Physical Findings

Vascular Laboratory and Treatment

Soak Solutions

Topical Oxygen Therapy

Wound Classification

Classification of Ischemia

Treatment Options with the Circulator Boot Systems

Illustrative Examples of Patients Treated with the Circulator Boot

Female Patient with Postoperative Lymphedema

Long-Lasting Relief from Chronic Lymphedema with Eight Outpatient Treatments (Case 139)

Type 1 Diabetic with Multiple Complications

Combined Disease—Heart, Venous, Cellulitis, and Osteomyelitis with 14-Year Follow-up (Case 2)

Outpatient Treatment of Osteomyelitis

Necrotizing Cellulitis in Diabetic Foot (Case 1)

References

LOWER-EXTREMITY AMPUTATIONS

Lower-Extremity Amputations (LEA) in Diabetics and Nondiabetics

In the United States, the most common cause of amputation of the lower extremity is disease (about 70%) and that disease is most frequently diabetes, which has been increasing in prevalence along with obesity. The 1997 age-adjusted rates of hospital discharges among persons with lower-extremity amputations (LEA) who had diabetes were 28 times that of those without diabetes.[1] In developed countries, like Germany, the same high relative risk is seen, 22.2 in the report of Trautner et al.[2] In the Veterans Health Administration system during the period 1989–1998, rates of major and minor amputation declined an average of 5% each year, but the number of diabetes-associated amputations remained the same.[3] Diabetes-related amputation rates do exhibit high regional variation in the United States, however, even after adjustment for age, sex, and race.[4] Trauma (22%), congenital or birth defects (4%), and tumors (4%) are less frequent causes for LEA. On the other hand, causes of amputation vary greatly throughout the world, as do the incidence of smoking, the state of nutrition, and the incidence of diabetes. In countries at war, amputations due to trauma and land-mine accidents are much more frequent.

Lower-Extremity Amputations (LEA) Associated with Diabetes

A. Incidence of Amputations in Diabetics

The number of the various types of lower-extremity nontraumatic amputations associated with diabetes in the United States increased almost every year from 1980 to 2001; as shown in Fig. 13–1, minor decreases were seen in only 4 of the 22 years. Likewise, the age-standardized amputation rate increased during the same time period; as shown in Fig. 13–2, minor decreases were seen in only 6 of the 22 years. The average amputation rate per thousand diabetic population for the years 1980 to 1983 was 3.44 for age 0–64 years, 6.9 for age 65–74, and 12.1 for age over 75. For the period 1994 to 1996, these rates increased, respectively, to 6.7, 10.6, and 16.6.[5] African Americans fared worse than whites during the 1980 to 2001 time period; the age-standardized rate of hospital discharges for nontraumatic LEA per thousand diabetics varied from approximately 0.05–2.4 of that for whites; in 2001, it was 5.2 among blacks and 4.4 among whites. Men in the United States fared worse than women; the average age-standardized LEA rate from 1980 to 2001 increased most years from 1980 to its peak in 1996, while in women it was relatively constant during the time period. In 2001, it was 6.9 for men and 4.0 for women per thousand diabetics.

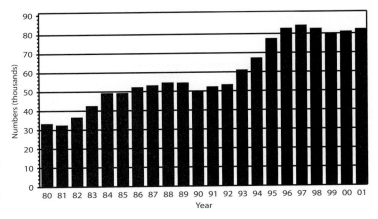

Fig. 13-1. Number of hospital discharges for nontraumatic lower-extremity amputation with diabetes as a listed diagnosis in the United States, 1980–2001. Source: Centers for Disease Control and Prevention, National Center for Health Statistics, Division of Health Care Statistics, data from the National Hospital Discharge Survey. Data computed by the Division of Diabetes Translation, National Center for Chronic Disease Prevention and Health Promotion, Centers for Disease Control and Prevention.

Mortality and Morbidity of Partial Amputations of the Foot

In Table 13–1, it is seen that amputations below the knee were more common in diabetics than nondiabetics in the National Hospital Discharge Surveys of 1989 to 1992. In the Hospital Discharge Data for the year 2000, the age-adjusted LEA rate for diabetics was 2.8 at the level of the toe, 0.9 for the foot, 1.9 below the knee, and 0.8 above the knee. Nondiabetics suffering above-the-knee amputations (AKA) have other risk factors, such as smoking (see below). The prognosis of those diabetics having distal amputations is guarded. Thirty years ago, the Joslin Clinic reported the fate of their diabetic patients having transmetatarsal amputations: 78, 70, 66, and 60% were living and 63, 57, 51, and 46% still had healed incisions at 2, 3, 4, and 5

years, respectively after amputation.[6] Gianfortune et al.[7] in reviewing 37 ray resections in 1985 found an overall success rate of 34%; 25% developed chronic ulcers and 41% required more proximal amputations.[7] Santi et al.[8] examined the fate of 94 partial foot resections, which had initially healed: 53.8% developed ulceration or needed local reoperation; the chance of completely avoiding any surgery after an initially healed partial foot amputation was 71% at 4 years after operation and 52% at 8 years after operation.[8] More recent reviews continue the same theme. The patients need follow-up and continued care. Initial healing may be seen with 58–69% with ultimate healing in up to 83%.[9–11] Later tissue breakdown is common, occurring in 27% by 3 weeks and up to 42% at 1 year.[12,13] Repeated operations may be necessary in 20–41%.[9,10]

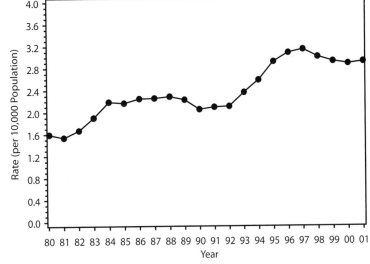

Fig. 13-2. Age-standardized rate of hospital discharge for nontraumatic lower-extremity amputation with diabetes as a listed diagnosis per 10,000 population, United States, 1980–2001. Source: Centers for Disease Control and Prevention, National Center for Health Statistics, Division of Health Care Statistics, data from the National Hospital Discharge Survey. Data computed by the Division of Diabetes Translation, National Center for Chronic Disease Prevention and Health Promotion, Centers for Disease Control and Prevention.

Table 13–1. Average annual number and percent distribution of hospital discharges listing lower extremity amputations by amputation level and presence of diabetes on the discharge record, United States, 1989–1992*

Amputation level	No diabetes		Diabetes		Totals	
	No.	%	No.	%	No.	%
Toe	12,427	24.1	21,671	40.3	34,098	32.3
Foot/ankle	2,967	5.8	7,773	14.5	10,740	10.2
Below knee	11,084	21.4	13,484	25.1	24,527	23.3
Knee disarticulation	778	1.5	704	1.3	1,482	1.4
Above knee	20,028	38.8	8,612	16.0	28,640	27.2
Hip/pelvis	386	0.7	87	0.2	473	0.5
Not specified	3,971	7.7	1,378	2.6	5,349	5.1
Total	51,605	100.0	53,709	100.0	105,309	100.0

*Reiber GE, Boyko EJ, Smith DG. *Diabetes in America,* 2nd ed. Bethesda, Maryland: National Diabetes Data Group of the National Institute of Diabetes and Digestive and Kidney Diseases, National Institute of Health; Table 18.4, p. 409.

Eventual leg amputation may be required in 12–46%, depending on the length of follow-up.[8–10,12–14] In a series collected over 6 years,[11] mortality rates again depend on follow-up, with perhaps 7% dying in the hospital[9] and 22.9% dying overall.

Successful distal procedures have advantages compared to below-the-knee amputations (BKA): ease of rehabilitation, retention of body image, ability to walk without gait-assisting devices, and increased ease of walking based on stride length, cadence, and oxygen consumption. The need for follow-up care after these surgical procedures, however, is frequently not emphasized to the patients or appreciated by some surgeons. In like fashion, patients undergoing treatment with the end-diastolic pneumatic boot require follow-up; relapse after a course of boot treatment does not require surgery in most patients, as healing is common after a second course of booting.[15] Again, failure to heal after a distal amputation has been a common reason for referral to our boot clinic.

Distal surgery reduces the plantar walking surface and itself produces deformities that predispose the feet to new lesions.[16] Attempts to lessen the detrimental effects of surgical deformities with the prescription of special shoes are largely unsuccessful, at least, in the inner cities studied.[17] It would appear to be appropriate to make every effort to keep the foot intact before resorting to deforming procedures.

Incidence, Morbidity, and Mortality of Major Amputations of the Lower Extremity and Risk to Remaining Leg

Of the 55,122 average annual major amputations in the 1989–1992 Hospital Discharge Surveys, 41.5% were in diabetics, who compromise perhaps 3% of the United States population. There are perhaps 350,000 amputees living in the United States. The number of amputees worldwide is not currently tracked by any organization. Persons with sufficient vascular disease in the leg to warrant leg amputation also have significant systemic vascular disease. Their prognoses both for life (Table 13–2) and maintenance of the other leg (Table 13–3) have remained guarded for the last 50 years in spite of the introduction of new therapies.

Reviews of lower-limb amputation statistics for populations, including both diabetics and nondiabetics, are equally grim.[30–34] At major centers like the Mayo Clinic, the amputation rate for peripheral arterial disease, but not the overall number of amputations, has declined since 1974.[31] While their patients since 1974 were more likely to have a BKA, the rate of successful prosthetic fitting in the geriatric population did not change significantly over 40 years. Concomitant cerebrovascular disease and discharge to a nursing home were more common since 1974. Buzato et al.[32] pointed out that in their clinic not only was the mortality rate (54.2%) considerable after 2 years, but that only 40.9% of their living patients (18.8% of all patients) were fully rehabilitated. Preoperatively, 31% had had an independent life style, 44% could walk 500 m, 15% required a wheelchair or crutches, and 10% were bedridden. Time and amputation had taken a major toll. In Finland, Eskelinen et al.[35] have found that chronic limb ischemia (79.1%) and acute ischemia (13.9%) were the major reasons for leg amputation with an increasing percentage of AKA being done as the amputees tended more often to be institutionalized and immobile, reconstruction was not an alternative, and BKA was impossible or useless.[35] Kuukasjarvi and Salenius[36] looked specifically at the risk of acute ischemia due to thrombosis or embolism.

Table 13–2. Mortality associated with leg amputations in diabetics

Author (year)	Postoperative	1 Year	2 Years	3 Years	4 Years	5 Years	7 Years
Silbert (1952)(17a)				35%		59%	
Hoar (1962)(18a)	7%				30%		
Cameron (1964)(19a)						65%	
Braddeley & Fulford (1965)(18)	15.1%						
Whitehouse et al. (1966)(19)							80%
Ecker & Jacobs (1970)(20)	23% Inpatient				39%	58%	
Roon et al. (1970)(20a)	3% Inpatient					55%	
Kahn et al. (1974)(21)	9%						
Kolind-Sorensen (1974)(21a)	25%						
Ebskov & Josephson (1980)(22)	16.3%, at 3 months				22.4%		
Haynes & Middleton (1981)(23)	16.4%, of 2 weeks & 25.5% Inpatient						
Rozin (1987)(24)	23.8%						
Enroth & Persson (1992)(25)	38% at 6 months			72%			
Deerochanawong et al. (1992)(26)	10%	40%	50%				
Apelqvist et al. (1993)(27)	20%				41%	73%	
VanBuskirk et al. (1994)(28)	10.1% in hospital						
Pohjolainen & Alaranta (1998)(29)		38%	53%		80%		

Significant risk factors for thrombosis included previous major amputation or vascular surgery and smoking. The overall amputation rate was 16% during the postoperative period. The amputation rate and mortality rate were significantly higher for acute thrombosis (26 and 16%) than for embolism (10 and 11%), respectively. The high amputation rate associated with acute thrombosis was related to the need for additional operations and thromboembolectomy rather than reconstruction. Fusetti et al.[34] reported that 36% of their amputees died in the hospital and only 28% were able to go home, while 44% were dead at 1 year. Seventy-eight percent were initially fitted with prostheses and 30% were fully independent. Only 35% were satisfied at the end of treatment, their satisfaction being influenced by the level of amputation, residual pain, and mobility. For most surviving patients the quality of life was poor.

Statistics from Veterans Hospitals on the mortality and morbidity among both diabetics and nondiabetics are equally dismal. Feinglass et al.[30] reviewed the experience of 119 Veterans Affairs (VA) hospitals from 1991 to 1995. Thirty-day postoperative mortality was 6.3% for 1909 below-knee and 13.3% for 2152 above-knee amputees. Surviving patients had 10,827 subsequent VA hospitalizations during a median 32-month follow-up. Survival probabilities for below- and above-knee amputees were 77 and 59% at 1 year, 57 and 39% at 3 years, and 28 and 20% at 7.5 years. Toursarkissian[33] reported in more detail on their current experience with 113 major lower-extremity amputations secondary to vascular disease

Table 13–3. Incidence of contralateral limb amputation in diabetic leg amputees

Author (year)	1 Year	2 Years	3 Years	4 Years	5 Years
Silbert (1952)(17a)		30%			51%
Goldner (1960)(22a)			40%		66%
Hoar (1962)(18a)			36%		50%
Cameron et al. (1964)(19a)	8.5%				
Baddeley & Fulford (1965)(18)			20%		
Ecker & Jacobs (1970)(20)		26%			
Roon et al. (1977)					36.6%
Ebskov & Josephson (1980)(22)		18%	27%	44%	
Apelquist et al. (1993)(27)	13%		35%		48%

among 99 diabetic and nondiabetic men over a 3-year period at their Veterans Affairs institution. Seventy-five percent were diabetic and above- to below-knee amputation ratio was 3:2, which was directly related to diabetic status: for BKA diabetics 43% and nondiabetics 26%. The in-hospital (2.6%) and 30-day (8%) mortality rates were not related to amputation level. Postoperative complications, most frequently wound related (22%), occurred in 40% and were more frequent with BKAs than AKAs. At an average follow-up of 10 (+/− 8 months) 35% had died. Fifty-one percent were discharged to rehabilitation units, but only 26% regularly wore a prosthesis with 23% ambulating. Significant differences were seen in those capable of ambulation: 34% of BKA patients versus 9% of AKA patients; and 25% of nondialysis patients versus 5% of dialysis patients. The contralateral limb later required amputation in 17% or bypass surgery in 7%. Significant differences in complication rates were seen among African Americans (59%), Hispanics (45%), and whites (23%).

Length of hospitalization for leg amputations— Patients undergoing leg amputation commonly have multiple medical problems significantly adding to their hospital length of stay. Cameron noted stays of 77 days for above-the-knee amputations and 55 days for below-the-knee-amputations in 1964. At a inner-city university hospital, Ecker[20] reported in 1970, stays of 5.9 months for AKAs and 6.7 months for BKAs if no further surgery was performed; 10.2% of his patients had died under 30 days, 32% healed by 30 days, 19.5% healed between 30–60 days, 30% healed after 60 days, and 10.2% did not heal. Haynes and Middleton[23] reported a mean postoperative stay of 65 days for their combined diabetic and nondiabetic group in 1981; failure to obtain immediate satisfactory healing of the stump occurred in 18.4% and reamputation was required in 5.6%. It is likely that amputees heal no faster in 2003 than they have over the years, but pressures in the United States to hasten discharges from the hospital and transfers to nursing facilities are greater. Thus, while the age-adjusted incidence of diabetes-related lower-extremity amputations (LEAs) was significantly higher in 1996 in the state of California than in the Netherlands (49.9 versus 36.1 per 10,000 diabetics, $p < 0.01$), the length of hospital stay was significantly higher in the Netherlands: 40.8 versus 16.0 ($p < 0.01$).[37] Economic pressures have resulted in decreased length of hospital stays both in city and suburbs in the United States. For the years 1980 to 1983, African Americans averaged 40.5 days per hospitalization and whites 33.1 days. By the 1994 to 1996 period, these numbers were reduced to 13.9 and 14.8 days, respectively. Over the entire 1980 to 1996 period, African Americans averaged 23.7 days and whites 22.1 days. In countries where the patients are not

transferred from the hospital before their recovery, the length of stay remains considerable—109 days in Switzerland, for example.[34] Length of stay is a major variable in the cost of care of peripheral vascular disease and its complications.

Causes of Amputations in Diabetics

Multiple risk factors are associated with vascular disease and leg amputations and their correction is important in the prevention of both the beginning and progression of vascular disease. Both the risk factors present and the risk factors likely explaining the need for leg amputation in their patients were reported by Pecoraro et al.[38] (Table 13–4). The main problems were neuropathy, gangrene, and infection. Most reports do not differentiate between the gangrene produced by necrotizing cellulitis and isolated ischemia. Clinically, combinations, of course, exist, but the two extremes are easily separated. A tight string around a toe, for example, produces dry gangrene with a sharp demarcation line between the normal and dead skin. A toe elevated above its perfusion pressure may also blacken and dry out. The weight of the foot pressing the heel into the bedding with a pressure higher than the arterial perfusion pressure may produce a black, dry heel eschar. Dry gangrene tends to be distal at the end of the vascular tree. In contrast, necrotizing cellulitis produces drainage and is surrounded by erythrema, where the infection is invading adjacent tissue; photoelectricplethysmographic tracings over the reddened areas commonly show bounding pulses. Tissue distal to necrotizing cellulitis may be healthy. Ischemic gangrene may be painful while the tissue is dying; after demarcation in the absence of infection, pain may be minimal. Necrotizing cellulitis continues to hurt while the infection is active; transcutaneous gas studies reveal the urgency of the cellulitic process: the transcutaneous

Table 13–4. Proportion of diabetic limb amputations due to individual causes and final component cause*

Factor	Present	Main problem
Ischemia	40%	5%
Neuropathy		61%
Gangrene	55%	40%
Infection	59%	41%
Ulceration	84%	
Minor trauma	81%	
Faulty wound healing	81%	14%

*Pecoraro RE, Reiber GE, Burgess EM. Pathways to diabetic limb amputation. Basis for prevention. *Diabetes Care.* 1990;13:513–521.

PO_2 may be zero and the PCO_2 level very high. Arrest of the infectious process with effective antibiotic therapy may relieve the pain. Such instantaneous pain relief is commonly seen with the local injection of antibiotics into the tissue and its dissemination with the end-diastolic pneumatic boot. Infection and neuropathy are the most important factors leading to amputations and are interrelated.

Monetary Costs and Social Effects of Amputations

While the monetary costs of peripheral vascular disease can be tabulated, the social costs are not immediately apparent. Leg amputation, the worst case outcome, robs most patients of their independence. Amputation of a limb can affect almost all aspects of the life of the individual and to fully recover from limb loss all of these areas need to be addressed. Issues of simple mobility and self-care are the initial problems that most amputees and their families face. Participation in a comprehensive rehabilitation program may help the amputees recover some function, but like nursing home care, loss of work and income are additional expenses to society not commonly initially considered. Costs may not be fully appreciated from case reports, which list the costs of care delivered by the authors and neglect previous and later care. Waugh[39] points out that diabetic patients requiring amputations do not limit themselves to the records and services of a single physician; they have a multiplicity of admissions to different specialties and utilize hospital beds at a cost equivalent at least to 1.2% of all hospital costs. Further costs may be underestimated and the benefits of treatment overestimated in reports using life-table analyses in their calculations. Jensen et al.[40] compared the patency and survival rates of their infrainguinal bypass procedures using life-table methods with the results based on their vascular registry accumulated in their clinical trial. They found a marked discrepancy between the calculated figures: primary (68% in the registry and 52% in the trial) and secondary patency rates (90 versus 63%), limb survival (97 versus 77%), as well as patients survival rates (95 versus 85%). The differences could be explained by a substantial number of patients being lost to follow-up according to the vascular registry database and the fact that these patients turned out to have a significantly increased rate of graft thrombosis, limb amputation, and death. Medicare claims provide a more global viewpoint including care wherever the Medicare beneficiary seeks care. Medicare claims data for 1995 and 1996 showed $1.5 billion expenditures in 1995 for lower-extremity ulcer patients. These were, on average three times higher than those for Medicare patients in general ($15,309 versus $5,226) and 73.7% of these costs were for inpatient care with

proportionately smaller amounts for physicians and nursing home facilities.[41] Such costs can be somewhat broken down by race and degree of disease. In California in 1991, the mean hospital charge per patient with all ethnic groups combined was $27,930; the mean length of stay was 15.9 days.[42] Hospital charges and length of stay for toe amputations were less than those for higher amputations. One-quarter of the patients had multiple amputations during their hospital stay and had significantly higher hospital charges ($44,731) and longer hospital stays (23.4 days) than those receiving only a single amputation. African Americans had significantly higher mean charges ($32,383) and longer stays (17.3 days) compared to all other ethnic groups, perhaps because of more advanced disease.

Studies from Europe and elsewhere provide similar themes. The population of Sweden (about 9 million) is 10% larger than the city of New York (over 7 million) and differs in climate, homeogeneity of population, and extremes in wealth. Among the 341 foot-ulcer patients in Sweden followed by the multidisciplinary foot-care team of Apelqvist et al.,[43] 11.7% died without healing and 62.7% healed primarily at an average cost of 14.8% of the 24.5% of patients that healed after amputation. The percentage of total costs for inpatient care was 37% for those primarily healed and 82% for the amputation group. The costs for topical treatment of the ulcers in outpatient care were 45% of the total average cost for primary healed and 13% for patients who healed with amputation. Health costs, however, do not cease with healing of a primary ulcer. Apelqvist reported that significant costs were incurred during a 3-year follow-up period after healing.[44] Their patients who healed primarily, in spite of ankle systolic blood pressures under 80 and toe pressures under 45 mm Hg, incurred $26,700 additional health and social care costs, while those with better blood flow still required $16,100 additional care. Their patients who healed after amputations below the ankle required $43,100 follow-up care and those with higher amputations required $63,100 additional care. They subsequently extended their analysis to the period from the time of the first operative procedure until death or 6 years of follow-up.[45] Of their 321 patients presenting with ankle systolic blood pressures under 80 and toe pressures under 45 mm Hg, 29.9% had a reconstructive vascular procedure with one-third having an ipsilateral amputation, 34.6% had a restorative vascular procedure with half having an ipsilateral amputation, and 35.5% had an initial major amputation (amputations above the ankle). The patients underwent a mean of three procedures (range 1–19). Their average length of hospital stay was 117 days (range 1–1097) with less than half in the surgery department, 10% in acute care, and about half in rehabilitation and nursing home facilities. After death, patients, of course, incurred no additional expenses. The mean costs for all patients over the course of their study was $47,000.

Restoration of blood flow to the extremity obviating need for leg amputation is a major goal and one with potential benefits in monetary costs and quality of life. Over a median follow-up period of 15.4 months, Panayiotopoulos et al.[46] found that primary amputation was 68.8% more expensive than femorodistal reconstruction in diabetics and 89.6% more expensive than in nondiabetics. Primary amputation itself was 28.7% more expensive in diabetics. However, revascularization procedures not infrequently require later costs in patient comfort and money because of need for revisions. Wixon et al.[47] found that among their 155 consecutive autogenous infrainguinal bypass grafts performed for chronic leg ischemia, 61 grafts required 86 revisions. Their mean 5-year cost of graft maintenance ($16,318) approached that of the initial bypass graft ($19,331) and the sum of the initial cost of bypass graft and 5-year graft maintenance cost ($35,649) was similar to the cost of amputation ($36,273). The costs of follow-up revascularization might be lessened if it is not performed in asymptomatic patients. Tangelder et al.[48] found that quality of life in patients with asymptomatic occluded grafts was similar to quality of life in patients with patent grafts. Revascularization of symptomatic occluded grafts, on the other hand, improved quality of life to a certain extent. However, the costs of both revascularization procedures and amputations are significant and their benefits occasionally limited. Hunink et al.[49] noted that initial angioplasty increased quality-adjusted life expectancy by 2–13 months and resulted in decreased lifetime expenditures compared with bypass surgery for their example of 65-year-old men with disabling claudication and a femoropopliteal stenosis or occlusion and/or with chronic critical ischemia and a femoropopliteal stenosis. Conversely, they reported that initial bypass surgery increased quality-adjusted life expectancy by 1–4 months and resulted in decreased lifetime expenditures for patients with chronic critical ischemia and femoropopliteal occlusion compared with angioplasty. A procedural mortality rate of 0–7.4% for angioplasty and 0.6–9.7% for bypass was noted. Major procedural cardiopulmonary, renal, or cerebrovascular complications occurred in 0.2–11% of angioplasty patients and 2.7–13% of bypass patients. Estimated costs in 1990 dollars were $2,443–11,809 for angioplasty and $9,331–33,367 for bypass. Amputation costs plus rehabilitation were estimated at $22,346. Annual costs postamputation were estimated at $88,765 for treatments and $23,000 for nursing care (based on the estimate that 29% of all amputees required nursing care at an average cost of $1,520 per week), conservative estimates for amputees becoming immobilized and dependent on nursing care is 29–38%. In comparison, boot therapy has no mortality or morbidity. It may suffer, however, from a longer duration of treatment. One can do a lot of booting for these costs.

INTERMITTENT CLAUDICATION AND ISCHEMIC DISEASE

Claudication and Its Prognosis

Arterial noninvasive testing has shown rates of peripheral arterial disease of 2.5% at ages 40–59, 8.3% at ages 60–69, and 18.8% at ages 70–79, all associated with increased risk for stroke and coronary disease.[50] When the disease becomes advanced enough to cause leg pain with walking, intermittent claudication is said to be present (Table 13–5). The risk of developing claudication in both sexes is increased two- to threefold by

Table 13–5. Differential diagnosis of claudication and rest pain

Arteriosclerosis obliterans	Degenerative joint disease in back, hips, knees, ankles, or feet
Spinal stenosis	
Ataxias	Weakness
Lymphedema	Venous stasis
Thrombophlebitis	Arterial emboli
Stress fractures	Plantar fasciitis
Reflex sympathetic dystrophy	Erythromelalgia
Gout	Compartment syndromes
Raynaud's syndrome	Cellulitis
Baker's cyst	Cold damage
Popliteal artery entrapment	Nerve entrapment syndromes
Endofibrosis in athletes	

diabetes.[51] Further progression of disease may result in rest pain. Symptoms are related to the ankle-brachial index (ABI); a 0.3 improvement in ABI is associated with an average improvement of 5.6% in physical functioning or 10.3% in a walking impairment questionnaire.[52] The risk for death and leg amputation increases with the progression through the stages of asymptomatic laboratory disease, claudication to rest pain. Criqui et al.[53] found 11.9% of 565 men and women, with an average age of 66, to have abnormal studies of segmental blood pressure and determination of flow velocity by Doppler ultrasound. After 10 years, 61.8% of the men and 33.3% of the women had died, as compared with 16.9% of the men and 11.6% of the women without abnormal vascular tests. Additional analyses revealed a 15-fold increase in rates of mortality due to cardiovascular and coronary heart disease among subjects with large-vessel peripheral arterial disease that was both severe and symptomatic. For individuals with modest intermittent claudication, the disease may run a variable course dependent on the management of risk factors. Overall, Dormandy et al.[54] note 1–3% of claudicants will require major amputation over a 5-year period. Indeed, perhaps 50% of claudicants become symptom-free during 5 years follow-up. About one fourth of patients with claudication will ever significantly deteriorate and that deterioration is most frequent during the first year after diagnosis (6–9%) compared with 2–3% per annum thereafter. Smoking is the most important risk factor for the progression of local disease in the legs, with an amputation rate 11 times greater in smokers than nonsmokers. Diabetes, male gender, hypertension, and the number of stenoses on an arteriogram are also important risk factors for progression. Jonason and Ringqvist[55] found that over 6 years, 86% of patients with single stenosis were free of rest pain versus 70% of those with multiple stenoses after adjustment for smoking (Table 13-6).

Table 13–6. Checklist for risk factors

Risk factor	Goal
Smoking	None
Glycohemoglobin	Normal
Endocrine visits	Enough to normalize HgbA1c
Systolic blood pressure	<130 mm Hg
Total cholesterol	<200 mg/dl, lower better
Body mass index	Male <27; female <26
Shoewear	Appropriate fit
Drugs and other diseases	Minimal use of steroids and vasoconstrictors

Treatment of Claudication

Goals of treatment include improvement in pain-free walking, normalization of risk factors, initiation of antiplatelet therapies to decrease cardiovascular ischemic events, and avoidance of limb injury and amputation. Commonly listed modalities of therapy include: exercise training and Cilostazol for mild to moderate claudication and, when the anatomy and health of the patient allows, endovascular procedures and surgical bypass in more severe cases. Dillon[15] has had little experience with Circulator Boot therapy in mild-to-moderate degrees of claudication as most patients referred for boot therapy were inoperable and had walking distances limited to, perhaps, 20 feet or less or had rest pain and were wheelchair-bound.[15] Thus, among his 139 male patients nondiabetic legs, 134 female patients nondiabetic legs, 176 diabetic male patients legs, and 116 diabetic female patients legs in the Wagner class one category (intact skin and only bony deformities) most had advanced claudication or rest pain; 72.7, 78.4, 81.8, and 84.5%, respectively, significantly improved with boot therapy. Of the 69 patients referred for inoperable rest pain, 34 were nondiabetic, 16 had type 1 diabetes, and 18 had type 2 diabetes; 84% were cured or markedly improved. Major amputations were performed early in two nondiabetic patients, after an initial relapse in one nondiabetic patient and one type 1 diabetic patient, and, finally, later, in another institution, again in one nondiabetic and one type 1 diabetic patient—overall 6 or 8.7% among the 69 patients. Forty-five of the 68 had lived 7.09 ± 4.82 years since presentation for treatment when the study was closed. Such patients have too much disease to participate in an exercise program. It has long been appreciated that active people have larger vessels than inactive people and that a plaque of given size in a large artery may not obstruct flow as it would in a small artery. Exercise programs hopefully might increase the lumen of the arteries, increase collateral flow, and/or improve the exercise capacity to a given amount of oxygen. There is little vascular test data showing the benefits of exercise in claudicants, however. Gerrits et al.,[56] however, have shown that paralyzed patients with spinal cord injuries increased the diameter of their femoral arteries along with inflow volumes and velocity index after 6 weeks of cycling using a functional electrically stimulated leg cycle ergometer. Typical supervised exercise programs require the performance of treadmill or track-based exercise for 45–60 minutes performed 3 or more times a week for a minimum of 12 weeks.[57] The possibility of exertional compartment syndromes must always be considered before prescribing exercise as surgical decompression by fasciotomy rather than exercise would be the proper therapy.[58] Cilostazol (Pletal) is an inhibitor of phosphodiesterase III and increases intracellular cyclic adenosine monophosphate levels in platelets and vascular smooth muscle cells, thereby decreasing platelet aggregation and inducing microvascular vasodilation. Its standard dosage of 100 mg twice daily may be reduced to 50 mg twice daily if side effects are apparent. It is expensive ($80–100/month) and is approved by the FDA for relief of symptoms of intermittent claudication. It is contraindicated if the possiblility of hypersensitivity is suspected or in the presence of any degree of congestive failure as drugs in this class have decreased survival in patients with class III-IV failure. It may be associated with a 98% increase in pain-free walking distance (versus 55% for placebo) and a 54% increase in maximal walking distance (versus 34% for placebo).[59] Its onset of efficacy is slow (2–4 weeks) and it may take up to 12 weeks to assess its full effectiveness. Furthermore, therapy must be continued to maintain increases in walking distance. Its list of adverse effects is considerable (versus percentage for placebo): headache 34% (14%), diarrhea 19% (7%), abnormal stools 15% (4%), palpitation 10% (1%), dizziness 10% (6%), pharyngitis 10% (7%), and infection 10% (8%). Drug interactions may be expected with drugs involving cytochrome CYP3A4 (eg, ketoconazole, erythromycin, diltiazem) or cytochrome CYP2C19 (omeprazole). Pentoxiflline (Trental) has also been approved for the treatment of claudication. It likewise poses a significant expense. Ernst[60] notes that not all health care providers agree that it is effective, but concludes that the collective published data does show that it prolongs walking distance in patients with intermittent claudication. The multiple actions of the drug are intriguing. Unfortunately, it takes several weeks before benefit is to be expected and then the benefit is generally small, perhaps a 20% increase in walking distance (a patient capable of taking 20 steps can now take 24 steps). The author has not prescribed the drug in his boot patients, but will continue it if their own physician had previously prescribed it and the patient believed it was beneficial. Beta-blockers and angiotensin-converting enzyme (ACE) inhibitors are commonly prescribed for the hypertension accompanying claudication in some patients and may have an adverse effect on the claudication. Roberts et al.,[61] for example, found that atenolol, labetolol, and pindolol decreased maximum walking distances on a treadmill and postexercise calf blood flow availability, but that captopril did not and possibly preserved collateral blood supply. The technical aspects of bypass and angioplasty are not reviewed in this chapter. Perkins et al.[62] have compared the benefits of exercise-training with angioplasty. While significant increases in the ABI were seen at each time period in the angioplasty group, the most significant changes in claudication and maximum walking distances were seen in the exercise training group and, at long-term follow-up, there were no significant

differences between the groups. Their subgroup analysis showed greater functional improvement in those patients with disease confined to the superficial femoral artery treated by exercise training. Whyman et al.[63] likewise found no long-term functional benefit to angioplasty in their randomized controlled trial. They further noted that most of the claudicants they screened for angioplasty were not candidates; only 10% of their 600 patients had discrete lesions suitable for percutaneous transluminal angioplasty (PTA).[64] Feinglass et al.[65] have compared the functional status and walking ability after bypass and angioplasty and compared them to the results obtained with exercise training in a nonrandomized prospective study. Of their 526 study patients, 20% chose to undergo revascularization procedures (60 surgical bypass grafting and 44 angioplasty only) and benefited with modest improvements in their ABI (0.20 for bypass surgery and 0.09 for angioplasty). Patient questionnaires showed that the patients had significant physical improvements in mean physical functioning, 17% for bypass and 14% for angioplasty, bodily pain (18 and 13%), and walking distance (28 and 27%) scores. In contrast, the conditions of the 277 unmatched patients who underwent medical management declined on all outcome measures, and the conditions of the 145 matched patients who underwent medical management improved only 5% on walking distance score. The greatest improvement was seen in those with the greatest improvements in ABI. Lundgren et al.[66] studied 75 patients with intermittent claudication, blood pressure in the great toe over 30 mm Hg, maximum walking distance under 600 m, and no rest pain or ischemic ulcers. Surgery most effectively increased walking distance, but training improved results even further. Age, symptom duration, and history of myocardial disease correlated negatively with walking distance after treatment. Fifty-eight operations were performed in 48 patients; the rest underwent exercise training. The surgical group had significant complications within the first month of surgery: wound hematomas evacuated in 3 patients, thrombectomies and re-reconstructions in 3 patients, myocardial infarctions in 2 patients, and pulmonary embolus in 1 patient. Late reoperations were performed in 2 patients and 2 patients died before follow-up. In the training group, no complications due to training were seen, but life-threatening ischemia developed in 2 patients who underwent operation and another 2 developed cardiac insufficiency of a degree preventing training. In contrast, Dillon[15] experienced no complications in his Wagner class 1 patients who were largely treated as outpatients. In athletes, the diagnosis of claudication may not be suspected. In cyclists, pain and a powerless feeling in the leg may indicate flow limitations in the iliac arteries caused by functional lesions (kinking and/or excessive length of vessels) and/or intravascular lesions (endofibrosis).[67,68] The external iliac artery is involved in over 90% of cases. A bruit in the inguinal region with the thigh maximally flexed may be the only physical finding pointing to the diagnosis. Provocative testing on a bicycle ergometer with high intensity of exercise, combined with postexercise blood pressure measurements (at the ankle of both legs, or the ankle to arm pressure ratio) may help confirm the diagnosis. Therapy first is the conservative advice that the athlete might change sports activity. Schep et al.[67] advise that angioplasty and intravascular stent are contraindicated because of high risks for dissection and reactive intimal hyperplasia, respectively, and that long-term follow-up of surgical procedures is lacking. Abraham et al.[69] note, however, that most surgically treated patients are able to return to competition.

Estrogen Replacement Therapy a Risk Factor?

In recent years, the desirability of replacement with female sex hormones has been under review. The Rotterdam study suggested hormone replacement therapy (HRT) has a protective influence: HRT given for a year or more was associated with a decreased risk of peripheral arterial disease among postmenopausal women.[70] Further, it showed that any use of HRT was associated with a decreased thickness of the intima in the common carotid artery in elderly women.[71] Others, however, have found no benefit of HRT on the heart or the intima of the carotids and support the recommendation of the American Heart Association that women with established coronary disease should not initiate hormone therapy, with an expectation of atherosclerotic benefit.[72,73] Again, Timaran et al.[74] have shown that in their femoropopliteal bypass patients, HRT was the only independent predictor of reduced primary graft patency. The interested reader might consult the multiple reviews on the effect of estrogen therapy on arteriosclerotic disease for more information. It would appear that women might take estrogens for their bones and menopausal symptoms but would do well not to start in later life in hopes of a cardiovascular benefit.

DIABETIC NEUROPATHY

Incidence and Diagnosis

While the most common cause of peripheral neuropathy in the United States is diabetes, there are many other causes (Table 13–7) that must be considered in the diabetic, especially when the diabetes has been of short duration and well controlled, as suggested by normal or minor elevation in the glycohemoglobin level. Among diabetic patients, peripheral neuropathy is common. Defining "neuropathy" as abnormal sensory or motor

Table 13–7. Neuropathic diseases, Charcot feet, and dysesthesias

Poorly controlled diabetes (most common cause of neuropathic foot ulcers seen in the United States)	Poisoning due to heavy metals or organic chemicals
Pernicious anemia	Drug toxicity
Chronic alcoholism	Inflammatory states
Old spinal cord injuries	Collagen diseases
Myelodysplasia	Uremia
Syringomyelia	Porphyia
Tabes Dorsalis	Acromegaly
Lyme Disease	Beriberi
Leprosy	Pyridoxine deficiency or excess
Hereditory sensory syndromes	Entrapment syndromes
Small vessel disease	Tendon shortening

signs, symptoms, or decreased deep dendon reflexes, Maser et al.[75] found among 400 diabetic subjects that 18% of those 18–29 years old and 58% of those over 29 years old were afflicted. In motor conduction studies, virtually all diabetics may be found to have some neuropathy. Vinik et al.[76] found the combination thermal and vibratory to give optimum sensitivity (92–95%) and specificity (77–86%) compared to the sensitivity of warm (78%), cold (77%), vibration (88%), tactile-pressure (77%), 5 Hz-current perception (52%), 250-Hz perception (48%), and 2000-Hz current perception when examining the dominant hallux.

Hyperglycemia and Glycosylation in Neuropathy

Hyperglycemia may damage nerves through three pathways: glycosylation, the polyol pathway (hyperglycemia → increased sorbitol-fructose→decreased myoinositol in Schwann cell→abnormal energy metabolism and damage,[77]) and vascular abnormalities. The glycohemoglobin test has found its way into common usage as a means to determine the adequacy of glucose control. HgbA is normally glycosylated slowly, nonenzymatically, and relatively irreversibly into HgbA1c at a rate detemined by the average glucose level. The glycosylation process may link proteins together into larger "advanced glycosylation products" that may alter function and structure. In the case of the red cell, for example, oxygen transport by hemoglobin is diminished. The red cell membrane is stiffened and an increased capillary perfusion pressure is required to push it through the capillary bed. The increased pressure may force other large proteins into the pores in the capillary wall where they may become trapped and thicken the capillary membrane. Leukocytes are likewise glycosylated altering their deformability and function. Glycosylation of various serum proteins and blood elements may result in platelet dysfunction, a hypercoagulable state, abnormal fibrinolysis, and in increased blood viscosity.

Neuropathy and Nerve Compression Syndromes

Glycosylation of tendons and ligments may increase their size and promote peripheral nerve compression syndromes or tendon contractures.[78,79] Perhaps, however, lessening enthusiasm for this glycosylation-nerve compression syndrome hypothesis is the report of Becker et al.[80] In studying 791 cases with carpal tunnel syndrome and 981 controls, they found that diabetes was not significantly associated with the carpal tunnel syndrome when the patients were stratified by body mass index. Still, surgical decompression procedures have produced marked improvement in nerve function in patients appearing to have typical diabetic peripheral neuropathy.[81–83] That factors other than external compression are operative in the diabetic with the carpal tunnel syndrome, for example, is likely as the improvement after decompression in the diabetic is less than that seen in the nondiabetic.[84] Alternatively, some of the patients not benefiting from decompression may have more than one area of nerve compression.[85] Likewise, lengthening the Achilles tendon may improve gait and motor function.[86,87]

Vascular Aspects of Diffuse Diabetic Neuropathy

The multiple derangements above have been shown in human and animal models to be associated with reduced nerve perfusion, endoneurial hypoxia, and structural changes in nerve microvasculature, including basement membrane thickening, pericyte degeneration, and endothelial cell hyperplasia. These vascular changes strongly correlate with clinical defects and nerve pathology[88] and in laboratory animals may precede slowing of motor nerve conduction.[89] Damage to the sympathetic and cholinergic nerve supply to the legs may result in further vascular abnormalities, again decreasing effective and appropriate tissue perfusion. Damage to the sympathetic nerves may promote orthostatic hypotension and opening of the arteriovenous shunts. The latter operate normally in thermal regulation allowing warm blood to flow near the skin surface without having to traverse the capillary beds, thus producing a warm pink foot. The warmth may increase tissue oxygen requirements without the provision of needed oxygen supply. Thus, sympathectomy has been shown to decrease skin PO_2 levels as the shunts open.[90]

Conversely, closing the shunts with the administration of ephedrine has been shown to increase subcutaneous PO_2 levels.[91] (The use of ephedrine is not encouraged. It may raise blood pressure, potentiate glaucoma, oppose the release of insulin by the pancreas, and increase arterial vasoconstriction. Indeed, susceptible patients, such as those with Raynaud's phenomenon, may develop peripheral cyanosis and ulcers with the regular use of ephedrine-containing nosedrops.) Even in patients screened to have an ABI over 1 and absent major vascular calcifications, arteriovenous shunts may be demonstrated to have significant clinical adverse associations. Thus, Uccioli et al.[92] found that radioactive albumen microspheres injected into the femoral artery escaped, presumably through shunts, entrapment in the capillary circulation of the leg, and found their way to the lung in increasing amounts, depending on the clinical status of the patients: 3.8% in healthy nonneuropathic patients, 6.8% in neuropathic patients free of foot ulcers, and 10.4% in patients with recurrent foot ulcers. At the bedside, the presence of significant shunting is suggested by continuous Doppler arterial flow heard between the pulse waves. Such continuous flow is associated with the presence of vascular calcifications in the foot. In like fashion, Chew et al.[93] found their neuropathic patients to have Doppler velocities from popliteal to big toes the same as controls, but triphasic flow was lost and replaced by monophasic flow with prolonged diastolic flow at level of dorsalis pedis and posterior tibial arteries and distally. Toe pressures were reduced approximately one third with a linear correlation between degree of neuropathy and decrease in toe pressure.[93] Vayssairat and Le Devehat[94] have emphasized the importance of the falloff in toe pressure, finding it present in about 15% of all diabetic patients without trophic changes and in 35% of those with trophic changes; they found it closely related to neuropathy. Zimny et al.[95] noted significant differences among their neuropathic diabetics (no history of foot ulcer), nonneuropathic diabetics and healthy controls regarding transcutaneous oxygen tension both supine and in the sitting/supine ratio in spite of their having normal Doppler ultrasound studies. In supine position, $TcPO_2$ was significantly reduced (means $+/-$ SE) in diabetic neuropathic patients (6.04 $+/-$ 0.52 kPa) compared with nonneuropathic diabetic (7.14 $+/-$ 0.43 kPa, $p = 0.035$) and nondiabetic (8.10 $+/-$ 0.44 kPa, $p = 0.01$) control subjects. The sitting/supine $TcPO_2$ difference was higher in diabetic neuropathic subjects (3.13 $+/-$ 0.27 kPa) compared with both nonneuropathic diabetic (2.00 $+/-$ 0.18, $p = 0.004$) and nondiabetic (1.77 $+/-$ 0.15 kPa, $p = 0.0003$) control subjects. The mean sitting/supine ratio was 1.70 $+/-$ 0.12 in diabetic neuropathic patients, 1.32 +/− 0.04 in diabetic control subjects, and 1.25 +/− 0.03 in nondiabetic control subjects ($p = 0.007$). The clinical value of possibly producing such deficits with sympathectomy is questionable. Repelaer-an-Driel et al.[96] found lumbar sympathectomy had no benefit in their patients with arm/ankle indices under 0.3; all required major amputation.

Cholinergic Neuropathy

Loss of cholinergic innervation in the diabetic foot might be considered separately. It has adverse cutaneous and circulatory effects. Absence of the cholinergic innervation to the sweat glands cause dryness of the skin, thus promoting cracks and fissures that are potential portals for infection. Release of acetylcholine in the tissues stimulates endothelial nitric acid synthase to make nitric oxide and prostacyclin, both vasodilators. At the bedside, local injections of cholinergic agents causes local erythema and increased capillary photoelectricplethysmographic pulse (PPG) waves. Acetylcholine, hence, may increase flow in the nutrient vessels, thus potentially delivering leukocytes, platelets, antibiotics, and growth factors. Conversely, the local injection of atropine blanches the skin and decreases the PPG pulse waves. These PPG changes are associated with alterations in wound healing: local injection of atropine delaying healing and local methacholine speeding healing in the neuropathic patient.[97] In like fashion, Cooke et al.[98] have reported an endogenous cholinergic pathway for angiogenesis mediated by endothelial nicotinic cholinergic receptors and found that stimulation of the receptor-accelerated wound healing in diabetic mice.[98] (For more on Dr. Cooke's work, see effects of smoking and nitric oxide below.) In patients with small nerve fiber injury, the rises in blood flow and transcutaneous oxygen tension are both reduced following stimulation with acetylcholine and mild thermal injury.[99] Ryder et al.[100] in finding an abnormal sweat test in all of their neuropathic patients with foot ulcers suggest that autonomic denervation may be a prerequisite for diabetic neuropathic foot ulceration. Thus, both sympathetic and cholinergic neuropathy adversely affect peripheral blood flow (Fig. 13–3).

Vascular Aspects of Acute Painful Diabetic Neuritis

Symmetrical painful peripheral neuritis is occasionally seen both in patients who have grossly uncontrolled diabetes and in those whose uncontrolled hyperglycemia is suddenly brought to near normal levels. The mechanism for the pain is not clear. Likewise, unusually rapid progression of diabetic retinopathy may be seen under similar circumstances.[101,102] In both situations, the reason for the deterioration is not clear and with continued tight control of the diabetes, the patients improved. Kihara et al.[103] have shown that intravenous insulin infusion resulted in a dose-dependent reduction in endoneurial oxygen tension in the nerves of normal rats and in hyperglycemic rats once their hyperglycemia was controlled; there was a reduction in nerve nutritive blood flow and an increase in arteriovenous shunt flow. Tesfaye et al.[104] studied five subjects with acute painful neuritis and found severe abnormalities in the epineurial nutrient vessels including arteriolar attenuation, tortuosity, and arteriovenous shunting in all subjects. Proliferating neural new vessels, which bore striking similarities to those found in the retina and were more leaky to fluorescein than normal vessels, were observed in three subjects. Venous distension and/or tortuosity

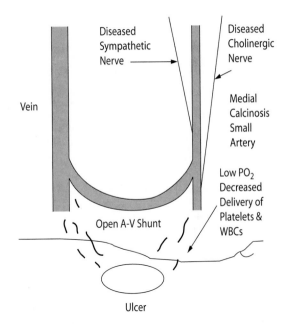

Fig. 13–3. In the diabetic neuropathic foot, decreased sympathetic tone results in an open A-V shunt and occasionally a warm pink foot. Increased flow rates are perhaps causally related to the commonly associated medial calcinosis of the arteries; kinks in the calcified vessel occasionally results in obstruction and decreased flow. A loss of cholinergic tone results in a decrease in sweating, dry skin and a decrease in flow through the nutrient vessels; in the presence of injury or infection, blood flow does not appropriately increase, and leukocytes, platelets, growth factors, antibiotics etc. are deficient. Essentially, the body behaves as if it did not know the lesion was there.

were also observed and this was most marked in the subject with severe autonomic neuropathy. They hypothesized that the presence of epineurial arteriovenous shunting and a fine network of vessels resembling the new vessels of the retina, may lead to a "steal" effect rendering the endoneurium ischemic. Dillon[105] has seen three patients with poorly controlled diabetes, retinopathy, and acute painful peripheral neuritis. Two were treated with the end-diastolic pneumatic boot relieving the pain acutely. The pain relief lasted perhaps 1 hour, but with repeated therapies disappeared. In two with palpable pedal pulses, subcutaneous PO_2 levels were measured and found to be low; the values returned to normal after their boot therapy. One of the two had a ^{31}P nuclear magnetic resonance (NMR) spectroscopy study in which the relative concentrations of intracellular phosphorylated metabolites [including adenosine triphosphate (ATP), phosphocreatinines (PCr), inorganic phosphate (P_i), and phosphomonoesters (PME)] in the living cell are examined. An anoxic pattern was seen especially after exercise. Therapy with the Circulator Boot normalized the subcutaneous PO_2 levels and improved recovery of PME/ATP ratios (indicating anaerobic metabolism). The ophthalmology consultant advised this patient that blindness would soon ensue. After a 2-week course of boot treatments, the retinal abnormalities also improved. Patients also had significant orthostatic hypotension in association with their leg pain; it disappeared as the pain disappeared. Such patients and reports suggest that the peripheral nerves and retina may share similar vascular lesions and that in some acute relief may be obtained with the end-diastolic boot. Truly, multiple factors alter the peripheral circulation in the diabetic (Table 13–8).

Table 13–8. Multiple vascular impairments in the diabetic patient

---

Autonomic and arteriosclerotic cardiomyopathy

Arteriosclerosis of large vessels, but especially those below the knee

Medial sclerosis of small vessels and calcification of the pedal arteries

Arteriovenous shunting due to autosympathectomy

Decreased capillary flow associated with cholinergic autonomic neuropathy and decreased small fiber nociceptor function

Thickening of the capillary membrane

Abnormal hemorrheology—stiff red and white cells, increased viscosity and fibrinogen, hypercoagulability and decreased fibrinolysis

Endothelial dysfunction and abnormalities in reactive hyperemia and capillaroscopy

---

REACTIVE HYPEREMIA AND VASCULAR DYSFUNCTION

Reactive Hyperemia (Post–Tourniquet) and Use of Pneumatic Boots

Boots have been designed for the treatment of arterial diseases since 1812 (see Fig. 13–4). Many other boots have been designed for the treatment of lymphedema and venous stasis disease. All should be examined for their effects on tests of vascular function. Classically

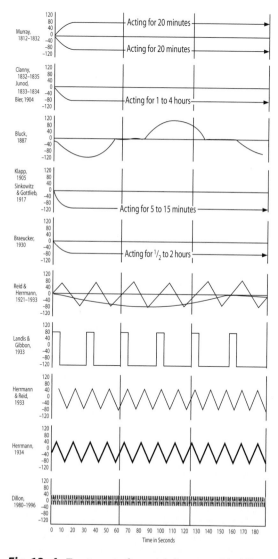

Fig. 13–4. Treatment of arterial diseases with different boot designs. From Dillon (340) and adapted from Hermann & Reid (341).

reactive hyperemia represents the increase in blood flow to a part that occurs when interrupted blood flow is restored, as with the removal of a tourniquet. The term commonly refers to increased cutaneous flow and its attendant rubor. Timing the reappearance of Doppler flow in the posterior tibial artery after the removal of a tourniquet left around the upper thigh for 3 minutes provides the basis of the standard reactive hyperemia test in the vascular laboratory.[106] No blood is delivered to the muscles of the thigh and calf during the placement of the cuff and anoxia of these tissues develops. When the cuff is removed in patients with circuitous blood flow, due to arteriosclerotic lesions, the metabolic needs of the proximal tissues are met before the blood flow reaches more distal tissues. In a normal leg with an open conduit between the thigh and a distal pulse, the distal pulse is quickly detected and the metabolic needs of the leg may be met more simultaneously. In the abnormal leg, however, it may take minutes before the distal pulse is detected. Such patients may be harmed with the use of pneumatic boots that inflate above the arterial pressure in the leg. While the boot is inflated, it may both block arterial flow into the leg and force the column of arterial blood back out of the leg, collapsing the arterial vessels. During the interval between boot compressions, the arterial tree must again refill and the metabolic needs of the leg be met before distal flow is detected. High-pressure cardiac external pneumatic counterpulsation devices (ECP anginal boots), because of their reversing blood flow in the ischemic leg, and boots used for lymphedema, venous stasis, and postoperative prophylaxis of thromboembolism, because of compressions lasting 10–45 seconds, must be used with care in such patients. In contrast, the Circulator Boot is designed for such patients and compresses the leg in end-diastole at pressures close to normal diastolic blood pressure and may be timed to compress the leg after each, every second, or every third heartbeat as needed to ensure that the arterial volumes are restored before boot compression (see later discussions with (Figs. 13-6 and 13-7).

Other Stimuli and Reactive Hyperemia

In a more general way, reactive hyperemia may refer to the increase in blood flow occurring in reaction to stimuli other than the removal of a tourniquet. Thus, Krsel et al.[107] noted that both maximal blood flow postocclusive reactive hyperemia and during thermal hyperemia was significantly decreased in type 1 diabetes and showed that the decrease was not clearly related to IGF-1 (somatomedin C).[107] Clarkson et al.[108] found that both reactive hyperemia (increased flow caused by endothelium-dependent dilation) and the vasodilatory response to sublingual glyceryltrinitrate (causing endothelium-independent dilation) were impaired in the systemic arteries of asymptomatic young adults with insulin-dependent diabetes, the impairment possibly representing early large-vessel disease. The degree of impairment was related to the duration of diabetes and low-density lipoprotein (LDL) cholesterol, the latter even at levels considered acceptable in nondiabetic subjects. Karnafel et al.[109] studied postocclusive reactive hyperemia in insulin-dependent diabetic patients without overt complications. Their best data was obtained from the hallex and the base of the little toe. Again, the maximum hyperemic response was significantly lower in the diabetic patients, especially the males in whom the time to peak flow was higher and the half-time for hyperemia was significantly longer. Skrha et al.[110] compared postocclusive reactive hyperemia and thermal hyperemia in normal controls and insulin-dependent diabetics both with and without ophthalmological findings and microalbuminuria. They found significantly lower postocclusive hyperemia and thermal hyperemia were accompanied by higher serum N-acetyl-β-glucosaminidase activity (NAG) in diabetic patients with microangiopathy as compared to healthy persons. Further, some of the diabetic patients without renal or ophthalmological abnormalities had reduced hyperemia associated with elevation of at least one of their biochemical markers for endothelial dysfunction (NAG, serum E-selectin, or intercellular adhesion molecule-1). Stansberry et al.[111] using laser Doppler techniques compared postocclusive hyperemia, thermal hyperemia, and the effects of raising and lowering the arm in type 2 diabetics and normal controls. Basal flow and reactive hyperemia did not differ in either the pulp of the index finger or the skin of the dorsum of the hand between groups. Vasodilation in response to heat and limb lowering (the latter a means to test vessel distensibility) were significantly diminished in the hairy skin of the dorsum of the hand but not in the finger pulp in the diabetic group. Small heat-sensitive C-fiber peripheral neurons (small-fiber polymodal nociceptors) signal vasodilation to heat and other noxious agents. While the initial vasodilation is due to relaxation of sympathetic tone, the primary nociceptive afferents then release several peptides (substance P, calcitonin gene-related peptide, and ATP), which then cause a more intense vasodilation.[112] Akbari et al.[113] found that the ingestion of a glucose load significantly impaired endothelium-dependent vasodilatation (changes in the vessel diameter) of the brachial artery induced with reactive hyperemia and endothelial function in the microcirculation assessed by changes in the erythrocyte flux after acetylcholine iontophoresis. They suggested that prolonged hyperglycemia and attendant endothelial dysfunction may be related to the early and accelerated atherosclerosis of diabetes. Veves et al.[114] also found that reactive hyperemia was diminished in both the macrocirculation and the microcirculation of their diabetic patients and was not improved by exercise training. Iwatsubo et al.[115] studied the impairment of endothelial function in patients with essential hypertension without diabetes mellitus, hyperlipidemia, coronary heart disease, or cerebrovascular disease. Forearm vasodilatory response to reactive hyperemia was decreased in the hypertensive patients and improved with the administration of the angiotensin-converting enzyme inhibitor temocapril but not with the calcium-channel blocker amlodipine. Erythema in reaction to exposure to ultraviolet B radiation has a different mechanism. Rhodes et al.[116] found increased amounts of both prostaglandin E_2 and nitric oxide in blister fluid from patients with ultraviolet B-induced erythema. The application of 1% indomethacin gel immediately after irradiation both reduced the blister fluid content of prostaglandin E_2 and the degree of erythema. Inhibition of nitric oxide synthesis in a dose-related fashion both decreased blister fluid content of nitric oxide and with complete inhibition abolished the ultraviolet B-induced erythema. (See below for more discussion on nitric oxide and prostacyclin.) Thus, the presence of diabetes with and without obvious neuropathy may diminish reactive hyperemia postvessel occlusion in response to heat and noxious stimuli. Kennedy et al.[117] have shown the converse is true in diabetic streptozotocin rats. While baseline nerve blood flow between diabetic and nondiabetic uninjured nerves, vessel number, density, and area were unaltered, after transection of the sciatic nerve, there were greater rises in blood flow in proximal stumps of nondiabetic nerves than in diabetic animals associated with a higher number, density, and caliber of epineurial vessels. Hyperemia also developed in distal stumps of nondiabetic nerves, but did not develop in diabetic nerves. The circle is complete: diabetes is associated with neuropathy, which may alter both baseline and reactive hyperemia, which may diminish repair of damaged nerves.

Capillaroscopy has also been utilized to assess the diabetic microcirculation. Thus, Meyer et al.[118] found capillary density, width, and arterial limb diameter were similar in the dorsal middle phalangeal area of the left ring finger of type 1 and 2 diabetic patients compared to their controls, while capillary diameters of the apical part and the venous limb were enlarged. Tortuous capillaries were significantly more often observed in type 1 and 2 diabetic patients than in controls. Capillary blood cell velocities (CBV) were significantly inversely related to capillary density in type 1 diabetics. In type 2 diabetic patients, peak CBV correlated significantly with capillary apex diameter. Disease duration significantly correlated inversely with arterial limb diameter and width of the capillaries in type 2 diabetic patients. Jorneskog and Fagrell[119] investigated CBV in the nailfolds of the great toe and left fourth finger with videophotometric capillaroscopy, and total skin microcirculation with laser Doppler fluxmetry (LDF) during rest, and following a

1-min arterial occlusion at the proximal phalanx of the digit. Their diabetic patients showed normal CBV and LDF values in skin microcirculation of the fingers, while a significantly reduced CBV was found during reactive hyperemia in the toes. The ratio between CBV and LDF was significantly decreased, indicating a maldistribution of blood between skin capillaries and subpapillary vessels in the toes of diabetic patients. They hypothesized that these disturbances may be of importance for the development of foot complications in diabetic patients. Lawall et al.[120] note that increases in erythrocyte rigidity, erythrocyte and platelet aggregation, plasma viscosity, and leukocyte adhesion may be associated with perfusion defects and that all may be improved with the administration of insulin and the metabolic state of the patient. However, they could not find a strong correlation between hemorheological parameters and capillary perfusion. Further, while they found the groups of patients with neuropathic lesions, macroangiopathic ulcers, and mixed neuropathic–angiopathic lesions had significant differences in capillary density, their microcirculatory examinations did not yield additional information to clinical and Doppler sonographic results.[121] They concluded that microcirculation evaluation techniques have a limited clinical role for diabetic foot syndrome. On the other hand, Ubbink et al.[122] found microcirculatory investigations helpful in determining the prognosis of patients with nonreconstructible chronic rest pain or small ulcers and an ankle blood pressure of 50 mm Hg or less or an ankle-to-brachial pressure index of 0.35. Classifying their patients into "poor" (capillary density less than $20/mm^2$, absent reactive hyperemia in capillary microscopy and laser Doppler perfusion measurements, and TcPO$_2$ less than 10 mm Hg), "good" (capillary density of $20/mm^2$ or more, present reactive hyperemia in capillary microscopy and laser Doppler perfusion measurements, and TcPO$_2$ of 30 mm Hg or more), and "intermediate" groups, they found a significant correlation between the risk of leg amputation and their microcirculatory classification, but not of the Fontaine stage, ankle blood pressure, or the presence of diabetes mellitus. After maximum conservative therapy from the surgeon, the cumulative limb survival at 6 and 12 months was 42 and 17% in the poor microcirculatory group, 80 and 63% in the intermediate microcirculatory group, and 88 and 88% in the good microcirculatory group.

EFFECTS OF SMOKING AND BUERGER'S DISEASE

Risks of Smoking and Vascular Disease

The adverse cardiovascular effects of smoking have been summarized by Simoni et al.[123] Tobacco use commonly represents a most powerful chemical addiction, which has been defined as "the inability to discontinue smoking." It is one of the main cardiovascular risk factors producing alterations in platelet activity, blood viscosity, and the vascular wall. Clinical signs and symptoms vary according to the degree of vasospastic, inflammatory, and arteriosclerotic disease present in different vascular circulations. The probability of carotid lesions increases up to 32% for 10 years of smoking and the progression of the disease is proportional to tobacco consumption; on the other hand, smoking cessation may be associated with slowing of progression and even regression of disease. Smoking increases the risk of peripheral arteriosclerosis obliterans two- to nine-fold, irrespective of the number of cigarettes and significantly decreases the long-term patency of the femorodistal reconstructions. It also decreases the benefits of end-diastolic boot therapies.[15] Data for major amputations (21 versus 2%) and the mortality rate for cardiovascular diseases (83 versus 33%) between smokers and nonsmokers are impressive. Smoking is the main independent risk factor for abdominal aortic aneurysms and the mortality rate rises 6- to 25-fold compared to the nonsmoking population. Variations in the incidence of smoking and its discontinuance confound studies on peripheral vascular disease. In the United Kingdom, black race was not detrimental in the study of Leggetter et al.,[124] unlike in the United States; they found no ethnic difference in diabetes-related amputation in women, while in men, amputation risk in African Caribbeans was one third that of Europeans, a finding that was wholly accounted for by low smoking, neuropathy, and peripheral vascular disease rates. As seen in Fig. 13–1, there have been some years showing a decline in amputation rates. Feinglass et al.[125] noted the decline in the early 1980s was significantly associated with reductions in the prevalence of smoking, hypertension, and heart disease, but not diabetes; a beneficial effect of vascular surgery was hard to ascertain. The benefits of stopping smoking have been long appreciated and its discontinuance may easily confound longitudinal vascular studies.[126–128]

Pathophysiological Effects of Smoking

The means whereby smoking produces its ill effects are multifactorial. Hemodynamic effects are well documented. A 10- to 20-mm Hg systolic or 5- to 15-mm Hg diastolic rise in blood pressure after smoking one to two cigarettes is common[129] and, rarely, increases up to 80 mm Hg may be seen.[130] In seemingly healthy young chronic smokers and nonsmokers, smoking one cigarette significantly increases both brachial and aortic blood pressure, augmentation index (a measure of arterial wave reflection in the aorta), pulse wave velocity, and arterial stiffness.[131] Cerebral blood flow velocity increases with smoking likely due to constriction of cerebral arteries possibly increasing the risk of stroke.[132] Chewing nicotine gum increases cardiac afterload and output, heart rate, and P wave duration.[133] Nicotine may contribute to smoking-induced endothelial dysfunction because of its ability to impair endothelium-dependent vasodilatation, such as hypotensive responses to bradykinin.[134] Nicotine and its metabolite cotinine are mitogenic for human vascular smooth muscle cells and thus have a potential role in the development of intimal hyperplasia and, ultimately, failure of vascular reconstructions.[135] Most studies regarding the acute effects of cigarette smoking refer to the higher sympathetic and adrenomedullary activity as a result of sympathetic ganglia and adrenal medulla nicotinic receptor activation. Yokotani et al.[136] found that the $\alpha 3\beta 4$ nicotinic receptors are predominantly involved in the release of catecholamines, at least from the rat adrenal gland. Smoking-induced lung disease may cause hypoxia. Hypoxia and modest chronic elevations in carbon monoxide may cause secondary polycythemia and increased blood viscosity.

Buerger's Disease or Thromboangiitis Obliterans (TAO)

Buerger's disease is an obliterative disease with inflammatory features involving the small and medium arteries and, less frequently, the veins most commonly in the lower legs. While the etiology of the disease is not clearly established, it has such a close association with cigarette smoking that many clinicians do not consider the possibility of the diagnosis in a nonsmoker. As cigarette smoking appears to have an undeniable link to the pathogenesis of vascular disease of many types, including the possibility of a strong causal connection to rheumatoid vasculitis,[137] it is possible that the pathological processes of Buerger's disease are unappreciated in the company of other diseases.

The occlusive nature of TAO does not prevent the development of collateral and anastomatic vessels that can be readily appreciated by arteriography.[138] Nicotine itself may play a role in angiogenesis. Heeschen et al.[139] have shown that nicotine, at concentrations that are pathophysiologically relevant, stimulates nicotinic acetylcholine receptors and the endothelial production of nitric oxide, prostacyclin, and vascular endothelial growth factor. They further provided anatomic and functional evidence that nicotine-induced angiogenesis accelerated the growth of tumor and atheroma, that it increased endothelial cell growth and tube formation *in vitro*, and that it accelerated fibrovascular growth *in vivo*.

While patients with TAO usually present with symptoms of ischemia of the lower extremities, the TAO process may involve the upper extremities and other vascular beds resulting in atypical presentations. Bozikas et al.[140] reported a patient with schizophrenic-like symptoms associated with deep and periventricular white matter lesions. Becit et al.[141] recovered an endarterectomy specimen that showed characteristic features of thromboangiitis obliterans from a 36-year old man with acute myocardial infarction and total occlusions of the proximal segment of the left anterior descending artery and right coronary artery. Hoppe et al.[142] found TAO in mammary arteries making them unavailable for coronary revascularization. Adem et al.[143] found histopathological features of TAO in a patient with a large mesenteric infarct with diffuse ischemic colitis and ischemia in the hepatic artery field.

Buerger's disease may be mimicked or aggravated by the use of cocaine or cannabis.[144–146] Both have vasoconstrictor properties and cannabis may have adverse effects on the immune system and host defense.[147] Chronic or acute fluctuations in endogenous catecholamines due to nicotine have been associated with TAO and may be important in its pathogenesis. In one study, patients with TAO had an impairment of sympathoadrenal function with an altered peripheral adrenergic response to cigarette smoking. Patients submitted to sympathectomy had high plasma epinephrine that was reversed after smoking (raising some question about the value of sympathectomy in TAO patients).[148] Vasospastic phenomena seem to be a feature of TAO, but lower sympathetic reactivity has been reported in Buerger's patients.[149] Thus, Singh et al.[149] noted increased basal heart rates and increased Valsalva ratios, decreased systolic blood pressure on the cold pressor test and a significant fall in blood pressure with head-up tilting in their TAO patients versus controls. Likewise, Iwase et al.[150] found their TAO patients to have significantly less vasoconstrictor skin sympathetic nerve activity than healthy controls. Moreover, they found no relationship between vasoconstrictor skin sympathetic nerve activity and skin blood flow in some patients, while they were well correlated in healthy subjects. There was no evidence for increased sympathetic activity in TAO patients and no evidence of a hypersensitive relationship was found between sympathetic activity and skin blood flow, all suggesting that TAO patients might not respond to sympathectomy.

Laboratory findings likely vary with the extent and activity of the TAO process. Patients with necrotic toes and cellulitis, for example, might be expected to have an increased sedimentation rate and a leukocytosis. Kroger et al.[151] found overall leukocyte counts (10839 +/− 782/nl versus 6205 +/− 414/nl for controls) along with absolute counts of granulocytes, monocytes, and lymphocytes were significantly different in their TAO patients versus their controls. Relative counts of naive helper T cells were significantly lower in the patient group, however, and HLA-DR expression on B cells was lower on the patients' lymphocytes. The concentrations of IgA, IgG, and IgM in circulating immune complexes were higher in the thrombangitis patients compared to the control group. Halacheva et al.[152] reported ultrastructural immunohistochemistry studies that revealed contacts between mononuclear blood cells and intercellular adhesion molecule-1 and E-selectin-positive endothelial cells. The latter showed morphological signs of activation. They interpreted their data to indicate that endothelial cells are activated in TAO, that vascular lesions are associated with tumor necrosis factor α secretion by tissue-infiltrating inflammatory cells, that the process is associated with intercellular adhesion molecule-1, vascular cell adhesion molecule-1, and E-selectin expression on endothelial cells, and that leukocyte adhesion occurs via their ligands. They conclude that the preferential expression of inducible adhesion molecules in microvessels and mononuclear inflammatory cells suggests that angiogenesis contributes to the persistence of the inflammatory process in TAO. As noted above, nicotine may stimulate angiogenesis through nicotinic acetylcholine receptors.

Therapy of TAO beguns with the prohibition of smoking and any vasoconstricting substances the patient may be taking. The occlusion of distal leg vessels frequently makes vascular reconstruction difficult or impossible. Shindo et al.[153] noted that patent but diseased arteries should be avoided for reconstruction and found some success in bypassing to disease-free collaterals. Talwar and Choudhary[154] have reviewed the successful use of omentopexy in restoring blood flow to the legs in amounts adequate to improve claudication and heal ischemic ulcers. Dillon has had uniform success in healing ulcers and relieving rest pain and claudication with the Circulator Boot in patients who stop smoking.[15] Those who continue to smoke may also improve, but are expected to relapse.

DIFFUSE VASCULAR DISEASE AND OPERATIVE RISK ASSESSMENT

The multiple effects of diabetes and smoking increase significantly operative risk. Mangano et al.[155] examined the perioperative fate of 243 men with coronary disease and of 2331 others thought to be high risk because of previous or current vascular surgery or two of the following other factors: age 65 or over, hypertension, active smoking, cholesterol over 240 mg/dl, or diabetes. Eighteen percent had postoperative ischemic cardiac events in the hospital; 15 died or had a myocardial infarction or unstable angina, 30 developed congestive heart failure, and 38 had ventricular tachycardia. Post-operative myocardial ischemia occurred in 41% of monitored patients and was associated with a 2.8-fold increase in the odds for all adverse cardiac outcomes and a 9.2-fold increase in the odds for an ischemic event. Ischemic events were increased 3.4-fold in patients with claudication, 5.0-fold for serum creatinine over 2mg/dl, and 9.2-fold for post-operative ischemia on Holter monitor. Congestive heart failure was increased 2.4-fold in diabetics and 3.5-fold in patients undergoing vascular surgery. Patients with small vessel disease in the foot may have diffuse disease and are especially at high risk. Carter and Tate[156] found ankle pulse wave amplitudes of 4 mm or less to be associated with a 4.20-fold increased risk for leg amputation and toe pressures of 30 mm Hg or less to have a 2.63 increased risk. Both were associated with an increased total and cardiovascular mortality rate in all patients.[156] The stress of vascular surgery clearly provides a challenge for those who need and undertake it. Therapy with the end-diastolic boot, in contrast, is a supportive device and has no morbidity associated with its use.

INFECTED WOUNDS

Pecoraro (Table 13–4) found infection to be second to neuropathy as a cause for leg amputation in diabetics. The two problems are interrelated. Patients with insensate feet may not experience pain and may fail to recognize the presence of infection that nondiabetics would appreciate. They may fail to modify their behavior appropriately to remove a causative factor (tight shoe, foreign body in their shoe, etc) or to curtail activity that might extend or worsen the infection (ambulation, swimming, etc). Neuropathy may open portals for infection because of abnormal pressure points due to bony deformities and fissures in dry calluses due to loss of sweating function. Finally, neuropathy may diminish the vascular response to injury through the opening of AV shunts (sympathetic defect) and the loss of both the cholinergic and nocireceptor responses as described above.

Risk Factors in the Elderly

The elderly have multiple factors that may promote infection and delay its recognition.[157] Degenerative arthritis and gout may offer another explanation for pain. Peripheral ischemia associated with diabetes, lipid disorders, and hypertension is common. Isolation, depression, fatalism, confusion, and poor eyesight may delay treatment. Arteriosclerotic heart disease (ASHD), congestive heart failure (CHF), peripheral cyanosis, and edema, along with stasis disease, may result in discoloration of the feet and a tissue environment conducive to infection. The immune response to infection may be blunted. Decreases in the production of thymic hormones, the number of helper T cells, generation of cytotoxic lymphocytes, antibody production, and cell-mediated immunity, along with increased percentages of immature lymphocytes and suppressor T cells, have

been described in the elderly. Poor control of diabetes and hyperglycemia may alter immune response in both the young and the elderly. Thus, hyperglycemia may decrease the inflammatory response, granulocyte response, leukocyte mobilization, granulocyte adherence, phagocytosis, and intracellular killing.

Recognition of Infection

Infection in chronic wounds may be difficult to recognize in both diabetics and nondiabetics. Gardner et al.[158] found serous exudate, delayed healing, discoloration of granulation tissue, friable granulation tissue, pocketing at the base of the wound, foul odor, and wound breakdown (mean sensitivity of 0.62) were better indicators of chronic wound infection than the classic signs of pain, erythema, edema, heat, and purulence (mean sensitivity of 0.38). None of the signs or symptoms was a necessary indicator that cultures would produce a significant growth of a pathogen, but increasing pain and wound breakdown were both sufficient indicators with specificity of 100%.

Tissue Damage from Infection

Once established, the bacteria may produce exotoxins and endotoxins along with enzymes that digest protein, promote tissue destruction, and allow separation of tissue planes. Pressure from edema, thrombosis of damaged vessels, and bacterial endarteritis further decrease local blood flow and the delivery of immune cells and antibiotics. Ambulation may press the fluid containing the enzymes and bacteria along the tissue planes disseminating the infection. Large areas of "wet gangrene" may develop. As described below, *Staphylococcus aureus* is an especially troublesome organism and is frequently found in nasal cultures in 30–50% of healthy adults with either or both methicillin-resistant or sensitive organisms.[159] Such people may transfer infection from their nose to a foot sore with their home wound care. The frequencies of both community- and hospital-acquired staphylococcal infections have increased steadily with little change in overall mortality.

Osteomyelitis

Staphylococcus commonly spreads from superficial ulcers to infect adjacent bone. The organism may have receptors or adhesions for bone matrix and cartilage and a fibronectin adhesin allowing it to bind to implanted devices.[160] The organism can be internalized by cultured osteoblasts and possibly survive intracellularly, which explains the persistence of some infections. Signs of infection for more than 10 days suggest the development of necrotic bone and chronic osteomyelitis. The development of osteomyelitis adds to the morbidity of foot infections. Longer and more aggressive antibiotic therapy and more surgery are likely.

Diagnosis of Osteomyelitis and Its Pathophysiology

A diagnosis of osteomyelitis must be first be suspected. The presence of exposed pus-covered bone most certainly indicates osteomyelitis. Bone that may be probed through fissures is most likely infected.[161] Baseline x-rays may not show abnormalities while later films do; bacteria do not consume calcium and are not responsible for the changes seen on x-ray. The immune response of the patient with the resultant dissolution of dead bone and the deposition of new bone are the processes revealed by the x-ray. The results of scans and x-rays depend on the stage of the osteomyelitic process. In diabetics, the latter usually begins as an extension of a cellulitic process. The periosteum may be penetrated and eventually separated from the bone. The superficial osteoblasts may be killed and the bacteria enter the bone along the haversian canals and lacunar system, killing the osteocytes and disrupting the membrane that normally separates the bony matrix and minerals from the extracellular fluid. The denuded matrix becomes a foreign body or sequestrum that invites attack and resorption by the scavenger cells in the body. An adequate blood supply is necessary for the resorption process and, together with control of the infection, for the preservation of the periosteum. The latter retains osteogenic potential and may surround the inflamed bone with an involucrum, which may be remodeled in time to produce a normal bone outline. Hence, scans early in the process showing an increase in blood flow or the concentration of leukocytes may be positive. A technetium scan is a nonspecific test with a specificity too low to confirm the diagnosis of osteomyelitis in many clinical situations.[162] A leukocyte scan is more specific. Newman et al.[163] found osteomyelitis to underlie 68% of ulcers, as determined by bone biopsy and culture, and detected these by leukocyte scanning with Indium in 111-oxyquinoline with an 89% sensitivity. Sixty-seven percent had no evidence of inflammation. The image intensity decreased by 16–34 days of antibiotic therapy and normalized by 36–54 days. In another report, they detected 100% of biopsy-proven osteomyelitis with their ^{111}In scans, while with magnetic resonance imaging they detected only 29%.[164] Weinstein et al.[165] might not contest the superiority of leukocyte scans over MRI's, but they do report that the MRI is significantly more sensitive than x-rays and technesium and gallium scans. As the scans and sedimentation rate become normal, the x-rays may show bone destruction and resorption. Over the subsequent year, the bone may remodel and gain a sharp well-mineralized outline that may or may not conform to its original shape. Sequential changes on x-rays do not necessarily indicate advancing infection and in the presence of improvement in the inflammatory process, closing of the skin, and normalization of the white count and sedimentation rate, may be a normal part of the healing process.[166,167] Such bony changes are likewise seen with healing traumatic fractures when they commonly are allowed to heal without surgical intervention. The need for bone scans and biopsy is questionable in clinical practice. Bone biopsy compounds the injury to the wound. While bone biopsy cultures are more definitive than cultures of swabs of the ulcer or drainage fluid, the latter are not traumatic and repeated as necessary over time will include the organism found by biopsy. The scans are expensive and rarely alter treatment; the presence of osteomyelitis slows the healing of ulcers and cellulitis thus prolonging their treatment to a time when the plain x-ray will be abnormal.

Problems with Antibiotic Therapy

Effective antibiotic therapy may be difficult, especially in the elderly. The latter have an increased incidence of drug allergies, gastrointestinal problems affecting proper nutrition and drug tolerance, cardiac problems affecting volume and solute overload, and nephrotoxicity associated with diabetes and use of diuretics. In all patients, an effective antibiotic must have activity against the invading bacteria and must reach the infected tissues in sufficient concentration. The neuropathic disease described above may decrease the delivery of antibiotics and, once sufficient vascular occlusions exist, tissue destruction is frequently found to progress in spite of adequate serum levels of appropriate antibiotics.

Morbidity of Foot Infections

The morbidity of foot infections can be considerable. Among 100 diabetic patients with an area of cellulitis over 2 cm across, with extensive tissue and/or bone destruction, with systemic toxicity or threatened limb loss, 36% underwent multiple operations, 67% had forefoot amputations, and over one third had a leg amputation at the Joslin Clinic in Boston.[168] Bamberger et al.[169] likewise had a significant amputation rate in their study of osteomyelitis. Of their 51 diabetic patients, 15 patients had a BKA and 9 had a toe amputation. The absence of necrosis and/or gangrene, the presence of swelling, and the use of antimicrobial therapy active against the isolated pathogens for at least 4 weeks intravenously or combined orally and intravenously for 10 weeks predicted a good outcome. Fejfarova et al.[170] found 26% of their 191 diabetic foot ulcer patients underwent amputations (88 minor and 12% major). Compared to their patients not having amputations, those having amputations were significantly more likely to have resistant organisms, especially resistant *Staphylococcus*, in their foot cultures (43 versus 14%) and to have osteomyelitis (69 versus 13%) and peripheral vascular disease (79 versus 60%). Taylor and Porter[171] emphasized local aggressive surgery on their vascular surgery service in the care of acute foot problems among their 114 diabetic patients (138 limbs); they performed 212 urgent or emergent operations and, over 0–86 months after presentation, 36 major amputations in 33 patients. Venkatesan et al.[172] prescribed oral antibiotics over a range of 5 to 72 weeks (median 12 weeks) to 22 diabetic patients with overt osteomyelitis with resolution of the osteomyelitis in 17 patients over 5–73 months (median 27); four patients did not respond and had amputations, while one patient had a recurrence of osteomyelitis at the same site 6 years later.

Antibiotics and Surgery for Foot Infections

The therapeutical approach to diabetic foot infections for the last 40 years is seen in the 1966 paper of Smith, Daniels, and Bohnen.[173] They first classified soft tissue infections as "local" or "spreading." The latter are considered potentially life-threatening conditions, requiring prompt diagnosis and treatment. Next, they estimated the level of infection (skin, fascia, and muscle) and whether necrosis was present. They noted that bacteriology of these infections is varied and of secondary importance. They recommended antibiotics alone for the treatment of skin infections in the absence of necrotic tissue. They considered débridements and adjuvant antibiotics as necessary for infections at the fascial or muscle level and for those with necrosis at any level. They noted that the feet of diabetic patients are prone to plantar forefoot ulcers associated with tissue destruction and infection, which for the vast majority are caused by mechanical factors and, in the presence of adequate immune defenses, are associated with bacterial colonization without infection. Antibiotics and debridement, hence, are required in infected or deep ulcers, or when the ulcer does not respond to relief of pressure with total contact casting. Chantelau et al.[174] agree; they found antibiotics to have no benefit as a supplement to standard therapy in uncomplicated neuropathic foot ulcers, provided pressure relief is complete and wound care is strictly supervised. Ha Van et al.[175] emphasized the addition of their conservative surgery (limited resection of the infected part of the phalanx or metatarsal bone under the wound with no other resection, associated with a removal of the ulcer site) to their improved therapeutic results between two time periods 1986–1993 and 1993–1995. Healing improved from 57 to 78% and the duration of healing was reduced from 462 ± 98 days

to 181 ± 30 days. Again, when infection has progressed to a state of foot "sepsis" (soft tissue infection with wet gangrene, necrotizing cellulitis or fasciitis and abscess and with or without osteomyelitis), surgery has been more emphasized than antibiotics. Scher and Steele[176] reviewed 65 amputations over 3 years in their patients with septic feet: 14 open partial foot, 4 closed partial foot, 17 guillotine transmetatarsal or BKA, 24 closed BKA, and 6 closed AKA. Ten of the 14 partial foot amputations healed with revision or grafting. They concluded that their surgical procedures were more important than antibiotic coverage. The average of 5.8 bacteria species isolated per patient potentially complicated their antibiotic program. Anaerobic antibiotic coverage did not alter outcome. Chronic planter ulcer preceded the sepsis in 52% of their patients. Other causes included ischemic gangrene (arm/ankle index less than 0.5 in 32.3%), trauma, and web-space fissures. When closed amputation was done 23.5% died and 35.3% stumps failed while no deaths and 12.9% stump failures were found when open amputations were done. They recommended guillotine transmalleolar amputation with later BKA for highest success. Others have pointed out that other procedures might still save the leg when most of the foot is lost. Grady and Winters[177] suggest a Boyd amputation be considered as an alternative to a Syme amputation; it preserves the function of the plantar heel pad and provides a more solid weight-bearing surface than a Syme amputation because a portion of the calcaneus is left and fused to the tibia. Smith et al.[178] suggest a partial calcanectomy be considered for the treatment of large ulcerations of heel and calcaneal osteomyelitis. In this author's boot clinic, these procedures are rarely needed.[15,166,167]

Choice of Antibiotics

Proper choice for the diabetic foot is dictated most accurately by reliable culture data, which may take 4–5 days to return, and, initially, by expectations of such data. Sapico et al.[179] in their study of the microbiology and clinical features of 32 amputated diabetic limbs, found 6 limbs with only aerobes, 1 with only anerobes, and 25 with a mixture of aerobes and anerobes. There was a mean of 4.81 species isolated per leg. Cultures obtained by curettage of the base of the ulcers correlated better with deep tissue cultures than did needle aspiration or swabs of the ulcer. The anaerobes were associated with higher frequency of fever and foul-smelling lesions. Prior antibiotic therapy did not appear to influence the nature of the microorganisms isolated. Wheat et al.[180] found cultures taken from contact with the ulcer or open draining lesions to be contaminated and "unreliable." In contradistinction, "reliable" cultures were obtained by aspiration of bullae or abscesses or by surgical biopsy of bone or soft tissue and had minimal contact with ulcers or a draining lesion. The reliable aerobes they recovered included staphylococcal species, enterococcal species, cornybacterial species, and various Enterobacteriaceae. Their reliable anaerobes included *Peptostreptococcus magnus* and *prevotii* and *Bacteroides* species. Reliable and unreliable cultures were in agreement in 27% of 26 patients while antibiotics selected to cover the unreliable results would have covered the reliable cultures in 93% of cases. Their empirical coverage possibilities included: (1) clindamycin/ampicillin/gentamicin; (2) cefoxitin/pipercillin/gentamicin; (3) clindamycin/pipercillin/gentamicin; (4) moxalactam/ampicillin; (5) third-generation cephalosporin/clindamycin/ampicillin; and (6) imipenem—all potentially effective in 90% of patients. Aminoglycosides alone were poor coverage for gram-negative bacteria because of low concentrations in infected tissues. Pathare and Sathe[181] evaluated synergistic potential of antibiotic combinations against pathogenic microorganisms isolated from 272 patients with diabetic foot wounds in India. Four combinations appeared especially useful: amikacin/piperacillin, ampitum–sulbactum in combination with either piperacillin or cefoperazone and ofloxacillin/cefotaxime. Grayson et al.,[182] in a study supported by Pfizer Pharmaceutical at the New England Deaconess Hospital, found ampicillin/sulbactum and imipenem/cilastatin equally efficacious in their treatment of "limb-threatening" foot infections in diabetic patients (infections associated with any degree of cellulitis with or without ulceration or purulent discharge). Reactions attributed to the drugs occurred in 18.4% of the former and 23.6% of the latter (most commonly, diarrhea, rash, and nausea). In keeping with their aggressive surgical approach, amputations were performed in 69% of the patients treated with ampicillin/sulbactum and in 58% of those treated with imipenem/cilastatin. Except for four BKAs, all were distal amputations. Finally, in considering therapy, the possibility of tetanus should be recognized. Thordarson et al.[183] reported a case of tetanus complicating a polymicrobial diabetic foot infection; their patient ran a difficult hospital course ending in a BKA. The authors point out that left untreated, 80% of these patients would die, while with appropriate therapy (aggressive débridement of toxin-containing tissue, tetanus toxoid, tetanus immune globulin, appropriate antibiotics that also include penicillin, and support of vital functions, as needed, in an intensive care unit) 10–20% may die, with the higher rates occurring in the elderly.

Home Intravenous Therapy

The cost-savings of outpatient parenteral antimicrobial-drug therapy have been emphasized by Gilbert et al.[184]

Of their patients, 8% had need for hospitalization. Potential complications were many: sterile phlebitis in 2–10%, large vein thrombosis soon after or many months after catheter placement, pulmonary emboli, superior vena cava syndrome, air embolism (potentially fatal), catheter fragment embolization, catheter tip migration to the right atrium or the jugular vein, catheter erosion through a vein or the right atrium (producing pericardial tamponade), intracatheter clots, fluid leaks through small holes in the catheter causing fluid extravasation or contiguous mass formation, rare idiosyncratic hypersensitivity reactions to the catheter substance, and exit-site infections, tunnel infections, and catheter-related bloodstream infections. Finally, a rare form of infective endocarditis may occur when a malpositioned catheter traumatizes the tricuspid valve resulting in platelet-fibrin thrombi that become infected. It should be noted that the authors point out that infusions should not be prescribed if there is an equally effective and safe oral antibiotic regimen. These same complications, of course, can occur if parenteral antibiotics are given in the hospital. Central venous catheters may account for an estimated 90% of all nosocomial bloodstream infections with multiple lumen catheters, especially having a high risk. The risk of such infections can be reduced at added expense with the use of antiseptic- or antibiotic-coated catheters.[185,186]

Tissue Levels of Antibiotics

The question of antibiotic penetration into ischemic tissue has been approached over many years. Spittell et al.[187] in 1961, concluded that multiple high doses of erythromycin and tetracyclines did reach ischemic tissue. In 1993, Duckworth et al.[188] found that 9 of 11 tissue samples taken from four diabetics having débridements or amputations for foot infections had clindamycin levels that exceeded the MICs reported for many commonly involved pathogens. Seabrook et al.[189] concluded that initial intravenous antibiotic therapy provided inadequate tissue antibiotic concentrations to treat diabetic foot infections; of their 26 patients given one dose of gentamicin/clindamycin, ticarcillin/clavulanate, or ampicillin/sulbactam 1 hour before surgical débridement when serum and tissue levels were measured, adequate antibiotic levels were reached in the serum in 16 patients and in the tissues in only 6 patients. Raymakers et al.[190] compared transcutaneous oxygen pressure measurements with tissue levels of ceftazidime in different tissues 30 minutes after its intravenous administration before leg amputation. They found that diabetes alone had little effect on the penetration of the antibiotic while the level of tissue perfusion did. Taken together, such studies along with the continued loss of limb, suggest that early intravenous or oral antibiotic therapy may not achieve

Table 13–9. Advantages of the circulator boot and local antibiotic techniques

---

Effects of the Circulator Boot
Thrombolytic effects
Delivery of erythrocytes and oxygen
Reduction of swelling
Delivery of systemic antibiotics and granulocytes
Dissemination of locally injected antibiotics

Use of Locally Injected Antibiotics
Ensured immediate high local concentration
Decreased total body exposure
No gastrointestinal upset or complications
No renal, liver, CNS, or inner ear toxicity
Decreased costs
Decreased amount of drug
Outpatient use in doctor's office
No visiting nurse
No complications from indwelling catheter

Use of Antibiotic Solutions within the Boot
Use of expensive antibiotics in a small volume of
    electrolyte solution
Débridement of necrotic tissue
Use of systemically toxic antibiotics with little or no
    untoward effects (aminoglycosides & amphotericin B)

---

tissue antibiotic levels sufficient to prevent significant tissue necrosis (necrotizing cellulitis). The advantages of the Circulator Boot and local antibiotic injections are summarized in Table 13–9.

Local Injection of Antibiotics

Local injection ensures that antibiotics in high concentration reach the site of infection immediately. Intraincisional antibiotics has proved effective in reducing the incidence of skin infections after dermatologic surgery.[191] Galandiuk et al.[192] showed that placement of polyglycolic acid beads containing antibiotics into experimental contaminated wounds of guinea pigs were more successful in reducing wound infection than were systemically administered antibiotics. Nelson et al.[193] showed that implantation of calcium sulfate tobramycin pellets into the lesions of rabbits with experimental osteomyelitis significantly eradicated infection (11/13) better than débridement only (5/12), placebo pellets and intramuscular tobramycin (5/14), or placebo pellets (3/13). Walenkamp et al.[194] treated 100 patients having osteomyelitis with debridement and gentamicin–PMMA beads and followed them for 5 (1–12) years. Of the infections, 66 were chronic, 18 cases had

osteomyelitis combined with arthritis, and in 3 cases with pseudarthrosis. They underwent 117 "treatment periods," consisting of one or more operations (total 152), in most cases with an interval of 2 weeks. No systemic antibiotics were necessary besides the local antibiotic treatment in 52 of the treatment periods. Healing was achieved in 92 patients, in 78 after a single treatment period, which included one to five operations, and in 14 after two or three treatment periods. Healing was more difficult to achieve when the infection was chronic, especially with a duration of more than 6 years or when caused by elective surgery. Local antibiotic treatment with gentamicin–PMMA beads has the advantage that the wound can be closed primarily and that a higher local antibiotic concentration in the tissues can be achieved, often making systemic antibiotic treatment unnecessary.

Historically, past reports of local antibiotic usage included the addition of antibiotics to peritoneal dialysis fluids, chest aerosols, bone cement after hip arthroplasty and irrigation fluids for infected arterial grafts and joint infections.[195–198] More recently, the dental profession has found local injection of antibiotics to have a role in the treatment of periodontitis[199,200] and as an intracanal medicament for the treatment of post-treatment pain in endodontically involved teeth with vital pulp–test readings.[201]

Topical Antibiotics

Antibiotic ointments, creams, suspensions and solutions are available for for the treatment of infections in the eyes, ears, nose, mouth, skin, and vagina. Kaplan and Gibson[202] found topical metronidazole (generally active against most obligately anaerobic bacteria and many protozoa) benefited a patient with an ischemic ulcer. The application of topical antibiotic creams and gels has been shown to significantly reduce infection in skin wounds presenting to the emergency room or school nursing office.[203,204] Potential drawbacks to the use of such topical agents include the development of local allergic reactions, the evolution of resistant organisms, and an inhibition of angiogenesis and wound healing. Wilson et al.[205] found positive patch allergy tests in 67% of their venous leg ulcer patients with a high incidence to lanolin and topical antibiotics. Multiple allergies were found in 58% of the patients. In addition, a new problem of allergy to cetearyl alcohol, a constituent of commonly used creams and paste bandages, was identified in 16%. While there is no proof that contact dermatitis reduces wound healing, the authors believed it was an adverse factor. Certainly, redness, swelling, and oozing due to allergy might be mistaken for infection and lead to inappropriate treatments. In Dillon's experience, resistant organisms are commonly found in patients using topical antibiotic agents over time. When local agents are desirable in such patients, physical agents such as local ultraviolet radiation, brief dilute hydrogen peroxide washes, and dilute silver nitrate preparations (Silvadene Cream) have been used. Hu[206] has reported that neomycin inhibits nuclear translocation of human angiogenin in human endothelial cells, an essential step for angiogenin-induced angiogenesis. Proliferation of human endothelial cells is inhibited in a dose-dependent manner. Other aminoglycoside antibiotics, including gentamicin, streptomycin, kanamycin, amikacin, and paromomycin, have no effect on angiogenin-induced cell proliferation. This report raises concern that the commonly used Neosporin creams might impede healing when applied to ischemic ulcers.

Sepsis and Septic Shock

Sepsis remains a major cause of morbidity and mortality in critically ill patients and in those with immune deficits or lack of a spleen. Antiinflammatory drugs have had little benefit. The pathophysiology of septic shock involves increased coagulation, diminished fibrinolysis, and an excessive and dysregulated inflammatory response. Generalized coagulopathy, microvascular thrombosis, and, ultimately, acute organ failure and death may ensue. Mavrommatis et al.[207] studied the activation of the fibrinolytic system and utilization of coagulation inhibitors in varying degrees of sepsis. They concluded that fibrinolysis is strongly activated and antithrombin III is utilized in sepsis and progressively more so in severe sepsis and septic shock. While in sepsis only, antithrombin III is decreased. In severe sepsis and particularly in septic shock, they found that plasminogen and the main coagulation inhibitors (ie, antithrombin III, and protein C) are depleted, indicating exhaustion of fibrinolysis and coagulation inhibitors. Identical impairments were found whether the infection was due to Gram-positive, Gram-negative, and other micro-organisms. Freeman and Buchman[208] have reviewed the efforts targeting the derangements in the clotting and fibrinolytic system as a means of therapy. They note that three agents have undergone extensive study in humans: recombinant human-activated protein C (rhAPC, drotrecogin-α), antithrombin III, and tissue factor pathway inhibitor (TFPI). One study has shown a potential survival benefit with rhAPC, but Freeman and Buchman feel more data is needed because of concern about the methodology of the study, the potential toxicity of rhAPC, and the questionable efficacy of this agent in patients with low mortality risk. Antithrombin III has failed to show clinical benefit in the treatment of sepsis. Despite early hopeful studies, one completed phase 3 trial of recombinant tissue factor pathway inhibitor in severe sepsis likewise failed to show

a reduction in mortality.[209] In short, the safety and benefit of these agents in the treatment of sepsis remains to be proved. Circulator Boot therapy has been used successfully to support the circulation of small numbers of patients with septic shock.[210] For example, one diabetic patient with infected peritoneal dialysis fluid and another diabetic with a blocked ureter were supported until their infections were controlled. The effect of end-diastolic booting on heart function and fibrinolysis are discussed below. Many patients referred for boot therapy due to cellulitis of the foot had been toxic and unresponsive to appropriate systemic antibiotics. An infective arteritis and thrombosis of small vessels have been partial explanations why such patients had not responded to their intravenous antibiotics; the antibiotics just did not get to the infection. Our local injection of antibiotics and pumping on the infected tissue improved both the systemic status and the status of the infected limb rapidly 15.[210] Additional studies are needed to ascertain the role of boot therapy in septic shock.

Circulator Boot and Local Antibiotic Therapy of Soft-Tissue Infections and Osteomyelitis

Boot therapy of early patients with foot infections were treated with sleeves allowing the infected part to protrude from the compression bag and escape boot compressions lest septic embolization occur. The Circulator Boot compresses the foot with a force varying from 1.1 (Long Boot) to 1.5 pounds (Miniboot) psi. In contrast, the standard 150-pound man may place his full weight on a square inch of his heel or first metatarsal head in walking and the forces and pressures generated by his muscles as they operate the pullies and levers with their reverse mechanical advantage in locomotion and lifting are far higher pressures than the boot generates. In practice, the author has not seen an embolus created by boot therapy and now takes no precautions in treating patients who are ambulatory. However, the inclusion of the cellulitic area within the boot bag improved their success; still patients were given either oral or intravenous antibiotics to lessen the possibility of septic emboli. Two patients with inoperable peripheral arteriosclerosis obliterans, cellulitis, and osteomyelitis whose cellulitis and ischemia were treated and improved with Long-Boot therapy. However, their osteomyelitis continued to drain organisms sensitive to the administered antibiotics after 6 weeks of intravenous therapy in the hospital. The man refused amputation of his toe unless the surgeons would promise him it would heal and no further surgery would be necessary. He was offered no promise, but he had had more than standard therapy offered in other hospital centers. We observed that we had done everything, but place antibiotics directly into his foot. He accepted the idea, which seemed to make sense to him. With the injection of antibiotics directly into his toe, the draining stopped and healing took only a few weeks. The female patient learned of the success of the male patient and also wanted to try local therapy. Her infection contained two organisms in the second metatarsal head which were sensitive to different antibiotics. After the injection of one antibiotic, her subsequent cultures were negative for the sensitive organism, but her foot pain continued. Several days later and within a few minutes of the injection of the second antibiotic, she exclaimed that her foot had suddenly stopped hurting. She also healed and thus, our local antibiotic technique was born. Subsequently, this author published two reports on the successful treatment of osteomyelitis and soft-tissue infections in ischemic diabetic legs by local antibiotic injections and the end-diastolic pneumatic compression boot.[166,167] In the first report, thirty-four legs at risk of amputation due to peripheral arterial insufficiency associated with ischemic necrosis, soft-tissue infections, osteomyelitis, and variable degrees of peripheral neuropathy were reported in 28 diabetic patients. Leg amputation had been considered in 27 legs for which standard therapies had failed for the current illness and in two legs in which standard therapy had failed for previous illnesses. Local therapy was the initial form of therapy for five legs in which standard therapy appeared likely to fail. Infection was controlled in all patients with the use of local antibiotics and compression boot therapy. Early leg amputation was avoided in all but one patient. Late leg amputation occurred in two patients who were lost to follow-up care. Osteomyelitis, ischemic necrosis, and advanced soft-tissue infection were shown not to be clear-cut indications for amputation in the ischemic diabetic foot. In the second report, a prospective study, our experience with local antibiotic therapy and the Circulator Boot in 35 consecutive diabetic patients having 42 episodes of osteomyelitis in the distal extremity was described. The patients largely had failed standard therapy elsewhere and had a mean duration of illness and previous therapies prior to presentation for boot therapy of 132.5 ± 162.5 days. Ischemia was documented in 62% of the feet by the absence of the distal pulses and widened low Doppler tracings in the metatarsal artery of the involved ray. Septic patients were hospitalized while less sick patients were largely treated as outpatients. Reliance was placed on the local antibiotics. Systemic antibiotics were used to prevent septic emboli and to help control the infection in the foot. The systemic antibiotics were given by the oral route alone in 16 episodes, by both oral and parenteral routes in 22 episodes, and by the parenteral route alone in 4 episodes. Sterilization of the drainage, healing of the associated ulcers, and normalization of the sed rate pointed to a successful outcome, regardless of

what the x-ray was showing. With enough time (weeks to months), the involved bone healed without surgery. All but two patients were spared amputations. One had presented with mummified second and third toes, which were amputated, along with osteomyelitis of the first proximal phalanx and metatarsal, which healed with treatment. The other healed his ulcers and the sites of osteomyelitis in the proximal phalanx of his big toe, in the third metatarsal head, and in the proximal phalanx and metatarsal head of the fourth toe. Unfortunately, several months later, the patient developed a Charcot foot and had a BKA. It was concluded that osteomyelitis does not dictate a need for surgery, that the clinical status of the foot is frequently more important than the x-ray, that the foot and its function can be maintained in such patients, and that effective care can be accomplished in the boot clinic rather than the hospital, in most patients.

CHOLESTEROL EMBOLI AND "TRASH FEET"

In a prospective evaluation of 1,000 coronary cases, Keeley et al.[211] found that some emboli debris was scraped from the aorta by placement of the large-lumen guiding catheters in more than 50% of procedures. The presence of debris, however, was not found to be associated with in-hospital ischemic complications. Eggebrecht et al.[212] examined the backflow from their catheters during cardiac catheterization of 7,621 patients and found visible debris in only 0.54%. Again, none had in-hospital embolic ischemic events. Still, clinically important cholesterol embolization does occur after such procedures. It may occur spontaneously and is well described after direct dislodgement of cholesterol crystals from atherosclerotic plaques on the walls of arteries by surgery, angiogram, and trauma. It may complicate anticoagulant and thrombolytic therapy presumably because fibrin clot that stabilizes the atheromas in place is weakened.[213] The manifestations of cholesterol emboli depend on the site from which they are loosened and the size of the embolic mass. Stroke, blindness, renal failure, intestinal gangrene, scrotal and penile gangrene, skin necrosis, livido reticularis, and gangrene of the foot and toes may all be seen. Significant emboli to the lower extremities may complicate surgery on the aorta and iliac arteries producing "trash feet." Nitecki et al.[214] noted that postoperative emboli on the abdominal aorta may occur in 7–29% or more of the cases; two of their three patients required BKA, while the third patient died. Thompson et al.[215] ultrasonically monitored the repair of aortic aneurysms by conventional surgery in 18 patients and by endovascular repair in 20 patients; significantly more particulate and gaseous emboli were seen in the endovascular group. None of their patients suffered massive embolization, but one patient in the conventional group required a femoral embolectomy and three patients undergoing endovascular repair developed self-limiting trash feet postoperatively. Gruss[216] encountered 15 patients with postoperative trash feet over 16 years. Thirteen had had infrarenal aortic aneurysms. Three patients died, two had thigh amputations (one of the deaths), and another had both legs amputated. Some of the patients were given postoperative E_1 (PGE$_1$) with possible benefit. Others have reported some therapeutic success with corticosteroids, especially in those patients with acute renal failure.[217,218] Dillon[219] has treated 14 patients (25 legs) with the Circulator Boot for trash feet. One male patient had the major vessels of both legs occluded following replacement of his aorta and iliac arteries. Embolectomies and heparin therapy were ineffective in restoring his blood flow. On the second postoperative day, he had focal gangrene of his scrotum, cool paralyzed mottled legs, and no measurable blood pressure at the ankle level. He was toxic and had significant elevations of his leukocyte count and serum transaminases. The possibility of high bilateral leg amputation was considered. He was referred for Circulator Boot therapy and spent the greater part of the next 30 hours in the boot. After that time, warmth and color had been restored to both his legs except for the distal portions of his feet. Two months later, his right foot was intact except for a small area of focal necrosis of his big toe, which autoamputated. The distal portions of the toes of the left foot had become well demarcated giving him the option of autoamputation or surgical amputations; he chose the latter to speed his return to work. Among the 14 patients were eight nondiabetics and all former smokers; half had involvement of both feet. Five type 2 diabetics, 4 former or active smokers, had both legs involved. The one type 1 diabetic was a nonsmoker and the only patient who had had streptokinase therapy prior to his embolization episode. The other patients had had repair of aortic aneurysms (2 patients and 4 legs), coronary angioplasty (2 patients and 2 legs), renal artery angioplasty (2 patients and 2 legs), heart catheterization (2 patients and 4 legs), aortoiliac bypass (1 patient and 2 legs), coronary artery bypass grafts (1 patient and 2 legs), coronary angioplasty and bypass grafts (1 patient and 2 legs), arteriography and hemodialysis (1 patient and 2 legs), arteriography alone (1 patient and 1 leg), and spontaneous without obvious cause (1 patient and 1 leg). Most patients had been given expectant care for several weeks prior to referral for boot therapy in hopes the lesions would spontaneously improve. At the time of referral, three patients could walk up to one half-block and 11 were wheelchair-bound. All had severe pain. Most arrived with advanced ischemic lesions: Wagner class 0 (1 patient), Wagner class 2 (1 patient), Wagner class 4 (7 patients),

and Wagner class 5 (5 patients). Blood flow was restored with booting to one female patient with incipient necrosis of the distal foot who had undergone bilateral lumbar sympathectomies, femoropopliteal bypass, tibial end embolectomy, and a patch-graft angioplasty before referral for boot; the booting produced "rubor mortis" (the distal necrotic foot remained red as it could not utilize oxygen, while the more proximal foot became dusky after booting as the tissue could utilize the oxygen). She underwent a BKA. The other patients all healed (17 legs) or were improved when lost to follow-up (5 legs; one patient dying 3 months after last boot therapy).

VASCULAR HORMONES AND CLOTTING FACTORS

Relationship to *in vitro* Studies

The vessel wall from the adventitia to the endothelium may respond to humoral signals changing the function of the vessel and the endothelial phenotype in health and disease.[220] Garcia-Cardena et al.[221] have shown that changing the biomechanical environment of cultured endothelial cell from one with no flow, to one with laminar flow, and finally to one with turbulent flow alters gene expression and remodeling of cytoskeletal elements. Dai et al.[222] designed an *in vitro* system to simulate the effect of intermittent pneumatic boot action on the endothelium. They found that pulsatile flow, more than vessel compression, upregulated expression of tissue plasminogen activator and nitric oxide synthase. The effects of boot therapies described below may be related to such *in vitro* studies.

Collecting Blood Samples

A clean stick, tourniquet technique and sample preservation are important in obtaining accurate data both for clinical studies and research. Venous occlusion by the tourniquet itself, for example, may raise fibrinolytic activity.[223] The following are technical considerations of note:

Euglobulin lysis time: A collection tube containing citrate is used and within 30 min, the blood sample is centrifuged at 4°C to obtain plasma for the test.

Clot lysis time: Whole blood is used. The test is a nonspecific indicator of overall fibrinolysis. In patients with disseminated intravascular coagulation (DIC), the test may be normal if plasminogen depleted.

Plasmin (fibrinolysis): Serum is collected in presence of a plasmin inactivator such as ε-aminocaproic acid. The test may be done immediately or the serum may be stored at 4°C for later analysis.

Plasminogen activator inhibitor: Blood is collected in a citrated tube and centrifuged rapidly to obtain platelet poor plasma. The latter is stable for 6 hours at 4°C. Morning values may be twice as high as afternoon values.

Thromboelastography: The test is done on whole blood and is readily incorporated into a clinical laboratory setting. It provides information on clotting dynamics, both clotting and fibrinolysis, and may identify both hypercoagulability and lack of fibrinolysis.[224]

Hypercoagulability States

Stasis, bed rest, congestive heart failure, and surgery especially in the hip, prostate, and pelvic regions are commonly associated with an increased incidence of thromboembolic disease. Venous hypertension associated with obesity, standing occupations, pregnancy, corsets, Baker's cysts, along with dominantly inherited clotting disorders (deficiency of protein C, protein S, and antithrombin III) are commonly associated with venous stasis disease and thrombophlebitis. About one of five patients of European descent who present with venous thromboembolism have a specific genetic defect in their anticoagulant pathway.[225] These and other factors described below may also be associated with peripheral arterial occlusive disease.

Other texts may be consulted for the drug and diet treatments of hyperlipidemias. The latter lead to the accumulation of subendothelial lipid deposits, which may be asymptomatic in the peripheral and coronary circulations for years. Calcification of devitalized tissue may develop, which may function as a firm hard patch in the vessel wall, an outcome preferable to the development of an aneurysmal dilatation. The fibrous cap over the lipid depositis may, however, break, exposing the blood to the thrombogenic lipid material (tissue factor, a small-molecular-weight glycoprotein) that initiates the extrinsic clotting cascade and may trigger an acute coronary syndrome or an acute deterioration in previously stable claudication.[226,227] Regression of the lipid deposits in vulnerable plaques with anticholesterol drug therapy may explain the early decrease in the incidence of coronary events seen after the start of such therapy. Both to prevent the progression of peripheral thromboarteriosclerotic disease and because of the strong association of claudication with coronary disease, patients with claudication should take steps to normalize their lipid abnormalities. Clotting abnormalities may also forewarn cardiovascular events. Thogersen et al.,[228] for example, found that plasma levels of plasminogen activator inhibitor-1 (PAI-1), tissue plasminogen inhibitor (tPA), and von Willebrand factor are associated with subsequent development of a first acute myocardial infarction independent of established risk factors.

Patients with advancing peripheral obstructive arterial disease have been shown to have platelet hyper-reactivity, hemostatic dysbalance of pro- and anticoagulant proteins, and a counterregulatory increase of fibrinolytic activity (fibrinogen and von Willebrand factor are increased and antithrombin III and the PAI-1/tPA ratio are decreased).[229] Patients who present with arterial thrombosis usually develop their disease as a complication of atherosclerosis. However, these patients may also have a form of hypercoagulability, manifested primarily by high fibrinogen levels and elevated factor VII activity.[224] In one study, patients who presented with central and branch retinal artery occlusion without an apparent embolic source had a thrombophilia in 43% of patients in the absence of other risk factors and in 50% of patients with diabetes, hypertension, or hypercholesterolemia.[230] Alagozlu et al.[231] found positive tests for anticardiolipin antibodies in 10% of diabetics without foot problems, 34.3% of diabetics with foot problems, and in 8.6% of healthy nondiabetic controls. Anticardiolipin antibodies (G and M) are found in sera of some patients with systemic lupus erythematosus and are associated clinically with spontaneous abortion, placental infarction, and thrombotic episodes. In the laboratory, they are frequently associated with the lupus anticoagulant, another antiphospholipid antibody. These antibodies are commonly measured in patients with peripheral vascular disease (PVD) when there is no obvious explanation for the clinical picture. They are not commonly measured in patients with diabetic foot problems in whom the possibility of a thrombophilia is rarely considered.

Diabetes through various mechanisms has been associated with a hypercoaguable state. Glycosylation of proteins induced by hyperglycemia is one such mechanism. Elevated levels of PAI-1 with and without reduction of tPA in plasma have been frequently found in patients with diabetes. Glycation enhances low-density lipoprotein (LDL)-induced production of PAI-1 and further decreases tPA generation in vascular endothelial cells, effects blocked by treatment with antioxidants, vitamin E, or cotreatment with native or glycated high-density lipoprotein (HDL).[232] Increased lipoprotein(a) [Lp(a)] in plasma is an independent risk factor for premature cardiovascular diseases and perhaps proliferative retinopathy.[233] Elevated Lp(a) levels, especially if combined with other factors, such as antiphospholipid antibodies, has been associated with massive thrombotic disease in nondiabetics.[234] The levels of glycated Lp(a) are elevated in diabetic patients and, as with glycosylated LDL, enhance Lp(a)-induced production of PAI-1, and decrease the generation of tPA by arterial and venous endothelial cells.[235] Tissue levels, like serum levels, of PAI-I have been found to be increased in diabetics. Sobel et al.[236] found substantially more PAI-1 and substantially less of urokinase-type plasminogen activator in atherectomy samples from subjects with diabetes compared to nondiabetics. PAI-1 detected in the atheroma may contribute *in vivo* to accelerated or persistent thrombosis underlying acute occlusion and to vasculopathy exacerbated by clot-associated mitogens in the vessel wall. E-selectin is another protein whose levels are altered by hyperglycemia. E-selectin is one of the adhesion molecules that may play a role in the development of atherosclerosis and may stabilize the adhesion of leukocytes to endothelium and be involved in cellular interactions within the tissues. Albertini et al.[237] found that levels of E-selectin and vascular cell adhesion molecule-1 elevated in poorly controlled type 2 diabetic patients and to fall to normal with short-term improvement in glycemic control.

Neuropathy is another mechanism promoting coagulation. Peripheral nervous system adrenergic neurons synthesize, transport, and store the serine protease, tPA in axon terminals, many of which innervate vessel walls. Peng et al.[220] have provided evidence for a physiological infusion of tPA into the vessel walls, blood, and other innervated matrices by sympathetic neurons. Sympathoadrenal stimulation induces a surge of tPA from vessel walls into the blood. Sympathectomy induced 30–50% reductions in tPA release from both arterial and microvascular explants; an acute release induced by $\alpha 1$ adrenergic receptor stimulations was also strongly suppressed, as were basal levels of the circulating enzyme *in vivo*. Adventitial and endothelial nerve plexus ablations from normal large vessel explants produced greater reductions than small vessel endothelial ablations.

Patients with diabetes are subject to dehydration and hypovolemia in association with uncontrolled hyperglycemia, hemodialysis, and aggressive diuretic therapy, all stimulating the renin–angiotensin system and vasopressin. Lottermoser et al.[238] demonstrated that in normal volunteers, 10 days of treatment with hydrochlorothiazide significantly increased PAI-1 antigen and PAI-1 activity and this effect was blunted by angiotensin II receptor blockade. Nakamura et al.[239] have shown that PAI-1 is induced in a variety of tissues in the rat by angiotensin II directly through the angiotensin type 1 receptor, independent of its effects on blood pressure. Vasopressin, like angiotensin, is a vasoconstrictor and its blockade may increase skin blood flow in patients with arteriosclerosis obliterans.[240] Therapy with vasopressin injections may be indicated to control bleeding in patients with hemophilia A or von Willebrand's disease (type 1), while therapy in patients with diabetes insipidus is rarely complicated by thrombotic events. The feet of diabetic patients rendered hypotensive by aggressive hemodialysis are commonly elevated to improve cerebral blood flow at the same time decreasing and occasionally stopping arterial flow to the feet thus promoting acute occlusive events.

The two most common known hypercoagulable states are hyperhomocysteinemia and protein C resistance, which is genetically determined and is present in about 15% of the population. One form of protein C resistance is due to the Leiden gene. In homozygotes, venous thrombosis begins early in life; in heterozygotes, it usually begins after age 30 and may first occur in old age or during immobilization.[241] Homocysteine elevations are associated with elevations in PAI-1[242] and an increased incidence of thromboarteriosclerotic disease. Stern et al.[243] reported a case of a 42-year-old woman without significant underlying arteriosclerotic disease who had a fatal stroke along with thrombosis in the aortic arch and its major branches and in the mesenteric arteries and veins. They recommend checking homocysteine levels in all young people with thrombotic disease. Homocysteine levels rise as the renal function decreases in diabetics.[244] Fasting levels of homocysteine may be determined by remethylation (vitamin B_{12} and folate-dependent) while postload levels may be related to abnormalities in trans-sulfation (vitamin B_6 dependent). Therapy with simple vitamins (folate, vitamin B_{12}, and possibly vitamin B_6) is indicated if homocysteine levels are elevated and the possibility of elevations should be suspected in diabetics especially with nephropathy. Hypercoagulative and hypofibrinolytic states also increase with the degree of microalbuminuria in the diabetic: PA1-1, factor VII, and fibrinogen all significantly increase.[245]

Excessive alcoholic ingestion, like hypoglycemia, may result in stupor, immobility, stasis, and exposure to the elements. The development of hypothermia with the latter results in peripheral vasoconstriction and potential cold damage. Binge drinking also affects the hemostatic system and its circadian variation. Numminen et al.[246] found that an acute alcohol load in healthy people increased urinary excretion of the platelet thromboxane A_2 metabolite 2, 3-dinor-thromboxane B_2 significantly more during the night after an evening intake of alcohol than during the control night. A smaller increase was observed during the daytime after an intake of alcohol in the morning. A sevenfold increase in PAI-1 activity was observed after both morning and evening intakes of alcohol.

Cushing's syndrome is associated with an increase in plasma clotting factors, especially Factor VIII and von Willebrand factor complex, and with an impairment of fibrinolytic capacity due to PAI-1 excess. Prophylactic anticoagulation with heparin or Coumadin may significantly reduce perioperative mortality and thromboembolic events.[247] Patients on long-term steroid immunosuppression for renal transplants have likewise been found to have a similar prothrombotic state that is ameliorated by withdrawal of the steroids.[248]

Fibrinolysis and Fibrinolytic/ Anticoagulation Therapies

Normal Postoperative State

The clotting cascade is activated by surgery to stem bleeding. Clotting must be restrained to prevent propagation of clots beyond the traumatized area. Subsequently, fibrinolysis is needed to restore patency to thrombosed areas. Outcomes of surgeries are complicated and frequently disastrous if clotting and fibrinolytic processes are abnormal. For many years, surgery and trauma have been noted to alter blood coagulation and lysis. In 1937, MacFarlane [249] noted a dispersion of fibrin reticulum as a result of major surgery. Others noted that patients having some fibrinolytic activity preoperatively are more likely to have it postoperatively. Rapid fibrinolysis may occur immediately during or after surgery or trauma and subsequently disappear associated with a rise or fall in plasminogen activator. Fibrinolytic shutdown may contribute to the development of deep vein thrombosis in postoperative patients. [223] Fibrinolysis is increased by exercise somewhat in parallel to the degree of effort and exercise; the increase in fibrinolysis is due to a rise in tissue-type plasminogen activator and decrease in PAI. [250] Conversely, bed rest in the postoperative state is associated with a decrease in venous capitance and venous outflow in the lower extremities. [251] Stasis is necessary for thrombus development and reduces inflow of fibrinolytic or antithrombotic substances. Stasis further promotes anoxia and the generation of oxygen-free radicals that may damage the endothelium. [252] Experimentally, general anesthesia combined with abdominal surgery can induce vasodilatation of the great veins away from the site of the surgery. [253] Separation of the endothelial cells may accompany the vasodilatation, in turn, thus exposing the subendothelial connective tissue and providing a focus for platelet aggregation. Means to prevent stasis during and after surgery along with rapid mobilization are desirable.

Fibrinolysis and Biguanide Therapy

The biguanide derivatives (phenformin and metformin) are hypoglycemic agents that have been recognized since 1959 as promoting fibrinolytic activity. [254–258] Thus, phenformin, especially in combination with ethylestrenol, has been shown to increase the level of plasminogen activator in the blood [255] and increase the serum concentration of fibrin breakdown products in patients with occlusive vascular disease or rheumatoid arthritis. [256] In diabetics, phenformin has been shown to return lysis time to normal when it was pathologically increased [257] and to be beneficial in a patient with recurrent pulmonary emboli and refractory deep vein thromboses and leg ulcers. [258]

Heparin and Coumadin Therapy

Heparin—Anticoagulation with heparin is indicated for the treatment and prophylaxis of acute venous thrombosis; with low-dosage regimens for the prevention of postoperative deep vein thrombi and prevention of pulmonary emboli in high-risk patients undergoing thoracic, abdominal, pelvic, and hip surgeries; for the prevention and treatment of pulmonary or peripheral arterial embolism; for the prevention of and subsequent embolization of mural thrombi in patients with atrial fibrillation; and for the diagnosis and treatment of consumptive coagulopathies. Limited studies have shown a role for heparin in wound healing. Heparin and growth factors have been associated with rapid and effective endothelial cell repair in cell culture studies. Patients with burns and diabetic foot ulcers have shown an increase in capillary circulation and deceased healing time. [259]

Small amounts of heparin in combination with antithrombin III can inhibit thrombosis by inactivating activated Factor X and inhibiting the conversion of prothrombin to thrombin. In the presence of recent thrombosis, larger amounts of heparin may inhibit further coagulation by inactivating thrombin and blocking the conversion of fibrinogen to fibrin. These events may be accompanied by changes in fibrinolytic activity. Minnema et al. [260] found that heparinization of patients with and without pulmonary emboli led to elevated tPA/Ag levels without enhancing fibrinolysis, as reflected by levels of plasmin-α 2-antiplasmin complexes and D-dimer, which actually decreased. Prisco et al. [261] gave either heparin or saline (controls) subcutaneously to patients with a previous myocardial infarction. Four hours after the first heparin administration tPA antigen levels significantly increased with respect to saline administration. After 15-day heparin treatment, a significant decrease in euglobulin lysis time and significant increases in tPA activity and antigen in comparison with placebo were observed before venous occlusion. No statistically significant changes in PAI-1 levels were found. The variations of fibrinolytic system activity induced by heparin treatment were more marked when evaluated after venous occlusion. Procedures like venous occlusion do make a difference in study results. Upchurch et al., [262] in a simulation of cardiopulmonary bypass, gave increasing doses of intravenous heparin to five adult baboons for over 60 minutes and found evidence of activation of the fibrolytic activity, an increase in plasmin activity and immunoreactive plasmin light chain, as well as an increase in immunoreactive fibrinogen fragment E *in vitro*. Lojewski et al. [263] gave low-molecular heparin to nonhuman primates over a 12-week period and found increasing activity of the fibrinolytic system. After 2 weeks, tPA increased twofold, but returned to baseline at 6 weeks, while the PAI-1 activity increased gradually over the entire study period. Psuja et al.[264] found that both subcutaneous and inhaled heparin decreased the euglobulin lysis time when given preoperatively in their abdominal surgery patients.

Heparin therapy may be complicated by thrombocytopenia and the development of white clot syndrome, new thrombi resulting from irreversible aggregation of platelets induced by the heparin. Severe thromboembolic complications may be associated varying from skin necrosis, stroke, and leg amputations to death.

Coumadin—Coumadin takes a few days to achieve effective anticoagulation and is commonly begun along with and continued after heparin. It is indicated in the treatment and prophylaxis of venous thrombi, pulmonary emboli, thromboembolic complications associated with atrial fibrillation and/or cardiac prosthetic valves, inoperable cerebrovascular insufficiency, and to reduce thromboembolic events after acute and recurrence of myocardial infarction. Therapy can be complicated by hemorrhage and rarely necrosis or gangerene of the skin or other tissues, which have resulted in death or permanent disabilities. Coumadin therapy may enhance the release of atheromatous plaque material resulting in emboli and necrosis of any tissue (spinal cord, penis, kidneys, spleen pancreas, etc). The "purple toe syndrome" may commonly develop 3–10 weeks after the start of therapy. The sides and plantar surfaces of the toes have a purplish or mottled color that blanches on pressure or elevation of the legs. The toes may be painful and tender. The syndrome may be reversible with discontinuance of the Coumadin, but some cases progress and require toe amputation.

Fibrinolytic Therapy in Specific Diseases and Situations

Livedoid vasculitis—This entity is a hyalinizing vasculopathy associated with extensive microthrombi in mid-dermal vessels and epidermal infarction. Associated laboratory abnormalities may include the presence of anticardiolipin antibodies, lupus anticoagulants, increased levels of plasminogen activator inhibitor and low levels of endogenous tPA activity. Klein and Pittelkow[265] administered 10 mg tPA over 4 hours daily for 2 weeks with a dramatic effect in 5 of their 76 patients. The sixth patient rethrombosed but responded to retreatment with concurrent anticoagulation.

Arterial graft occlusions—Intra-arterial thrombolytic therapy can be regarded as a possible consideration in the initial management of acute lower-extremity arterial and synthetic graft occlusions, especially in patients with multiple prior vascular reconstructions. Unsuccessful thrombolysis results in a poor outcome despite surgical reconstruction in the majority of cases.

Bhatnagar et al.[266] had best results with high-dose urokinase infusions among their 55 patients, when the infusions had no residual defects that required surgical reconstructions or angioplasty: 46 versus 8% patent at 3 years and 82 versus 76% limb salvage rates. Failure of thrombolysis was associated with a 37% limb salvage rate at 3 years. Complications of lytic therapy occurred in 43% of their patients. Lang[267] found a high rate of complications among 35 patients treated with injection of streptokinase into a bypass graft or a native artery treated for thrombotic or thromboembolic occlusions. Five patients had massive myoglobinuria following restoration of flow to ischemic and necrotic tissue. Acute tubular necrosis developed in two patients. One patient died as a result of renal shutdown, electrolyte imbalance, hypofibrinogenemia, and mediastinal and retroperitoneal hemorrhage. Massive myoglobinuria was also noted in five out of 13 patients with compartment syndrome, but no evidence of ischemic necrosis. Sniderman et al.[268] tried catheter-directed low-dose therapy with either streptokinase or urokinase on 42 separate occasions in 36 patients for recent lower-extremity thromboembolic occlusion. Their cumulative success rate was 44% ± 9% at 24 months. Complications occurred on 17 occasions and included hemorrhage (6), distal embolization (3), compartment syndrome (1), retrograde thrombosis during infusion (5), hypotension (1), and systemic fibrinogenolysis (1). Law et al.[269] administered intra-arterial urokinase in the immediate postoperative period to 12 patients with the "no-reflow" phenomenon (the loss of distal tissue perfusion sufficient for limb salvage following restoration of inflow to an acutely ischemic extremity). The procedure was complicated by bleeding sufficient to require transfusions in seven patients. One patient required reoperation for a groin hematoma. Limb salvage resulted in seven of the 12 patients. Six patients had viable functional limbs at follow-up 6.4 to 49.7 months later. Lang[267] pointed out that a tissue pressure of 30 mm Hg existing for 8 hours or longer may be the critical point at which tissue necrosis ensues and compartment syndrome may develop. His group apparently, however, did not use pressure measurements as a guide as to the need for fasciotomy. Among thousands of boot patients, we have not recognized reperfusion complications due to boot therapy. Among our web case reports, one patient (#182) developed renal shutdown after fasciotomy. Boot therapy may have helped restore the patient's kidney function. Fasciotomy was considered in another case (#122), but Long-Boot therapy was used successfully instead, which also supported the heart. On occasion we have successfully combined boot therapy both with systemic intravenous lytic therapy and with catheter-directed low-dose infusions.

Boot Therapy and Fibrinolysis

Pneumatic boots have been utilized for decades for the prevention of postoperative deep vein thrombosis. Knight and Dawson[270] provided early evidence that booting did more than prevent venous stasis; it had a systemic effect on fibrinolysis (Fig. 13–5). By pumping on arms, they showed a decrease in the euglobulin lysis time and a decreased incidence of positive I-125 labeled fibrinogen leg scans for deep vein thrombi.

Dai et al.[222] designed an *in vitro* cell culture system to study the influence of external pneumatic compression on endothelial function. They found that both pulsatile flow and, to a lesser degree, vessel compression, influenced endothelial cell morphology and function up-regulating expression of tPA and nitric oxide synthase. Elastic stockings, lacking a pulsative function and an action delivering shear forces to the leg, have been shown to have no fibrinolytic potential.[271] Multiple-bladder sequential boots have not demonstrated a significant advantage over single-bladder apparatuses.[272] Tarnay et al.[273] showed intermittent compression increases fibrinolytic potential locally and the effect can be demonstrated systemically with greater responses accompanying greater volumes of

tissue compressed. Watanabe[274] showed the euglobulin lysis times in both the antecubital vein and femoral vein decreased after bilateral intermittent sequential leg compression, while the mean blood velocity (183%) and peak velocity (178%) increased in the femoral vein. Inada et al.[275] had similar results and emphasized that pneumatic leg compressions should begin preoperatively to prevent postoperative deep vein thromboses because venous return is apt to be lower at the beginning of anesthesia. Fibrinogen uptake tests have shown that deep vein thromboses develop during surgery and in the early postoperative period.[275] Jacobs et al.[276] in studying the time consequences of hemodynamic and fibrinolytic changes associated with sequential gradient intermittent pneumatic leg compression noted that even the catheter placement caused elevations in PAI-1 and tPA–PAI, which took 4 hours to stabilize. Leg compressions induced prompt significant increases in degradation products of fibrin, fibrinogen, and tPA–PAI and decreases in euglobulin lysis times and PAI-1, all of which quickly reverted to baseline on termination of compression. This led them to conclude that noncontinuous pumping may result in suboptimal thromboembolic prophylaxis. Comerota et al.[277] used five different leg compression devices to study both normal volunteers and patients with a history of thrombotic events. They found a significant striking elevation in fibrinolytic activity after pumping the legs 180 min with all devices in normal subjects and, to a lesser degree, in post-thrombotic patients. The tPA-activity increased only in normal subjects, despite a significant decrease in plasma tPA-antigen, which was observed in both normal subjects and patients. PAI-1-antigen and activity significantly decreased in both normal subjects and patients. They concluded that the mechanism of increased fibrinolytic activity was likely a reduction in PAI-1, with a resulting increase of tPA activity.[277] Their study shows the importance of measuring fibrinolytic activity in addition to antigen levels. Thus, Christen et al.,[278] while finding similar venous flow increases with a foot impulse device and a full leg low pressure device (the former pumping on limited tissue and the latter being low pressure and lacking vigorous shear forces), found no changes of tPA or PAI-1 antigens with either device. They concluded that the antithrombotic effect of mechanical prophylaxis is probably mainly due to its ability to increase venous peak velocity. The concomitant use of heparin may have confounded the effects of pumping on fibrinolysins in some studies. Thus, Kosir et al.[279] compared the effects of heparin and sequential leg compression therapy on tPA antigen, PAI-1, and D-dimer. Among their 136 patients, there were three thrombotic events in the heparin group and one in the leg compression group. Fibrinolysis studies in the subjects without thrombosis showed parallel increases in D-dimer and tPA antigen levels. PAI-1

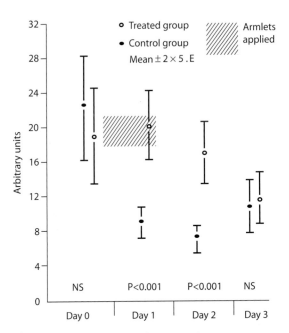

Fig. 13–5. In the control group, there was a pronounced decrease in fibrinolytic activity immediately postoperatively with a rise to normal levels by day 3. The effect of the armlets lasted 18 hours after their removal.
From: Knight MTN, Dawson R. Effect of intermittent compression of the arms on deep vein thrombosis in the legs. *Lancet* 1976; II: 1265–1267.

levels increased in both groups, but severalfold more in the compression devices group. Some studies are hard to interpret. Killewich et al.[280] examined the possibility that thigh-length sequential compression boots might enhance regional fibrinolysis when no systemic effects are noted. They measured the activities of tPA and PAI-1 in three groups: one given heparin only, one with leg compression only, and one given both heparin and leg compression treatments. Blood samples from the femoral vein showed no changes in fibrinolysins within any group and there was no difference between groups attributed to leg compressions. The authors concluded that leg compression devices do not appear to prevent deep vein thrombosis (DVT) with fibrinolytic enhancement; effective and safe prophylaxis is provided only when the devices are used in a manner that reduces lower-extremity venous stasis. They might equally conclude that their dosage of heparin also had no fibrinolytic effect. The study of Guyton et al.[281] complicates the fibrinolysin issue further. They applied external compression therapy to one leg and obtained blood samples from both femoral arteries and the right arm. At 30 min, they found modest increases in endogenous PA in both the control leg and arm while PA activity decreased progressively in the leg receiving compression therapy. They noted that *in vitro,* PA activity varies directly with the concentration of fibrin and hypothesized that the progressive decline in activity in this study may, therefore, represent a decline in substrate (molecular fibrin) as a result of increased venous blood flow. Likewise, the increased blood flow may have washed out and diluted any increase in the production of PA that may have occurred.

Many studies have shown benefit in the prophylaxis of deep vein thromboses and pulmonary emboli with the use of leg compression devices. Blackshear et al.[282] showed that venous function is improved with the use of leg compression devices. They measured venous capacitance and outflow in a series of general surgical patients. In control patients, preoperative values for venous capacitance significantly decreased 35% postoperatively and venous outflow significantly decreased 33% at the same time. In patients who began compression therapy on one leg preoperatively and continued for 24 hours postoperatively, leg compression therapy prevented significant changes in both venous capacity and outflow both in the pumped and in the unpumped limb.

Prostacyclin (PGI)

Prostaglandins are compounds with a five-carbon ring with two extending fatty acid chains. The prostaglandin A (PGA) and prostaglandin B (PGB) compounds both have a ketone group and double bond in the ring, but the latter differs in position. In the prostaglandin E (PGE)

and prostaglandin F (PGF) compounds, the double bond in the ring is gone. A hydroxyl group is added to the ring in the PGE compounds and another replaces the ketone in the PGF compounds. Subscripts indicate the number of double bonds in the fatty acid side chains. Prostaglandins are found in minute quantities in nearly all animal cells. They are derived from essential polyunsaturated fatty acids in the cells where they act. They have many actions beyond this review. Bradykinin may have vascular regulating effects mediated through prostaglandins; it promotes the synthesis of PGE in arterial walls causing vasodilation, while in veins it activates 9-ketoreductase and promotes PGF synthesis, which can cause vasoconstriction. The number of double bonds in the side chains can have profound effects on the action of the parent compound. Thus, PGE_1 increases erythrocyte deformability and inhibits platelet aggregation, while PGE_2 decreases erythrocyte deformability and increases platelet aggregation. PGE and PGA compounds play a role in local inflammation. They increase histamine-mediated vascular permeability and prolong the delayed phase of the acute inflammatory response associated with the ingress of leukocytes. Inhibitors of the enzymes producing prostaglandins (cyclo-oxygenases, COX-1 and COX-2) have found their way into the treatment of arthritis where their usage may be complicated by gastrointestinal injury. The selective inhibition of either COX-1 or COX-2 does not elicit gastrointestinal damage; inhibition of both enzymes is necessary for gastrointestinal mucosal damage to develop. Prostaglandins generated by both enzymes contribute to normal renal function by regulating the vascular tone and the normal blood flow; COX inhibitors may promote fluid retention and a decrease in renal function. The synthesis of endothelial prostacyclin is mainly driven by COX-2, so that the selective COX-2 inhibition may bias vascular prostaglandin synthesis in favor of COX-1-derived thromboxane A_2 in platelets, leading to a prothrombotic outcome. Moreover, prostaglandins formed by COX-2 appear to have a major role in myocardial protection.[283] Prostacyclin is the major product of arachidonic acid metabolism formed in the macrovascular endothelium. It is a potent vasodilator, antithrombotic, and antiplatelet agent that mediates it effects through a membrane-associated receptor termed the isoelectric point (i.p). The latter is a member of the G protein-coupled receptor superfamily.[284] Various neurohumoral substances (eg, bradykinin or acetylcholine) and physical stimuli (eg, cyclic stretch, fluid shear stress, and pneumatic boot therapy) stimulate the endothelium to synthesize and release prostacyclin and nitric oxide.[285–287] Aspirin is the most commonly used inhibitor of prostaglandin production. Aspirin interferes with arachidonic acid metabolism both in platelets and endothelial cells and thereby reduces thromboxane A_2

and prostacyclin. It also has other mechanisms of action, including antiinflammatory roles, protection from oxidative stress, enhancement of fibrinolysis, and suppression of plasma coagulation, and platelet-dependent inhibition of thrombin generation.[288] It has been used for primary and secondary prevention of myocardial ischemia and for primary and secondary prevention of cerebrovascular ischemia. Isolated suppression of COX-2 might have a role in preventing arteriosclerotic disease. Cyclooxygenase-2 is up-regulated in activated monocyte/macrophages, which play a key role in the pathogenesis of atherosclerosis. Linton and Fazio[289] found that pharmacological inhibition of COX-2 in LDL-receptor deficient mice reduced early atherosclerosis after 6 weeks on a Western-type diet.

Prostaglandin E$_1$ has found its way into clinical research and therapies. Schellong et al.[290] examined muscle blood flow in the legs with a positron emission tomography (PET) scanner. They concluded that the pharmacodynamic profile of intra-arterial PGE$_1$ differs clearly from intravenous PGE$_1$; the flow-enhancing property is lost during metabolization in the lung. They noted, however, that since no difference exists between the therapeutic efficacy of intra-arterial and intravenous PGE$_1$, the impact on muscular blood flow is not as important as suggested previously. Matsumoto et al.[291] have studied the effect of PGI$_2$ on hepatocyte growth factor (HGF), which has many protective functions against endothelial damage by high d-glucose and might be a trigger of endothelial injury. They found that treatment with a prostaglandin I$_2$ (PGI$_2$) analog restored endothelial dysfunction in their diabetic rats and restored the induction of vascular HGF (restoration was inhibited, however, if nitric oxide synthesis was simultaneously inhibited). Kamper et al.[292] demonstrated the interrelationships between prostacyclin and nitric oxide-mediated vasodilatation in the human forearm. They found that sodium nitroprusside-induced vasodilation (a drug stimulating nitric oxide effect independent of nitric oxide synthase [NOS]) was not influenced by inhibition of either NOS or COX. The vasodilatation induced by iloprost, a prostacyclin analog, was significantly attenuated by inhibition of NOS, but not affected by inhibition of COX. Both acetylcholine and 5-hydroxytryptamine can induce release of both nitric oxide and PGI. The vasodilator responses of both agents were significantly attenuated by COX inhibition, but not further influenced by a concomitant inhibition of NOS. Prostacyclin infusions have been attempted with mixed results in the treatment of patients with primary pulmonary hypertension. The treatment may be complicated by massive pulmonary edema, pulmonary veno-occlusive disease, and death.[293,294] Chang et al.[295] found that PGE$_1$ infusions improved the vascular studies of patients with modest vascular impairment

and/or small foot ulcers, but had no effect in patients with ulcers over one half centimeter or gangrenous changes.

Nitric Oxide

Nitric oxide is a relative newcomer to discussions of vascular physiology, having been identified in the late 1980s as a vascular relaxing factor.[296,297] It acts as an endogenous nitrovasodilator, stimulating soluble guanylate cyclase to increase cyclic guanosine monophosphate (GMP) levels in vascular smooth muscle and platelets, with consequent relaxant and antiaggregatory effects. Subsequently, it has been shown to be a vascular hormone with many functions. Boykin et al.[298] reported that low urine levels portend poor wound healing in the diabetic patient and a poor response to the application of topically applied platelet-derived growth factor (PDGF). In their discussion on wound healing, they list the many roles and actions of nitric oxide: promotion of angiogenesis and cellular migration, increased wound collagen deposition and collagen cross-linking, promotion of vasodilatation, inhibition of platelet aggregation and endothelial–leukocyte adhesions, modulation of endothelial proliferation and apoptosis, increase in the viability of random cutaneous flaps, and enhancement of cellular immunomodulation and bacterial cytotoxicity.

Infusion of L-arginine produces systemic vasodilatation via stimulation of endogenous nitric oxide (NO) formation. The basic amino acid arginine, of course, is well known in endocrinology literature as an important component in the urea cycle (Krebs–Henseleit cycle) where it is cleaved to form isourea and ornithine. Clinically, the endocrinologist has used infusions of arginine in doses of 0.5 mg/kg up to 30 gm as a potent stimulus for the secretion of insulin, glucagon, and growth hormone. Obviously, much happens with the infusion of arginine. Schellong et al.[299] have shown that intravenous L-arginine enhances nutritive capillary muscular blood flow in patients with peripheal vascular disease via the NO–cyclic GMP pathway in a dose-related manner. Schmetterer et al.[300] showed that administration of L-arginine increased pulsations in the ophthalmic artery and decreased blood pressure in both normal and diabetic subjects and that inhibition of nitric oxide synthase with NG-monomethyl-L-arginine decreased fundus pulsations and increased blood pressure. (This study is included because it may be related to the effects of booting on diabetic retinopathy; we may be seeing an improvement in retinal blood flow with booting possibly mediated by increases in circulating NO and/or other factors.) Maxwell et al.[301] have carried arginine therapy to the practical world in devising a food bar enriched with L-arginine and a combination of other nutrients known to enhance the activity of endothelium-derived nitric oxide. Use of their nutrient bar improved pain-free and total walking distance as well as quality of life in individuals with intermittent claudication. On the other hand, a beneficial effect of arginine on the incidence of coronary heart disease has not been seen; Venho et al.[302] found no association between dietary arginine intake and the risk of acute coronary events in middle-aged men in eastern Finland.

In the case of exercise-induced muscular hyperemia, factors in addition to nitric oxide, are operative. Blood flow increases in spite of systemic inhibition of nitric oxide synthase. Hillig et al.[303] demonstrated that cytochrome P450 2C9 also plays a role in the regulation of hyperemia and oxygen uptake during exercise. Since inhibition of neither NOS nor CYP 2C9 alone affect skeletal muscle blood flow, inhibition of both together do decrease blood flow. An interaction between CYP 2C9 and NOS appears to exist so that a CYP-dependent vasodilator mechanism takes over when NO production is compromised.

As with prostacyclin (above), acetylcholine and physical stimuli (eg, cyclic stretch, fluid shear stress, and pneumatic boot therapy) stimulate the endothelium to synthesize and release nitric oxide.[285,286,304,305] Nitric oxide is generated also by acetylcholine. Cholinergic neuropathy has been discussed above as part of diabetic peripheral neuropathy. Nitric oxide is involved with the reactive hyperemia associated with reperfusion injury in skeletal mucle in rats in whom neutrophil extravasation and edema may be reduced with the administration of the selective nitric oxide inhibitor 1400W. The negative effects of ischemia/reperfusion on vessel diameter and muscle blood flow are likewise reduced.[306] In the mouse heart, neuronal nitric oxide synthase appears to be a key protein in generating the cardiac vagal gain of function elicited by exercise training.[307] Transgenic mice that overexpress endothelial NOS (eNOS) exclusively in cardiac myocytes and have high levels of NO/cyclic guanosine monophosphate (cGMP) are strongly protected against ischemia/reperfusion injury, likely related to reduced preischemic performance.[308] Cooke's laboratory has shown that nitric oxide induces synthesis of vascular endothelial growth factor by rat vascular smooth muscle cells[309] and that angiogenesis is impaired by hypercholesterolemia.[310] The latter effect is related to nitric oxide through the endogenous inhibitor of NOS, ADMA. ADMA or asymmetric dimethylarginine is an arginine analog that competes with arginine for NOS. The effect of ADMA is reversed by supplemental arginine. Elevated plasma levels of ADMA and an impairment of the NOS pathway potentially adversely affecting angiogenesis are seen in hypertension, hyperglycemia, hyperhomocysteinemia, hypertriglyceridemia, and insulin resistance. The effects of nicotine and cholinergic agents on wound healing that Cooke's group has reported is discussed further in sections on Neuropathy and Buerger's disease above.

VEGFs (Vascular Endothelial Growth Factors)

Tissue anoxia results in the elaboration of nitric oxide, prostacylin, and vascular endothelial growth factors (VEGFs) in an attempt to restore tissue perfusion. VEGF itself may promote the production of nitric oxide and prostacyclin.[311] In the absence of some pulsatile flow, however, angiogenesis may not occur. Levy[312] showed that the hypoxic induction of VEGF is reduced by chronic anoxia. Hemodynamic forces play a fundamental role even in the regulation of endothelial cell survival. Urbich[313] showed that fluid shear stress in microvascular and large-vessel derived endothelial cells upregulate endothelial VEGF receptor-2 expression and endothelial cell survival. Thus, the amount of VEGA in anoxic tissue might be reduced and the effect of any produced might be blunted in the absence of pulsatile flow, explaining, perhaps, the inadequate amount of compensatory angiogenesis seen in many chronic ischemic disorders. On the other hand, in the case of the coronary circulation, a marked angiogenesis is known to occur with chronic bradycardia; pulsatile flow may be important but it need not be rapid. Zheng et al.[314] showed that bradycardia induced with alinidine in rats increased VEGF and promoted angiogenesis and that the angiogenesis could be blocked by the administration of VEGF-neutralizing antibodies. The authors postulated that the mechanism underlying this VEGF-associated angiogenesis may be an increase in stretch, due to enhanced diastolic filling. (Treatment with the Circulator Long-Boot increases venous return, preload and diastolic filling, and decreases afterload. The treatment is commonly associated with a slowing of the heart rate. When the heart rate of the patient is 90–120 per min, the clinician may choose to either slow the heart rate with the use of beta blockers or digitalis or pump the legs on every second or third heartbeat. Could such maneuvers increase VEGF and myocardial angiogenesis?) Various investigators have administered VEGA and other growth factors to ischemic limbs and hearts with variable success. The therapy is not without hazard. High dosages or repeated administration may produce hypotension, proteinuria, and atherosclerotic plaque instability. The potential harm VEGA therapy might have in producing angiogenesis near tumors or other sites, where it it not wanted, remains to be seen. Both virial and nonvirial vectors have been used to transfer the angiogenic genes. Vale et al.[315] have published some early optimistic studies treating both hearts and legs. The TRAFFIC investigators administered placebo, one intra-arterial dose of recombinant fibroblast growth factor-2 (rFGF-2) or two doses of intra-arterial rFGF-2 to patients with claudication due to infrainguinal arteriosclerotic disease.[316] The patients were free of rest pain and sufficient baseline tissue flow was present to allow over 1 minute of exercise on the treadmill. Peak walking time at 90 days was increased by 0.60 min with placebo, by 1.77 min with single dose, and by 1.54 min with double dose. Paired comparison showed a significant difference between placebo and single dose, but placebo and double dose did not differ by much ($p = 0.45$). Nitta et al.[317] have shown that recombinant human erythropoietin stimulates VEGF release by glomerular endothelial cells and had a proliferative effect, which was inhibited by anti-VEGF antiserum. Chae et al.[318] have shown that the coadministration of angiopoietin-1 and VEGF enhances collateral vascularization in a rabbit ischemic hindlimb model more than either agent alone. Recombinant technology may also play a role in the treatment of the infected diabetic foot. The efficacy of recombinant human granulocyte colony-stimulating factor (G-CSF) (lenograstim) as an adjunctive therapy for the standard treatment of diabetic foot infection was investigated by de Lalla et al.[319] in 20 patients and 20 controls. While at the 3- and 9-week assessments, no significant differences between the two groups could be observed, additional studies may be warranted as the the cumulative number amputation was significantly lower in the treated group. Whether such studies will result in effective and practical therapies for people with ischemic disease remains to be seen. For example, there has been no role for the administration of recombinant insulin to people without an insulin deficit. The studies do further understanding of pathophysiology and should be related to clinical medicine, where possible. Patients with rest pain, no Doppler pulses, and very low transcutaneous PO_2 levels might not be expected to respond to VEGF. Many such patients have responded to therapy with the Circulator Boot and developed Doppler pulses and collaterals on arteriography. These patients have gone on to heal their lesions,[320,321] suggesting that VEGF will work if pulsative flow is provided.

Erythrocyte Sedimentation Rate and C-Reactive Protein—Guides of Healing

The sed rate is a nonspecific test that is commonly increased in the presence of infection, inflammatory disease, tissue damage, and conditions associated with increased plasma fibrinogen or globulins. Rouleau formation, flattening of the red cells, and anemia increase the sed rate, while polycythemia, sickle cell disease, and spherocytosis may decrease it. The test is commonly used in the diagnosis and monitoring of temporal arteritis and polymyalgia rheumatica. The test is commonly employed by rheumatology consultants who may interpret an elevation as proof that leg lesions may be the result of collagen disease and an arteritis. On this basis, corticosteroids may be prescribed with devastating results when the lesions are the result of diabetes complicated by osteomyelitis. The sed rate is useful in

following the course of patients with osteomyelitis. Normalization of the sed rate may presage eventual healing of osteomyelitis in spite of apparent progression of x-rays. Missov et al.[322] found that insulin therapy was associated with higher levels of fibrinogen and higher sed rates in type 2 diabetics. The deleterious effect of insulin therapy was lessened when the fructosamine level was considered as a measure of glycemic control. C-reactive protein (CRP) likewise increases with inflammation, tissue necrosis, and trauma. Treatment with corticosteroids lowers CRP. Very high levels may be associated with infection and may fall with appropriate antibiotic therapy. The test is also used to follow patients with collagen diseases, arteritic syndromes, and coronary artery disease. Matzke et al.[323] have observed that, in their series of 143 femoropopliteal reconstructions, the preoperative CRP was the only predictor of postoperative major amputation ($p = 004$): mean CRP for those with no amputation was 13.0 mg/l, 47.5 mg/l for those with an amputation after graft occlusion, and 115.0 mg/l for those with an amputation despite a patent bypass graft.[323]

HYPERINSULINEMIA AND INSULIN RESISTANCE

Insulin is an anabolic hormone, which is necessary for wound healing and the storage of all food stuffs: protein, fat, and carbohydrates. Excessive intake, stuffed fuel depots or a relative lack of insulin all result in increased serum lipids and glucose. Cholesterol, a modern-day villain in abundant societies, is necessary for steroidogenesis and the synthesis of the lipid mosaic of cell membranes. Decreased caloric intake in states of starvation or weight-reduction programs, increased caloric requirements as with physical training or illness, or increased need for cholesterol as in the synthesis of new erythrocytes after blood loss are all associated with low serum levels of cholesterol. Likewise, wide spread weight reduction as occurred in Western Europe during the World War II is associated with a marked reduction in the incidence of type 2 diabetes. Except for smoking, all of the common risk factors for arteriosclerotic cardiovascular diasease are related to excessive weight gain. Hyperlipidemia, hypertension, and type 2 diabetes are all either avoided or lessened with weight control.

Weight Gain and Hyperinsulinemia

The Metropolitan Life Insurance Company provided a large well-known data base on the detrimental effect of weight gain on the incidence of arterial hypertension and death. When their tables for desirable weights are converted to body mass indices (BMI), they show ranges across all heights of 20.6 to 22.7 for light-framed men, 21.4–24.4 for medium-framed men, and 22.7–26.7

heavy-framed men. The corresponding values for women were 19.6–22, 20.5–24, and 22–26.7.[324] The observations made on the morbidity and mortality of adult-onset obesity in the Build and Blood Pressure Study are quite pertinent to the concept of insulin resistance and its risks. Unadjusted average blood pressure for successive life insurance rate groups for each height and weight category increased in both systolic and diastolic blood pressure more or less regularly with the increase in weight. Mortality rates also increased with weight. The risk imposed by obesity varied with the age of onset and the degree of obesity. Moderately obese people insured under the age of 20 had no apparent increase in mortality rate and moderately obese women issued policies from ages 15 to 39 even had a decreased mortality rate with the duration of their moderate obesity. Subjects of both sexes who acquire their obesity after the age of 30 and had pronounced obesity also had greater increased mortality rates. The concepts of body frame and potential hazard of weight gain after maturity have been lost in recent years as the body mass index as been commonly used to define weight categories. Thus, Reaven[325] has used a BMI equal to 30 as the dividing line between obese and normal weight individuals. Note that some persons at their desirable weights at age 25 might gain 50% in weight, if small framed, and 11–12% in weight, if at the upper limits of heavy frame, to reach a BMI of 30! The concepts of body frame and the importance of the weight history for the individual are missing from the literature on hyperinsulinism and syndrome X, which share with obesity increased incidences of hypertriglyceridemia, high free fatty acid levels, low serum levels of HDL-cholesterol, diabetes, hypertension, increased serum levels of inflammatory markers,[326] and arteriosclerotic cardiovascular disease. Paris et al.[327] illustrated the importance of varying degrees of obesity in their study of the characteristics of U.S. military personnel at entry who develop type 2 diabetes over time. They found that the incidence of diabetes increased threefold for persons with a BMI of 30 or more and twofold for those with BMI's between 25.0 and 29.9. Again, mortality data shows that there is no cutoff BMI to define obesity; mortality increases progressively above a BMI of 24. Thus, adjusted mortality ratios, taking 100% for persons with a BMI of 20, increase exponentially to 115% for a BMI of 24, to 130% for 27, to 155% for 30, to 250% for 34, and to 300% for a BMI of 36.[328] Obesity is found to precede hyperinsulinemia in all age groups independently of baseline insulin levels, sex, or race.[329] Healthy light-framed individuals may differ from healthy heavy-framed individuals of the same height by differences in the mass of their bones, muscle, and fat. The mass of bone and muscle that the growing body attains is strongly related to exercise, work levels,

and nutrition. The number of fat cells attained is related to the amount of overnutrition enjoyed during the growth years. The size of the fat cell in the adult is related to the degree of overnutrition. Old literature on the subject of fat cell hyperplasia versus hypertrophy is pertinent here.[330–332] One learns that the number of fat cells does not decrease with weight reduction, but the amount of fat per cell does. Weight reduction of the superobese to "normal" weight may reduce fat cell content such that biopsy specimens appear to come from starved individuals. Packing extra fuel into cells comes with a price. The skeleton does not increase in size with weight gain in the adult and weight gain is clearly associated with postural strain and the development of degenerative arthritis. The highest triglyceride and cholesterol values are not in the most obese patients, but in those with the highest percentage weight gain since the age of 25.[333] The Framingham Study emphasized the importance of obesity in the genesis of hypertension. An eightfold increased incidence was found in subjects who were 20% or more overweight compared to the group who were 10% underweight. The incidence of hypertension in men who maintained a desirable weight was 20% of that in those with a significant weight gain. Of those who gained 29 pounds or more since their 25th birthday, 20% were hypertensive.[334] On the other hand, 75% of overweight patients given weight-reduction diets but no medications or salt restriction may be able to normalize their blood pressures.[335] It is not the purpose of this chapter to review all of the metabolic relationships between diet and hyperinsulinemia. The reader might see the review of Kraegen et al.[336] for more recent references on the subject. They point out that with the development of hyperinsulinemia, increased fat is found outside of the adipose cell significantly infiltrating muscle. Increased fat may be more than a weight burden. It produces estrogens in women. Visceral fat may overproduce PAI-1.[337] However, we include this discussion to make the points: (1) the concept of hyperinsulinemia and obesity is old; (2) hyperinsulinemia is a normal accompaniment to overfeeding; (3) hyperinsulinemia disappears or is lessened by weight reduction achieved by calorie restriction and/or exercise; (4) hyperinsulinemia is likely but a marker of chronic overfeeding in most subjects; (5) the current epidemics of type 2 diabetes, hyperlipidemia, and hypertension in the Western world are more likely related to chronic overfeeding than any mysterious insulin abnormalities; (6) studies relating surgical and medical mortality and morbidity to insulin levels and resistance are misleading; and (7) inadequate insulin therapy and hyperglycemia increase risk for infection and death in the postoperative period and the intensive care unit. One might also observe that detracting from the importance of diet and exercise does public harm. A drug like metformin, which generally is associated with weight loss, may reduce the incidence of new diabetes 31%, but an intensive lifestyle change is both more economical and effective (58% reduction in new cases).[338]

THE CIRCULATOR BOOT AND ITS DIFFERENCES FROM OTHER BOOTS

History of Vascular Boots and Effects on Vascular Tests

Pneumatic boots for the treatment of arterial diseases have evolved over the last 191 years (see Fig 13–4). Proof of their efficacy was limited by the vascular laboratory methods of their era. Improvement in blood flow with the suction pressure boots of the 1930s was documented largely by thermocouples, a technique that becomes very powerful when performed in a constant-temperature room under standard conditions.[339] Thus, patients are warmed under blankets with toes bare in a 20°C constant-temperature room. Toe temperatures then reflect the degree of vascular impairment of the patient: none over 30, slight 28–30, moderate 25–28, and severe 21–25°C. Amputation is seldom necessary with results over 26°C. The suction-pressure boots found their way into clinical practice in a limited number of centers and enjoyed a success that might seem remarkable for the preantibiotic era.[341, 342] In 1956, Allwood[343] pumped on the lower calf and documented an increase in blood flow in the foot with a plethysmographic method. In 1959, Loane[344] rhythmically inflated a cuff around the ankle in the seated position and noted an increase in blood flow in the foot by three methods: venous occlusion plethysmography, heat flow, and calorimetry. Henry and Winsor,[345] in 1965, pumped from the head of the fibula to the malleoli and documented increased flow in the foot by measuring a decrease in counts from injected I131. Gaskell and Parrott,[346] in 1978, pumped on the foot and ankle and documented an increased clearance of 133 Xe from the dorsum of the foot. Agerskov et al.[347] in 1990, applied 35–45 mm Hg negative pressure (suction) around the thighs of patients with occluded femoral arteries and rest pain or claudication and measured increases in toe blood pressures and 133 Xe washout in the first toe interstice. Their use of suction was similar to that used in the 1930s; it requires an air seal against the thigh and produces a modest shear force that over time can cause skin breakdown. Their 30 mm Hg of suction is equivalent to about 17 inches of water pressure, about the distance from the aortic valve to the midthigh in the sitting position. Merely by sitting up during therapy with the Circulator Long-Boot, one gains the benefits of gravity and an equivalent of about 30 mm Hg negative pressure. Abu-Own et al.[348] measured transcutaneous oxygen pressure and laser Doppler flux in evaluating the acute effects of an impulse pump (a mini-pump device limited to the foot) on the microcirculation of the big toe. After 10 minutes of pumping, they found significant increases in both $TcPO_2$ (8% for patients and 10% for controls) and laser Doppler flux (57% for patients and 66% for controls), but the latter briefly faded away within 20 seconds of stopping the foot pump. Eze et al.[349] studied the effects of intermittent calf and foot compressions on the Duplex scans of the popliteal artery and laser flux on the big toe of normal volunteers and patients with occluded superficial femoral arteries; both groups had similar tibial vessels. Their patients had ABIs ranging from 0.55 to 0.75 mm Hg (ankle blood pressures perhaps varying from 77 to 105 mm Hg supine and, perhaps, 132 to 160 mm Hg sitting with their foot lowered 30 inches to a low stool— 30 inches of water pressure equals 55 mm Hg). A 22-cm calf cuff and a 12-cm foot cuff were used to inflate to a pressure of 120 mm Hg over 0.3 seconds; the pressure was held 10 seconds and then released. The cuffs then remained deflated for 20 seconds. Measurements were averaged over six cycles in each of three combinations: compressions of (1) calf alone, (2) foot alone, and (3) both calf and foot. Baseline flow was greater in both the popliteal and toe in the patients. Flow increased in the popliteal in the three combinations, respectively: 124% controls versus 76% patients, 54% controls versus 13% patients, 173% controls versus 50% patients. Likewise skin perfusion increased, respectively: 260% controls versus 116% patients, 500% controls versus 246% patients, and 328% controls versus 188% patients. The flow in the popliteal was increased more by calf compressions, than foot compressions, while the flow in the toe was more increased by foot compressions. These results could be explained, in part, if the 10-second compression impeded flow through the calf in some patients; an empty calf would welcome popliteal flow and an empty foot would not respond as well to foot compressions. The data in Fig. 13–6 shows what happens, however, when a leg is very ischemic and has a progressive drop in systolic pressure from the groin to the foot.

Dillon studied the persistent effects of courses of end-diastolic full-leg compression treatments with diastolic blood pressure in normals subjects and patients with ischemic leg disease.[320] Significant beneficial effects were documented by subcutaneous PO_2 levels, pulse volume measurements, ankle blood pressure measurements, and Doppler ultrasound tracings. Of the 25 severely ischemic legs, 22 benefited clinically from therapy. In an individual patient, the effects of end-diastolic pumping on the pulsatile flow in the toes may be demonstrated at the bedside (see Fig. 13–7).

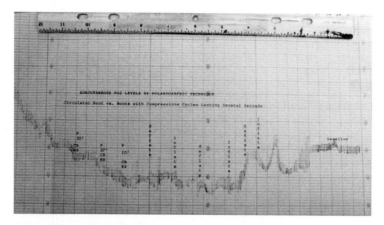

Fig. 13–6. Subcutaneous PO_2 changes in an ischemic leg as influenced by end-diastolic compressions versus compressions lasting a few seconds. A boot encompassing the leg from the groin to the ankle was used and the boot was inflated to 55 mm Hg for periods of several seconds. These tracings were obtained from a patient referred to the Bryn Mawr Circulator Boot Clinic after his leg had deteriorated elsewhere after treatments with a boot designed for treating lymphedema and venous stasis. In obtaining this study, a Circulator Boot was utilized setting the delay time to zero and the compression time to 1 second; in effect, the boot continued to compress the leg until the boot switch was manually turned off. Thus, the boot could be alternately inflated and deflated for any desired time period. The graph reads from right to left. A baseline period is followed by a series of compressions and decompressions lasting several seconds each. The subcutaneous PO_2 level is seen to progressively drop. The boot was then set to deliver end-diastolic compressions and the PO_2 tension is seen to progressively rise. Such measurements are not necessary in clinical practice as improper pumping will produce pain and numbness in the distal extremity. If such pain occurs with end-diastolic pumping, the Circulator Boot is set to allow more arterial inflow by decreasing the compression rate from 1:1 to 1:2 or 1:3.

Pneumatic Leg Devices and Their Differences

There are many pneumatic leg devices. Most of the full-leg devices are designed for the treatment or prevention of venous stasis disease and lymphedema (see Table 13–10). Delis et al.[351] have shown that foot pumps may also improve arterial disease. Like Eze et al.[349] however, they found that pumping on both foot and calf was more effective.[352] A different application for external boots is cardiac assist. The External Counterpulsation devices (ECP systems and the Circulator Boot systems) fall into this category and differ from other systems in being cardiosynchronous.

Circulator Boot Versus ECP Devices

The Circulator Boot systems differ from the ECP devices in being both end-diastolic in timing and pres-

sure. Both key off the electrocardiogram, but the ECP devices begin compression with the end of the T-wave and the closure of the aortic valve and apply a square wave of pressure for perhaps 250 to 340 msec, not paying attention to the moment of deflation unless it coincides with the next electrocardiographic wave (QRS) complex.[353] In contrast, the monitor of the Circulator Boot systems averages the R-R intervals of the last ten beats and applies a formula to predict the appearance of the next QRS complex.[354,355] The monitor then places its calculated delay time after the QRS complex so that the operator-preset compression time (commonly 340 msec in the Miniboots and 380 to 450 msec in the Long Boots) will end 40 msec before the next QRS complex, allowing boot deflation to maximally decrease cardiac afterload. The ECP devices may deflate well before the next QRS complex. For example, with a pulse rate of

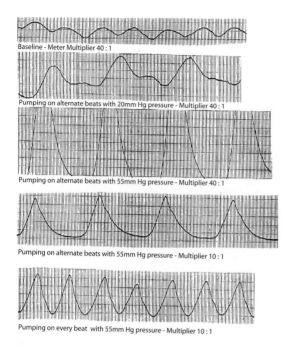

Baseline - Meter Multiplier 40 : 1

Pumping on alternate beats with 20mm Hg pressure - Multiplier 40 : 1

Pumping on alternate beats with 55mm Hg pressure - Multiplier 40 : 1

Pumping on alternate beats with 55mm Hg pressure - Multiplier 10 : 1

Pumping on every beat with 55mm Hg pressure - Multiplier 10 : 1

Fig. 13–7. A photoelectricpletysmography probe was on the dorsum of big toe. A boot bag was adjusted to compress leg from groin to ankle. Baseline tracings (top line) multiplied 40:1were but 5 mm in this arteriosclerotic patient. On the 2nd to 4th tracings the boot pumped on alternate beats with 20 mm Hg pressure (40:1), 55 mm Hg pressure (40:1) and 55 mm Hg pressure (10:1). The baseline beats are barely seen on the 2nd line. On the 4th line, the waveform is 25 mm high . . . correcting for the multiplier, 20 times higher than on the baseline. On the bottom line, the boot is pumping on every beat at 55 mm Hg with a waveform about 18x baseline.

100, a QT interval of 320 msec, and a compression time of 280 msec, the ECP device will deflate in end-diastole, but if the pulse rate were to slow to 60, it might deflate 400 msec before the end of diastole. Thus, the timing of the Circulator Boot differs from that of the ECP devices in that it allows additional time for the pulse wave to travel distally to prime the legs with blood and it deflates regularly close to the next QRS to maximize the decrease in afterload. The devices also differ in the height of their compression pressures and the number of compression bags. The ECP devices are designed to increase diastolic blood pressure in hopes of maximizing coronary blood flow during diastole at the expense of the legs. Thus, they utilize three compression bags beginning calf compression with a pressure of 280 mm Hg, followed by thigh compression, perhaps at 240 mm Hg, and finishing with compression of the buttocks at a pressure per-

haps of 180 mmHg—all pressures greater than systolic pressure and acting to drive arterial blood back out of the legs. Occlusive peripheral vascular disease is one contraindication to treatment with ECP devices. Finally, the Circulator Boot may be timed to compress the leg after *each* heartbeat, *every other* heartbeat, or *every third* heartbeat and its monitor automatically signals these options at rapid heart rates, when there might not be enough time for significant arterial inflow to the legs. It does *not* compress the leg during the moments of heart contraction and arterial inflow into the leg. In these options, it stands alone. Timed with the heartbeat, both the Circulator Boots and the ECP devices deliver far more energy and compressions to the legs than do compression boots approved for use in lymphedema or venous stasis, which commonly take 20 to 30 seconds to inflate, remain inflated perhaps one minute, and then deflate over a few seconds. During their inflated periods, they potentially may block blood flow into the ischemic leg and cause damage. The Circulator Boot system is highly flexible allowing the operator to treat *any desired portion* of the leg according to the needs of the patient: high groin to toes, midthigh to toes, high groin to ankle, knee to ankle or toes, calf to toes etc. Last, the Circulator Boot system readily lends itself to treatment of infected ulcerated legs, which may be treated while immersed in bags containing multielectrolyte and antibiotic solutions. Such treatments may help not only help restore blood flow but débride and sterilize the ulcers.

Circulator Boot Therapy for PVD Versus Invasive Procedures

In comparison with bypass surgery and angioplasty, Circulator Boot therapy stands well. Therapy can be initiated without delay immediately in the outpatient arena or the hospital; invasive procedures require scheduling in the hospital. Booting provides pulsatile flow to the ischemic leg hypothetically allowing angiogenic growth factors stimulated by anoxia to develop collateral flow; rapid restoration of tissue oxygen levels removes the anoxic drive for collateral flow. Treatment with the Circulator Boot systems may be discontinued at any time if the therapy appears to be ineffective without harm to the patient; the interruption of an invasive procedure is generally for some complication or an inability to finish the procedure and leaves the patient with a wound of varying size. One FDA-approved indication for Circulator Boot therapy is an attempt to improve runoff either before or after bypass; boot therapy may enhance the success of subsequent invasive procedures should it fail itself. The performance of invasive procedures lessens the success of both subsequent invasive procedures and boot therapy. Boot therapy has few if any complications; invasive procedures have a definite risk of morbidity and mortality. Boot therapy supports high-risk patients with

Table 13–10. Some commercially available devices for venous disease prevention and treatment*

Device	Manufacturer	Pressure range (mm Hg)	Cycle time[a]
Sequential multichambered leggings			
Thrombogard	Graymar Industries	45	16 sec infl/60 sec defl
Lymphatron	HNE Healthcare	20–98	90 sec infl/30 sec defl
FlowPlus	HNE Healthcare	30–70	50 sec infl/70 sec defl
FlowPress	HNE Healthcare	30–100	2 min infl/1 min defl
Lympha Press	Global Med. Imports	30–200	30 sec infl/3 sec hold
Kendal SCD	Kendal Healthcare P	30–55	11 sec infl/60 sec hold
Jobst Extr. Pump	Beierdorf-Jobst Inc.	10–120	190 sec infl/50 sec defl
Single-chamber leggings			
Flowtron HC	HNE Healthcare	30–90	90 sec infl/90 sec defl
Venodyne	Lyne-Nicholson Inc	40–45	12 sec infl/48 sec hold
PAS	American Hamilton	40–45	5 sec infl/15 sec hold/60 sec defl
Foot pumps			
AV Impulse	Kendal Healthcare P	60–200	0.4 sec infl/3 sec hold/20 sec defl
Plexipulse	NuTech	140–180	1-5 sec infl/hold/20–60 sec

*Adapted from Koch (350).
[a] sec, second; infl, inflate; defl, deflate.

coronary heart or renal disease; invasive procedures involve a challenge. Boot therapy may be planned on the basis of physical findings and the noninvasive vascular laboratory; invasive procedures require an arteriogram. Boot therapy has no risk of blood loss; invasive procedures require blood bank support. Boot therapy may enhance male potency (especially if the penis is included in the treated area); bypass may provide a denervated runoff and angioplasty of the common iliac has the potential of showering emboli to the internal iliac, both diminishing or destroying potency. Boot therapy may be utilized in patients with or without a patent saphenous vein, with focal of diffuse occlusive disease and with or without runoff. Bypass requires a patent saphenous vein (for distal bypass), a healthy segment of artery both to initiate and end the bypass and runoff, while angioplasty requires focal lesions and runoff. While all three modalities of treatment have been shown to improve noninvasive vascular tests,[320] prospective controlled studies in the diabetic leg are limited to those of Dillon who used the patients as their own controls; first, they had failed standard therapy and, second, their other leg deteriorated while their treated leg was healed.[15] The one bypass study in the literature, in which the bypassed leg was compared to the non-bypassed leg with serial arteriograms, showed that the bypassed leg deteriorated faster than the non-bypassed leg.[356] Finally, Circulator Boot therapy lends itself to the use of local antibiotics and

invasive procedures have not. On the other hand, the benefits of therapy with invasive procedures are realized the day of the procedure while boot therapy may take many days or weeks to achieve a successful outcome. Invasive procedures, their techniques, and success are covered elsewhere in this book. It is to be appreciated that there are reports of great success for both angioplasty and bypass in salvaging legs. Balmer et al.[357] found that among 60 consecutive patients with technically successful balloon angioplasty for infrainguinal chronic critical ischemia, 25% were dead at 1 year, restenosis rates correlated with the length of the segment treated (65% at the femoropopliteal and 56% at the infrapopliteal level), while by 1 year over 90% of survivors avoided major amputations.[357] Axisa et al.[358] found angioplasty to be both safe and effective in their series of 988 patients undergoing 1377 interventional procedures. Major medical morbidity complicated 2.4% procedures. Emergency surgical intervention was required in 2.3%. The amputation rate following angioplasty for critical limb ischemia was 2.2%. Overall, the risk of death and/or major medical complication and/or requiring emergency surgical intervention was 3.5%. Neufang et al.[359] emind us of the earlier reports of Pomposelli et al.[360] that pedal bypass may help salvage over 80% of patients with the diabetic foot. In spite of reports of such success, however, the incidence of diabetic amputations has continued to increase.

Cardiosynchronous External Compression Boots and the Heart

Developmental Considerations for the Adult

During embryonic development, the heart is one of the few organs that must function almost as soon as it is formed and begins to beat and pump blood through the embryo around day 22 of gestation. The contractions arise spontaneously within the myocardium itself and propagate from cell to cell. The ability to beat is an intrinsic property of these cells and is seen in tissue cultures. Beats are seen even before structures, such as valves and septa, have formed. For beats to occur, cardiac myocytes must have contractile proteins, such as actin and myosin, which are properly assembled into a scaffold or sarcomere. In addition, these cells must have specialized structures called gap junctions, which allow them to communicate so they can beat together in a synchronized fashion. Still, it is not yet known what stimuli initiate contraction. It is possible that the pulsations of a maternal capillary may be a factor inducing beats in the embryo. In the adult with ischemic heart disease, the myocytes may be stunned and cease to beat. With prolonged immobility, they may be replaced by fibrocytes. Regular electric stimulation of skeletal muscle may convert skeletal muscle into a fatigue-resistant power source.[361-363] There are anecdotal reports in which synchronized mechanical support has restored function in stunned myocardium.[364] Heart function commonly seems to improve in patients receiving Circulator Boot therapy. Soran et al.[365] have shown that enhanced external counterpulsation has benefited their patients with congestive failure. Future research will be needed to show if mechanical support devices have a definite role in treating patients with congestive heart failure and in restoring contractions to the stunned myocardium complicating some myocardial infarction and cardiac surgery procedures.

External Devices Versus the Intra-Aortic Balloon

The hemodynamic effects of external cardiac-assist devices should be compared with those of the intra-aortic balloon. The latter suffers from its invasive character, its vascular complications,[366,367] the need for specialized individuals to insert it, its obstruction of distal aortic blood flow, and the fact that it commonly changes hemodynamic data little. Williams et al.,[368] for example, were appropriately able to place their thermodilution catheter in the coronary sinus and obtain meaningful pulsations with the balloon in six of nine patients studied; five of the six had an insignificant 5% fall in systolic blood pressure, a 17% rise in mean diastolic blood pressure, and a 14.1% drop in myocardial oxygen consumption. They theorized that coronary flow and oxygen consumption were diminished because heart work was decreased. Cohen et al.[369] compared the sequential external counterpulsation with the intraaortic balloon before and after cardiogenic shock; the sequential device increased cardiac output 25 and 17% before and after the induction of shock compared to 4 and 10% for the intra-aortic balloon, respectively.[369] Others have reported the changes seen in cardiac output with external counterpulsation: negative[370], no change[371], to positive changes of 15 to 60%.[372,373] Improvement in coronary blood flow seen with counterpulsation may be mediated through the vasodilatory effects of nitric oxide stimulated by increased diastolic–systolic oscillations and shear on the coronary endothelium associated with the counterpulsation. Toyota et al.[374] observed coronary blood flow with a videomicroscope in dogs. The stimulatory effect on coronary flow of counterpulsation was significantly blocked by inhibiting the generation of nitric oxide with Nomega-nitro-L-arginine.[374]

Starling's Law Versus Boot Hemodynamics

External cardiac assist increases venous return to the heart. Starling's Law would dictate that an increase in cardiac output would then occur. In the normal person, an elastic network in the walls of the ventricles is deformed during systole. During diastole, the mitral valve opens when the pressure in the left ventricle has fallen below the pressure in the atrium and blood enters the ventricle. The pressure in the ventricle continues to fall after the valve opens as the collapsed elastic network regains its shape; the ventricle seems to be sucking blood into itself. Atrial contraction then further primes and distends the ventricles in preparation for systole. Historically, rotating venous tourniquets and elevation of the head of the bed have been used to diminish venous return to the heart in patients with congestive heart failure. The use of some boots, especially those for the treatment of lymphedema, are thought to be contraindicated in patients with heart disease lest they promote congestive heart failure. Dillon[375] reported the hemodynamic effects of Circulator Boot therapy in five situations: (1) baseline before pumping; (2) during end-diastolic pumping on both legs after every heartbeat, (3) on one leg after every heartbeat; (4) on both legs on alternate beats; and (5) during pumping on both legs during every systole. Both an increase in venous return and a reduction in afterload likely contributed to significant increases in cardiac output (51.1 ± 33.6%), stroke volume (52.1 ± 35.6%), dZ/dT (72.0 ± 68.1%), cardiac index (51.2 ± 33.8%), and acceleration index (50.7 ± 62.2%) during end-diastolic pumping on both legs after every heartbeat. A crucial role for afterload reduction was implicated by opposite effects on CO, CI, *dZ/dT*, and SV during systolic pumping when venous return was also increased. Again, reductions (or lack of an increase) in ventricular ejection time and/or the

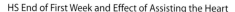

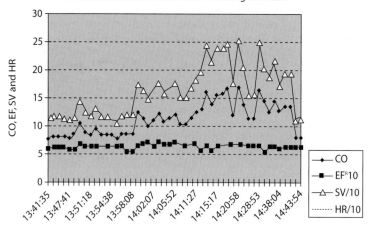

HS End of First Week and Effect of Assisting the Heart

Fig. 13–8. End-diastolic treatments: baseline values for cardiac output, ejection fraction (multiplied by 10), and stroke volume and heart rate (both divide by 10) were followed for 15 minutes before both legs were pumped in end-diastole in the Circulator Boot. Stroke volume and cardiac output then gradually increased over the next 40 minutes during treatment (373).

preejection period suggested a decrease in afterload during end-diastolic pumping (see Fig. 13–8). Pumping on one leg after every heartbeat and on both legs on alternate heartbeats was also effective—but less so. After the initial study, the patients were given 14 additional end-diastolic treatments to both legs over 3 weeks. A clinical benefit was shown by symptomatic improvement in all patients along with a significant reduction in the amount and duration of the RST abnormalities in their ambulatory heart monitoring. It is instructive to compare these effects of counterpulsation with the work of Frank in 1895 and Starling in 1914. Frank noted that an increase in preload increased the force of contractions of the isolated frog heart. Starling utilized a canine heart–lung preparation in which the lungs were artificially ventilated (potentially preventing pulmonary congestion as right atrial-filling pressures were increased). While allowing aortic pressure to increase about 5%, he found perhaps a 70% increase in stroke volume after a 53% increase in right atrial-filling pressure and provided us with the now classic concept that cardiac output increases to a point as the heart fibers are stretched with increases in ventricular filling.[376] Again, he noted increases in stroke volume, albeit less prominently when ventricular volume was increased by increasing peripheral vascular resistance and aortic blood pressure. Two potentially detrimental effects of his experiment are to be noted, however. First, ventricular dilatation significantly increases the force each heart fiber must exert to obtain a given intraventricular pressure; heart work increases and heart efficiency decreases. Second, coronary artery perfusion occurs predominantly in diastole and increased diastolic ventricular pressures decrease coronary perfusion. While therapy with the Circulator Boot does increase preload, the increase in preload is shown not to be crucial. In contrast to Frank and Starling, Circulator Boot therapy increases stroke volume by decreasing after-

load, while at the same time decreasing heart work and maintaining or possibly increasing coronary perfusion. Therapy has been both safe and beneficial in patients with congestive heart failure and angina. The clinical implications of these observations are obvious. It is apparent, for example, that the failing patient in intensive care may be better served with Circulator Boot therapy than a fluid challenge and that the benefit may be easily documented both rapidly and noninvasively with an electrical impedance monitor. Further, ECP treatments, while improving cardiac output, have also been shown to improve arterial flow to both the head and kidneys.[377] Circulator Long Boot therapy, likewise, has been associated with improvement in renal function and improvement in vision.[210] Yu et al.[378] have reviewed the use of external counterpulsation in China where, in 1990, there were 1,800 clinics. Besides success in treating angina, they claimed success in treating ischemic cerebral disease, sudden deafness, and thrombus of the retinal artery.

Afterload reduction may also be seen in pulse volume tracings of the arms and in some patients photoplethysmographic tracings of the fingers (see Fig. 13–9).

METHOD OF TREATMENT AND HOW THE BOOT WORKS

Effect of Booting on Hemodynamic Variables

Effective blood flow (EBF) to the foot is a function of many variables [$f(V)$] and most all are affected by Circulator Boot therapy. An adequate cardiac output (CO) is the only consistent positive factor. Patients with low output may have peripheral cyanosis in spite of patent peripheral arteries. Circulator Boot therapy increases cardiac output. Some factors, like gravity (G), can be

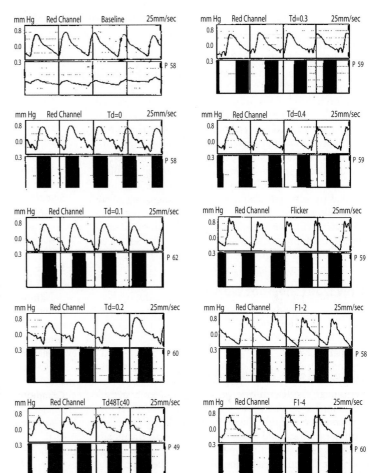

Fig. 13–9. Brachial pulse volume curves (PV) are shown in the upper part of each segment of the figure. The upper left shows the PV curve without pumping. The black bars show the time of pumping and are followed shortly by a sudden falloff in the PV curve. The timing of the leg compressions is moved slowly through systole to late diastole where it is buried in the ensuing pulse wave. Maximum alteration of the ensuing waveform was seen when the leg was released 0.04 seconds before the QRS complex. The heart monitor of the Circulator Boot is programmed to anticipate the next QRS complex and to release the leg 0.04 seconds before it.

either positive or negative. Dependency increases the effect of gravity, improving arterial inflow. However, increased venous pressure (*VP*) with dependency is a negative factor. Conversely, a factor decreasing venous pressure without elevation is a positive factor. The muscular pumps in the extremities may function as peripheral hearts when the venous valves are intact and force venous blood back to the heart with each step (calf systole) leaving the venous pressure significantly reduced between steps (calf diastole). Patients with incompetent venous valves, however, may pump blood from the deep venous system to their superficial varices and increase the back pressure on the capillary bed. Circulator Boot therapy presses on both the deep and superficial veins forcing blood back to the heart. Patients with a history of phlebitis may have a decreased venous velocity in the superficial femoral vein after a standard leg cuff compression due to incomplete recanalization with resulting stenosis or valvular incompetence in the calf.[379] Such

patients may have swollen, indurated, pigmented, and ulcerated legs. Circulator boot therapy may decrease the swelling, induration, and pigmentation and heal the ulcerations of such patients.[340] Bed rest and stasis in the postoperative patient may be associated with decreased venous capacitance and outflow.[282] Both are improved with compression boot therapy. Increased interstitial fluid pressure (*IFP*) and edema fluid may press on the capillary circulation and impede flow, leading the physician to order diuretics and foot elevation. The latter in patients with advanced arterial disease may decrease foot perfusion perhaps replacing rubor with pallor and, in time, tissue breakdown. Diuretics may contract blood volume, lower systemic blood pressure, and increase plasma viscosity. Circulator Boot therapy reduces edema without these complications. Decreased stimulation of the endothelium accompanying decreased flow associated with the postoperative state, bed rest, arteriosclerosis obliterans, and advanced ischemia alters the tissue sensitivity to and endothelial elaboration of nitric oxide, prostacyclin, VEGF, and fibrinolysins (endothelial factors or *EF*). Arteriosclerosis obliterans (ASO) may critically decrease blood flow. The improvement in noninvasive vascular tests and arteriographic changes following boot therapy have been attributed to rechannelization of arteriosclerotic lesions, thrombolysis, and new collateral flow. Altered peripheral flow with neuropathy (*Neur*) has been attributed to metabolic and vascular abnormalities. Circulator Boot therapy has been associated with improved sensation and healing of recalcitrant neuropathic ulcers. Infection (*Inf*) or necrotizing cellulitis may increase the metabolic needs of the tissue, consume needed oxygen, and elaborate enzymes digesting tissue and obliterating vessels. Circulator Boot therapy, along with with the use of locally injected antibiotics, may reverse these processes, even in patients with advanced lesions that are progressing in spite of maximum standard care. Examples are to follow.

How Does the Boot Work?

$$EBF = f(V)(CO)(G)(EF)/(VP)(IFP)(Neur)(ASO)(Inf)$$

Patient Data

Historical data and occupation

Peripheral vascular disease commonly makes a significant impact on the ability of the patient to meet the obligations of the job. The physician will be required to supply employers and disability agencies with the details of the capabilities of the patient. First, one must supply the job title and a description of the job and supply the dates for full-time, part-time, and day of last employment. A statement as to why the patient had to stop work and why he/she cannot work now or in the future is then supplied. What is the effect of the disability on job performance? What is the effect of work on the disability? What are the requirements of the job that aggravate the disability? Could the patient return to lesser demanding work either part or full time? What restrictions might you impose before recommending that the patient can return to work? What follow-up is recommended? What is the prognosis of the illness? These same items should be discussed with the patient to be sure he/she understands the significance of the illness.

General presentation—While the patient may present to a boot clinic or vascular surgeon because of a foot problem, many factors may mimic or aggravate the condition of the patient and may be suspected from the general appearance and motor activity of the patient (see Table 13–5 and Table 13–11). Older patients may be expected to pay some price for their obesity. Patients with heart or lung disease may not be able to walk very far and may have peripheral cyanosis in spite of patent arteries.

Table 13–11. General presentation and clues to current pathology

Obesity	
Degenerative joint disease	
Hyperlipidemia	Gout
Hypertension	Diabetes mellitus
History arteriosclerotic heart disease and/or congestive failure:	
Concomitant diffuse arteriosclerosis	
Diminished tissue perfusion	
Smoking	
Cyanosis due to pulmonary insufficiency	
Buerger's disease	Osteoporosis
Stroke	
Gait imbalance and trauma	
? Emboli	
Neurovascular changes and stasis	
Renal failure	
Dehydration and hypotension	
? Calciphylaxis	
Collagen disease	
Rheumatoid arteritis	Lupus anticoagulant
Adverse effects of steroids	

Some patients may claim to walk any distance without pain but have learned to walk slowly to avoid pain. Stroke patients may benefit more from a walker or leg brace than extra-depth shoes with molded inserts. Stasis and neurovascular skin changes after stroke may result in a cool ruborous immobile leg suggesting advanced arterial insufficiency. Excessive dialysis may promote hypotension and markedly decrease blood flow to the feet when they are elevated. Calciphylaxis may develop in some chronic renal failure patients; it a special type of life-threatening metastatic calcinosis characterized by the abrupt onset of painful ischemic skin ulcers and necrosis characterized by calcium deposition in tissues and small- and medium-sized vessels.[380–385] Ultraviolet light therapy and the ingestion of calcium salts to bind phosphorus have been considered as precipitating factors, which has also been described with cryofibrinogenemia and Crohn's disease.

History of current illness—The presenting problem and when it began should be clearly stated. Note any history of similar previous difficulties. Does the patient or family have a theory or concern about precipitating factors? Commonly, for example, they may blame their family doctor or podiatrist for having débrided a foot lesion that subsequently did not heal. List and record possible reasons why such lesions might not heal, débrided or non-débrided, so that these factors can be addressed and appreciated in the future. List the names of previous physicians and their therapies. Obtain the results of laboratory and x-ray procedures and a copy of reports of operative procedures. Prominently list allergies in your chart. List and discuss the therapeutic options offered by other physicans. The walking capacity of the patient is commonly estimated far differently by the patient and his/her family. Further, as they leave their wheelchair and begin to walk good distances, especially the elderly may forget their recent limitations and, recalling their youthful athletic capacities, claim that they are not improved with their therapy. The Walking Questionnaire of Regensteiner et al.[386] (Table 13–12) is helpful both for baseline and follow-up data and may best be filled out in the presence of a family member. A timed walk in the hospital or office corridor also provides simple documentation.

Physical Findings

Baseline and follow-up physical findings should be documented and interpreted for the patient and family. They are important to establish the proper diagnosis and therapy. They provide legal evidence and are occasionally required by insurance carriers. Properly understood, they provide prognostic information.

Pulses

These should be graded in a fashion so that most examiners would arrive at the same numbers. Thus, "0" is easy for all; no pulse can be found. "Trace" may indicate a pulse that may be there or may not be there; something seems to be there but it is not distinct. A "1+" is a distinct pulse that is faint and hard to find, while "2+" is a pulse that is strong but requires firm palpation to find. A "3+" is a pulse that is easily found with light palpation and a "4+" is a visible pulse. The firmness of and calcifications in the femoral and popliteal vessels should be noted, if obvious. Bruits over the femoral pulse and popliteal pulses should also be noted. A common error in a patient's chart is the recording of a pulse that is not there; the examiner is feeling his own pulse. Again the rhythmic movement of tendons in patients with tremor may be mistaken for a pulse. The presence of strong pulses in the feet is strong evidence against diagnoses of ischemic disease in the extremities and makes formal vascular testing unnecessary, in most situations.

Skin and nail changes

Rubor and blanching indicate inadequate tissue perfusion. Capillaries normally open intermittently to meet the oxygen needs of the tissue. It may be helpful to explain to the patient that when the flow through the capillary is so slow that the needs of the tissue are not met, all of the capillaries may remain open giving the skin the color of the circulating blood, ranging from a dusky ruborous color to deep purple. When the blood pressure, in inches of water (30 inches = 55 mm Hg) at the ankle, is less than the height a foot is lifted above the examining table, the foot blanches and oscillations of a PPG apparatus, for example, cease. Feet should not be raised for any prolonged period to any height that causes blanching. Skin color normally returns within 10 seconds of lowering blanched feet from an elevated to a dependent position and a superficial vein on the foot should be found to fill by 15 seconds. Areas of skin with no blood flow and incipient gangrene may remain white on dependency and require immediate steps for revascularization. Extravasation of blood may occur in extremely ischemic tissue giving a red or blue color that does not blanch on pressure; such tissue commonly breaks down in spite of successful appropriate steps to improve blood flow; such breakdown does not mean the foot cannot be saved, but that it may take a little longer. Confluent petechiae have the same significance while occasional petechiae over the lower leg and foot may signify thrombocytopenia. Mottling, coldness, and blistering, the latter in the absence of edema, are also signs of severe ischemia, as are complaints of numbness and paralysis. Loss of hair on the toes and feet and trophic nail changes, on the other hand, are common with modest loss of arterial flow to the feet.

Signs of neuropathy at the bedside

Deep tendon reflexes are first affected distally and decrease with the duration of diabetes. Loss of light touch, pain, position or temperature sensation, loss of sweating and dry feet, callus over pressure points, foot ulcers, and abnormally shaped feet (hammertoes, bunions, flat feet, or Charcot joints), all are easily noted. The mass and presence of the extensor digitorum brevis may be noted while dorsiflexing the toes against resistance.[387] Reduced or absent mass is more common in type 1 (44%) and type 2 (48%) diabetics than controls (12%). In type 1 diabetics, abnormal mass is associated with age, duration of diabetes mellitus (DM), smoking, dry feet, and foot ulcers and, along with the loss of mass, are significant elevations in sensory thresholds for vibration, perception, and pain. Anatomically, small nerve fiber dysfunction may be assessed by the measurement of thermal and pain perception thresholds and large-fiber disturbances evaluated by means of vibration perception threshold and two-point discrimination, which may be evaluated with the blunt wooden end of Q-tips or with the help of a Tacticon (a device with a series of protruding rods of increasing size).[388] In both normal and neuropathic patients, the cutaneous pressure threshold is inversely related to the

Table 13–12. Walking impairment questionnaire*

A. Walking distance: For each of the following distances, report the degree of difficulty that best describes how hard it was for you to walk WITHOUT stopping to rest.

During the past week how much physical difficulty did you have ...

	Degree of difficulty				Score × distance = factor
	None	**Some**	**Much**	**Did not do**	
1. Walking indoors, such as around your home?	3	2	1	0	_____ × 20 = _____
2. Walking 50 feet?	3	2	1	0	_____ × 50 = _____
3. Walking 150 feet?	3	2	1	0	_____ × 150 = _____
4. Walking 300 feet?	3	2	1	0	_____ × 300 = _____
5. Walking 600 feet?	3	2	1	0	_____ × 600 = _____
6. Walking 900 feet?	3	2	1	0	_____ × 900 = _____
7. Walking 1,500 feet? (5 blocks or more)	3	2	1	0	_____ × 1,500 = _____

Sum of factors = _____

Patient impairment distance score = sum of factors/10,560 (10,560 = no impairments)

B. Walking Speed: These questions refer to HOW FAST you were able to walk ONE CITY BLOCK. Tell us the degree of difficulty required for you to walk at EACH OF THESE SPEEDS WITHOUT STOPPING TO REST.

During the past week how much physical difficulty did you have ...

	Degree of difficulty				Score × distance = factor
	None	**Some**	**Much**	**Did not do**	
1. Walking 1 block slowly?	3	2	1	0	_____ × 1.5 = _____
2. Walking 1 block at average speed?	3	2	1	0	_____ × 2 = _____
3. Walking 1 block quickly?	3	2	1	0	_____ × 3 = _____
4. Running or jogging 1 block?	3	2	1	0	_____ × 5 = _____

Sum of factors = _____

Patient impairment speed score = sum of factors/34.5 (34.5 = no impairments)

*After Regensteiner et al. (386).

static distance between the sticks.[389] Vinik et al.[390] noted that when specificity of tests are held greater than 90%, the diagnostic sensitivity for diabetic neuropathy varied considerably: vibration 88%, warm 78%, cold 77%, tactile-pressure 77%, 5-Hz current perception 52%, and 250-Hz current perception 48%; they conclude that vibratory and thermal testing should be the primary screening tests for diabetic peripheral neuropathy and that other modalities may be of use only in specific situations. Autonomic cardiovascular neuropathy is suggested by a lack of beat-to-beat variation in heart rate,[391] systolic orthostatic hypotension of 20 mm Hg or more, and failure of sustained handgrip at 30% maximal contraction to raise diastolic blood pressure by 16 mm Hg.[392] The presence of A-V shunting in the legs is related to the duration of diabetes and is associated with abnormalities in postural hypotension, sustained handgrip, deep breathing, and lying-to-standing pulse ratios.[92]

Vascular Laboratory and Treatment

The vascular laboratory should be used to document the pathology and therapeutic needs of the patient, if needed, after a careful physical examination.

Venous disease patients

A family history of venous disease may suggest hereditary change in the vein wall or dominantly inherited clotting disorders (deficiency of protein "C" or "S" or deficiency or antithrombin III). More common is the family tendency to underactivity and overnutrition promoting obesity. Other factors promoting venous hypertension should be considered and noted: pregnancy, thrombophlebitis, standing occupations, Baker's cyst, and use of garters or corsets. The symptoms of varicose veins are many and may suggest other ailments; Lofgren[393] lists aching 71%, swelling 60%, heaviness 47%, cramps 37%, itching 30%, cosmetic dissatisfaction 25%, stasis dermatitis 16%, pigmentation 16%, burning 16%, ulcers 8%, and cellulitis 6%. Hematologic studies appropriate for the venous patient might include complete blood count and differential, protein C, protein S, antithrombin III, cold agglutinins, and serum viscosity. Studies in the vascular laboratory might include: venous reflux test for venous valvular incompetency (normal ≥20 seconds); maximum venous outflow to assess both venous capacitance and maximum venous outflow (normal ≥0.61); Doppler studies to document respiratory variation, spontaneous flow, reflux, and augmentation maneuvers; photoelectricpletysmography (PPG) to document pulsatile arterial flow in and around ulcers; transcutaneous oxygen pressure (TcPO$_2$) to assess the adequacy of the arterial supply; and a Duplex scan to evaluate the risk for thromboembolism. The presence of pulsatile flow on the PPG, and low TcPO$_2$ and high TcPCO$_2$ is diagnostic of cellulitis with aerobic organisms.

Such patients may rapidly be relieved of pain and their TcPO$_2$ improved with the injection of local antibiotics and Circulator Boot therapy. One insurance company lists a paper by Comerota[394] as reason not to cover boot therapy in venous patients; the paper points to a failure to properly apply the boots rather than a failure of the boots properly applied. Various authors have shown that intermittent compression boots hasten the healing of venous ulcers.[395–397] Dillon[340] used the Circulator Boot to successfully treat the venous ulcers of 17 patients with difficult or refractory stasis dermatitis and ulcers and noted decreases in induration, pigmentation, and palpable thrombi. In the outpatient treatment of stasis ulcers, the Long Circulator Boot is used with the legs straight out on the treatment table. Locally injected antibiotics are used if cellulitis is a problem and wet-to-dry dressings with multielectrolyte solutions (with antibiotics if the surface of the ulcer is clearly infected or a culture shows a worrisome pathogen) are applied within the boot. Daily treatments are continued until progress of the ulcer and the comfort of the patient make less frequent treatments feasible.

Arterial testing

In the past, a modest investment in a Directional Doppler and pulse volume equipment allowed us to do segmental blood pressure and pulse volume determinations, along with mapping of the Doppler velocity wave forms in the groin, midthigh, popliteal area, midcalf, ankle, foot, and toes for the superficial femoral, popliteal, tibial arteries, dorsalis pedis, and involved metatarsal or digital arteries, respectively. Such studies are helpful in predicting the results of arteriograms[398] and in considering invasive procedures or boot therapy—but these are time-consuming. The segmental pressure and pulse volume studies are easily mastered by the office nurse. The Doppler waveform studies require the attention of a trained technician or physician. The tests were also helpful in following the response of patients to their therapies and in providing encouragement to those with severe disease and a slow course. Duplex scans may be helpful in evaluating flow through the superficial femoral and popliteal. The Moor Laser Doppler Scan can provide a picture measuring the adequacy of cutaneous flow in the foot and toes.[399] In recent years, however, the emphasis on cost-saving has limited the quality and number of tests being reimbursed by insurance carriers. In Table 13-13, one method to meet the needs of the patient in an economical fashion is shown. Bedside care during the assessment and treatment periods remain important. Routine orders to avoid common pitfalls in care are listed in Table 13-14.

Soak Solutions

Lesions may be immersed in soak solutions (baths) or covered with dampened dressings. Industry has provided

Table 13–13. Vascular assessments

1. Initial history and physical: Is significant arterial insufficiency a possibility? What is the nature and likely location of vascular occlusions?
2. Determination of urgency of treatment and danger of immediate tissue breakdown:
   a. Toe photoplethsmography tracings (PPG)
      Normal tracings usually eliminate possibility of arterial disease sufficient to prevent wound healing and additional testing is commonly not necessary; flat tracings point to danger of tissue breakdown
   b. Transcutaneous PO_2 and PCO_2 levels
      $TcPO_2$ levels below 20 mm Hg are said to be associated with nonhealing. Levels below 10 may be commonly associated with progressive tissue necrosis. Very low $TcPO_2$ and high $TcPCO_2$ levels associated with clear-cut PPG waveforms point to cellulitis, which may be quickly sterilized with infiltration of the tissues with appropriate antibiotics, administration of oral broad-spectrum antibiotics, and boot therapy (Refs. 164, 165). Early treatment is desirable.
3. Noninvasive determination of pathological vascular anatomy if proper prescription of boot therapy in doubt or need to determine possible benefit of bypass surgery or angioplasty (recent arteriograms not available), segmental blood pressure, pulse volumes, and Doppler arterial mapping are considered. If renal function in doubt and still a possible candidate for bypass, MRI arteriogram then obtained.
4. Arteriograms to provide road map for invasive procedures. Never performed as a routine test in patients not disabled enough to consider vascular reconstruction or in patients with other disabilities severe enough to rule out invasive procedures.

Table 13–14. Routine orders for patients with arterial insufficiency*

Routine orders	Explanation
1. Bed position: Raise head of bed on blocks. Pubic area should be higher than the toes.	Blood does not run uphill. The toes may not get blood if they are elevated. Maximum flow in the foot is obtained with a 10 degree slant*
2. Pressure sores: Pressure should be removed from the heels and malleoli by some means (Podus splint, towels taped in place smoothly around the calf, etc.) Pad side-rails if the patient is at risk of catching the foot in them.	In patients with low blood pressure in the feet, the weight of the foot itself against the bed may be sufficient to block blood flow into the skin and, thus, cause skin breakdown.
3. Foot boards or pillows: Placed under the blankets to keep weight off the toes.	The weight of bedding on ischemic toes can be painful and decrease blood flow in the skin of both the toes and heels.
4. Blankets: Make sure the patient is adequately covered so that his/her own blood can warm the legs.	Even normal legs have a decrease in blood flow when the body core temperature drops. Healing speed is decreased in cold tissue.
5. Bandages: Change bandages as needed to minimize dampness due to drainage, 1–4 times a day. Bandages should not be tight. Do not wedge gauze between toes.	Bacteria can grow in wet bandages. The wet bandage macerates the skin. Drainage can contaminate the bed, the room, and the attending nurse or aide. Blood does not nourish skin compressed by tight bandages.
6. Bathing: Open lesions are not to be wetted in a tub or shower. Carefully bag such lesions for a quick whole-body shower (patient willing). The area of and around the lesions should be separately washed with sterile soap and water and rinsed with sterile water or electrolyte solution.	Bacteria such as *Pseudomonas* may commonly be cultured from the water nozzles of baths and showers. The fecal organisms, which may become increasingly resistant during antibiotic therapy, may be expected to get into a bath.
7. Cultures: In addition to initial cultures, weekly cultures should be obtained if lesions continue to drain or if there appears to be any deterioration in the physical status of the lesions.	Deterioration of a foot under treatment is more likely to be due to infection with an untreated organism or abuse of the foot than a decrease in blood flow (except in dialysis patients).
8. Hot and cold: Avoid exposing ischemic tissue to hot or cold environments.	External heat (hot pads or sun from the window) increases tissue metabolism and need for oxygen and blood flow. Heat may promote death of borderline ischemic tissue.

*Montgomery H, Horwitz O. Oxygen tension of tissue by the polarograph method. *J Clin Invest.* 1950; 21:1120.

a myriad of soaks and creams to hasten healing. Foot soaks are commonly used to cleanse draining lesions with necrotic elements. Antibiotics or physical agents (silver nitrate or hydrogen peroxide) may be added. Saline (0.9%) has been given the name, "physiologic saline solution" or PSS as it is isotonic with serum and does not alter the shape of erythrocytes. PSS, unfortunately, is commonly a basic ingredient of many agents and functions as a control substance in many studies. However, PSS is a toxic substance; sodium chloride has been used for centuries as a food preservative. Even in a normal electrolyte environment, it is estimated that cells expend as much as 60% of their energy in maintaining the Na^+/K^+ gradient across the cell wall.[400] For industry to maintain their tissue banks and cell cultures, multielectrolyte solutions containing all of the trace elements in the serum have been derived.[401] The brief application of saline soaks is not crucially harmful when applied to tissue that has vigorous blood flow that can supply the normal electrolyes in the serum and cells. However, saline left for hours in cups superglued around standard leg incisions in normal people impedes wound healing.[97] Likewise, repeated saline wet-to-dry dressings may have a similar adverse effect. In general, bacteria derived from the colon thrive in a moist environment, while those derived from the skin do not. With these thoughts in mind, hence, the author uses a multielectrolyte solution similar in composition to culture media and the primordial sea (Sea Soaks) as a basic soak solution both in the basin at home and in the compression bag during Miniboot treatments. During the Miniboot treatments appropriate antibiotics may be added to the solution. During home soaks in a basin, dilute hydrogen peroxide may be added to help clean and sterilize the wound. High concentrations of peroxide or iodine or prolonged exposure to either may damage even normal tissue and are best avoided. The costs of foot soaks can be kept to a minimum using the following technique: A large basin is filled with tap water of any desired temperature. A small clean (sterile) plastic bag is placed over the water and a puddle of the therapeutic soak solution is placed on top of the plastic bag. The foot is then placed in the puddle on the top of the bag and the bag is pulled up around the leg as the foot is lowered to the bottom of the basin. The tap water contours the plastic bag and therapeutic solution against the foot.[402] The foot lesions can be safely massaged through the bag. A moist environment with Sea Soaks may be created by wet-to-dry dressings that are changed every few hours to discourage significant bacterial growth in the dressings. Such dressings are not used if coliforms are cultured from the ulcer. Maggot therapy might be considered early in shaggy ulcers growing resistant organisms. Maggot suppliers can be found on the Internet.

Topical Oxygen Therapy

Patients with threatened and progressing skin breakdown may temporarily benefit from topical oxygen therapy. Just as oxygen may diffuse from the subcutaneous tissue to the surface probe of the transcutaneous oxygen electrode, oxygen can diffuse from the atmosphere into the superficial few millimeters of skin; the skin does breathe. Topical oxygen therapy can prolong the life of the skin envelope and allow additional time for revascularization with boot therapy or invasive means. In considering topical oxygen therapy, it is helpful to review the potential gains from the treatment. The partial pressure of atmospheric oxygen is about 152 mm Hg or 20% of the total 760 mm Hg atmospheric pressure. Placing the foot in a plastic bag containing 100% oxygen raises the partial pressure of oxygen fivefold to the 760 mm Hg. Placing the foot in an air-pressurized oxygen chamber, however, may add little, if any, benefit. For example, if the chamber is pressurized to 20 or 40 mm Hg, the gain would be 780/760 (2.5%) or 800/760 (5.3%), respectively, while, at the same time, the increased air pressure on the leg would oppose the arterial inflow pressure by the same amount; indeed, if the true ankle systolic blood pressure were 40 mm Hg and 40 mm Hg oxygen pressure were applied constantly to the foot, the effective systolic blood pressure would be zero. Further, the chamber must have a seal around the proximal leg to contain the pressure; those seals with elastic elements may have a tourniquet effect. Our application technique circumvents these problems.

Application of topical oxygen bag

The foot is washed first with mild soap and water to remove skin debris, dirt, caked blood or drainage. Then, the foot may be soaked in multielectrolyte solution (Sea Soaks) containing 40 mg/L gentamicin to reduce skin bacteria flora and to hydrate the skin. The foot is next wrapped with a single layer of sterile gauze to prevent the plastic air bag from sticking anywhere to the skin. A nasal oxygen catheter is placed around the foot with the nasal prongs under the arch pointing toward the toes. Protuberances and ridges in the tubing are padded to protect the skin from focal pressure. A thin clean plastic bag is placed over the foot and ankle to contain the oxygen around the foot. The plastic bag is loosely contoured against the foot with a second piece of wrapping gauze and tape applied as necessary to keep the gauze wrap in place. The portions of the plastic bag reaching the calf are rolled down and bunched up behind the Achilles tendon to provide a soft pad that elevates the heel slightly above the bed. Oxygen at a rate of 1 L/minute is then run through the nasal catheter. If the skin appears to dry out from the treatment, the oxygen can be bubbled through sterile water to saturate the oxygen stream with water. The bag may be left in place for many hours, changing it only as needed because of drainage or other concerns. The bagged foot may be placed inside either the Circulator Miniboot or the Long-Boot systems.

Results and warnings

Topical oxygen itself does not restore blood flow; other means are required. Previously mottled and cyanotic skin may appear relatively normal for several minutes after being removed from the oxygen bag. Some areas of skin may remain red, not even blanching with direct pressure, while more proximal tissue slowly regains its cyanosis; these red areas may represent "rubor mortis"—dead tissue that cannot consume oxygen once supplied. Such areas are likely to blister or blacken with time and mean that a prolonged course of booting will be necessary to salvage the foot. A visiting consultant unfamiliar with these techniques may mistakenly underestimate the severity of the ischemic process if he/she does not wait at least several minutes after removing the oxygen bag. The patient, family, and nurses need be reminded that the foot can be smothered and harm done if the oxygen flow is interrupted for any length of time while the plastic bag is in place.

Wound Classification

Classification systems are helpful in both describing wounds and predicting outcomes (Table 13-15). The wound descriptions provided by the Public Health Service are widely used especially in patients with decubiti. The Wagner classification has been related to both surgical procedures and outcomes. Thus, Calhoun et al.[403] in performing 855 procedures among 355 patients, found increasing need for major amputation (ankle disarticulation, Symes, BKA or AKA) and vascular reconstruction with an increasing Wagner grade: no major amputations or vascular procedures in category "0" patients, 3 and 1 in category "1", 8 and 4 in category "2", 26 and 4 in category "3", 75 and 22 in category "4", and 70 and 1 in category "5", respectively.[403] The Texas classification is included because it demonstrates the additive risks of increasing depth of the wound, infection, and ischemia on outcome.

Table 13–15. Methods of wound classification

A. Public Health Service[404]

1. Nonblanchable erythema of intact skin.
2. Partial thickness skin loss involving epidermis, dermis or both … commonly an abrasion, blister or shallow crater.
3. Full thickness skin loss involving damage to or necrosis of subcutaneous tissue maybe extending to but not through underlying fascia.
4. Deep ulcer to muscle, bone, tendon or joint capsule.

B. Wagner classification[405]

0. Intact skin (may have bony deformities)
1. Localized superficial ulcer
2. Deep ulcer to tendon, bone, ligament or joint
3. Deep abscess or osteomyelitis
4. Gangrene of toes or forefoot
5. Gangrene of whole foot

C. University of Texas Wound Classification System[406]

Stage	Grade "0"	Grade "1"	Grade "2"	Grade "3"
A	Pre- or postulcerative lesion completely epithelized—0 amp	Superficial wound not involving tendon, capsule or bone—0 amp	Wound penetrating to tendon or capsule—0 amp	Wound penetrating to bone or joint—0 amp
B	Infection— 12.5% amp	Infection— 8.5% amp	Infection— 28.6% amp	Infection— 92% amp
C	Ischemia— 25% amp	Ischemia— 20% amp	Ischemia— 25% amp	Ischemia— 100% amp
D	Infection and ischemia— 50% amp	Infection and ischemia— 50% amp	Infection and ischemia— 100% amp	Infection and ischemia— 100% amp

Classification of Ischemia

Ischemia has been classified separately from wounds. Fontaine described four main stages and two subclassifications: no adverse symptoms with demonstrable stenosis or lack of pulse (stage I), modest intermittent claudication or "shop window" disease (stage II), claudication allowing a distance over 200 m (IIa), claudication preventing a walking distance of 200 m (IIb), ischemic rest pain (Stage III), and finally necrosis or gangrene (Stage IV). Revised standards were published in the *Journal of Vascular Surgery* in 1986 and again in 1997.[407] Here a classification was provided both for acute and chronic ischemia. The acute ischemic group is classified on the basis of sensory changes, muscle weakness, and Doppler signals. Thus, legs in category I are viable, not immediately threatened, have neither sensory loss or muscular weakness, and have both audible Doppler arterial and venous signals. Legs in category IIa are marginally threatened, salvageable if promptly treated, and have minimal or no sensory loss in the toes, no muscular weakness, and audible venous Doppler sounds, but loss of arterial Doppler sounds. Legs in category IIb are immediately threatened, salvageable with immediate revascularization, and have sensory loss above and including the toes with rest pain and mild to moderate muscular weakness; again venous Doppler sounds are audible, while arterial Doppler sounds are not. Legs in category III are thought to have major irreversible damage that will require major amputation or suffer significant, permanent neuromuscular damage regardless of therapy; the legs have profound anesthesia and weakness or paralysis and all Doppler sounds are inaudible.

The clinical categories of the revised standards for chronic ischemia in the *Journal of Vascular Surgery* are based on symptoms and objective findings in the vascular laboratory.[407] Thus, grade "0" and category "0" are clinically asymptomatic and have no hemodynamic significant lesions; their treadmill and reactive hyperemia tests are normal. Patients with category 1 chronic ischemia suffer mild claudication; they are able to do 5 min of exercise on a treadmill with a 12% incline and have ankle pressures after exercise over 50 mm Hg, but at least 20 mm Hg less than their resting values. Patients with grade I and category 2 chronic ischemia are between categories 1 and 3. Patients with severe claudication in category 3 cannot complete the 5-min treadmill test and have ankle pressures below 50 mm Hg after exercise. Those in grade II and category 4 present with ischemic rest pain; their ankle pressures are under 40 and toe pressures under 30 mm Hg. Their pulse volume tracings are either flat or barely pulsatile at the ankle and transmetatarsal areas. Patients with grade III and category 5 present with minor tissue loss—nonhealing ulcer, focal gangrene with diffuse pedal ischemia; their resting pressures are under 60 mm Hg at the ankle and under 30 mmHg in the toes. Their PVR curves are flat or barely pulsatile at the ankle and metatarsal areas. Finally, those in category 6 present with major tissue loss—extending above transmetatarsal level and a functional foot is no longer salvageable; their vascular laboratory data is the same as in category 5. Grades II and III and categories 4, 5, and 6 are embraced by the term chronic critical ischemia. A scale for gauging changes in clinical status with treatment is also provided.[407]

Treatment Options with the Circulator Boot Systems

Patient Position

An attempt is made to maximize the effects of gravity in promoting arterial inflow into the legs. Patients are treated horizontally in the supine position only if they cannot tolerate a reverse Trendelenburg position in the bed or a sitting position (back up) in the bed, treatment table or chair. In the cases of venous stasis disease and lymphedema, where arterial inflow is not an issue, the legs are treated in a horizontal position to lessen reflux of fluid back into the legs between compressions.

Choice of Bags and Boots

A Long-Boot is chosen to match the length of the leg of the patient; the other dimensions of the Long Boots are adjustable. The Miniboot has one size for all, but adjustable fluted leggings allow a custom fit for therapy from the toes to the knees. A clean disposable compression bag is chosen to match the treatment needs of the patient: A Miniboot bag is used to treat patients with ischemic disease below the knee and in conjunction with the use of local antibiotic injections and antibiotic solutions. A sleeve from groin to midfoot or ankle is chosen for people with diffuse arteriosclerotic disease throughout the leg and pain in the foot that is troublesome if treated with a full leg bag. A full leg bag is chosen to benefit patient with angina, congestive heart failure, lymphedema, diffuse arteriosclerosis obliterans, and full-leg stasis disease. The Long-Boot bag may be rolled back to include the knee-to-toe area in patients with stasis disease of the calf and ankle.

Pressure Settings

Pressures are chosen considering patient comfort and expected diastolic pressure at the proximal portion of the treatment bag: 30 inches of water or 55 mm Hg for the Long-Boots and 45 inches water or 82 mm Hg for the Miniboot.

Monitor Settings

An internal pacemaker and "divide-by" switch (varying from 1:1, 1:2, to 1:3) may be used to initiate 2–120 compressions a min, independent of the EKG. Thus, patients with severe occlusive iliac disease might be given 10–20 full-leg compressions a min, preferably in a high reverse Trendelenburg position. Again patients with a very rapid irregular pulse rapid and modest ischemic leg disease might be given 70 leg compressions a min each lasting 0.42 seconds. The computer-assisted EKG pacer is most commonly chosen to place compressions automatically in the end-diastolic portion of the heart cycle. A compression time is chosen to overcome the inertia of the fluids in the vascular channels: 0.34 seconds for the Miniboot and 0.40–0.44 for the Long-Boots. The 1:1 setting of the "divide-by" switch is chosen for Long-Boot patients with modest arterial occlusive disease, stasis disease, lymphedema, angina, and congestive heart failure and for Miniboot patients with heart rates under 60. The 1:2 setting is used in most Miniboot patients and in Long-Boot patients with rapid heart rates and those with more advanced arterial occlusive disease who might develop leg discomfort with the 1:1 setting. The 1:3 setting is used in patients with rapid heart rates and in those who cannot tolerate the 1:2 setting (Table 13-16).

ILLUSTRATIVE EXAMPLES OF PATIENTS TREATED WITH THE CIRCULATOR BOOT

Female Patient with Postoperative Lymphedema

This 79-year-old woman was referred with complaints of pain and swelling in her left leg. She had had a right colectomy 2 months earlier for adenocarcinoma of the cecum. Postoperative complications included possible left iliofemoral arterial obstruction, an abdominal abscess, and a possible pulmonary embolus. A phleborheogram and a lung scan were normal. She was readmitted with shortness of breath and leg swelling. Diuretics and anticoagulants were prescribed but appeared not to affect the leg swelling. Her arterial Doppler studies were normal. Venous Doppler testing was normal except for a lack of respiratory variation in the lower leg easily explained by the swelling in her leg. She was referred for boot therapy. A Circulator Boot system was rolled to her bedside and she was treated 1:1 (in end-diastole of each heart cycle) with a compression pressure equal to 30 inches of water or 55 mm Hg. With her bed in high-reverse Trendelenburg and her legs extended flat horizonly. Her leg swelling and discomfort were relieved. Within a few weeks of discharge, however, her leg again swelled and became

Table 13–16. Method of treatment*

---

1. Hospitalize patient if septic, other medical or surgical necessities or initial need for multiple boot therapies
2. Drain any obvious abscesses; limit débridements to removal of clearly dead tissue and loose protruding bone fragments
3. Stop the cellulitic process immediately by:
    a. Administer either orally or parenterally antibiotics to prevent septic emboli
    b. Soak ulcerated lesions and/or irrigate fistulas and abscesses before first boot treatment with saline–dilute hydrogen peroxide solutions to remove pus and loose debris
    c. Infiltrate abscessed or cellulitic tissue and osteomyelitic bone with antibiotics usually once daily (eg, 40 mg gentamicin)
    d. If devitalized ulcerated area present, place foot in plastic bag of multielectrolyte solution (Sea Soaks) containing antibiotics; avoid prolonged contact with saline
    e. Place bagged foot in Miniboot and pump after each heartbeat (1:1) if a palpable pulse, after every other heartbeat (1:2) if no palpable pulse, after every third heartbeat (1:3) if very ischemic foot. Pump 40 minutes to disseminate the injected antibiotic throughout the cellulitic area, to scrub the infected ulcer, and breakup thrombi in the foot secondary to the cellulitic process
    f. Repeat steps d–e 3–4 times daily if advanced infection
4. Establish need for vascular reconstruction; avoid booting on a leg with no arterial inflow
5. Consider angioplasty of the iliac or femoral artery, brachial–femoral bypass or aorto–femoral bypass to establish flow into the leg
6. In patients with a flat pulse volume at the ankle or no detectable Doppler sounds at the ankle, consider obtaining an early arteriogram
7. Include in the area of the leg to be booted the ischemic area and a proximal 6 inches of well-vascularized leg. Patients with diffuse ASO and infected foot ulcers may receive the Miniboot therapy (3b–f) and Long-Boot treatments from groin to toes, groin to ankle or to midfoot as needed
8. Treatments are continued 3–4 times a day in the hospital or nursing home, and once daily as an outpatient; taper as healing progresses.

---

*From Dillon (210).

painful. Her walking became limited to 25–30 feet. Her doctor again referred her for outpatient boot therapy. Over 4 months, she was given 24 Long-Boot treatments, 76,800 compressions if her pulse rate averaged 80, successfully increasing her walking distance to 150-200 feet. Her leg did well until her death the next year. *Points to consider:* Her claudication-like leg pain and limitation was not associated with arterial abnormalities and disappeared with reduction of the leg size with pumping. The possibility of thromboembolism was considered but (1) she was ambulating; (2) her venous tests were normal, and (3) she had been given anticoagulants. Effective blood flow is inversely related to interstitial fluid pressure, which we reduced: *EFB* ∝ 1/*IFP*.

Long-Lasting Relief from Chronic Lymphedema with Eight Outpatient Treatments (Case 139)

At age 74, this male patient was referred by his family doctor for boot therapy for bilateral chronic lymphedema (see Fig. 13–10). He had seen many doctors over 40 years. A recent CAT scan of the abdomen revealed no intra-abdominal obstructive pathology. His cardiologist provided no assistance. Noninvasive vascular arterial and venous studies were normal. His legs no longer diminished in size at night. He found support stockings (Suphose) too painful to wear. His past surgical procedures, which were not closely associated in time with his lymphedema, included prostatic surgery, a

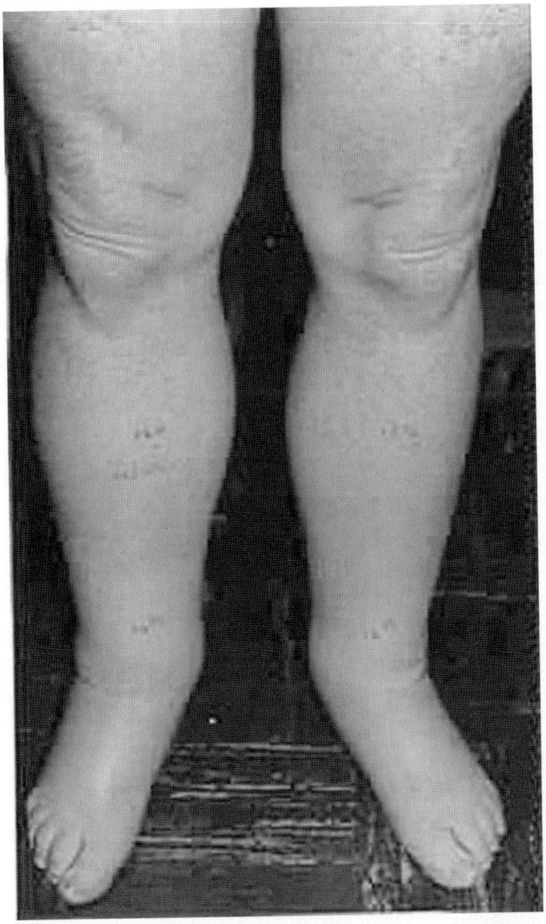

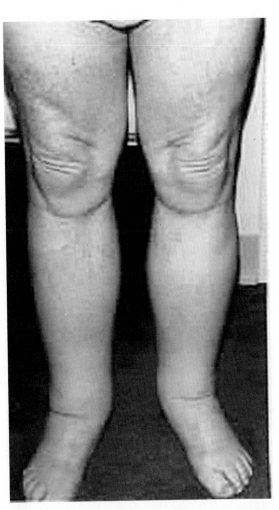

Fig. 13–10. Both legs were swollen with the circumferences of the right larger than the left: 13 1/8 vs 12 1/2 inches at the ankle, 18 vs 17 1/4 inches at the calf and 22 1/2 vs 22 inches at the thigh.

Fig. 13–11. He returned for a few treatments in 1987 reporting that his legs were then just beginning to swell again.

vasectomy, and thyroid surgery. His medicines included Synthroid (L-levothyroxine), furosemide 40 mg daily, Hygroton 50 mg, and 3–4 ounces of whiskey daily.

The circumference of both the right and left legs diminished after eight treatments given to the right leg only: $11\frac{3}{8}$ and $11\frac{1}{2}$ inches at the ankle, $16\frac{1}{4}$ and $16\frac{1}{8}$ inches at the calf, and $22\frac{1}{8}$ and $21\frac{1}{8}$ inches at the thigh, respectively. One-to-one Long-Boot (the boot bag extending from his groin to his big toe) treatments were only given to the right leg, because it was larger and more symptomatic. After his course of therapy, he was referred to our physical therapy department for additional treatments with a lymphedema boot. We sought to ascertain if additional reduction in his leg size would result (it did not) and if he could benefit from the purchase of the less expensive lymphedema home boot. He found the Circulator Boot had a massaging and softening action that the lymphedema boot did not have. The approximate 25,600 compressions (8 treatments × 40 minutes per treatment × pulse rate of 80) his leg received apparently had altered the pathophysiology of his lymphedema. The benefit from his pumping lasted 5 years (Fig. 13–11).

We hypothesized that we had decreased an obstruction in his pelvic lymphatics. *Points to consider:* Swelling begins just below the point of obstruction. Here, as the whole leg was swollen, treatment was chosen to compress the leg as high as possible, and long-term benefit was achieved.

Type 1 Diabetic with Multiple Complications

The treatment and course of patient JM has been described in detail.[210] Over 9 years, he was successfully treated with Circulator Boot therapy for recurrent foot lesions, renal failure, septic shock, and congestive heart failure. The cardiac-assist action of the boot raised his blood pressure during his episode of sepsis and on a chronic basis improved his urine output and renal function tests. The effect of boot therapy on his carotid waveforms shows a simple, noninvasive means of demonstrating afterload reduction with boot therapy (see Fig. 13–12). The heart monitor was set to 1:1 when treating congestive heart failure associated with a pulse under 100 and 2:1 with faster rates. The 2:1 setting was also used in treating his foot lesions. *Points to consider:* A vascular assist device has many potential uses in the intensive care unit. Effective blood flow in the limbs is proportional to cardiac output: $EBF \propto CO/IFP$.

Combined Disease—Heart, Venous, Cellulitis, and Osteomyelitis with 14-Year Follow-up (Case 2)

Born on August 17th, 1920, this female patient presented 180 cm in height and 109 kg in weight. She had no palpable distal pulses since 1981 and had retinal hemorrhages since 1982. She received boot treatments in 1986 for stasis disease and cellulitis of both legs and

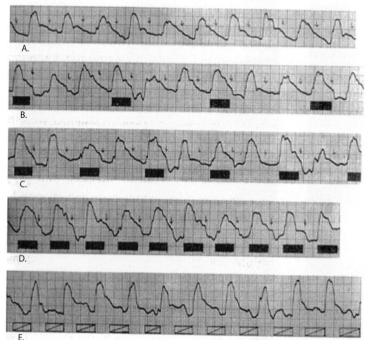

Fig. 13–12. Patient JM: Doppler tracings of carotid artery are shown. The top tracings were taken before boot therapy. Boot compressions (black rectangles) were timed to coincide with cardiac systole on every third beat (second line), every other beat (third line) and on every beat (fourth line). Small arrows mark the moment of expected boot decompression and are associated with a sudden dropoff in blood velocity when actually occurring after a boot pulsation (after end of black rectangle). Boot compressions were timed in late diastole (hatched rectangle) in the bottom line; here the dropoff in velocity is buried in the next waveform which is narrowed.

did well. She had hypertensive arteriosclerotic heart disease and episodes of congestive heart failure. High-risk heart surgery was under consideration. She presented January 7th, 1988 in a wheelchair with cellulitis and osteomyelitis of her left fifth toe and metatarsal head secondary to an insulin needle under her proximal phalanx (Figs. 13-13 and 13-14).

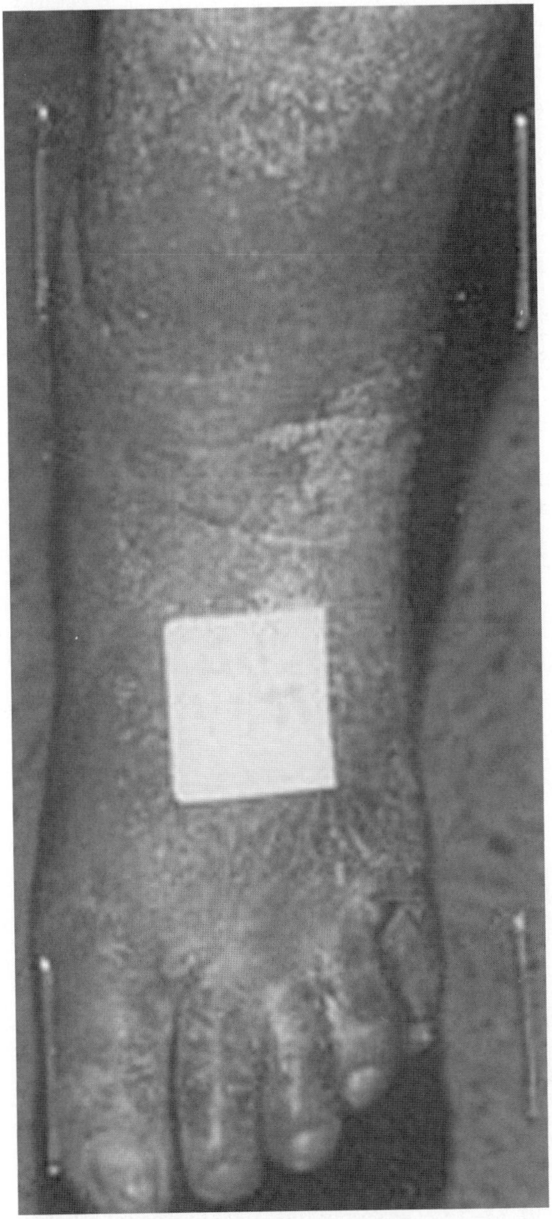

She was treated with local antibiotic injections and both Long-Boot and Miniboot therapies. Her foot and leg did well (Fig. 13-15). As she attributed her sense of well-being to her boot treatments, she hired a nurse from our boot clinic and purchased a boot system to take home. She has continued to receive daily boot treatments to both legs. A compulsive eater, however, she has been unable to control her diabetes; her blood glucose levels have varied from 170 to 350 mg/dl. Nonetheless, her heart and eyes stabilized allowing cataract surgery and a vitrectomy. Her cardiologist dismissed her from his immediate care.

She did well in spite of her dietary non-compliance and poorly controlled diabetes until November 10th, 1995, when she returned to the boot clinic for routine follow-up and was found to have an asymptomatic bradycardia (pulse rate 40) and first-degree AV heart block (PR interval 0.26). She was referred back to her cardiologist who obtained a Holter monitor study, which showed four instances of sinus arrest. An A–V pacemaker was subsequently inserted. She then appeared to develop angina and underwent coronary catheterization. On January 18th, 1996, she had bypass grafts to her left anterior descending and proximal obtuse marginal arteries with her saphenous veins. Postoperatively, she had edema and

Fig. 13–13. Cool, edematous and pigmented leg with ulcer and pus at base of 5th toe.

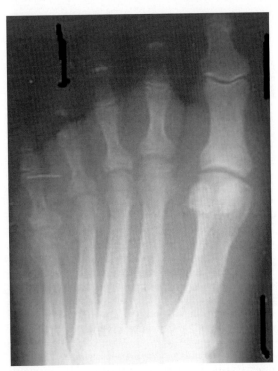

Fig. 13–14. Needle embedded in 5th toe and osteomyelitis of 5th MP joint.

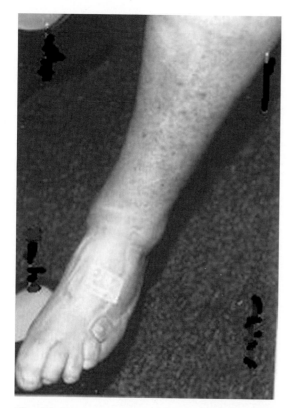

Fig. 13–15. Five year follow-up ... ambulatory all the while.

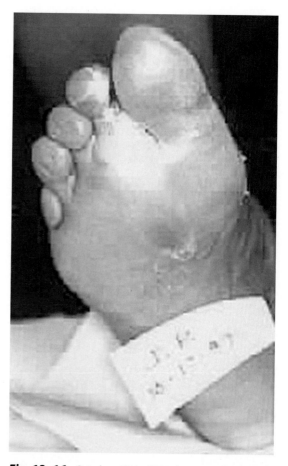

Fig. 13–16. October 17th, 1997: her proximal toe was still swollen and the skin soft and macerated.

cellulitic changes from her ankle to her midcalf. She was discharged to our boot clinic where her leg did well with local antibiotic injections and Long-Boot therapy. In June of 1996, she returned again with an ingrown toenail and a ulcer that penetrated through callus over her second left hammer toe; *Enterococcus* was cultured from the ulcer, which was treated quickly and successfully in the Miniboot with local gentamicin injections. She continued with her business ventures which, on the 24th of September, 1997, took her to a building site where she unfortunately stepped on a nail that penetrated the middle phalanx of her second toe (Figs. 13-16 and 13-17). Her many drug allergies (clindamycin, sulfa, ciprofloxacin, amoxicillin/clavulanate, and cephalexin) were to limit her therapies. Her photoelectricplethysmography tracings showed minimal pulsatile flow in her toes. Local gentamicin was injected into the nail hole and Miniboot therapy and oral doxycycline were prescribed. Cultures eventually grew out yeast, coagulase-negative staphylococci, and *Pseudomonas aeruginosa*. The latter proved to be resistant to gentamicin. Her antibiotic treatment, hence, became local injections of ceftazidime and gentamicin, and oral fluconazole.

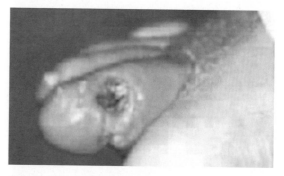

Fig. 13–17. December 10th, 1997: the toe cellulitis was largely controlled but the nail track through the infected bone remained to be healed.

Her x-rays showed osteomyelitis of the body and proximal head of the second proximal phalanx. She returned September 5, 2000 for a routine visit for evaluation of her diabetes. Her feet and legs were found to be doing well. A healed indentation of her second toe marked the episode of osteomyelitis (Fig. 13–18). She continues her home boot treatments because she has found that it increases her comfortable walking distances. *Points to consider*: This patient has benefited from boot therapy in (1) greatly improving her venous stasis disease ("VP"), the stasis disease being one early contraindication to consideration by her physicians of leg bypass surgery for her ischemic leg disease ("ASO"); (2) in supporting her heart ("CO"); (3) in healing two episodes of osteomyelitis associated with foreign bodies (a needle and a nail); (4) in healing her cellulitic leg after heart surgery (Inf); (5) and in improving her overall mobility—all done as an outpatient. Other therapeutic options were few. Now in the year 2004, she still has intact feet and vision and is functioning well.

$$EBF \propto (CO)/(IFP)(VP)(ASO)(Inf)$$

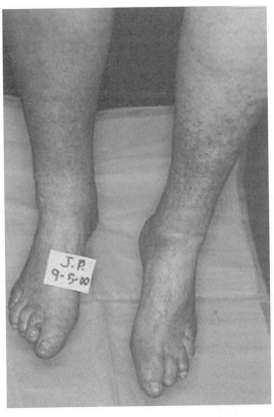

Fig. 13–18. September 2000.

Outpatient Treatment of Osteomyelitis

The osteomyelitis in the first toe and metatarsal head of this 47-year-old (female patient, a diabetic since age 15, had failed to heal in spite of two hospitalizations elsewhere for débridements and parenteral antibiotic therapy. She came to Bryn Mawr to be treated as an outpatient mainly with local measures. First, small punctures were made with a scalpel over the dorsal–medial aspect of the swollen area and in the scab between the first and second toes (Fig. 13–19). Appropriate cultures were made (Fig. 13–20). X-rays showed advanced osteomyelitis (Fig. 13–21). The puncture sites were irrigated with a multielectrolyte solution (Sea Soaks) containing gentamicin, which removed modest amounts of clot and debris. A similar irrigation was performed on day two. Each day for the rest of her stay, the infected area was injected with 40 mg (1 ml) gentamicin, particularly targeting the swollen areas with an attempt to infiltrate the infected joint. She was given oral Cipro for systemic coverage. The injections were followed by Miniboot therapy pumping 2:1. One month later, her sed rate was normal, her drainage had gone, and her fistulas closed. A postinflammatory rubor persisted and she was discharged. Four years later, she was kind enough to send us some follow-up photographs (Fig. 13–22).

Points to consider: The technique described here has been very helpful for us in curing most of the cases of osteomyelitis referred to us. It should be noted that we did not do extensive débridements. We did not do a ray resection. We did irrigate out loose bodies. We did get the antibiotics where they were needed. The patient did not require hospitalization. She did not require home-visiting nurses. We did not put the patient at the risk of

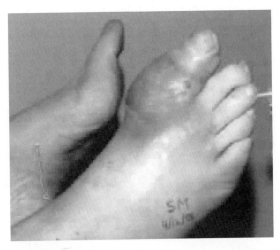

Fig. 13–19. Her proximal toe and first metatarsal head were pigmented and swollen.

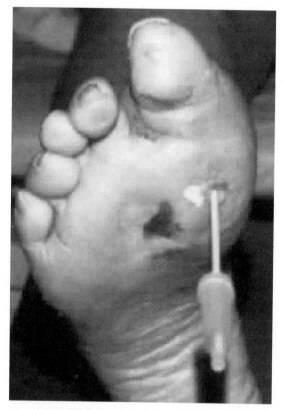

Fig. 13–20. The culturette stick easily entered the metatarsal-phalangeal joint space.

complications from central catheters and eventually restored a functional foot.

Necrotizing Cellulitis in Diabetic Foot (Case 1)

A 33-year-old bride with type 1 diabetes, developed plantar callus while on her honeymoon. She was appropriately given oral cephradine and prescribed bed rest

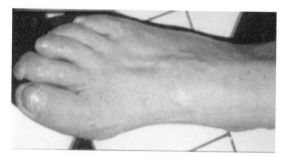

Fig. 13–22. Four year follow-up: walking and hiking daily.

which proved ineffective in arresting spread of cellulitis. She was hospitalized for 12 days and given intravenous tobramycin and cefobid, again appropriate antibiotics for the beta *Streptococcus* and *Eikenella* species cultured from her foot. This therapy was ineffective in arresting her cellulitis. A bone scan showed ostemyelitis of her third, fourth, and fifth metatarsal heads. An incision and drainage procedure showed advanced tissue necrosis. Peroxide soaks, whirlpool treatments, and blood transfusions neither helped her foot or her general condition. Her attending physicians unanimously recommended a BKA because she had: (1) uncontrolled soft-tissue and bone infection; and (2) persisting systemic toxicity with spiking fevers, uncontrolled diabetes, loss of veins and poor access for intravenous treatments, vaginal and rectal yeast infections. She refused amputation and requested another opinion, ignoring the five opinions of her family doctor, diabetologist, infectious disease consultant, and general and vascular surgions. She then requested another hospital and was transferred to Bryn Mawr.

On transfer to Bryn Mawr, her foot was found to be heavily pigmented. A large ulcer with a necrotic base occupied the dorsum of the foot over the third, fourth, and fifth metatarsals. Rubber drains exited the webbing between the first and second toes and the fourth and fifth toes. Necrotic tissue was seen under the flap of skin over the first and second metatarsal bones and

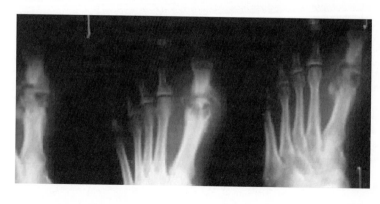

Fig. 13–21. Destruction of first metatarsal head and proximal phalanx.

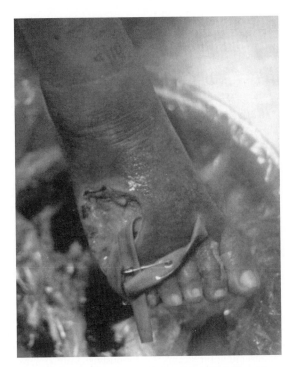

Fig. 13–23. Her pulseless foot on arrival at Bryn Mawr.

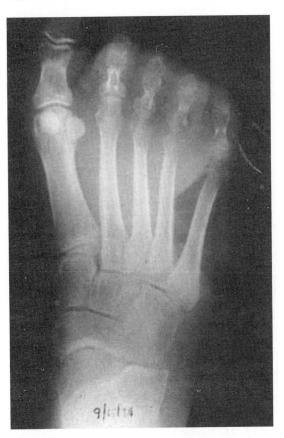

Fig. 13–24. Foot X-ray on admission to Bryn Mawr showed the outline of her ulcer in the lateral foot. The 3rd, 4th and 5th metatarsal heads were demineralized and reported by the roentgenologists as being destroyed by osteomyelitis.

protruded through the webbing between the first and second toes. The toes had a slight hammer-toe deformity, but were intact. (Fig. 13–23) No pulses were detected in the foot. Her foot x-ray showed multiple sites of osteomyelitis (Fig. 13–24). Standard therapy called for a BKA.

Her foot and leg were salvaged (Fig. 13–25). Her treatment and its rationale were as follows: Her infection began as an aggressive cellulitis. Early in her course, there was no abscess to drain. Such a procedure would have produced a large hole in already inflamed tissue. There was no place for surgery at that time and none was performed. The bacteria had produced various digestive enzymes (collagenases, elastases, etc) that had moved through the tissue planes and lymphatics in the foot damaging the tissue and small vessels, leaving the inflamed tissue with a diminished blood supply. Her antibiotics were appropriate in kind and quantity, but were not reaching the crucial areas in the foot. The cultures from her home hospital showed her bacteria was sensitive to erythromycin. The latter was given orally with her Circulator Boot therapy to block septic emboli from her feet. Intravenous antibiotics were stopped; her arms were swollen and sore and she had no veins. Oral nystatin and vaginal mycostatin were prescribed for her yeast infections. Her foot was placed in a plastic bag with multielectrolyte solution (Sea Soaks) and dilute iodine (Betadine) was used to rinse off loose pus and debris.

Such a soak began each day. Her foot was then injected at multiple sites with gentamicin using an insulin needle. The osteomyelitic areas between the metatarsal heads and the necrotic areas were especially infiltrated. Such injections were performed daily the first 10 days of her

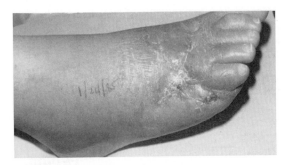

Fig. 13–25. Intact foot four months later.

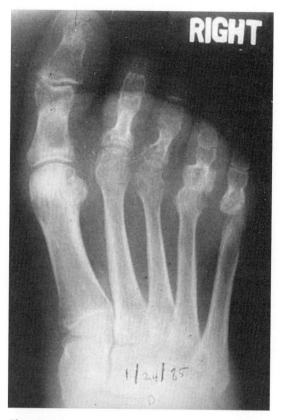

Fig. 13-26. Healed osteomyelitis.

treatments. Her foot was then placed within another plastic bag containing 40 mg genamicin in approximately 200 ml of multielectrolyte solution (Sea Soaks) and pumped within the Miniboot after alternate heartbeats. After the boot treatment, the fluid in the bag was cloudy with debris. During her 10-day hospitalization, her foot was pumped in the antibiotic–Sea Soaks solution four times daily for 40 min each. She was transferred to a nursing home for further treatment and shortly thereafter to her own home where she performed the treatments herself, having rented a Miniboot. Follow-up x-rays showed her bones had healed (Fig. 13–26).

REFERENCES

1. Hospital discharge rates for nontraumatic lower–extremity amputation by diabetes status—United States, 1997. *MMWR Morb Mortal Wkly Rep.* 2001;50(43):954–958.

2. Trautner C, Haastert B, Giani G, et al. Incidence of lower limb amputations and diabetes. *Diabetes Care.* 1996;19:1006–1009.

3. Mayfield JA, Reiber GE, Maynard C, et al. Trends in lower limb amputation in the Veterans Health Administration, 1989–1998. *J Rehabil Res Develop.* 2000;37:23–30.

4. Wrobel JS, Mayfield JA, Reiber GE. Geographic variation of lower-extremity major amputation in individuals with and without diabetes in the Medicare population. *Diabetes Care* 2001;24:860–864.

5. Centers for Disease Control and Prevention, National Center for Health Statistics, Division of Health Care Statistics, data from the National Hospital Discharge Survey. Data computed by the Division of Diabetes Translation, National Center for Chronic Disease Prevention and Health Promotion, Centers for Disease Control and Prevention.

6. Wheelock FC, Marble A. Surgery and diabetes *Joslin's Diabetes Mellitus,* 11th edition. Marble A, ed. Philadelphia: Lea & Febiger; 1971;599.

7. Gianfortune P, Pulla RJ, Sage R. Ray resections in the insensitive or dysvascular foot: a critical review. *J Foot Surg.* 1985; 24:103–107.

8. Santi MD, Thoma BJ, Chambers RB. Survivorship of healed partial foot amputations in dysvascular patients. *Clin Orthop.* 1993;292:245–249.

9. Turnbull AR, Chester JF. Partial amputations of the foot for diabetic gangrene. *Ann R Coll Surg Engl.* 1988;70:330–331.

10. Hodge MJ, Peters TG, Efird WG. Amputation of the distal portion of the foot. *S Med J.* 1989;82:1138–1142.

11. Sanders LJ, Dunlap G. Transmetatarsal amputation: a successful approach to limb salvage. *J Am Podiat Med Assoc.* 1992; 82:129–135.

12. Sage R, Pinzur MS, Cronin R, et al. Complications following midfoot amputations in neuropathic and dysvascular feet. *J Am Podiatric Med Assoc.* 1989;79:277–280.

13. Mueller MJ, Allen BT, Sinacore DR. Incidence of skin breakdown and higher amputation after transmetatarsal amputation: implications for rehabilitation. *Arch Phys Med Rehab.* 1995;76:50–54.

14. Quigley FG, Faris IB, Xiouruppa H. Transmetatarsal amputation for advanced forefoot tissue loss in elderly patients. *Aust NZ J Surg.* 1995;65:339–341.

15. Dillon RS. Fifteen years of experience in treating 2,177 episodes of foot and leg lesions with the Circulator Boot—Results of treatments with the Circulator Boot. *Angiology* 1997;48:S17–S34.

16. Quebedeaux TL, Lavery LA, Lavery DC. The development of foot deformities and ulcers after great toe amputations in diabetes. *Diabetes Care.* 1996;19:165–167.

17. Sobel E, Japour CJ, Giorgini RJ, et al. Use of prostheses and footwear in 110 inner-city partial-foot amputees. *J Am Podiatr Med Assoc.* 2001;91:34–49.

17a. Silbert S: Amputation of the lower extremity in diabetes mellitus. Diabetes 1952; 1:297–99.

18. Braddeley RM, Fulford JC. A trial of conservative amputations for lesions of the feet in diabetes mellitus. *Br J Surg.* 1965;52:38–43.

18a. Hoar CS Jr, Torres J: Evaluation of below-the-knee amputation in the treatment of diabetic gangrene. N Engl J Med 1962;266:440–3.

19. Whitehouse FW, Jurgenson C, Block MA. The later life of the diabetic amputee: another look at the fate of the second leg. *Diabetes* 1968;17:520–521.

19a. Cameron HC, Lennard-Jones JE, Robinson MD: Amputations in the diabetic, outcome and survival. Lancet 1964;2:605–607.

20. Ecker ML, Jacobs BS. Lower extremity amputation in diabetic patients. *Diabetes* 1970;19:189.

20a. Roon AJ, Moore WS, Gladstone J: Below-knee amputation: a modern approach. Am J Surg 1977;134(1)153–8.

21. Kahn O, Wagner W, Bessman AN. Mortality of diabetic patients treated surgically of lower limb infection and or gangrene. *Diabetes* 1974;23:287–292.

21a. Kolind-Sorensen V: Follow-up of lower limb amputees. Acta Orthop Scand 1974;45(1):97–104.

22. Ebskov B, Josephson P. Incidence of reamputation and death after gangrene of lower extremity. *Prosth Ortho Int.* 1980; 4:77–80.

22a. Goldner MG: The fate of the second leg in diabetic amputee. diabetes 1960;9:100–3.

23. Haynes IG, Middleton MD. Amputation for peripheral vascular disease: experience of a district general hospital. *Ann R Coll Surg Engl.* 1981;63:342–344.

24. Rozin, RR. Gangrene of the lower limbs in diabetic patients: A malignant complication. *Am J Surg.* 1987;154:305–308.

25. Enroth M, Persson BM. Amputation for arterial occlusive disease. *Int Orthopaed.* 1992;16:383–387.

26. Deerochanawong C, Home PD, Alberti KGMM. A survey of lower limb amputations in diabetic patients. *Diabetic Med.* 1992;9:942–946.

27. Apelqvist J, Larsson J, Agardh C. Long-term prognosis of diabetic patients with foot ulcers. *J Internal Med.* 1993;233: 485–491.

28. VanBuskirk A, Barta PJ, Schlossbach NJ. Lower extremity amputations in New Jersey. *New Jersey Med.* 1994;91: 260–263.

29. Pohjolainen T, Alaranta H. Ten-year survival of Finnish lower limb amputees. *Prosth Ortho Int.* 1998;22:10–16.

30. Feinglass J, Pearce WH, Martin GJ, et al. Postoperative and late survival outcomes after major amputation: findings from the Department of Veterans Affairs National Surgical Quality Improvement Program. *Surgery* 2001;130:21–29.

31. Fletcher DD, Andrews KL, Hallett JW, Jr, et al. Trends in rehabilitation after amputation for geriatric patients with vascular disease: implications for future health resource allocation. *Arch Phys Med Rehab.* 2002;83:1389–1393.

32. Buzato MA, Tribulatto EC, Costa SM, et al. Major amputations of the lower leg. The patients two years later. *Acta Chir Belg.* 2002;102:248–252.

33. Toursarkissian B, Shireman PK, Harrison A, et al. Major lower-extremity amputation: contemporary experience in a single Veterans Affairs institution. *Am Surg.* 2002;68: 606–610.

34. Fusetti C, Senechaud C, Merlini M. Quality of life of vascular disease patients following amputation. *Ann Chir.* 2001;26: 434–439.

35. Eskelinen E, Eskelinen A, Hyytinen T, et al. Changing pattern of major lower limb amputations in Seinajoki Central Hospital. 1997–2000.

36. Kuukasjarvi P, Salenius JP. Perioperative outcome of acute lower limb ischaemia on the basis of the national vascular registry. The Finnvasc Study Group. *Eur J Vasc Surg.* 1994;8: 578–583.

37. Van Houtum WH, Lavery LA. Outcomes associated with diabetes-related amputations in The Netherlands and in the state of California, USA. *J Int. Med.* 1996;240:227–231.

38. Pecoraro RE, Reiber GE, Burgess EM. Pathways to diabetic limb amputation. Basis for prevention. *Diabetes Care.* 1990; 13:513–521.

39. Waugh NR. Amputations in diabetic patients—A review of rates, relative risks and resource use. *Community Med* 1988; 10:279–288.

40. Jensen LP, Nielsen OM, Schroeder TV. The importance of complete follow-up for results after femoro-infrapopliteal vascular surgery. *Eur J Vasc Endovasc Surg.* 1996;12(3): 282–286.

41. Harrington C, Zagari MJ, Corea J, et al. A cost analysis of diabetic lower-extremity ulcers. *Diabetes Care* 2000;23: 1333–1338.

42. Ashry HR, Lavery LA, Armstrong DG, et al. Cost of diabetes-related amputations in minorities. *J Foot Ankle Surg.* 1998; 37:186–190.

43. Apelqvist J, Ragnarson-Tennvall G, Persson U, et al. Diabetic foot ulcers in a multidisciplinary setting. An economic analysis of primary healing and healing with amputation. *J Intern Med.* 1994;235:463–471.

44. Apelqvist J, Ragnarson-Tennvall G, Larson J, et al. Long-term costs for foot ulcers in diabetic patients in a multidisciplinary setting. *Foot Ankle Int.* 1995;16:388–394.

45. Eneroth M, Apelqvist J, Troeng T, et al. Operations, total hospital stay and costs of critical leg ischemia. A population-based longitudinal outcome study of 321 patients. *Acta Orthop Scand.* 1996;67:459–465.

46. Panayiotopoulos YP, Tyrrell MR, Arnold FJ, et al. Results and cost analysis of distal [crural/pedal] arterial revascularisation for limb salvage in diabetic and non-diabetic patients. *Diabet Med.* 1997;14:214–220.

47. Wixon CL, Mills JL, Westerband A, et al. An economic appraisal of lower extremity bypass graft maintenance. *J Vasc Surg.* 2000;32:1–12.

48. Tangelder MJ, McDonnel J, Van Busschbach JJ, et al. Quality of life after infrainguinal bypass grafting surgery. Dutch Bypass Oral Anticoagulants or Aspirin (BOA) Study Group. *J Vasc Surg.* 1999;30:1162–1163.

49. Hunink MGM, Wong JB, Donaldson MC, et al. Revascularization for femoropopliteal disease. A decision and cost-effectiveness analysis. *JAMA* 1995;274:165–171.

50. Criqui MH. Epidemiology and prognostic significance of peripheral arterial disease. In: Hirsch AT, ed. Primary Care Series: Peripheral Arterial Disease and Intermittent Claudication. *The American Journal of Medicine Primary Care Series.* Hillsborough, NJ. Excerpta Medica, 2001.

51. Brand RN, Abbott RD, Kannel WB. Diabetic intermittent claudication and risk of cardiovascular events. The Framingham Study. *Diabetes* 1989;38:504.

52. Feinglass J, McCarthy WJ, Slavensky R, et al. Effect of lower extremity blood pressure on physical functioning in patients who have intermittent claudication. *J Vasc Surg.* 1996;24: 503–511.

53. Criqui MH, Langer RD, Fronek A, et al. Mortality over a period of 10 years in patients with peripheral arterial disease. *N Engl J Med* 1992;326:381–386.

54. Dormandy J, Heeck L, Vig S. The natural history of claudication: risk to life and limb. *Semin Vasc Surg.* 1999;12: 123–137.

55. Jonason T, Ringqvist I. Factors of prognostic importance for subsequent rest pain in patients with intermittent claudication. *Acta Med Scand.* 1985;218;27–33.

56. Gerrits HL, de Haan A, Sargeant AJ, et al. Peripheral vascular changes after electrically stimulated cycle training in people with spinal cord injury. *Arch Phys Med Rehab* 2001;82: 832–839.

57. Gardner AW, Poehlman ET. Exercise rehabilitation programs for the treatment of claudication pain. A meta-analysis. *JAMA* 1995;274:975–980.

58. Schepsis AA, Lynch G. Exertional compartment syndromes of the lower extermity. *Curr Opin Rheumatol.* 1996;8: 143– 147.

59. Dawson DL, Cutler BS, Hiatt WR, et al. A comparison of cilostazol and pentoxifyline for treating intermittent claudication. *Am J Med.* 2000;109:523–530.

60. Ernst E. pentoxifylline for intermittent claudication: a critical review. *Angiology* 1994;45:339–345.

61. Roberts DH, Tsao Y, McLoughlin GA, et al. Placebo-controlled comparison of captopril, atenolol, labetalol and pindolol in hypertension complicated by intermittent claudication. *Lancet* 1987;2:650–653.

62. Perkins JMT, Collin J, Creasy TS, et al. Exercise training versus angioplasty for stable claudication. Long and medium term results of a prospective, randomised trial. *Eur J Vasc Endovasc Surg.* 1996;11:409–413.

63. Whyman MR, Fowkes FGR, Kerracher EMG, et al. Is intermittent claudication improved by percutaneous transluminal angioplasty? A randomized controlled trial. *J Vasc Surg.* 1997; 26:551–557.

64. Whyman MR, Fowkes FG, Kerracher EM, et al. Randomised controlled trial of percutaneous transluminal angioplasty for intermittent claudication. *Eur J Vasc Endovasc Surg.* 1996; 12(2):167–172.

65. Feinglass J, McCarthy WJ, Slavensky R, et al. Functional status and walking ability after lower extremity bypass grafting or angioplasty for intermittent claudication: results from a prospective outcomes study. *J Vasc Surg.* 2000;31:93–103.

66. Lundgren F, Dahllof AG, Ludhjolm K, et al. Intermittent claudication-surgical reconstruction or physical training. *Ann Surg.* 1989;209:346–355.

67. Schep G, Bender MH, Kaandorp D, et al. Flow limitations in the iliac arteries in endurance athletes. Current knowledge and directions for the future. *Int J Sports Med.* 1999; 20:421–428.

68. Abraham P, Saumet JL, Chevalier JM. External iliac artery endofibrosis in athletes. *Sports Med.* 1997;24:221–226.

69. Abraham P, Chevalier JM, Leftheriotis G, et al. Lower extremity arterial disease in sports. *Am J Sports Med.* 1997; 25:581–584.

70. Westendorp IC, in't Veld BA, Grobbee DE, et al. Hormone replacement therapy and peripheral arterial disease: the Rotterdam study. *Arch Intern Mesd.* 2000;160:2498–2502.

71. Westendorp IC, in't Veld BA, Bots ML, et al. Hormone replacement therapy and intima-media thickness of the common carotid artery: the Rotterdam study. *Stroke* 1999;30: 2562–2567.

72. Byington RP, Furberg CD, Herrington DM, et al. The Heart and Estrogen/Progestin Replacement Study Research Group. Effect of estrogen plus progestin on progression of carotid atherosclerosis in postmenopausal women with heart disease: HERS B-mode substudy. *Arterioscler Thromb Vasc Biol.* 2002; 22:1692–1697.

73. Waters DD, Alderman EL, Hsia J, et al. Effects of hormone replacement therapy and antioxidant vitamin supplements on coronary atherosclerosis in postmenopausal women: a randomized controlled trial. *JAMA* 2002;288:2432–2440.

74. Timaran CH, Stevens SL, Grandas OH, et al. Influence of hormone replacement therapy on graft patency after femoropopliteal bypass grafting. *J Vasc Surg.* 2000;32:506–518.

75. Maser RE, Steenkiste AR, Dorman JS, et al. Epidemiological correlates of diabetic neuropathy. Report from Pittsburgh epidemiology of diabetes complications study. *Diabetes* 1989; 38:1456–1461.

76. Vinik AI, Suwanwalaikorn S, Stansberry KB, et al. Quantitative measurement of cutaneous perception in diabetic neuropathy. *Muscle Nerve* 1995;18:574–584.

77. Finegold D, Lattimer SA, Nolle S, et al. Polyol pathway activity and myoinositol metabolism: a suggested relationship in the pathogenesis of diabetic neuropathy. *Diabetes* 1983; 32:988–992.

78. Grant WP, Sullivan R, Sonenshine DE, et al. Electron microscopic investigation of the effects of diabetes mellitus on the Achilles tendon. *J Foot Ankle Surg.* 1997;36:272–278.

79. Reddy GK, Stehno-Bittel L, Enwemeka CS. Glycation-induced matrix stability in the rabbit achilles tendon. *Arch Biochem Biophys.* 2002;399:174–180.

80. Becker J, Nora DB, Gomes I, et al. An evaluation of gender, obesity, age and diabetes mellitus as risk factors for carpal tunnel syndrome. *Clin Neurophysiol.* 2002;113:1429–1434.

81. Aszmann OC, Kress KM, Dellon AL. Results of decompression of peripheral nerves in diabetics: a prospective, blinded study. *Plast Reconstr Surg.* 2000;106(4):816–822.

82. Hollis Caffee H. Treatment of diabetic neuropathy by decompression of the posterior tibial nerve. *Plast Reconstr Surg.* 2000; 106(4):813–815.

83. Dellon AL. Preventing foot ulceration and amputation by decompressing peripheral nerves in patients with diabetic neuropathy. *Ostomy Wound Manage.* 2002;48:36–45.

84. Ozkul Y, Sabuncu T, Kocabey Y, et al. Outcomes of carpal tunnel release in diabetic and non-diabetic patients. *Acta Neurol Scand.* 2002;106:168–172.

85. Zahir KS, Zahir FS, Thomas JG, et al. The double-crush phenomenon—an unusual presentation and literature review. *Conn Med.* 1999;63(9):535–538.

86. Lormeau B. The "short Achilles tendon" syndrome: a new entity of the diabetic foot. *Diabetes Metab.* 1997;23(5): 443–447.

87. Hastings MK, Mueller MJ, Sinacore DR, et al. Effects of a tendo-Achilles lengthening procedure on muscle function and gait characteristics in a patient with diabetes mellitus. *J Orthop Sports Phys Ther.* 2000;30(2):85–90.

88. Cameron NE, Eaton SE, Cotter MA, et al. Vascular factors and metabolic interactions in the pathogenesis of diabetic neuropathy. *Diabetologia* 2001;44:1973–1988.

89. Coppey LJ, Davidson EP, Dunlap JA, et al. Slowing of motor nerve conduction velocity in streptozotocin-induced diabetic rats is preceded by impaired vasodilation in arterioles that overlie the sciatic nerve. *Int J Exp Diabetes Res.* 2000;1(2): 131–143.

90. Davis MT, Greene NM. Polarographic studies of skin oxygen tension following sympathetic denervation. *J Appl Physiol.* 1959;14:961–965.

91. Wollersheim H, et al. Ephedrine improves the microcirculation in the diabetic neuropathic foot. *Angiology* 1989;40: 1030–1033.

92. Uccioli L, Mancini L, Giordano A, et al. Lower limb arteriovenous shunts, autonomic neuropathy and diabetic foot. *Diabetes Res Clin Pract.* 1992;16:123–130.

93. Chew J T-H, Tan S-B, Sivathasan C, et al. Vascular assessment in the neuropathic diabetic foot. *Clin Orthopaed Related Res.* 1995;320:95–100.

94. Vayssairat M, Le Devehat C. Diabetic angiopathy: the role of microvascular exploration in routine practice. Consequences of a new algorithm for care of the diabetic foot. *J Mal Vasc.* 2001;26(2):126–129.

95. Zimny S, Dessel F, Ehren M, et al. Early detection of microcirculatory impairment in diabetic patients with foot at risk. *Diabetes Care.* 2001;24:1810–1814.

96. Repelaer-an-Driel OJ, et al. Lumbar sympathectomy for severe lower limb ischemia: results and analysis of factors influencing outcome. *J Cardiovasc Surg* (Torino) 1988;29:310–314.

97. Dillon RS. Role of cholinergic nervous system in healing neuropathic lesions: preliminary studies and prospective, double-blinded placebo-controlled studies. *Angiology* 1991; 42:767–778.

98. Cooke JP. Novel mechanisms of angiogenesis/smoking and angiogenesis trials. *13th Annu Meet Soc Vasc Med Biol.* Boston, 2002.

99. Pfutzner A, Forst T, Engelbach M, et al. The influence of isolated small nerve fibre dysfunction on microvascular control in patients with diabetes mellitus. *Diabetic Med* 2001;18: 489–494.

100. Ryder REJ, Kennedy RL, Newrick PG, et al. Autonomic denervation may be a prerequisite of diabetic neuropathic foot ulceration. *Diabetic Med.* 1990;7:726–730.

101. The KROC Collaborative Study Group: diabetic retinopathy after two years of intensified insulin treatment: follow-up of the KROC Collaborative Study. *JAMA* 1988;260:37–41.

102. The Diabetes Control and Complications Trial Research Group: The effect of intensive treatment of diabetes on the development and progression of long-term complications in insulin-dependent diabetes mellitus. *N Engl J Med.* 1993; 329:977–986.

103. Kihara M, Zollman PJ, Smithson IL, et al. Hypoxic effect of exogenous insulin on normal and diabetic peripheral nerve. *Am J Physiol.* 1994;266:E980–985.

104. Tesfaye S, Malik R, Harris N, et al. Arterio-venous shunting and proliferating new vessels in acute painful neuropathy of rapid glycaemic control (insulin neuritis). *Diabetologia.* 1996; 39:329–335.

105. Dillon RS. Case 143: Peripheral neuritis and retinopathy following rapid control of diabetes treated successfully with boot? http://www.circulatorboot.com/casehistory/case143.html

106. Barnes RW. *Noninvasive Diagnostic Techniques in Peripheral Vascular Disease.* St Louis: Mosby; 1980:41–43.

107. Krsek M, Prazny M, Skrha J, et al. The relationship between the IGF-I system and its binding proteins and microvascular reactivity in type 1 diabetes mellitus. *Physiol Res.* 2002;51: 379–385.

108. Clarkson P, Celermajer DS, Donald AE, et al. Impaired vascular reactivity in insulin-dependent diabetes mellitus is related to disease duration and low density lipoprotein cholesterol levels. *J Am Coll Cardiol.* 1996;28:573–579.

109. Karnafel W, Juskowa J, Maniewski R, et al. Microcirculation in the diabetic foot as measured by a multichannel laser Doppler instrument. *Med Sci Monit.* 2002;8MT137–144.

110. Skrha J, Prazny M, Haas T, et al. Comparison of laser-Doppler flowmetry with biochemical indicators of endothelial dysfunction related to early microangiopathy in type 1 diabetic patients. *J Diabetes Complications.* 2001;15:234–240.

111. Stansberry KB, Peppard HR, Babyak LM, et al. Primary nociceptive afferents mediate the blood flow dysfunction in non-glabrous (hairy) skin of type 2 diabetes: a new model for the pathogenesis of microvascular dysfunction. *Diabetes Care* 1999;22:1549–1554.

112. Lawson SN. Peptides and cutaneous polymodal nociceptor neurons. In: Kumazawa T, Krugger L, Mizumura L, eds. *Progress in Brain Research, Vol. 113, The Polymodal Receptor: A Gateway to Pathological Pain.* Elsevier, Amsterdam, 1996.

113. Akbari CM, Saouaf R, Barnhill DF, et al. Endothelium-dependent vasodilatation is impaired in both microcirculation and macrocirculation during acute hyperglycemia. *J Vasc Surg.* 1998;28:687–694.

114. Veves A, Saouaf R, Donaghue VM, et al. Aerobic exercise capacity remains normal despite impaired endothelial function in the micro- and macrocirculation of physically active IDDM patients. *Diabetes.* 1997;46:1846–1852.

115. Iwatsubo H, Nagano M, Sakai T, et al. Converting enzyme inhibitor improves forearm reactive hyperemia in essential hypertension. *Hypertension.* 1997;29:286–290.

116. Rhodes LE, Belgi G, Parslew R et al. Ultraviolet-B-induced erythema is mediated by nitric oxide and prostaglandin E_2 in combination. *J Invest Dermatol.* 2001;117:880–885.

117. Kennedy JM, Zochodne DW. Influence of experimental diabetes on the microcirculation of injured peripheral nerve: functional and morphological aspects. *Diabetes.* 2002;51: 2233–2240.

118. Meyer MF, Pfohl M, Schatz H. Assessment of diabetic alterations of microcirculation by means of capillaroscopy and laser-Doppler anemometry. *Med Klin.* 2001;96:71–77.

119. Jorneskog G, Fagrell B. Discrepancy in skin capillary circulation between fingers and toes in patients with type 1 diabetes. *Int J Microcirc Clin Exp.* 1996;16:313–319.

120. Lawall H, Angelkort B. Correlation between rheological parameters and erythrocyte velocity in nailfold capillaries in patients with diabetes mellitus. *Clin Hemorheol Microcirc.* 1999;20:41–47.

121. Lawall H, Amann B, Rottmann M, et al. The role of microcirculatory techniques in patients with diabetic foot syndrome. *Vasa* 2000;29:191–197.

122. Ubbink DT, Spincemaille GH, Reneman RS, Jacobs MJ. Prediction of imminent amputation in patients with non-reconstructible leg ischemia by means of microcirculatory investigations. *J Vasc Surg.* 1999;30:114–121.

123. Simoni G, Baiardi A, Galleano R, et al. Smoking as a risk factor in arteriopathies. *Minerva Cardioangiol.* 1994;42: 245–248.

124. Leggetter S, Chaturvedi N, Fuller JH, et al. Ethnicity and risk of diabetes-related lower extremity amputation: a population-based, case-control study of African Caribbeans and Europeans in the United kingdom. *Arch Intern Med.* 2002;162:73–78.

125. Feinglass J, Brown JL, LoSasso A, et al. Rates of lower-extremity amputation and arterial reconstruction in the United States, 1979 to 1996. *Am J Public Health.* 1999;89: 1222–1227.

126. Quick CRG, Cotton LT. The measured effect of stopping smoking on intermittent claudication. *Br J Surg* 1982; 69 Suppl :s24–s26.

127. Jonason T, Bernstrom R. Cessation of smoking in patients with intermittent claudication. *Acta Med Scand*. 1987;221:253–260.

128. Faulkner KW, House AK, Castleden AM. The effect of cessation of smoking on the accumulative survival rates of patients with symptomatic peripheral vascular disease. *Med J Austr*. 1983;5:217–219.

129. Smoking and Health. Report of the Advisory Committee to the Surgeon General of the Public Health Service, U.S. Dept. of Health, Education and Welfare, Public Health Service. *PHS Publ*. 1964;No. 1103:318.

130. Hines EA, Jr. The effects of tobacco on blood pressure and in peripheral vascular diseases. *Proc Staff Meet Mayo Clin*. 1960;35:337.

131. Mahmud A and Feely J. Effect of smoking on arterial stiffness and pulse pressure amplification. *Hypertension*. 2003;41:183–187.

132. Terborg C, Birkner T, Schack, B, et al. Acute effects of cigarette smoking on cerebral oxygenation and hemodynamics: a combined study with near-infrared spectroscopy and transcranial Doppler sonography. *J Neurol Sci*. 2002;205:71–75.

133. Jolma CD, Samson RA, Klewer SE, et al. Acute cardiac effects of nicotine in healthy young adults. *Echocardiography*. 2002;19:443–448.

134. Paganelli MO, Tanus-Santos JE, Toledo JC, et al. Acute administration of nicotine impairs the hypotensive responses to bradykinin in rats. *Eur J Pharmacol*. 2001;413:241–246.

135. Carty CS, Huribal M, Marsan BU, et al. Nicotine and its metabolite cotinine are mitogenic for human vascular smooth muscle cells. *J Vasc Surg*. 1997;25:682–688.

136. Yokotani K, Okada, S, Nakamura K. Characterization of functional nicotinic acetylcholine receptors involved in catecholamine release from the isolated rat adrenal gland. *Eur J Pharmacol*. 2002;446:83–87.

137. Albano SA, Santana-Sahagun E, Weisman MH. Cigarette smoking and rheumatoid arthritis. *Semin Arthritis Rheum*. 2001;31:146–159.

138. McKusick VA, Harris WS, Ottesen OE, et al. The Buerger syndrome in the United States: arteriographic observations, with special reference to involvement of the upper extremities and the differentiation from atherosclerosis and embolism. *Bull John Hopkins Hosp*. 1962;110:145–176.

139. Heeschen C, Jang JJ, Weis M, et al. Nicotine stimulates angiogenesis and promotes tumor growth and atherosclerosis. *Nat Med*. 2001;7(7):833–839.

140. Bozikas VP, Vlaikidis N, Petrikis P, et al. Schizophrenic-like symptoms in a patient with thrombo-angiitis obliterans (Winiwarter–Buerger's disease). *Int J Psychiatry Med*. 2001;31:341–346.

141. Becit N, Unlu Y, Kocak H, Ceviz M, et al., Involvement of the coronary artery in a patient with thromboangiitis obliterans. A case report. *Heart Vessels*. 2002;16:201–203.

142. Hoppe B, Lu JT, Thistlewaite P, et al. Beyond peripheral arteries in Buerger's disease: angiographic considerations in thromboangiitis obliterans. *Catheter Cardiovasc Interv*. 2002;57:363–366.

143. Adem C, Benamouzig R, Royer I et al. Buerger's disease or thromboangiitis obliterans revealed by an enteric ischemia. Case report and literature review. *Gastroenterol Clin Biol*. 2002;26:409–411.

144. Marder VJ, Mellinghoff IK. Cocaine and Buerger disease: is there a pathogenetic association? *Arch Intern Med*. 2000;160:2057–2060.

145. Disdier P, Granel B, Serratrice J, et al. Cannabis arteritis revisited—ten new case reports. *Angiology*. 2001;52:1–5.

146. Schneider F, Abdoucheli-Baudot N, Tassart M, et al. Cannabis and tobacco: cofactors favoring juvenile obliterative arteriopathy. *J Mal Vasc*. 2000;25:388–389.

147. Roth MD, Baldwin GC, Tashkin DP. Effects of delta-9-tetrahydrocannabinol on human immune function and host defense. *Chem Phys Lipids*. 2002;121:229–239.

148. Roncon-Albuquerque R, Serrao P, Vale-Pereira R, et al. Plasma catecholamines in Buerger's disease: effects of cigarette smoking and surgical sympathectomy. *J Vasc Endovasc Surg*. 2002;24:338–343.

149. Singh K, Sood S. Autonomic functions in Buerger's disease. *Indian J Physiol Pharmacol*. 2001;45:470–474.

150. Iwase S, Okamoto T, Mano T, et al. Skin sympathetic outflow in Buerger's disease. *Auto Neurosci*. 2001;87:286–292.

151. Kroger K, Kreuzfelder E, Moser C, et al. Thrombangitis obliterans: leucocyte subpopulations and circulating immune complexes. *Vasa*. 2001;30:189–194.

152. Halacheva K, Gulubova MV, Manolova I, et al. Expression of ICAM-1, VCAM-1, E-selectin and TNF-alpha on the endothelium of femoral and iliac arteries in thromboangiitis obliterans. *Acta Histochem*. 2002;104:177–184.

153. Shindo S, Matsumoto H, Ogata K, et al. Arterial reconstruction in Buerger's disease: bypass to disease-free collaterals. *Int Angiol*. 2002;21:228–232.

154. Talwar S, Choudhary SK. Omentopexy for limb salvage in Buerger's disease: indications, technique and results. *J Postgrad Med*. 2001;47:137–142.

155. Mangano DT, Browner WS, Hollenberg M, et al. Association of perioperative myocardial ischemia with cardiac morbidity and mortality in men undergoing noncardiac surgery. *N Engl J Med*. 1990;323:1781–1788.

156. Carter SA, Tate RB. The value of toe pulse waves in determination of risks for limb amputation and death in patients with peripheral arterial disease and skin ulcers or gangrene. *J Vasc Surg*. 2001;33:708–714.

157. Dillon RS. Management of soft-tissue infections in elderly persons with diabetes. *Geriatric Med Today*. 1987;6:21–35.

158. Gardner SE, Frantz RA, Doebbeling BN. The validity of the clinical signs and symptoms used to identify localized chronic wound infection. *Wound Repair Regen*. 2001;9:178–186.

159. Lowy FD. Staphylococcus aureus infections. *N Engl J Med*. 1998;339:520–532.

160. Lew DP, Waldvogel FA. Current concepts: Osteomyelitis. *N Engl J Med*. 1997;336:999–1007.

161. Grayson ML, Gibbons GW, Balogh K, et al. Probing to bone in infected pedal ulcers: a clinical sign of underlying osteomyelitis in diabetic patients. *JAMA* 1995;273:721–723.

162. Littenberg B, Mushlin AI and the Diagnostic Technology Assessment Consortium. Technetium bone scanning in the diagnosis of osteomyelitis. A meta-analysis of test performance. *J Gen Inter Med*. 1992;7:158–163.

163. Newman LG, Waller, J, Palestro J, et al. Unsuspected osteomyelitis in diabetic foot ulcers. Diagnosis and monitoring by leukocyte scanning with Indium in 111-oxyquinoline. *JAMA* 1991;266:1246–1251.

164. Newman LG, Waller J, Palestro CJ, et al. Leukocyte scanning with 111-In is superior to magnetic resonance imaging in diagnosis of clinically unsuspected osteomyelitis in diabetic foot ulcers. *Diabetes Care* 1992;15:1527–1530.

165. Weinstein D, Wang A, Chambers R, et al. Evaluation of magnetic resonance imaging in the diagnosis of osteomyelitis in diabetic foot infections. *Foot Ankle* 1993;14:18–22.

166. Dillon RS. Successful treatment of osteomyelitis and soft tissue infections in ischemic diabetic legs by local antibiotic injections and the end-diastolic pneumatic compression boot. *Ann Surg.* 1986;204:643–649.

167. Dillon RS. Treatment of osteomyelitis in the diabetic foot with systemic and locally injected antibiotics and the end-diastolic pneumatic compression—Case studies. *Vasc Surg.* 1990;24: 683–696.

168. *Joslin's Diabetes Mellitus,* 12th ed. Philadelphia: Lea & Febiger; 1971:717–718.

169. Bamberger DM, Daus GP, Gerding DN. Osteomyelitis in the feet of diabetic patients: long-term results, prognostic factors and the role of antimicrobial and surgical therapy. *Am J Med.* 1987;83:653–660.

170. Fejfarova V, Jirkovska A, Skibova J, et al. Pathogen resistance and other risk factors in the frequency of lower limb amputations in patients with the diabetic foot syndrome. *Vnitr Lek.* 2002;48(4):302–306.

171. Taylor LM, Jr, Porter JM. The clinical course of diabetics who require emergent foot surgery because of infection or ischemia. *J Vasc Surg.* 1987;6:454–459.

172. Venkatesan P, Macfarlane RM, Fletcher EM, et al. Conservative management of osteomyelitis in the feet of diabetic patients. *Diabetic Med.* 1997;14:487–490.

173. Smith AJ, Daniels T, Bohnen JMA. Soft tissue infections and the diabetic foot. *Am J Surg.* 1966;172 (Suppl 6A):7S–12S.

174. Chantelau E, Tanudjaja T, Altenhofer F, et al. Antibiotic treatment for uncomplicated neuropathic forefoot ulcers in diabetes: a controlled trial. *Diabetic Med.* 1996;13: 156–159.

175. Ha Van G, Siney H, Danan J-P, et al. Treatment of osteomyelitis in the diabetic foot. *Diabetes Care.* 1996;19: 1257–1260.

176. Scher KS, Steele FJ. The septic foot in patients with diabetes. *Surgery.* 1988;104:661–666.

177. Grady JF, Winters CL. The Boyd amputation as a treatment for osteomyelitis of the foot. *J Am Podiatr Med Assoc.* 2000; 90(5):234–239.

178. Smith DG, Stuck RM, Ketner L, et al. Partial calcanectomy for the treatment of large ulcerations of the heel and calcaneal osteomyelitis. *J Bone Joint Surg.* 1992;74A:571–576.

179. Sapico FL, Witte JL, Canawati HN, et al. The infected foot of the diabetic patient: quantitative microbiology and analysis of clinical features. *Rev Infect Dis.* 1984;6 (Suppl 1): S171–S176.

180. Wheat LJ, Allen SD, Henry M, et al. Diabetic foot infections: bacteriologic analysis. *Arch Intern Med.* 1986;146: 1935–1940.

181. Pathare NA, Sathe SR. Antibiotic combinations in polymicrobic diabetic foot infections. *Indian J Med Sci.* 2001;55(12): 655–662.

182. Grayson ML, Gibbons GW, Habershaw GM, et al. Use of ampicillin/sulbactam versus imipenem/cilastatin in the treatment of limb-threatening foot infections in diabetic patients. *Clin Infect Dis.* 1994;18:683–693.

183. Thordarson DB, Perry JR, Patzakis J. Tetanus complicating a polymicrobial diabetic foot infection: case presentation and review of current treatment. *Foot Ankle Int.* 1995;16:97–99.

184. Gilbert DN, Dworkin RJ, Raber SR, et al. Outpatient parenteral antimicrobial-drug therapy. *N Engl J Med.* 1997;337: 829–838.

185. Maki DG, Stolz SM, Wheeler S, et al. Prevention of central venous catheter-related bloodstream infection by use of an antiseptic-impregnated catheter. A Randomized, controlled trial. *Ann Intern Med.* 1997;127:257–266.

186. Bach A. Efficacy of antibiotic-coated central venous catheters. *Crit Care Med.* 1999;27:1217.

187. Spittell JA, et al. Concentration of orally administered erythromycin and tetracycline in ischemic tissue. *Proc Staff Meet Mayo Clinic.* 1961;36:11.

188. Duckworth C, Fisher JF, Carter SA, et al. Tissue penetration of clindamycin in diabetic foot infections. *J Antimicrobial Chem* 1993;31:581–584.

189. Seabrook GR, Edminston CE, Schmitt DD, et al. Comparison of serum and tissue antibiotic levels in diabetes-related foot infections. *Surgery* 1991;110:671–677.

190. Raymakers JT, Houben AJ, van der Heyden JJ, et al. The effect of diabetes and severe ischaemia on the penetration of ceftazidime into tissues of the limb. *Diabetic Med.* 2001;18: 229–234.

191. Griego RD, Zitelli JA. Intra-incisional prophylactic antibiotics for dermatologic surgery. *Arch Dermatol.* 1998;134: 688–692.

192. Galandiuk S, Wrightson WR, Young S, et al. Absorbable, delayed-release antibiotic beads reduce surgical wound infection. *Am Surg.* 1997;63:831–835.

193. Nelson CL, McLaren SG, Skinner RA, et al. The treatment of experimental osteomyelitis by surgical débridement and the implantation of calcium sulfate tobramycin pellets. *J Orthop Res.* 2002;20:643–647.

194. Walenkamp GH, Kleijn LL, de Leeuw M. Osteomyelitis treated with gentamicin-PMMA beads: 100 patients followed for 1-12 years. *Acta Orthop Scand.* 1998;69:518–522.

195. Maxwell D. The role of antibiotics given by inhalation on chronic chest disease. *J Antimcrob Chemother.* 1983;11: 203–206.

196. Hinton PJ, Bryant LR. Preservation of an infected arterial graft with combination systemic-topical antibiotic therapy. *Am Surg.* 1981;47:511–514.

197. Compere EL, Metzger WI, Mitra RW. The treatment of pyogenic bone and joint infections by closed irrigation (circulation) with a non-toxic detergent and one or more antibiotics. *J Bone Joint Surg.* 1967;49A:614.

198. Josefsson G, Lindberg L, Wiklander B. Systemic antibiotics and gentamicin-containing bone cement in the prophylaxis of postoperative infections in total hip arthroplasty. *Clin Orthop.* 1981;159:194–200.

199. Garrett S, Johnson L, Drisko CH, et al. Two multi-center studies evaluating locally delivered doxycycline hyclate, placebo control, oral hygiene, and scaling and root planing in the treatment of periodontitis. *J Periodontol.* 1999;70: 490–503.

200. Stabholz A, Nicholas AA, Zimmerman GJ, et al. Clinical and antimicrobial effects of a single episode of subgingival irrigation with tetracycline HCl or chlorhexidine in deep periodontal pockets. *J Clin Periodontol.* 1998;25:794–800.

201. Negm MM. Intracanal use of a corticosteroid-antibiotic compound for the management of posttreatment endodontic pain.

Oral Surg Oral Med Oral Pathol Oral Radiol Endod. 2001; 92: 435–439.

202. Kaplan B, Gibson LB. Topical metronidazole for arterial insufficiency ulcers. *JAOA* 1995;95:201–203.

203. Dire DJ, Coppola M, Dwyer DA, et al. Prospective evaluation of topical antibiotics for preventing infections in uncomplicated soft-tissue wounds repaired in the ED. *Acad Emerg Med.* 1995;2:4–10.

204. Langford JH, Artemi P, Benrimoj SI. Topical antimicrobial prophylaxis in minor wounds. *Ann Pharmacother.* 1997;31: 559–563.

205. Wilson CL, Cameron J, Powell SM, et al. High incidence of contact dermatitis in leg-ulcer patients—implications for management. *Clin Exp Dermatol.* 1991;16:250–253.

206. Hu GF. Neomycin inhibits angiogenin-induced angiogenesis. *Proc Natl Acad Sci USA.* 1998;95:9791–9795.

207. Mavrommatis AC, Theodoridis T, Economou M, et al. Activation of the fibrinolytic system and utilization of the coagulation inhibitors in sepsis: comparison with severe sepsis and septic shock. *Intensive Care Med.* 2001;27:1853–1859.

208. Freeman BD, Buchman TG. Coagulation inhibitors in the treatment of sepsis. *Expert Opin Investi Drugs* 2002;11: 69–74.

209. Doshi SN, Marmur JD. Evolving role of tissue factor and its pathway inhibitor. *Crit Care Med.* 2002;30(Suppl 5): S241–250.

210. Dillon RS. Patient assessment and examples of a method of treatment—Use of the Circulator Boot in peripheral vascular disease. *Angiology.* 1997;(Suppl 48):s35.

211. Keeley EC, Grines CL. Scraping of aortic debris by coronary guiding catheters: a prospective evaluation of 1,000 cases. *J Am Coll Cardiol* 1998;32:1861–1865.

212. Eggebrecht H, Oldenburg O, Dirsch O, et al. Potential embolization by atherosclerotic debris dislodged from aortic wall during cardiac catheterization: histological and clinical findings in 7,621 patients. *Catheter Cardiovasc Interv.* 2000; 49(4):389–394.

213. Pennington M, Yeager J, Skelton H, et al. Cholesterol embolization syndrome: cutaneous histopathological features and the variable onset of symptoms in patients with different risk factors. *Br J Dermatol.* 2002;146:511–517.

214. Nitecki S, Schramek A, Torem S. Trash foot following abdominal aortic surgery. *Harefuah.* 1992;122:16–18.

215. Thompson MM, Smith J, Naylor AR, et al. Ultrasound-based quantification of emboli during conventional and endovascular aneurysm repair. *J Endovasc Surg.* 1997;4:33–38.

216. Gruss JD. Experience with PGE$_1$ in patients with postoperative trash foot. *Vasa Suppl.* 1989;28:57–60.

217. Stabellini N, Cerretani D, Russo G, et al. Renal atheroembolic disease: evaluation of the efficacy of corticosteroid therapy. *G Ital Nefrol.* 2002;19:18–21.

218. Mann SJ, Sos TA. Treatment of atheroembolization with corticosteroids. *Am J Hypertens.* 2001;14:831–834.

219. Dillon RS: http://www.circulatorboot.com/casehistory/case5.html.

220. Peng T, Jiang X, Wang Y, et al. Sympathectomy decreases and adrenergic stimulation increases the release of tissue plasminogen activator (t PA) from blood vessels: functional evidence for a neurologic regulation of plasmin production within vessel walls and other tissue matrices. *J Neurosci Res.* 1999;57: 680–692.

221. Garcia-Cardena G, Comander J, Anderson KR, et al. Biomechanical activation of vascular endothelium as a determinant of its functional phenotype. *Proc Natl Acad Sci USA.* 2001; 98(8):4478–4485.

222. Dai G, Tsukurov O, Orkin RW, et al. An *in vitro* cell culture system to study the influence of external pneumatic compression on endothelial function. *J Vasc Surg.* 2000;32: 977–987.

223. Lee BY, Thoden WR, Trainor FS. Fibrinolytic activity of intermittent pneumatic compression. *Contemp Surg.* 1981;18: 77–86.

224. Lee BY, Thoden WR, Del Guercio LRM, et al. Monitoring coagulation dynamics with thromboelastography. *Contemp Surg.* 1984;24:19–24.

225. Thomas DP, Roberts HR. Hypercoagulability in venous and arterial thrombosis. *Ann Intern Med.* 1997;126:638–44.

226. Toschi V, Gallo R, Lettino M, et al. Tissue factor modulates the thrombogenicity of human atherosclerotic plaques. *Circulation* 1997;95:594–599.

227. Toussaint J-F, LaMuraglia GM, Southern JF, et al. Magnetic resonance images lipid, fibrous, calcified, hemorrhagic, and thrombotic components of human atherosclerosis in vivo. *Circulation.* 1996;94:932–938.

228. Thogersen AM, Jansson JH, Boman K, et al. High plasminogen activator inhibitor and tissue plasminogen activator levels in plasma precede a first acute myocardial infarction in both men and women: evidence for the fibrinolytic system as an independent primary risk factor. *Circulation* 1998;98:2241–2247.

229. Koksch M, Zeiger F, Wittig K, et al. Haemostatic derangement in advanced peripheral occlusive arterial disease. *Int Angiol.* 1999;18:256–262.

230. Salomon O, Huna-Baron R, Moisseiev J, et al. Thrombophilia as a cause for central and branch retinal artery occlusion in patients without an apparent embolic source. *Eye.* 2001;15: 511–514.

231. Alagozlu H, Bakici Z, Gultekin F, et al. Anticardiolipin antibody positivity in diabetic patients with and without diabetic foot. *J Diabetes Complications.* 2002;16:172–175.

232. Ren S, Shen GX. Impact of antioxidants and HDL on glycated LDL-induced generation of fibrinolytic regulators from vascular endothelial cells. *Arterioscler Thromb Vasc Biol.* 2000;20: 1688–1693.

233. Kim C-H, Park H-J, Park J-Y, et al. High serum lipoprotein(a) levels in Korean type 2 diabetic patients with proliferative diabetic retinopathy. *Diabetes Care.* 1998;21:2149–2151.

234. Levy PJ, Cooper CF, Gonzalez MF. Massive lower extremity arterial thrombosis and acute hepatic insufficiency in a young adult with premature atherosclerosis associated with hyperlipoprotein(a)emia and antiphospholipid syndrome. A case report. *Angiology.* 1995;46:853–858.

235. Zhang J, Ren S, Shen GX. Glycation amplifies lipoprotein(a)-induced alterations in the generation of fibrinolytic regulators from human vascular endothelial cells. *Atherosclerosis.* 2000; 150:299–308.

236. Sobel BE, Woodcock-Mitchell J, Schneider DJ, et al. Increased plasminogen activator inhibitor type 1 in coronary artery atherectomy specimens from type 2 diabetic compared with nondiabetic patients: a potential factor predisposing to thrombosis and its persistence. *Circulation* 1998;97: 2213–2221.

237. Albertini J-P, Valensi P, Lormeau B, et al. Elevated concentrations of soluble E-selectin and vascular cell adhesion Molecule-1 in NIDDM. Effect of intensive insulin treatment. *Diabetes Care.* 1998;21: 1008–1013.

238. Lottermoser K, Hertfelder HJ, Vetter H, et al. Fibrinolytic function in diuretic-induced volume depletion. *Am J Hypertens*. 2000;13:359–363.

239. Nakamura S, Nakamura I, Ma L, et al. Plasminogen activator inhibitor-1 expression is regulated by the angiotensin type 1 receptor *in vivo*. *Kidney Int*. 2000;58:251–259.

240. Toba K, Ouchi Y, Akishita M, et al. Improved skin blood flow and cutaneous temperature in the foot of a patient with arteriosclerosis obliterans by vasopressin V1 antagonist (OPC21268): a case report. *Angiology* 1995;46:1027–1034.

241. Ridker PM, Glynn RJ, Miletich JP, et al. Age-specific rates of venous thromboembolism among heterozygous carriers of factor V Leiden mutation. *Ann Intern Med*. 1997;126: 528–531.

242. Midorikawa S, Sanada H, Hashimoto S, et al. Enhancement by homocysteine of plasminogen activator inhibitor-1 gene expression and secretion from vascular endothelial and smooth muscle cells. *Biochem Biophys Res Commun*. 2000;272: 182–185.

243. Stern JM, Saver JL, Boldy RM, et al. Homocysteine associated hypercoagulability and disseminated thrombosis, a case report. *Angiology*. 1998;49:765–769.

244. Hofmann MA, Kohl B, Zumbach MS, et al. Hyperhomocyst(e)inemia and endothelial dysfunction in IDDM. *Diabetes Care*. 1998;21:841–848.

245. Gruden G, Cavallo-Perin P, Bazzan M, et al. PA1-1 and factor VII activity are higher in IDDM patients with microalbuminuria. *Diabetes*. 1994;43426–43429.

246. Numminen H, Syrjala M, Benthin G, et al. The effect of acute ingestion of a large dose of alcohol on the hemostatic system and its circadian variation. *Stroke*. 2000;31:1269–1273.

247. Boscaro M, Sonino N, Scarda A, et al. Anticoagulant prophylaxis markedly reduces thromboembolic complications in Cushing's syndrome. *J Clin Endocrinol Metab*. 2002;87: 3662–3666.

248. Sartori MT, Patrassi GM, Rigotti P, et al. Improved fibrinolytic capacity after withdrawal of steroid immunosuppression in renal transplant recipients. *Transplantation* 2000;69: 2116–2121.

249. MacFarlane RG. Fibrinolysis following operation. *Lancet* 1937;1:10–12.

250. El-Sayed MS, Sale C, Jones PG, et al. Blood hemostasis in exercise and training. *Med Sci Sports Exercise* 2000;32:918–925.

251. Tripolitis AJ, Bodily KD, Blackshear WM, Jr, et al. Venous capacitance and outflow in the postoperative patient. *Ann Surg*. 1979;190:634–637.

252. Sacks T, Moldow CF, Craddock PR, et al. Oxygen radicals mediate endothelial cell damage by complement-stimulated granulocytes. *J Clin Invest*. 1978;61:1161–1167.

253. Stewart GJ, Stern HR, Schaub RG. Endothelial alterations, deposition of blood elements and increased accumulation of [131] I-albumen in canine jugular veins following abdominal surgery. *Thromb Res*. 1978;12:555–563.

254. Back N, et al. Fibrinolytic studies with biguanide derivatives. *Ann NY Acad Sci*. 1969;148:691.

255. Fearnley GR, Chakrabarti R, Evans JF. Mode of action of phenformin plus ethyloestrenol on fibrinolysis. *Lancet* 1971; 1:723–735.

256. Fearnley GR, Chakrabarti R, Evans JF. Fibrinolytic and defibrinating effect of phenformin plus ethyloestrenol *in vivo*. *Lancet* 1969;1:910–914.

257. Fiaschi E, Barbui T, Previato G, et al. The effects of phenphormin on blood fibrinolysis in diabetes mellitus. *Arzneimittelforschung*. 1969;19:638–640.

258. Cunliffe WJ, Menon IS. Treatment of Behcet's syndrome with phenformin and ethyloestrenol. *Lancet* 1969;1:1239–1240.

259. Galvan L. Effects of heparin on wound healing. *J WOCN* 1966;23:224–226.

260. Minnema MC, ten Cate H, van Beek EJ, et al. Effects of heparin therapy on fibrinolysis in patients with pulmonary embolism. *Thromb Haemost*. 1997;77:1164–1167.

261. Prisco D, Paniccia R, gensini GF, et al. Effect of low-dose heparin treatment on fibrinolysis in patients with previous myocardial infarction. *Haemostasis*. 1993;23:308–313.

262. Upchurch GR, Valeri CR, Khuri SF, et al. Effect of heparin on fibrinolytic activity and platelet function *in vivo*. *Am J Physiol*. 1996;271:H528–H534.

263. Lojewski B, Backer P, Iqbal O, et al. Evaluation of hemostatic and fibrinolytic alterations associated with daily administration of low-molecular-weight heparin for a 12-week period. *Semin Thromb Hemost*. 1995;21:228–239.

264. Psuja P, Tokarz A, Turowiecka Z, et al. Activation of the fibrinolytic system following subcutaneous administration and inhalation of heparin. *Pol Tyg Lek*. 1993;48:105–108.

265. Klein KL, Pittelkow MR. Tissue plasminogen activator for treatment of livedoid vasculitis. *Mayo Clin Proc*. 1992;67: 923–933.

266. Bhatnagar PK, Ierardi RP, Ikeda Y, et al. The impact of thrombolytic therapy on arterial and graft occlusions: a critical analysis. *J Cardiovasc Surg*. 1996;37:105–112.

267. Lang EK. Streptokinase therapy: complications of intra-arterial use. *Radiology*. 1985;154:75–77.

268. Sniderman KW, Kalman PG, Odurny A, et al. Low dose fibrinolytic therapy for recent extermity thromboembolism. *J Can Assoc Radiol*. 1989;40:98–103.

269. Law MM, Gelabert HA, Colburn MD, et al. Continuous postoperative intra-arterial urokinase infusion in the treatment of no reflow following revascularization of the acutely ischemic limb. *Ann Vasc Surg*. 1994;8:66–73.

270. Knight MTN, Dawson R. Effect of intermittent compression of the arms on deep vein thrombosis in the legs. *Lancet* 1976; II:1265–1267.

271. Conchonnet PH, Mismetti P, Reynaud J, et al. Fibrinolysis and elastic compression; no fibrinolytic effect of elastic compression in healthy volunteers. *Blood Coagul Fibrinolysis* 1994; 5:949–953.

272. Salzman EW, McManama GP, Shapiro AH, et al. Effect of optimization of hemodynamics on fibrinolytic activity and antithrombotic efficacy of external pneumatic calf compression. *Ann Surg*. 1987;206:636–641.

273. Tarnay TJ, Rohr PR, Davidson AG, et al. Pneumatic calf compression, fibrinolysis, and the prevention of deep venous thrombosis. *Surgery*. 1980;88:489–496.

274. Watanabe H. Postoperative deep venous thrombosis prevention with intermittent sequential compression. *Nippon Geka Gakkai Zasshi*. 1985;86:1654–1663.

275. Inada K, Koike S, Shirai N, et al. Effects of intermittent pneumatic leg compression for prevention of postoperative deep venous thrombosis with special reference to fibrinolytic activity. *Am J of Surg*. 1988;155:602–605.

276. Jacobs DG, Piotrowski JJ, Hoppensteadt DA, et al. Hemodynamic and fibrinolytic consequences of intermittent pneumatic compression: Preliminary results. *J Trauma*. 1996;40: 710–716.

277. Comerota AJ, Chouhan V, Harada RN, et al. The fibrinolytic effects of intermittent pneumatic compression: Mechanism of enhanced fibrinolysis. *Ann Surg.* 1997;226:306–313.

278. Christen Y, Wutschert R, Weimer D, et al. Effects of intermittent pneumatic compression on venous haemodynamics and fibrinolytic activity. *Blood Coagul Fibrinolysis* 1997;3: 185–190.

279. Kosir MA, Schmittinger L, Barno-Winarski L, et al. Prospective double-arm study of fibrinolysis in surgical patients. *J Surg Res.* 1998;74:96–101.

280. Killewich LA, Cahan MA, Hanna DJ, et al. The effect of external pneumatic compression on regional fibrinolysis in a prospective randomized trial. *J Vasc Surg.* 2002;36: 953–958.

281. Guyton DP, Khayat A, Schreiber H, et al. Endogenous plasminogen activator and venous flow: therapeutic implications. *Crit Care Med.* 1987;15:122–125.

282. Blackshear WM Jr, Prescott C, LePain F, et al. Influence of sequential pneumatic compression on postoperative venous function. *J Vasc Surg.* 1987;5:432–436.

283. Parente L, Perretti M. Advances in the pathophysiology of constitutive and inducible cyclooxygenases: two enzymes in the spotlight. *Biochem Pharmacol.* 2003;65:153–159.

284. Smyth EM, FitzGerald GA. Human prostacyclin receptor. *Vitam Horm.* 2002;65:149–165.

285. Busse R, Edwards G, Feletou M, et al. EDHF: bringing the concepts together. *Trends Pharmacol Sci.* 2002;23:374–380.

286. Guyton DP, Khayat A, Husni EA, et al. Elevated levels of 6-keto-prostaglandin-F_1a from lower extremity during external pneumatic compression. *Surg Gynecol Obstet.* 1988;166: 338–342.

287. Rubanyi GM, Romero JC, Vanhoutte PM. Flow-induced release of endothelium-derived relaxing factor. *Am J Physiol.* 1986;250:1145–1149.

288. Mehta P. Aspirin in the prophylaxis of coronary artery disease. *Curr Opin Cardiol.* 2002;17:552–558.

289. Linton MF, Fazio S. Cyclooxygenase-2 and atherosclerosis. *Curr Opin Lipidol.* 2002;13:497–504.

290. Schellong SM, Burchert W, Boger RM, et al. Prostaglandin E_1 in peripheral vascular disease: a PET study of muscular blood flow. *Scand J Clin Lab Invest.* 1998;58:109–117.

291. Matsumoto K, Morishita R, Tomita N, et al. Impaired endothelial dysfunction in diabetes mellitus rats was restored by oral administration of prostaglandin 12 analogue. *J Endocrinol.* 2002;175:217–223.

292. Kamper AM, Paul LC, Blauw GJ. Prostaglandins are involved in acetylcholine- and 5-hydroxytryptamine-induced, nitric oxide-mediated vasodilation in human forearm. *J Cardiovasc Pharmacol.* 2002;40:922–929.

293. Humbert M, Maitre S, Capron F, et al. Pulmonary edema complicating continuous intravenous prostacyclin in pulmonary capillary hemangiomatosis. *Am J Respir Crit Care Med.* 1998;157:1681–1685.

294. Palmer SM, Robinson L J, Wang AD, et al. Massive pulmonary edema and death after prostacyclin infusion in a patient with pulmonary venoocclusive disease. *Chest.* 1998; 113:237–240.

295. Chang CH, Yu HS, Wang MT, et al. Study on blackfoot disease: with special reference to evaluating its cutaneous microcirculatory status. *Kaohsiung J Med Sci.* 1993;9: 559–566.

296. Palmer RMJ, Ferrige AG, Moncada S. Nitric oxide release accounts for the biological activity of endothelium-derived relaxing factor. *Nature.* 1987;327:524–526.

297. Griffith TM, Lewis MJ, Newby A. et al. Endothelium derived relaxing factor. *J Am College Cardiol.* 1988;12:797–806.

298. Boykin JV, Jr, Kalns JE, Shawler LG, et al. Diabetes-impaired wound healing predicted by urinary nitrate assay: a preliminary, retrospective study. *Wounds.* 1999;11:62–69.

299. Schellong SM, Boger RM, Burchert W, et al. Dose-related effects of intravenous L-arginine on muscular blood flow of the calf in patients with peripheral vascular disease: a H215O positron emission tomography study. *Clin Sci.* 1997;93: 159–165.

300. Schmetterer L, Findl O, Fasching P, et al. Nitric oxide and ocular blood flow in patients with IDDM. *Diabetes.* 1997; 46:653–658.

301. Maxwell AJ, Anderson BE, Cooke JP. Nutritional therapy for peripheral arterial disease: a double-blind, placebo-controlled, randomized trial of HeartBar. *Vasc Med.* 2000;5:11–19.

302. Venho B, Voutilainen S, Valkonen VP, et al. Arginine intake, blood pressure, and the incidence of acute coronary events in men: the Kuopio Ischaemic Heart Disease Risk Factor Study. *Am J Clin Nutr.* 2002;76:359–364.

303. Hillig T, Krustrup P, Fleming I, et al. Cytochrome P450 2C9 plays an important role in the regulation of exercise-induced skeletal muscle blood flow and oxygen uptake in humans. *J Physiol.* 2003;546:307–314.

304. Morgan RH, Carolan G, Dsaila JV, et al. Arterial flow enhancement by impulse compression. *Vasc Surg.* 1991;25: 8–15.

305. Arnal JF, Dinh-Xuan AT, Pueyo M, Darblade B, Rami J. Endothelium-derived nitric oxide and vascular physiology and pathology. *Cell Mol Life Sci.* 1999;55:1078–1087.

306. Zhang L, Looney CG, Qi WN, et al. Reperfusion injury is reduced in skeletal muscle by inhibition of inducible nitric oxide synthase. *J Appl Physiol.* 2003;94:1473-1478.

307. Danson EJ, Paterson DJ. Enhanced neuronal nitric oxide synthase expression is central to cardiac vagal phenotype in exercise-trained mice. *J Physiol.* 2003;546:225–232.

308. Brunner F, Maier R, Andrew P, et al. Attenuation of myocardial ischemia/reperfusion injury in mice with myocyte-specific overexpression of endothelial nitric oxide synthase. *Cardiovasc Res.* 2003;57:55–62.

309. Dulak J, Jozkowicz A, Dembinska-Kiec A, et al. Nitric oxide induces the synthesis of vascular endothelial growth factor by rat vascular smooth muscle cells. *Arterioscler Thromb Vasc Biol.* 2000;20:659–666.

310. Jang JJ, Ho HK, Kwan HH, et al. Angiogenesis is impaired by hypercholesterolemia: role of asymmetric dimethylarginine. *Circulation.* 2000;102:1414–1419.

311. He H, Venema VJ, Gu X, et al. Vascular endothelial growth factor signals endothelial cell production of nitric oxide and prostacyclin through flk-1/KDR activation of c-Src. *J Biol Chem.* 1999;274:25130–25135.

312. Levy AP. A cellular paradigm for the failure to increase vascular endothelial growth factor in chronically hypoxic states. *Coron Artery Dis.* 1999;10:427–430.

313. Urbich C, Stein M, Reisinger K, et al. Fluid shear stress-induced transcriptional activation of the vascular endothelial growth factor receptor-2 gene requires Sp1-dependent DNA binding. *FEBS Lett.* 2003;535:87–93.

314. Zheng W, Brown MD, Brock TA, et al. Bradycardia-induced coronary angiogenesis is dependent on vascular endothelial growth factor. *Circ Res.* 1999;85:192–198.

315. Vale PR, Isner JM, Rosenfield K. Therapeutic angiogenesis in critical limb and myocardial ischemia. *J Interv Cardiol.* 2001; 14:511–528.

316. Lederman RJ, Mendelsohn FO, Anderson RD, et al. TRAF-FIC Investigators: therapeutic angiogenesis with recombinant fibroblast growth factor-2 for intermittent claudication (the TRAFFIC study): a randomised trial. *Lancet* 2002;359: 2053–2058.

317. Nitta K, Uchida K, Kimata N, et al. Recombinant human erythropoietin stimulates vascular endothelial growth factor release by glomerular endothelial cells. *Eur J Pharmacol.* 1999; 373:121–124.

318. Chae JK, Kim I, Lim ST, et al. Coadministration of angiopoietin-1 and vascular endothelial growth factor enhances collateral vascularization. *Arterioscler Thromb Vasc Biol.* 2000;20: 2573–2578.

319. de Lalla F, Pellizzer G, Strazzabosco M, et al. Randomized prospective controlled trial of recombinant granulocyte colony-stimulating factor as adjunctive therapy for limb-threatening diabetic foot infection. *Antimicrob Agents Chemother.* 2001;45:1094–1098.

320. Dillon RS. Effect of therapy with pneumatic end-diastolic leg compression boot on peripheral vascular tests and on the clinical course of peripheral vascular disease. *Angiology.* 1980; 31:614–638.

321. Vella A, Carlson LA, Blier B, et al. Circulator Boot therapy alters the natural history of ischemic limb ulceration. *Vasc Med.* 2000;5:21–25.

322. Missov RM, Stolk RP, van der Bom JG, et al. Plasma fibrinogen in NIDDM, The Rotterdam Study. *Diabetes Care.* 1996; 19:157–159.

323. Matzke S, Biancari F, Ihlberg L, et al. Increased preoperative creactive protein level as a prognostic factor for postoperative amputation after femoropopliteal bypass surgery for CLI. *Ann Chir Gynaecol.* 2001;90:19–22.

324. *Metropol Life Ins Co Stat. Bull.* 1959;40:11–12.

325. Facchini FS, Hua N, Abbasi F, Reaven GM. Insulin resistance as a predictor of age-related diseases. *J Clin Endocrinol Metab.* 2001;86:3574–3578.

326. Fernandez-Real JM, Broch M, Vendrell J, Ricart W. Insulin resistance, inflammation, and serum fatty acid composition. *Diabetes Care.* 2003;26:1362–1368.

327. Paris RM, Bedno SA, Krauss MR, et al. Weighing in on type 2 diabetes in the military: characteristics of U.S. military personnel at entry who develop type 2 diabetes. *Diabetes Care.* 2001;24:1894–1898.

328. Sjostrom L. In: Obesity, Theory and Therapy; 2nd ed New York: Raven Press; 1993:13.

329. Berenson GS, Srinivasan SR. Emergence of obesity and cardiovascular risk for coronary artery disease: the Bogalusa Heart Study. *Prev Cardiol.* 2001;4(3):116–121.

330. Salans LB, Wse JK. Metabolic studies in obesity. *Med Clin N Am.* 1970;54:1533.

331. Bray GA. Measurement of subcutaneous fat cells. *Ann Intern Med.* 1970;73: 565.

332. Stern JS, Batchelor BR, Hollander N, et al. Adipose cell size and immunoreactive insulin levels in obese and normal-weight adults. *Lancet* 1972;2:948–951.

333. Albrink MJ, Meigs JW, Granoff MA. Weight gain and serum triglycerides in normal men. *N Engl J Med.* 1962;266:484.

334. Kannel WB, Brand N, Skinner JJ, Jr, et al. The relationship of adiposity to blood pressure and development of hypertension. *Ann Intern Med.* 1967;67:48–59.

335. Reisin E, Abel R, Modan M, et al. Effect of weight loss without salt restriction on the reduction of blood pressure in overweight hypertensive patients. *N Engl J Med.* 1978; 298:1–6.

336. Kraegen EW, Cooney GJ, Ye J, et al. Triglycerides, fatty acids, and insulin resistance–hyperinsulinemia. *Exp Clin Endocrinol Diabetes.* 2001;109:S516–S526.

337. Matsuzawa Y, Funahashi T, Nakamura T. Molecular mechanism of metabolic syndrome X: contribution of adipocytokines adipocyte-derived bioactive substances. *Ann N Y Acad Sci.* 1999;892:146–154.

338. The Diabetes Prevention Program Research Group: *N Engl J Med.* 2002;346:393–403.

339. Horwitz O, Abramson DG. A modification of the vasodilatation test. *Am J Cardiol.* 1960;6:663.

340. Dillon RS. Treatment of resistant venous stasis ulcers and dermatitis with the end-diastolic pneumatic compression boot. *Angiology* 1986;37:47–57.

341. Hermann LG, Reid MR. The conservative treatment of peripheral vascular diseases. *Ann Surg* 1934;100:750–760.

342. Silverglade A. Peripheral vascular disease: diagnosis and treatment by passive vascular exercises. *Arch Phys Ther.* 1940;XXI: 100–110.

343. Allwood MJ. The effect of an increased local pressure gradient on blood flow in the foot. *Clin Sci.* 1957;16:231–239.

344. Loane RA. Effect of rhythmically inflating a pneumatic cuff at the ankle on blood flow in the foot. *J Appl Physiol.* 1959;14: 411–413.

345. Henry JP, Winsor T. Compensation of arterial insufficiency by augmenting the circulation with intermittent compression of the limbs. *Am Heart J.* 1965;70:79–88.

346. Gaskell P, Parrott JCW. The effect of a mechanical venous pump on the circulation of the feet in the presence of arterial obstruction. *Surg Gyn Obstet.* 1978;146:583–592.

347. Agerskov K, Tofft HP, Jensen FB, et al. External negative thigh pressure. Effect upon blood flow and pressure in the foot in patients with occlusive arterial disease. *Dan Med Bull.* 1990; 37:451–454.

348. Abu-Own A, Cheatle T, Scurr JH, et al. Effects of intermittent pneumatic compression of the foot on the microcirculatory function in arterial disease. *Eur J Vasc Surg.* 1993;7:488–492.

349. Eze AR, Comerota AJ, Cisek PL, et al. Intermittent calf and foot compression increases lower extremity blood flow. *Am J Surg.* 1996;172:130–135.

350. Koch CA. External leg compression in the treatment of vascular disease. *Angiology* 1997;(Suppl 49):s3–s15.

351. Delis KT, Nicolaides AN, Wolfe JH, Stansby G. Improving walking ability and ankle brachial pressure indices in symptomatic peripheral vascular disease with intermittent pneumatic foot compression: a prospective controlled study with one-year follow-up. *J Vasc Surg.* 2000;31:650–661.

352. Delis KT, Nicolaides AN, Labropoulos N, Stansby G. The acute effects of intermittent pneumatic foot versus calf versus simultaneous foot and calf compression on popliteal artery hemodynamics: a comparative study. *J Vasc Surg.* 2000;32: 284–292.

353. Zheng et al., US patent 4753226.

354. Dillon RS. Optimizing external cardiac-assist compressions in patients with atrial fibrillation by anticipating the next beat. *Angiology.* 1996;47:123–129.

355. Dillon RS. US patent 5514079.

356. Morris PE, Hessel SJ, Couch NP, et al. Surgery and the progression of the occlusive process in patients with peripheral vascular disease. *Radiology.* 1977;124:343–348.

357. Balmer H, Mahler F, Do DD, et al. Balloon angioplasty in chronic critical limb ischemia: Factors affecting clinical and angiographic outcome. *J Endovasc Ther.* 2002;9:403–410.

358. Axisa B, Fishwick G, Bolia A, Thompson MM, London NJ, Bell PR, Naylor AR. Complications following peripheral angioplasty. *Ann R Coll Surg Engl.* 2002;84:39–42.

359. Neufang A, Kraus O, Dorweiler B, et al. Pedal bypass surgery in diabetic foot syndrome: indications, technique and outcome. *Med Klin.* 2002;97:256–262.

360. Pomposelli FB, Jepsen SJ, Gibbons GW, et al. Efficacy of the dorsal pedis bypass for limb salvage in diabetic patients: short term observations. *J Vasc Surg.* 1990;11:745–752.

361. Majzoub RK, Bardoel JW, Maldonado C, et al. Analysis of fiber type transformation and histology in chronic electrically stimulated canine rectus abdominis muscle island-flap stomal sphincters. *Plast Reconstr Surg.* 2003;111:189–198.

362. Askew GN, Cox VM, Altringham JD, et al. Mechanical properties of the latissimus dorsi muscle after cyclic training. *J Appl Physiol.* 2002;93:649–659.

363. Trainini J, Cabrera Fischer EI, Barisani J, et al. Dynamic aortomyoplasty in treating end-stage heart failure. *J Heart Lung Transplant.* 2002;21:1068–1073.

364. Kooguchi K, Fukui M, Tsuruta H, et al. Mechanical supports for stunned myocardium after esophagectomy. *Masui* 2002; 51:1275–1279.

365. Soran O, Fleishman B, Demarco T, et al. Enhanced external counterpulsation in patients with heart failure: a multicenter feasibility study. *Congest Heart Fail.* 2002;8:204–208, 227.

366. Goldman BS, Hill TJ, Rosenthal GA, et al. Complications associated with use of intra-aortic balloon pump. *Can J Surg.* 1982;153–156.

367. Makhoul RG, Cole CW, McCann RL. Vascular complications of the intra-aortic balloon pump: an analysis of 436 patients. *Am Surg.* 1993;59:564–568.

368. Williams DO, Korr KS, Gewirth H, et al. The effects of intraaortic balloon counterpulsation of regional myocardial blood flow and oxygen consumption in the presence of coronary artery stenosis in patients with unstable angina. *Circulation.* 1982;66:593–597.

369. Cohen LS, Mullens CB, Mitchell JH. Sequenced external counterpulsation and intraaortic balloon pumping in cardiogenic shock *Am J Cardiol.* 1973;32:656–666.

370. Solignac A, Ferguson RJ, Bourassa MG. External counterpulsation: coronary hemodynamics and use in patients with stable angina. *Cathet Cardiovasc Diag.* 1977;3:37–45.

371. Kern MJ, Henry RH, Lembo N, et al. Effects of pulsed external augmentation of diastolic pressure on coronary and systemic hemodynamics in patients with coronary artery disease. *Am Heart. J.* 1985;110:727–735.

372. Parmley WW, Chatterjee K, Charuzi Y, et al. Hemodynamic effects of noninvasive systolic unloading (nitroprusside) and diastolic augmentation (external counterpulsation) in patients with acute myocardial infarction. *Am J Cardiol.* 1974;33: 819–825.

373. Amsterdam EA, Lee G, Tonkon MJ, et al. Noninvasive circulatory assistance by external counterpulsation. In: Mason DT. ed. *Advances in Heart Disease, Vol. I,* New York: Grune & Stratton; 1977.

374. Toyota E, Goto M, Nakamoto H, et al. Endothelium-derived nitric oxide enhances the effect of intraaortic balloon pumping on diastolic coronary flow. *Ann Thorac Surg.* 1999;67:1254–1261.

375. Dillon RS. Improved hemodynamics shown by continuous monitoring of electrical impedance during external counterpulsation with the end-diastolic pneumatic boot and improved ambulatory EKG monitoring after 3 weeks of therapy. *Angiology* 1998;49:523–535.

376. Patterson SW, Piper H, Starling EH. *J Physiol.* 1914;48:465.

377. Applebaum RM, Kasliwal R, Tunick PA, et al. Sequential external counterpulsation increases cerebral and renal blood flow. *Am Heart J* 1997;133:611–615.

378. Yu S, Da H, Zhen Z. External Counterpulsation, Review Article. *Chinese Med J* 1990;103:768–771.

379. van Bemmelen PS, Bedford G, Beach K, et al. Functional status of the deep venous system after an episode of deep venous thrombosis. *Ann Vasc Surg.* 1990;4:455–459.

380. James LR, Lajoie G, Prajapati D, et al. Calciphylaxis precipitated by ultraviolet light in a patient with end-stage renal disease secondary to systemic lupus erythematosus. *Am J Kidney Dis.* 1999;34:932–936.

381. Mawad HW, Sawaya BP, Sarin R, et al. Calcific uremic arteriolopathy in association with low turnover uremic bone disease. *Clin Nephrol.* 1999;52:160–166.

382. Zacharias JM, Fontaine B, Fine A. Calcium use increases risk of calciphylaxis: a case-control study. *Perit Dial Int.* 1999; 19:248–252.

383. Oh DH, Eulau D, Tokugawa DA, et al. Five cases of calciphylaxis and a review of the literature. *J Am Acad Dermatol.* 1999; 40(6):979–987.

384. Hafner J, Keusch G, Wahl C, et al. Calciphylaxis: a syndrome of skin necrosis and acral gangrene in chronic renal failure. *Vasa* 1998;27:137–143.

385. Sankarasubbaiyan S, Scott G, Holley JL. Cryofibrinogenemia: an addition to the differential diagnosis of calciphylaxis in end-stage renal disease. *Am J Kidney Dis.* 1998;32: 494–498.

386. Regensteiner JG, Steiner JF, Panzer RJ, et al. Evaluation of walking impairment by questionnaire in patients with peripheral arterial disease. *J Vasc Med Biol.* 1990;12:142–152.

387. Lithner F, Bergenheim T, Borssen B. Extensor digitorum brevis in diabetic neuropathy: a controlled evaluation in diabetic patients aged 15–50 years. *J Intern Med.* 1991;230:449–453.

388. Vileikyte L, Hutchings G, Hollis S, et al. The tactile circumferential discriminator. A new, simple screening device to identify diabetic patients at risk of foot ulceration. *Diabetes Care.* 1997;20:623–626.

389. Aszmann OC, Dellon AL. Relationship between cutaneous pressure threshold and two-point discrimination. *J Reconstr Microsurg.* 1998;14:417–421.

390. Vinik AI, Suwanwalaikorn S, Stansberry K, et al. Quantitative measurement of cutaneous perception in diabetic neuropathy. *Muscle Nerve* 1995;18:574–584.

391. Wheeler T, Watkins PJ. Cardiac denervation in diabetes. *Br Med J.* 1973;4:584–586.

392. Ewing DJ, Campbell IW, Burt AA, et al. Vascular reflexes in diabetic autonomic neuropathy. *Lancet* 1973;2:1354–1356.

393. Lofgren EP. Present-day indications for surgical treatment of varicose veins. *Mayo Clin Proc.* 1966;41:515–523.

394. Comerota AJ, Katz ML, White JV. Why does prophylaxis with external pneumatic compression for deep vein thrombosis fail? *Am J Surg.* 1992;164:265–268.

395. Smith PC, Sarin S, Hasty J, et al. Sequential gradient pneumatic compression hastens venous ulcer healing: a randomized trial. *Surgery.* 1990;108:871–875.

396. Mulder G, Robinson J. Seeley J. Study of sequential compression therapy in the treatment of non-healing chronic venous ulcers. *Wounds* 1990;2:111–115.

397. McCulloch JM, Marler KC, Neal MB, et al. Intermittent pneumatic compression improves venous ulcer healing. *Advan Wound Care.* 1994;7:22–26.

398. Fitzgerald DE, Carr J. Peripheral arterial disease: assessment by arteriography and alternative noninvasive measurements. *Am J Roentgenol.* 1977;128:385.

399. Brown RF, Rice P, Bennett NJ. The use of laser Doppler imaging as an aid in clinical management decision making in the treatment of vesicant burns. *Burns* 1998;24:692–698.

400. Ismail-Beigi F, Edelman IS. The mechanism of the calorigenic action of thyroid hormones. Stimulation of NA^+ and K^+ activated adenosinetriphosphatase activity. *J Gen Physiol.* 1971; 57:710.

401. Ham RG, McKeehan WL. Media and growth requirements. *Methods Enzymol.* 1979;58:44–93.

402. Dillon RS. Saving on soaks. Letter to the editor in *N Engl J Med.* 1984;311:540.

403. Calhoun JH, Cantrell J, et al. Treatment of diabetic foot infections: Wagner classification, therapy, and outcome. *Foot Ankle.* 1988;9:101–108.

404. U.S. Department of Health and Human Services, Public Health Service, Agency for Health Care Policy and Research. Clinical Practice Guideline, Number 15. Treatment of Pressure Ulcers, December. 1994, pp 12–13.

405. Wagner FW. The diabetic foot and amputations of the foot. In: Mann, R, ed. *Surgery of the Foot,* St Louis: Mosby; 1986; 423.

406. Armstrong DG, Lavery DA, Harkless LB. Validation of a diabetic wound classification system. The contribution of depth, infection, and ischemia to risk of amputation. *Diabetes Care.* 1998;21:855–859.

407. Rutherford RB, Baker JD, Ernst C, et al. Recommended standards for reports dealing with lower extremity ischemia: revised version. *J Vasc Surg.* 1997;26:517–538.

Intermittent Pneumatic Compression Devices in Critical Limb Ischemia

George Louridas

Introduction
Characterization of Critical Limb Ischemia
Mechanism of Action
  Mechanical Compression Effects
  Biochemical Compression Effects

Clinical Results
Conclusion
References

INTRODUCTION

The concept and development of external devices for improving circulation in the lower limbs originated in the 18th century. In 1812, Sir James Murray introduced the first suction device for improving lower-extremity circulation in a patient who had cholera.[1] There had been numerous reports of success with this suction device up until the 1930s.[2–4]

In 1887, Bluck[5] developed a combination suction and compression device. Herrmann further developed this device, but it was Reid, in 1932, who devised a boot-shaped pressure chamber to be applied around a lower limb. They postulated that the application of alternating pressure and suction would result in a passive vascular exercise and coined the term "PAVAEX."[6]

In the late 1950s, Allwood[7] and Loane[8] described the use of only compression therapy. They independently demonstrated that in a sitting position the arterial inflow of a leg could be improved after lowering the venous pressure.

In the late 1980s, Gardner and Fox,[9,10] while researching the physiology of venous return in the lower limb, discovered the significance of the venous foot pump. They showed that weight bearing on the sole of the foot generated enough pressure to dislocate a column of blood up to the heart against the forces of gravity. This increase in venous flow was shown to be protective in preventing deep venous thrombosis. Coincidentally, the arterial circulation was also noted to be affected. Consequent to each compression impulse, there followed a period of hyperemia, noticeably marked in the ischemic foot. This increase in arterial blood flow was particularly noted in situations where the veins had been previously filled as in the dependent position and then suddenly emptied by rapid compression of the foot venous pump.

CHARACTERIZATION OF CRITICAL LIMB ISCHEMIA

Critical limb ischemia (CLI) has been clinically defined as the presence of rest pain, ulceration or gangrene in a patient with underlying peripheral arterial occlusive disease. This is associated with an ankle pressure < 50–70 mm Hg, or a toe pressure < 30–50 mm Hg or a transcutaneous oxygen tension ($TcPO_2$) < 30– 50 mm Hg.[11]

The outcome of critical limb ischemia has been reported to be rather poor. After initial evaluation, 25% of these patients are treated medically, 25% are offered an amputation, and the remaining 50% undergo bypass surgery. At 1 year of follow-up, 25% will be cured, 20% will still have CLI, 25% will have undergone an amputation, and 25% will have died. However, the subgroup of patients with either a failed bypass graft or nonreconstructable vessels as per angiography, fare even worse—within 6 months, 20% will have died, 35% will have required an amputation, while only 45% will be alive without an amputation.[12]

The financial resources required for bypass surgery and/or amputations are formidable. Successful bypass surgery is less expensive than a primary amputation provided there are no major postoperative complications.[13–16] Amputations are themselves still very problematic. It can take up to 9 months to initially rehabilitate an amputee and, by 2 years, 30% of these patients are not using their prostheses.[17] The outcome of a below-knee amputation (BKA) has been summarized as follows. Early on, 60% heal primarily, 15% undergo secondary healing, 15% require an above-knee amputation (AKA), and 10% die perioperatively. After 2 years, only 40% will be mobile, 15% will have had a contralateral amputation, 15% will have been converted to an AKA and 30% will have died.[18] Any form of management that could be shown to successfully replace surgical intervention (especially amputation) would obviously present great benefits to both patients and healthcare systems.

Numerous elderly patients who have poor circulation in their legs, namely, very low ankle and toe pressures, but no symptoms, do not fulfill the criteria for CLI. When these patients injure their feet, they are unable to heal, as they do not have the blood supply needed to mount the inflammatory response needed to repair the injured tissues. It is suggested that if intermittent pneumatic compression devices (IPCD) were used early on in these patients, they might be able to avoid surgical interventions. A reasonable approach is to apply the IPCD to these patients for a 6 to 8-week period. If, at any time, the wound showed any sign of deterioration or of non-healing, these patients should undergo the surgical route

of angiography and intervention either radiologically or surgically.

One should be mindful of the publication Nicoloff et al.[19] from the late John Porter's group. The authors' reviewed 112 consecutive patients who underwent infrainguinal bypass surgery for limb salvage. Their results were very disconcerting. The mean patient age was 66 years. The mean postoperative follow up was 42 months (range 0–100.1 months). There were seven perioperative deaths (6.3%) and wound complications occurred in 27 patients (24%). By life table, the assisted primary graft patency and limb salvage rates of the index extremity 5 years after operation were 77 and 87%, respectively; the patient survival rate was 49%. Wound (operative and ischemic) healing required a mean of 4.2 months (range 0.4–48 months) and 25 patients (22%) had not achieved complete wound healing at the time of last follow-up or death. Repeat operations to maintain graft patency, treat wound complications, or treat recurrent or contralateral ischemia were required in 61 patients (54%). Twenty-six patients (23.2%) ultimately required major limb amputation of the index limb or contralateral extremity. Only 16 of 112 patients (14.3%) achieved the ideal surgical result of an uncomplicated operation with long-term symptom relief, maintenance of functional status, and no recurrence or repeat operation.

Intermittent pneumatic compression devices such as the ArtAssist device have been used for a long time to improve arterial inflow. The ArtAssist device is a small portable unit consisting of the pump, air tubing, and cuffs, which are placed around the foot and calf (Fig. 14–1). This form of IPCD applies very rapid, high

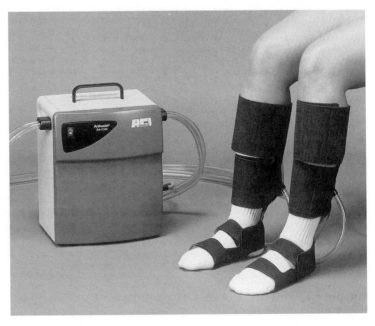

Fig. 14–1. The ArtAssist Device, showing how cuffs are placed around the foot and calf.

pressure pulses progressively up the limb and must be used with the patient in the sitting position. These devices must not be confused with those used for the prevention of deep vein thrombosis that slowly apply low pressure to patients in the supine position.

Their clinical value in chronic critical limb ischemia, however, has never been assessed by a randomized trial. In this chapter, I will attempt to review the evidence to support its use in patients with critical limb ischemia.

MECHANISM OF ACTION

Mechanical Compression Effects

When using the IPCD to improve the arterial circulation in a patient, the patient must be in a sitting position as compared to using these devices for prevention of deep vein thrombosis when the patient is placed in the supine position.[20–22] A cuff is applied with air bladders located at the foot, ankle and around the calf. Delis et al. showed that the sequential foot and calf compression was more effective in improving arterial calf blood flow than a cuff placed only around the foot or the calf.[23]

On activating the compression device (ArtAssist Model AA–1000, ACI Medical, San Marcos, CA), the foot cuff is rapidly inflated (within 300 ms) to a pressure of 120 mm Hg and after a 1-second delay, the calf cuff is then rapidly inflated (within 300 ms) to 120 mm Hg. After 3 seconds, the foot cuff deflates followed 1 second later by calf cuff deflation to complete the cycle. Inflation lasts approximately 3 seconds and deflation lasts 17 seconds. Each complete cycle is, therefore, approximately 20 seconds; there are three cycles per minute. At the completion of a cycle, the venous pressure has been decreased from about 70 mm Hg to almost zero, while arterial pressure is unaffected, thus creating a substantial increase in the arterio–venous gradient (Figs. 14–2 and 14–3). Flow is increased based upon the formula:

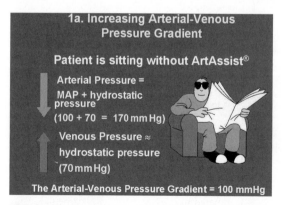

Fig. 14–2. Mechanism of action. Pressure gradients before inflation begins.

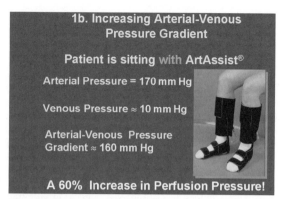

Fig. 14–3. Mechanism of action. Pressure gradients after compression has ended.

$$\text{Flow} = \frac{\text{Arterial} - \text{venous pressure}}{\text{Peripheral resistance}}$$

where the numerator and, therefore, flow, is increased with decreased venous pressure.

The most effective means of emptying the leg veins is by using intermittent pneumatic compression with the combination of a foot and calf cuff. A inflation pressure of 120 to 140 mm Hg at a frequency of 3 to 4 impulses per minute and a proximal inflation delay of 1 second, has been shown to be the optimal stimulus to achieve this.[24]

The ArtAssist Device should be used for a minimum of 3 months. Delis, in his claudication study, found maximal improvement in blood flow to the leg after 3 months on the pump; this effect lasted up to a year.[25]

It has been well demonstrated that pneumatic compression of the foot or foot and calf is associated with an increase in popliteal artery blood flow as shown by duplex scanning of the popliteal artery. There is also a marked increase in end-diastolic velocities, which is indicative of a decrease in peripheral vascular resistance stimulated by the biochemical factors discussed below.[25,26–28]

Increase in foot and toe perfusion has also been demonstrated after intermittent pneumatic compression.[22,29–31]

Intermittent pneumatic compression has also been shown to decrease the edema in lower extremities. The most likely mechanism is the result of decrease in venous pressure and hydrostatic pressure in the capillary beds.[27] Drainage of edema fluid by lymphatics is likely to be encouraged by intermittent pumping, although this form of IPCD is not optimized for lymphatic drainage.[28]

Biochemical Compression Effects

The application of an IPCD on the lower extremity results in a sudden rapid compression, which leads to emptying of the venous system beneath the cuff and a rapid onset of pulsatile blood flow in a forward direction. This sudden increase in flow causes an increase in shear stress on the endothelial cells of both veins and arteries.

This increase in shear force results in (Figs. 14–4 and 14–5):

1. The release of nitric oxide from the endothelium causing vasodilatation[32–34]

2. Release of prostacyclin, a potent vasodilator and antiplatelet agent[35,36]

3. Increase in fibrinolytic activity[34,37–42]

4. Relaxation of the venoarterial reflex[43–45]

5. The above factors lead to a decrease in peripheral vascular resistance and an increase in blood flow to the foot based upon the above flow equation wherein the denominator is decreased with a resultant increase in flow[20,23,30,46]

All data support the assertion that intermittent pneumatic compression does improve arterial circulation to the calf and foot in patients with peripheral arterial occlusive disease.

An overview of the effects of IPCD is shown in Fig. 14–6.

CLINICAL RESULTS

In the only prospective randomized trial published to date, Delis et al.[25] showed significant benefit in claudicants who were randomized to the intermittent compression group as compared to the control group. The maximal effect was seen at 3 months; the benefit lasted for at least 1 year.

Vella et al.[47] reported their experience in treating ischemic ulcers at the Mayo clinic with intermittent compression. Of the 96 patients treated, 19 (20%) had

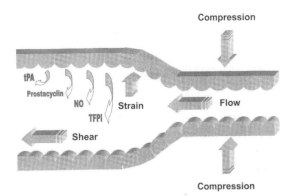

Fig. 14–5. The release of biochemical factors from the endothelium after rapid compression. tPA, tissue plasminogen activator; NO, nitric oxide; TFPI, tissue factor pathway inhibitor. Reproduced from Chen et al. (55) with permission of *Eur J Vasc Endovas Surg.*

an unfavorable outcome in that 17 needed amputation and the ulcer increased in size in 2 patients. It is important to note that all these patients had a TcPO$_2$ < 20 mm Hg. The remaining 77 (80%) patients had a favorable outcome, ie, either the ulcers healed, decreased in size or patients came to successful bypass. None of these patients in this group lost a limb. It is important to realize that out of the 77 patients with a favorable outcome, 19(24.6%) had TcPO$_2$ < 20 mm Hg. From this study it is difficult to predict which patients are likely to respond to the IPCD. Bacharach et al.[48] predicted that wounds with TcPO$_2$ < 20 mm Hg will not heal, however, in this study, 38 (39.5%) patients had TcPO$_2$ < 20 mm Hg of which 19 (50%) patients had favorable outcomes. One can only conclude from this study that all patients should be given the benefit of the IPCD and not selected out because of low TcPO$_2$ levels.

Van Bemmelen[49] treated 13 patients with 14 legs having critical limb ischemia. All his patients were non-surgical candidates as a result of no target outflow vessels, no autologous vein material available for bypass grafting, or not fit for surgery. Of the 14 legs, all had rest pain and 13 had tissue loss. Patients were advised to pump their legs for 4 hours a day for 3 months. At the end of the study, with a mean follow-up of 8.7 months (range 0.5–23 months), 70% of patients had saved their limb, while only 4 (30%) came to amputation. It is interesting to note that in patients in whom limb salvage was achieved, these patients used their compression devices for a longer period of time (mean 2.38 hours/day) as compared to those patients who came to amputation (mean 1.14 hours/day). Good compliance with using the IPCD resulted in better outcomes.

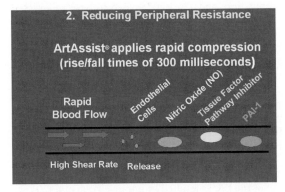

Fig. 14–4. The release of factors from the endothelial cells.

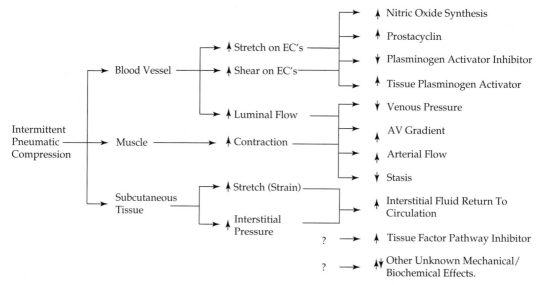

Fig. 14–6. Overview of the mechanical effects of intermittent pneumatic compression. Reproduced from Chen et al. (55) with permission of *Eur J Vas C Endovasc Surg.*

Louridas et al.,[50] in a prospective pilot study, treated 33 legs in 25 patients. All patients were considered to be nonsurgical candidates for bypass surgery. Patients were advised to use the IPCD for 3 hours a day for 3 months. Ten legs presented with rest pain, while 23 had tissue loss. Of the 10 legs presenting with rest pain, 3 came to amputation at a mean follow-up of 3 months and 7 were salvaged. At a mean follow-up of 9 months, one patient had acceptable ongoing rest pain, four improved to claudication, and the remaining two underwent bypass surgery and were cured. These two patients were initially felt to have very poor target vessels to bypass and were, therefore, not referred to surgery. When their symptoms deteriorated, surgery was attempted and was successful until the study ended. Twenty-three patients presented with tissue loss, of these, 11 came to amputation at a mean follow up of 3 months, and, of the remaining 12 legs, 1 ulcer healed, 8 improved, and 3 remained the same. At a mean follow-up of 9 months, three patients died, five ulcers healed spontaneously, two ulcers healed after undergoing inflow procedures, and two limbs have ongoing ulcers, which are being treated medically.

Overall, 40% of patients presenting with rest pain improved, whereas only 23% of ulcers healed on the IPCD. The study also confirmed that patients with $TcPO_2 > 29$ mm Hg healed their ulcers, however 4 out of 9 (44%) patients with $TcPO_2 < 29$ mm Hg also healed their ulcers. Of the patients who came to amputation, 80% were in chronic renal failure on dialysis. In this study, patients in renal failure and on dialysis did very poorly, amputation rate was 80%, whereas it was only 13% in the nonrenal failure patients.

Montori et al.[51] reporting from the Mayo clinic, have reviewed their latest experience using the IPCD. They reviewed 101 patients with ulcers in their lower limbs that underwent therapy with the IPCD. Patients were advised to pump for 6 hours per day. Follow-up was for 35 weeks. It is interesting to note that $TcPO_2$ did not help them differentiate between responders and nonresponders to the IPCD. Diabetics did as well as nondiabetics. Finally 56% of patients healed their wounds and, in this group, 86% had an intact limb, 16% had an amputation, and 1% were advised to have an amputation. Of the patients 44% did not heal their ulcers and, in this group, only 59% had an intact limb, 32% came to amputation, and 9% were advised to have an amputation. This study again confirms that there is benefit in using the IPCD in this high-risk group of patients.

Armstrong et al.,[52] in a prospective double blinded, randomized, placebo-controlled study, in diabetic patients showed that IPCD improved the edema in the foot and improved wound healing after these patients had undergone debridement of their foot infections. The study was performed in 115 patients. The authors again confirmed that increase in compliance with the use of the IPCD resulted in improved outcomes.

Dillon has reviewed his 15-year experience with a cardiosynchronous form of IPCD in treating patients with peripheral arterial occlusive disease and also patients who have leg ulcers. His results are very impressive, but, unfortunately, he never randomized any of his patients.[53,54]

To date, the role of IPCD in patients who have chronic wounds in well vascularized legs has not been investigated. One can only speculate that IPCD will increase the blood supply to the wound and this may accelerate the healing process.

CONCLUSION

Intermittent pneumatic compression devices have been shown to improve blood supply to the calf and the foot in patients who have peripheral arterial occlusive disease.

Prospective randomized controlled studies have proved the benefit of this mode of therapy in patients with intermittent claudication.

Numerous studies have shown the benefit of this form of therapy in patients with critical limb ischemia and nonhealing ulcers. It should be remembered that these patients have a generalized disease process called atherosclerosis and their life span is very limited by this process. Therefore, implementing therapy in an attempt to prevent limb loss, improve rest pain, and heal nonhealing ulcers should be undertaken. The advantage of this form of therapy is that it is very benign. It is simple, easy to use, and very portable, allowing the patient to use it wherever he is, ie, in the hospital, at home or on vacation.

What is needed is a randomized study to confirm the above results. This study is presently being conducted in the author's institution. However, until these results are available, patients with critical limb ischemia (rest pain, gangrenous patches on toes, and nonhealing ulcers) should be encouraged to use this device, as it can only be of benefit to them.

Patients who are good surgical candidates should still be advised to undergo bypass surgery in order to save their limbs. At present, the IPCD cannot be used as a replacement for surgical bypass in low-risk surgical candidates.

REFERENCES

1. Murray J. Nature and treatment of cholera—new method proposed. *London Med Surg J.* 1832;1:749–752.
2. Clanny WR. Apparatus for removing the pressure of the atmosphere from the body or limbs. *Lancet.* 1835;1:804–805.
3. Bier A. Veber einege Verbesserungen Hyperamisterender Apparate. *Munich Med Wochenschr.* 1904;5:241.
4. Sinkowitz SJ, Gottlieb I. Thromboangiitis obliterans—the conservative treatment by Bier's hyperemia suction apparatus. *JAMA.* 1917;68:961–963.
5. Bluck E. *Improvement Means or Appliances for Promoting or Modifying the Circulation of the Blood in a Living Body.* London: Darling and Sons, 1888.
6. Reid MR, Herrmann LG. Passive vascular exercise-treatment of vascular disease by rhythmic alternation of environmental pressure. *Arch Surg.* 1933;29:697–704.
7. Allwood MJ. The effect of increase local pressure gradient on blood flow in the foot. *Clin Sci* 1957;16:231–239.
8. Loane AR. Effect of rhythmically inflating a pneumatic cuff at the ankle on blood flow in the foot. *J Appl Physiol.* 1959; 14:411–413.
9. Gardner AMN, Fox RH. Reduction of post-traumatic swelling and compartment pressure by impulse compression of the foot. *J Bone Joint Surg.* (Br) 1990;72B:810–815.
10. Gardner AMN, Fox RH. *The Return of Blood to the Heart.* 2nd ed. London: John Libbey; 1993.
11. TransAtlantic Inter-Society Consensus Document. *J Vasc Surg.* 2000;31:1:S170.
12. TransAtlantic Inter-Society Consensus Document. *J Vasc Surg.* 2000;31:1:S25.
13. Cheshire NJW, Wolfe MS, Noone MA, et al. The economics of femorocrural reconstruction for critical leg ischaemia with and without autologous veins. *J Vasc Surg.* 1992;15:167–175.
14. Mackey WC, McCullough JL, Conlon TP, et al. The costs of surgery for limb threatening ischaemia. *Surgery.* 1986;99: 26–34.
15. Gupta SK, Veith FJ. Is arterial reconstruction cost effective compared with amputation? In: Greenhalgh RM, et al. eds. *Limb Salvage and Amputation for Vascular Disease.* Philadelphia, Saunders; 1988:447–452.
16. Panayiotopoulos YP, Tyrrel MR, Owen SE, et al. Outcome and cost analysis after femorocrural and femoropedal grafting for critical limb ischaemia. *Br J Surg.* 1997;84:207–212.
17. Kihn RB, Warren R, Beebe GW. The geriatric amputee. *Ann Surg.* 1972;176:305–314.
18. TransAtlantic Inter-Society Consensus Document. *J Vasc Surg.* 2000;31(1)S26.
19. Nicoloff AD, Taylor LM, McLafferty RB, et al. Patient recovery after infrainguinal bypass grafting for limb salvage. *J Vasc Surg.* 1998;27:256–266.
20. van Bemmelen PS, Mattos M, Faught WE, et al. Augmentation of blood flow in limbs with occlusive arterial disease by intermittent calf compression. *J Vasc Surg.* 1994;19:1052–1058.
21. Morgan RH, Carolan G, Psaila JV, et al. Arterial enhancement by impulse compression. *Vasc Surg.* 1991;25:8–15.
22. Abu-Own A, Cheatle T, Scurr JH, et al. Effects of intermittent pneumatic compression of the foot on the microcirculatory function in arterial diease. *Eur J Vasc Surg.* 1993;7:488–492.
23. Delis KT, Nicolaides AN, Labropoulos N, et al. The acute effects of intermittent pneumatic foot versus calf versus simultaneous foot and calf compression on the popliteal artery haemodynamics: A comparative study. *J Vasc Surg.* 2000;32:284–292.
24. Delis KT, Aziz ZA, Stevens RJG, et al. Optimum intermittent pneumatic compression stimulus for lower-limb venous emptying. *Eur J Vasc Endovasc Surg.* 2000;19:261–269.
25. Deils KT, Nicolaides AN, Wolfe JH, et al. Improving walking ability and ankle brachial pressure indices in symptomatic peripheral vascular disease with intermittent pneumatic foot compression: A prospective controlled study with one year follow up. *J Vasc Surg.* 2000;31:650–661.
26. Labropoulos N, Watson WC, Mansour MA, et al. Acute effects of intermittent pneumatic compression on popliteal artery blood flow. *Arch Surg.* 1998;133:1072–1075.

27. White JV, Zarge MD. The plantar venous plexus and applications of A-V impulse system technology. *Int Angiol.* 1996;15:3 (Suppl. 1) 42–50.

28. Gardner AMN, Fox RH, Lawrence C, et al. Reduction of post traumatic swelling and compartment pressures by impulse compression of the foot. *J Bone Joint Surg.* (Br) 1990;72-B: 810–815.

29. Gaskell P, Parrott JCW. The effect of a mechanical venous pump on the arterial circulation of the feet in the presence of arterial obstruction. *Surg Gynaecol Obstet.* 1978;146:583–592.

30. Eze AR, Comerota AJ, Cisek PL, et al. Intermittent calf and foot compression increases lower extremity blood flow. *Am J Surg.* 1996;172:130–135.

31. Delis KT, Husmann MJW, Nicolaides AN, et al. Enhancing foot skin blood flux in peripheral vascular disease using intermittent pneumatic compression: Controlled study on caludicants and grafted arteriopaths. *World J Surg.* 2002;26:861–866.

32. EDRF (Editorial). *Lancet* 1987:2;137–138.

33. Yin and Yang in vasomotor control. (Editorial). *Lancet* 1988; 2:19–20.

34. Dai G, Tsukurov O, Orkin RW, et al. An in vitro cell culture system to study the influence of external pneumatic compression on endothelial function. *J Vasc Surg.* 2000;32:977–987.

35. Guyton DP, Khayat A, Husni EA, et al. Elevated levels of 6-keto-prostaglandin–F 1a from a lower extremity during external pneumatic compression. *Surg Gynecol Obstet.* 1988:166; 338–342.

36. Frangos JA, Eskin SG, McIntire LV. Flow effects on prostacyclin production by cultured human endothelial cells. *Science* 1985;227:1477–1479.

37. Weitz J, Michelsen J, Gold K, et al. Effects of intermittent pneumatic compression on postoperative thrombin and plasmin activity. *Thromb Haemostasis* 1986;56:198–201.

38. Ida T, Shin T, Sonoda T, et al. Stimulation of endothelium secretion of tissue-type plasminogen activator by repetitive stretch. *J Surg Res.* 1991;50:457–460.

39. Iba T, Sumpio BE. Tissue plasminogen activator expression in endothelial cells exposed to cyclic strain in vitro. *Cell Transplant.* 1992;1:43–50.

40. Papadaki M, Ruef J, Nguyen KT, et al. Differential regulation of protease activated receptor-1 and tissue plasminogen activator expression by shear stress in vascular smooth muscle cells. *Circ Res.* 1998;83:1027–1034.

41. Comerota AJ, Chouhan V, Harada RN, et al. The fibrinolytic effects of intermittent pneumatic compression: Mechanism of enhanced fibrinolysis. *Ann Surg* 1997;226:306–313.

42. Jacobs DG, Piotrowski JJ, Hoppensteadt DA, et al. Hemodynamic and fibrinolytic consequences of intermittent pneumatic compression: preliminary results. *J Trauma* 1996; 40:710–716.

43. Henriksen O. Orthostatic changes of blood flow in subcutaneous tissue in patients with arterial insufficiency of the legs. *Scand J Clin Lab Invest.* 1974;34:103–109.

44. Henriksen O. Local nervous mechanism in regulation of blood flow in human subcutaneous tissue. *Acta Physiol Scand.* 1976;11:40–42.

45. Delis KT, Nicolaides AN, Wolfe JHN. Peripheral sympathetic autoregulation in arterial calf inflow enhancement with intermittent pneumatic compression. *Eur J Vasc Endovasc Surg.* 2001;22:317–325.

46. Delis KT, Labropoulos N, Nicolaides AN, et al. The effect of intermittent pneumatic foot compression on popliteal artery haemodynamics. *Eur J Vasc Endovasc Surg.* 2000;19:270–278.

47. Vella A, Carlson LA, Blier B, et al. Circulator boot therapy alters the natural history of ischemic limb ulceration. *Vasc Med.* 2000;5:21–25.

48. Bacharach JM, Rooke TW, Osmundson PJ, et al. Predictive value of transcutaneous oxygen pressure and amputation success by use of supine and elevation measurements. *J Vasc Surg.* 1992;15:558–563.

49. Van Bemmelen PS, Gitlitz DB, Rishad RM, et al. Limb salvage using high-pressure intermittent compression arterial assist devices in cases unsuitable for surgical revascularization. *Arch Surg.* 2001;136:1280–1285.

50. Louridas G, Saadia R, Spelay J, et al. The ArtAssist device in chronic lower limb ischaemia. A pilot study. *Int Angiol.* 2002; 21:28–35.

51. Montori VM, Kavros SJ, Walsh EE, et al. Intermittent compression pump for nonhealing wounds in patients with limb ischaemia. The Mayo Clinic experience (1998–2000). *Int Angiol.* 2002;21:360–366.

52. Armstrong DG, Hienvu DPM, Nguyen HC. Improvement in healing with aggressive edema reduction after debridement of foot infections in persons with diabetes. *Arch Surg.* 2000; 135:1405–1409.

53. Dillon RS. Fifteen years of experience in treating 2177 episodes of foot and leg lesions with a circulator boot. Results of treatment with a circulator boot. *Angiology* 1997:48: S17–S34.

54. Dillon RS. Patient assessment and examples of a method of treatment. Use of the circulator boot in peripheral vascular disease. *Angiology* 1997;48:S35–S58.

55. Chen AH, Frangos SG, Kilaru S, et al. Review Article. Intermittent pneumatic compression devices-physiological mechanisms of action. *Eur J Vasc Endovasc Surg* 2001;21: 383–392.

15 Dermagraft: Living, Bioengineered, Human Dermis for Healing Chronic Wounds

Gary D. Gentzkow

Introduction
Background
Dermagraft Manufacture
Wound Bed Preparation and Implantation
    of Dermagraft
Mechanism of Action
Clinical Studies

Diabetic Foot Ulcers
Venous Leg Ulcers
Other Chronic Wounds
Acute and Surgical Wounds
Summary
References

INTRODUCTION

Dermagraft is living human dermal replacement tissue used to heal a variety of chronic wounds, including diabetic, venous, and pressure ulcers. It has also been used in acute soft-tissue wounds created by surgery (oral cancer resection, Moh's micrographic surgery), in reconstructive soft-tissue surgeries, for specialized wounds such as epidermolysis bullosa, and as a replacement for palatal grafts in periodontal surgery.

It is clear that many chronic wounds have an abnormal, degraded dermal matrix that is unable to support keratinocyte migration, as well as senescent fibroblasts that are unable to produce the matrix proteins and growth factors necessary for healing. Dermagraft, a living human dermis grown using the science of tissue engineering, is a replacement tissue containing normal matrix and normal fibroblasts. It has been shown to overcome these defects in a wide variety of chronic wounds.

Dermagraft is grown from newborn human fibroblasts on a three-dimensional biodegradable scaffold using the science of tissue engineering. Invented by Dr. Gail Naughton and developed by the company she founded (Advanced Tissue Sciences, La Jolla, California), Dermagraft reached the United States market following FDA approval in 2001. Its initial indication was for the treatment of diabetic foot ulcers. It was available in

Canada, the United Kingdom and other countries outside the United States for several years prior to its approval in the United States. Published and ongoing research has demonstrated its ability to heal many different types of acute and chronic soft tissue wounds.

BACKGROUND

Chronic wounds have been extensively studied and compared to normally healing wounds and found to be different in many important respects.[1] First, they are "stuck" in a chronic inflammatory state with a high matrix metalloproteinase (MMP) environment. Second, the matrix (granulation tissue) of the chronic wound is abnormal, having been degraded by the MMPs. This degradation of matrix proteins is of critical importance, because the keratinocytes cannot attach and migrate to close the wound if the collagen and fibronectin in the wound bed are degraded. Fibronectin is especially important because it contains the RGD domain that serves as an attachment and binding site for the integrins on the surface of keratinocytes. Third, the fibroblast cells in chronic wounds have been shown to be senescent, meaning they no longer function correctly and cannot act to direct efficient wound healing. Normally, the fibroblasts fulfill several critical functions in wound healing. They synthesize collagen, fibronectin, and the other matrix proteins. They make and secrete the entire "orchestra" of growth factors and cytokines needed for wound healing, including angiogenic factors to promote new blood vessels (vascular endothelial growth factor [VEGF], hepatocyte growth factor [HGF]), TGF-β to stimulate matrix deposition, keratinocyte growth factor (KGF) to encourage keratinocyte migration and proliferation, and many others. They also act as the "conductor" of the growth-factor orchestra, responding to the wound environment by up- or down-regulating production as needed and delivering the right growth factors at the right place, in the right amounts, and at the right time to the microenvironment of the wound. The senescent fibroblasts of the chronic wound are not able to fulfill these functions and wound healing does not take place.[1]

Thus, it makes perfect sense to seek a replacement tissue to overcome the deficiencies found in chronic wounds. If such a tissue could be provided, it would be a more rational therapy than, for example, the use of supraphysiologic bolus doses of single exogenous growth factors. It could be hoped that by providing both a fully formed, normal human dermis with intact collagen and fibronectin, as well as young, fully functional fibroblasts capable of responding to the wound environment and secreting appropriate growth factors, one could overcome the barriers to healing that exist in chronic wounds.

Such replacement of diseased or damaged tissue with functioning tissues, able to fulfill all the requirements of the original native tissue, is what the new science called "tissue engineering" is all about. Tissue engineering seeks to generate, outside of the body, replacement tissues composed of living human cells seeded onto a suitable support scaffold, grown in specialized bioreactors, and fed appropriate nutrients to essentially "trick" the cells into acting as if they were in the body. The cells, in this case fibroblasts, then do what they are programmed to do by their DNA. They make what they know how to make: in this case, dermal tissue and wound healing growth factors. Dermagraft is such a replacement tissue.

DERMAGRAFT MANUFACTURE

Dermagraft is manufactured through the three-dimensional cultivation of human diploid fibroblast cells on a three-dimensional polymer scaffold composed of Vicryl suture material. The fibroblasts secrete a mixture of growth factors and matrix proteins to create a living dermal structure which, following cryopreservation, remains metabolically active after being implanted into the patient's wound bed.[2,3] The human fibroblast cell strains used to produce Dermagraft are established from newborn foreskins (surgically discarded after circumcision)[4,5] and cultured by standard methods. Maternal blood samples are tested for exposure to infectious diseases, and an initial screen is made of the cultured cells for sterility, mycoplasma, and for eight human viruses: adeno-associated virus, herpes simplex virus (HSV) 1 and 2, cytomegalovirus (CMV), human immuno virus (HIV) 1 and 2, and human T-cell leukemia virus (HTLV) I and II. Master Cell Banks (MCBs) and Manufacturer's Working Cell Banks (MWCBs) are created and tested according to applicable sections of the FDA "Points to Consider"[6] and the guidelines from the European Union Committee for Proprietary Medicinal Products (CPMP).[7] This testing provides a much more uniform and highly tested product than is available from cadaveric donors. It also provides a readily available "off the shelf" product immediately available for implantation.

The Dermagraft tissue is created by seeding the polymer scaffolds with human fibroblast cells. (Fig. 15–1)

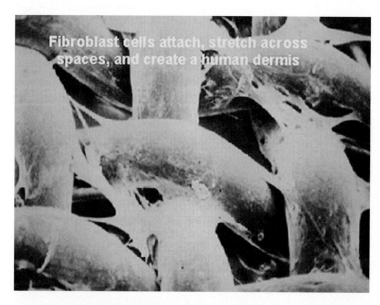

Fig. 15–1. This electron photomicrograph shows the three-dimensional scaffold (a mesh of Vicryl suture material) and, (lower left), a human newborn fibroblast seeded onto it. The fibroblast has attached and stretched across the interstices of the mesh.

The fibroblast cells have been expanded in cell culture to a population doubling level of approximately 30 (which is about half the life-span for this cell type). Because of the enormous number of cells obtained by such repeated doubling, a single donor foreskin provides sufficient cell seed to produce 250,000 ft^2 of finished Dermagraft tissue (enough to cover six football fields!). A closed bioreactor system is utilized for the manufacture of Dermagraft. This closed system offers major advantages, including the maintenance of sterility during manufacture, the ability to utilize in-process testing to maintain cell growth and matrix deposition, and the use of automated processes for tissue growth. The upscaled bioreactor systems manufacture hundreds of units of Dermagraft per lot.

The final product is extensively tested after manufacture for sterility as well as for specific levels of collagens and other matrix proteins. Since Dermagraft was designed to be a living tissue, remaining viable and delivering growth factors and matrix proteins into the wound bed after implantation, testing is performed pre-and post-cryopreservation to assess its metabolic activity. A routine MTT [3-(4,5-dimethylthiazol-2-y1)-2,5 diphenyl bromide assay] is utilized for this assessment both at time of manufacture and for testing of product stability over time.

The dermal implant is cryopreserved after growth in order to preserve tissue integrity and metabolic activity of the fibroblasts. Dermagraft is cryopreserved and stored at −70°C and shipped on Dry Ice to the clinical site. Manufacturing, cryopreservation, storage, shipping, and thawing protocols were all established to maintain integrity and metabolic activity of this tissue-engineered implant. The final product is a 2″ × 3″ tissue in a laser-welded EVA bioreactor (Fig. 15–2). A cross section of the dermal implant clearly shows the physiologic characteristics of this product, with human fibroblasts arranged in parallel and surrounded by naturally secreted human matrix proteins, including normal collagens and fibronectin.

Years of clinical experience, as well as laboratory testing, have demonstrated that this tissue is not rejected, despite the fact that it is an allograft containing "foreign" fibroblasts. Hundreds of patients were carefully followed for clinical signs of rejection, biopsies were examined for histological markers of rejection, and serum was analyzed for both humoral and cellular immunity. No rejection has been observed. It is known that fibroblasts, in general, and the fibroblasts in Dermagraft, in particular, do not normally express the (histocompatibility leukocyte antigen-DR) HLA-DR antigen on their surface. HLA-DR is thought to be the predominate antigen recognized by CD28 helper lymphocytes that results in tissue rejection. Because of the lack of expression of this antigen, tissues made from a pure culture of fibroblasts, as Dermagraft is, are relatively privileged and well-tolerated when implanted into a genetically distinct host.[8]

Because Dermagraft is made from male fibroblast cells, it is possible to determine how long the donor cells remain in female recipients. Biopsies can be taken after Dermagraft implantation and analyzed for the presence of the Y chromosome. If this male chromosomal marker is found in female recipients, it can be assumed that the donor DNA is still present. Such studies in patients with venous stasis ulcers have demonstrated that donor cells can be detected at 6 months.[9] There is, however, a gradual decline in the number of donor cells and a gradual replacement by host tissue. This phenomenon, sometimes dubbed "creeping substitution" is distinct from rejection. It probably represents either a low level of recognition of the foreignness of the donor cells or the replacement of these cells as they undergo programmed cell death (apoptosis) at the end of their life span.

WOUND BED PREPARATION AND IMPLANTATION OF DERMAGRAFT

Dermagraft is essentially a dermal skin graft that has been manufactured to be an "off-the-shelf" living tissue. As such, preparation of the wound bed to receive such a graft and the protection of the graft after implantation are of vital importance.

Fig. 15–2. The right-hand panel is an histological cross section of Dermagraft. The dots are fibroblast cells. The blue-staining material is the normal dermis secreted by the fibroblasts, including collagens, fibronectin, GAGs, etc. The left-hand panel shows the final product, a 2 × 3 inch piece of human dermis in its bioreactor bag, which is also the final package in which it is cryopreserved. After thawing and rinsing, the wound is traced and a piece of tissue is cut out to be implanted into the wound bed.

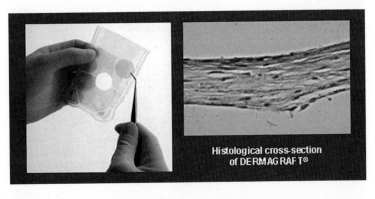

Histological cross-section of DERMAGRAFT®

Extensive débridement of the wound bed to remove all necrotic material (and in the case of diabetic ulcers, removal of surrounding callous) down to a viable, bleeding wound bed is essential. Treatment with an appropriate topical antibacterial (such as nanocrystalline silver [Acticoat]) to lower the bacterial burden of the wound is highly recommended. It has been shown that high levels of bacteria ($> 10^5$ CFU/g tissue), even in wounds that do not appear to be infected and are regarded by clinicians as "clean," will prevent wounds from healing and will cause skin grafts to fail.[10]

Prior to implantation, the Dermagraft is removed from its protective trilaminate foil pouch and thawed. Following the exact instructions for thawing is extremely important in order to ensure that the tissue will be living at the time of implantation. After a rapid thaw, the top of the bioreactor/product package is cut and the tissue is rinsed three times with sterile saline. The bioreactor containing the Dermagraft is translucent to allow tracing of the wound and precise trimming of the implant with sterile scissors. Dermagraft is cut to the wound size, removed from the EVA package, and placed into the wound bed. No sutures are required.

As with any skin graft, proper bolstering and dressing of the wound is required. A nonadherent dressing layer is placed immediately over the Dermagraft. A bolster of an appropriate absorbent dressing is then placed into the wound. It is common practice to use a layer of Acticoat silver dressing to guard against infection. Outer dressings are utilized to ensure that the dermal implant remains in place and is kept moist during integration into the patient's wound bed so that it functions as a replacement dermis. The specific dressing should be chosen according to the exudative status of the wound, with highly exudative wounds requiring highly absorptive dressings, such as alginates, foams, and specialty absorbents. It should be kept in mind that Dermagraft promotes extensive new capillary formation, which, in turn, provides a greater surface area for fluid transudation, and, therefore, may temporarily increase exudation. Finally, the outer dressings are secured in place with adhesive or tapes and then protected from sheer forces and compressive damage.

Off-weighting of plantar diabetic foot wounds is critically important. No skin graft can be expected to function properly if it is subjected to crushing forces as a patient walks on the implant over a bony prominence. Clinical studies with Dermagraft demonstrated that noncompliant patients who ambulated several hours per day still achieved much more healing than with comparable control patients,[11] but much higher levels of healing can be obtained with better off-weighting, such as total contact casting or removable cast boots.

Dermagraft was designed to be a multiapplication product. It was purposely grown as a relatively thin tissue (approximately 250 μm thick) so that it could live on nutrients in the wound fluid until it obtained a blood supply. If it were too thick, outer layers might die before the blood supply was obtained. Thus, it was designed to be implanted weekly, gradually building up the dermal base and providing a substrate for keratinocyte attachment and migration to close the wound. In addition to the volume of tissue implanted, Dermagraft, by secretion of appropriate growth factors, has the capacity to stimulate the host to produce additional dermal tissue to heal the wound.

MECHANISM OF ACTION

Current understanding of the mechanism of action of Dermagraft is represented in Fig. 15–3. Its actions can be thought of in two main categories: (1) implantation

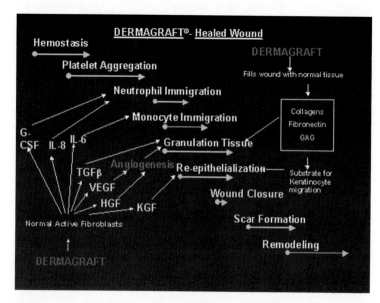

Fig. 15–3. This schematic of the wound healing process shows the multiple ways in which Dermagraft positively impacts the process to speed healing.

of a replacement dermal structure and (2) implantation of replacement living human fibroblasts.

Histological characterization of Dermagraft has shown that it has the structure of the papillary dermis of newborn skin. This dermal implant contains normal matrix proteins (Table 15–1) which play an integral role in providing structure, as well as enhancing cell growth. In addition, all of the glycosaminoglycans (GAGs) found in young healthy dermis are found in Dermagraft. These matrix components, vital for cell migration and for the binding of growth factors, are secreted by the newborn fibroblasts during the manufacturing process to yield a dermal implant with an appropriate complement of human GAGs.

The living fibroblasts, evenly dispersed throughout the tissue, remain metabolically active after implantation and deliver a variety of growth factors, which are key to neovascularization, epithelial migration, and differentiation, modulation of the inflammatory state, and integration of the implant into the patients' wound bed.[12] Growth factors expressed in Dermagraft are listed in Table 15–1. The most important of these factors may be the angiogenic factors, such as vascular endothelial growth factor (VEGF), which promote rapid and extensive development of new capillaries. Newton et al.[13] demonstrated, using laser Doppler imaging, that Dermagraft improved the blood flow in chronic diabetic foot ulcers by an average of 72%. Most chronic wounds have a deficit of blood flow and this particular action of Dermagraft may be key in its ability to heal a wide variety of wounds. In addition to angiogenic growth factors, the fibroblasts in Dermagraft secrete the entire "orchestra" of growth factors and

Table 15–1. Matrix proteins, glycosaminoglycans, and growth factors in Dermagraft.

Matrix proteins		Function
Collagens, type I and III		Major structural protein of dermis
Fibronectin		Cell adhesion, spreading, migration, mitogenesis
Tenascin		Induced in wound-healing, control of cell adhesion
Glycosaminoglycans		**Function**
Versican		Structural, binds hyaluronic acid and collagen
Decorin		Binds growth factors, influences collagen structure
Betaglycan		TGF-β type III receptor
Syndecan		Binds growth factors, enhances activity
Growth Factors	**Name**	**Function**
Matrix deposition factors		
Transforming growth factor β$_1$	TGF-β1	Stimulates matrix deposition
Transforming growth factor β$_3$	TGF-β3	Stimulates matrix deposition, antiscarring
Mitogenic factors		
Platelet-derived growth factor A chain	PDGF-A	Mitogen for fibroblasts, granulation tissue, chemotactic
Insulin-like growth factor 1	IGF-1	Mitogen for fibroblasts
Keratinocyte growth factor	KGF	Mitogen for keratinocytes
Heparin-binding epidermal growth factor-like growth factor	HBEGF	Mitogen for keratinocytes, fibroblasts
Transforming growth factor α	TGF-α	Mitogen for keratinocytes, fibroblasts
Angiogenic factors		
Vascular endothelial growth factor	VEGF	Angiogenesis
Hepatocyte growth factor	HGF	Angiogenesis
Basic fibroblast growth factor	bFGF	Angiogenesis
Secreted protein acidic and rich in cysteine	SPARC	Both anti- and proangiogenic
Interleukin 6	IL-6	Angiogenic, inflammatory cytokine
Interleukin 8	Il-8	Angiogenic, inflammatory cytokine
Inflammatory cytokines		
Interleukin 6	IL-6	Angiogenic, inflammatory cytokine
Interleukin 8	Il-8	Angiogenic, inflammatory cytokine
Granulocyte colony-simulating factor	G-CSF	Stimulates neutrophil production and maturation
Tumor necrosis factor α	TNF-α	Inflammatory cytokine

cytokines needed for wound healing, including TGF-β to stimulate matrix deposition and keratinocyte growth factor (KGF) to encourage keratinocyte migration and proliferation. They also make cytokines (granulocyte colony-stimulating factor [GCSF], inter leukin [IL]-6, IL-8) that modulate the inflammatory state to move the wound healing process forward. In effect, they act as the "conductor" of the growth factor orchestra, responding to the wound environment by up- or down-regulating production as needed and delivering the growth factors at the right place, in the right amounts, and at the right time to the microenvironment of the wound.

Taken together, these multiple activities have been demonstrated to result in enhanced healing in a wide variety of wounds.

CLINICAL STUDIES

Diabetic Foot Ulcers

Dermagraft has been most extensively studied in patients with diabetes who have chronic ulcerations of the feet. Several different studies have been published demonstrating the effectiveness and safety of Dermagraft in diabetic foot ulcers.

Following a pilot study[14] that determined that up to 8 weekly applications of single layers of Dermagraft was the most effective regimen studied, large pivotal trials were undertaken. All of these studies used the same primary endpoint of effectiveness—the percentage of wounds that were completely healed at week 12 of the trial. The studies were carefully controlled with explicit inclusion/exclusion criteria and patients were randomized to ensure comparable populations in the Dermagraft and control groups. Control (or standard) treatment consisted of extensive sharp debridement, infection control, saline-moistened gauze dressings remoistened several times daily to keep them moist, and carefully prescribed identical off-loading techniques for all patients. Those patients who were randomized to Dermagraft treatment received identical standard care, so that the only difference between the groups was whether or not they recieved the Dermagraft tissue implant.

The first trial showed a significant improvement in healing rates, with 51% of the Dermagraft patients completely healed at 12 weeks versus 32% of the control patients ($p = 0.006$).[15] The second trial, undertaken in a very difficult to heal population, showed 30% of the Dermagraft patients completely healed at 12 weeks versus 18% of the control patients ($p = 0.023$).[16] This trial also showed that the infection rate in the wounds treated with Dermagraft was half that of the control wounds (10 versus 18%), confirming the notion that faster healing ought to result in lower levels of infectious

complications. Another publication, by Hanft et al.[17] showed a dramatic difference in healing: 71% of Dermagraft treated wounds healed versus 14% of control treated wounds ($p = 0.003$).[17]

Venous Leg Ulcers

Studies have also been published in venous stasis ulcers. In these studies, venous ulcers, since they are usually less volumetric than diabetic ulcers, have required fewer applications of Dermagraft. The main dosage regimen has been up to four applications, applied at weeks 1 and 2, then weeks 4 and 8. Patients were treated with four-layer compression bandaging (Profore, Smith & Nephew) with or without Dermagraft. Brassard et al.,[18] in a randomized controlled trial in 53 venous stasis patients, reported complete healing by week 12 in 38% of Dermagraft-treated versus 15% of control patients.[18] Hjerppe et al.[19] conducted an open, noncomparative study in 151 leg ulcers of multiple etiologies, many of which were venous. These were very chronic wounds with a mean duration of 15 months (range 1–132) months and with an average size of > 10 cm^2. He demonstrated a mean reduction in size of the ulcers of 63% after a mean of 9 weeks of Dermagraft treatment, and 61% of the venous ulcers were completely healed.

Other Chronic Wounds

Individual case reports have been presented at medical meetings on the use of Dermagraft in uncommon difficult to heal chronic ulcers. Success (albeit anecdotal) has been reported in ulcers of arterial, rheumatic, sickle cell, pyoderma gangrenosum, necrobiosis lipoidica diabeticorum, and pressure etiology. Some of these ulcers were extremely resistant to healing, having been present for years, yet healed with Dermagraft treatment.

Acute and Surgical Wounds

Dermagraft has also been reported to heal wounds resulting from trauma, fasciotomy, and reconstructive surgery.[20–22] Patients with epidermolysis bullosa have been treated after surgery to correct "mitten hand" deformities with excellent results, including restoration of function.[23] Dermagraft has been used after skin cancer surgery and to heal large soft-tissue defects after oral cancer resection.[24] It has even been studied as an alternative to soft palate autografts in periodontal surgery.

SUMMARY

Understanding of the reasons why wounds become chronic and do not heal has been growing in the past two decades. It is clear that many chronic wounds have an abnormal, degraded dermal matrix that is unable to support keratinocyte migration as well as senescent fibroblasts that are unable to produce the matrix proteins and growth factors necessary for healing. Dermagraft, a living human dermis grown using the science of tissue engineering, is a replacement tissue containing normal matrix and fibroblasts. It has been shown to overcome these defects in a wide variety of chronic wounds. It has also shown the capacity to stimulate rapid healing of surgical soft-tissue defects. As researchers and clinicians continue to explore its applications in soft-tissue repair, it is expected to be beneficial in a wide variety of wounds. As such, it represents a major advance in the treatment of wounds, resulting in healing more wounds, healing them faster, and preventing infectious and other complications.

REFERENCES

1. Schultz GS, Sibbald RG, Falanga V, et al. Wound bed preparation: A systematic approach to wound management. *Wound Rep Reg* 2003;11:1–28.

2. Cooper ML, Hansbrough JF, Spielvogel RL, et al. *In vivo* optimization of a living dermal substitute employing cultured human fibroblasts on a biodegradable polyglycolic acid or polyglactin mesh. *Biomaterials.* 1991;12:243–248.

3. Landeen LK, Zeigler FC, Halberstadt C, et al. Characterization of a human dermal replacement. *Wounds* 1992;5: 167–175.

4. Kruse PF, Jr, Patterson MK, Jr, eds. *Tissue Culture Methods and Applications.* New York, Academic Press, 1973.

5. Jakoby WB, Pastan IH, eds. Cell Culture. *Methods Enzymol.* 1979;58.

6. U.S. Food and Drug Administration. *Points to Consider in the Characterization of Cell Lines Used to Produce Biologicals.* Bethesda, MD: U.S. Department of Health and Human Services, 1993.

7. Committee for Proprietary Medicinal Products: Ad Hoc Working party on Biotechnology/Pharmacy (1989). Notes to applicants for marketing authorizations on the production and quality control of monoclonal antibodies of murine origin intended for use in man. *J Biol Stand.* 1989;17:213.

8. Kern A, Liu K, Mansbridge J. Modification of fibroblast γ-interferon responses by extracellular matrix. *J Invest Dermatol.* 2001;117:112–118.

9. Mansbridge JN, Liu K, Pinney RE, et al. Growth factors secreted by fibroblast: Role in healing diabetic foot ulcers. *Diabetes, Obesity, Metab.* 1999;1:265–279.

10. Schultz GS, Sibbald RG, Falanga V, et al. Wound bed preparation: a systematic approach to wound management. *Wound Rep Reg.* 2003;11:1–28.

11. Marston WA, Hanft J, Norwood P, et al. The efficacy and safety of Dermagraft in improving the healing of chronic diabetic foot ulcers. *Diabetes Care.* 2003;26:1701–1705.

12. Mansbridge JN, Liu K, Pinney RE, et al. Growth factors secreted by fibroblast: Role in healing diabetic foot ulcers. *Diabetes, Obesity, Metab.* 1999;1:265–279.

13. Newton DJ, Kahn F, Belch JJ, et al. Blood flow changes in diabetic foot ulcers treated with dermal replacement therapy. *J Foot Ankle Surg.* 2002;41(4);233–237.

14. Gentzkow GD, Iwasaki I, Hershon KS, et al. Use of Dermagraft, a cultured human dermis, to treat diabetic foot ulcers. *Diabetes Care.* 1996;19(4):350–354.

15. Pollak RA, Edington H, Jensen JL, et al. A human dermal replacement for the treatment of diabetic foot ulcers. *Wounds.* 1997;9(6):175–183.

16. Marston WA, Hanft J, Norwood P, et al. The efficacy and safety of Dermagraft in improving the healing of chronic diabetic foot ulcers. *Diabetes Care.* 2003;26:1701–1705.

17. Hanft JR, Surprenant MS. Healing of chronic foot ulcers in diabetic patients with a human fibroblast-derived dermis. *J Foot Ankle Surg.* 2002;41(5):291–299.

18. Brassard A. A prospective, multicentre, randomized, controlled clinical investigation of Dermagraft in patients with venous leg ulcers: A feasibility study. *Can J Plast Surg.* 2002;10(Suppl. A):17A–22A.

19. Hjerppe, A, Hjerppe, M, Autio, V, et al. Treatment of chronic leg ulcers with a cultured human dermis—A case series of 114 patients. Wounds 2004;16(3)97–104.

20. Deckert CJ, Jordens LJ, VanWyk GL. Use of Dermagraft in the treatment of acute traumatic wounds. *Can J Plast Surg.* 2002;10(Suppl. A):31A–35A.

21. Omar AA, Mavor AI. Homer-Vanniasinkam S. Evaluation of Dermagraft as an alternative to grafting for open fasciotomy wounds. *J Wound Care.* 2002;11(3):94–97.

22. Gath HJ, Raguse JD. Use of Dermagraft in plastic and reconstructive surgery. *Can J Plast Surg.* 2002;10(Suppl. A): 23A–26A.

23. Williamson D, Coutts P, Sibbald RG. The role of dermal skin substitutes in the management of "hard to heal" unusual wounds. *Can J Plast Surg.* 2002;10(Suppl. A):27A–30A.

24. Gath HJ, Berthold H, Zarrinbal R, et al. Regeneration of intraoral defects after tumor resection with a bioengineered human dermal replacement (Dermagraft). *Plast Reconstr Surg.* 2002;109(3):889–893.

Marc E. Gottlieb

Introduction
  An Overview of Integra
  Integra and Chronic Wounds
Integra Biology
  Structure
  Acute Physiologic Effects
  Subacute Physiologic Effects
  Related Therapeutic Effects
Indications and Uses of Integra
  Integra General Indications
  Overview of Wound Repair Surgery
  Integra and Conventional Wound
    Surgery
**Integra for Chronic and
  Pathologic Wounds**
  The Problem of the Chronic Problem
    Wound

**Rationale and Indications for Integra on
  Chronic Wounds**
  Integra and Chronic Wound, Surgical
    Planning, Compared to Conventional
    Methods
  Use of Integra and Discussion by Diagnosis
    and Pathology
  Use of Integra and Discussion by Anatomy
Technique and Management
  Technique and Management
Review of Experience
  Patients and Ulcers
  Outcomes
  Summary of Author's Data
  Other Sources
  Other Indications
References

INTRODUCTION

Wounds, and especially chronic and pathologic wounds, are subjects which historically have received minor attention from organized, academic, and commercial medicine. However, since the last decade or two of the 20th century, there has been a burgeoning interest in the subject. Basic and clinical research has proliferated, and robust principles of pathology, therapeutics, and clinical care are evolving, practiced by cross-discipline physicians, allied health professionals, and manufacturers who make the products needed to support clinical practice. In prior years, the product base in this specialty consisted mostly of bandages and nonpharmacologic topical medications. As this chapter has currently been written, there are now a dozen or two legitimate pharmaceuticals and other products designed to facilitate or accelerate wound repair, including sophisticated manufactured devices,

living and nonliving. These contemporary products are the nascence of wound engineering and wound biotechnology, presumably presaging ever increasing capabilities for the hasty cure of chronic wounds. Among these modern technology products is Integra Dermal Regeneration Template (manufactured by Integra Life Sciences, Plainsboro, NJ; marketed by Ethicon, Somerville, NJ). Integra's structure and biologic effects are unique among contemporary wound and surgical devices. Originally developed as an artificial skin for treating burns, its special properties make it effective for treating many wounds, acute and chronic, traumatic and pathologic. It is often superior to any conventional surgical method and it is sometimes the only permissible option. It can solve problems simply not curable by customary modalities, thus extending the boundaries of successful care and curable wounds. This chapter will detail Integra, its biologic properties, the rationale for its use on various wounds, and its methods of use and related care. Because trauma wounds occur in usually healthy people, and because the art is already very dependable for trauma wounds, most of this chapter will focus on the exceptional ability of Integra to close chronic and pathologic wounds.

An Overview of Integra

Integra is a nonliving semibiologic spongy matrix composed of type 1 collagen and chondroitin-6-sulfate. It is manufactured as a thin bilaminate sheet, the deep layer being the sponge, which is placed in contact with the wound, and the top layer being a silicone rubber "epidermis" (Fig. 16–1). It has two main functions or modes of use. The first is as an artificial skin, effectively performing the barrier functions of normal skin while persuading the host that skin is actually present and that there is no injury or need for inflammation. Its second function is as an agent of tissue regeneration. The sponge has histoinductive and histoconductive properties, which attract mesenchymal cells and direct them to begin regenerating, within the sponge, a lamina of tissue comparable to embryonic dermis. Both the native and the regenerated material have desirable properties and beneficial effects on the recipient wound.

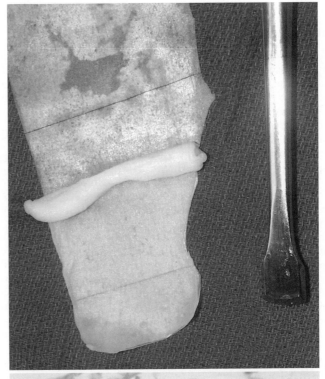

A

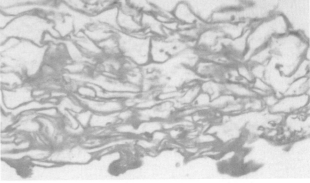

B

Fig. 16-1. **A.** This is a piece of Integra, silicone side down, from which the sponge has been partially separated. (While not the usual mode of use, the sponge can be used alone for bulk filling of small spaces. **B.** This is the structure of the spongy collagen-GAG matrix (missing the silicone which comes off in histology processing). It is somewhat flattened in this view, but the pore voids typically fill to capacity as histogenesis progresses.

As a surgical implant, Integra's use is comparable to ordinary skin grafts. Patients and wounds have a period of preparatory care. When ready for surgery, the wound is excised, and Integra is used to cover the exposed surfaces. Compression dressings and splints are applied. The regeneration process, which occurs over a period of several weeks, can be observed directly through the transparent outer silicone. When regeneration of the "neodermis" is complete, the silicone is discarded, and true epithelium is restored with thin epidermal autografts. Its spectrum of use includes: (1) acute wounds such as deglovings, fasciitis, and excisional defects, (2) reconstruction, such as controlling keloids and correcting contractures, and (3) chronic wounds due to many disorders.

Integra and Chronic Wounds

To anyone not familiar with the principles of reconstructive plastic surgery, an obvious question is "why the middle man, why not just stick the second-stage skin graft on the wound in the first place?" The answer is that certain wounds cannot support skin grafts, either because disease has rendered the host wound incompetent to heal, or because visceral or skeletal structures are exposed. Conventional principles teach that flaps are required in these situations. The art of conventional surgical wound closure—repairs, flaps, and grafts–is a detailed subject. Options are chosen individually based on size, location, acuity or severity, exposure of internal structures, patient history and comorbidities, and many other factors. Most surgery is done with the implicit faith that wound healing is competent and that the repair will heal. However, these assumptions and all of the usual art of surgical repair are challenged when caring for chronic and pathologic wounds. The various illnesses and risk factors which cause ulceration (arterial and venous diseases, immunopathies, hematopathologies, and many others) also conspire to eliminate the ordinary options for wound closure; they can impair the wound healing process itself. For these patients, disease and pathologic anatomy make them ineligible for the repairs that would be done for comparable defects in healthy trauma patients.

All treatment options, from topical care in support of natural contraction to simple rapair to elaborate reconstruction with autogenous living tissues, are all prone to fail when working with chronic and pathologic ulcers. This is reflected in the chronicity of the problems, the prolonged failed care, the multiple failed procedures, the incidence of amputation, and the loss of vocation, lifestyle, and well being. Integra can reliably close such ulcers. It not only withstands many disease-imposed risks, but it actually has a therapeutic effect on the wound to control local pathology. When applied to impaired wounds, injury, inflammation, and ulceration cease, conventional fibrous wound repair is inhibited, symptoms and nursing requirements abate, and tissue regeneration begins. It can succeed in healing chronic wounds when all other options are contraindicated or will fail, and it does so safely, without donor sites or risk to the patient.

It must be noted that good outcomes with Integra do not come automatically. No legitimate remedy for chronic wounds works in the absence of systematic and comprehensive good care. This includes a program of proper diagnosis, treatment or correction of underlying diseases and risks, diligent care of the wound and periwound, prudent treatment choices, thorough preoperative wound preparation, continuity of care from one treatment phase to the next, and long-term maintenance management. Used properly, Integra is, for many patients, the crucial component of care that solves otherwise unsolvable problems. Integra's favorable properties, its clinical utility, and its superiority for many wound repairs and reconstruction all derive from its unique structure and biologic properties.

INTEGRA BIOLOGY

Structure

Integra was first conceived in Boston in the 1970s in a collaboration between a burn surgeon Dr. John F. Burke and polymer scientist and engineer Dr. Ioannis V. Yannas. Biology, materials, and manufacturing were all foremost issues.[1-3] While the gamut of Integra indications were not perceived at that time, each detail of the product's design was important in creating the properties that now make it so versatile. Chemical composition and materials, microarchitecture and fabrication, and macroarchitecture and composite structure all contribute crucial effects that allow Integra to function first as an almost normal skin and then to act as a skin regenerant.

Chemical Composition

The Integra sponge or matrix is composed of two ingredients, type 1 collagen (acquired from bovine achilles tendon) and chondroitin-6-sulfate [chondroitin sulfate C, a glycosaminoglycan (GAG) from shark cartilage]. The raw materials are processed and chemically crosslinked in a proprietary process, resulting in a porous sponge with 8% chondroitin. The material is generically referred to as CGM, collagen–GAG matrix. There are many collagen products marketed for wound care, so it must be understood that Integra is *not* a "collagen product." The chemistry of Integra depends on both components. The collagen provides mainly structural form and stability. The chondroitin-6-sulfate is what confers key properties. Along with hyaluronan, dermatan, keratan, and heparan, the glycosaminoglycans are the large saccharide polymers which are key components of the extracellular matrix. Vertebrate cells cannot function without adhesion to these molecules, which have key roles in cell and tissue development and differentiation. In unproteinized embryonic tissues, they are the sole medium in which young cells develop, accumulating in fetal wounds which heal by regeneration without inflammation nor fibrosis.[4,5,6] As will be discussed, Integra histogenesis is highly analogous to normal embryonic dermatogenesis and the chondroitin is largely responsible for this effect. Another Integra property is that the chondroitin masks binding sites on the collagen, thereby preventing platelet adhesion and resulting inflammation. It is interesting that when the material was invented, chondroitin was used only for chemical engineering purposes of improving the mechanics and stability of "the collagen matrix," and it was serendipity that the combination had remarkable other effects on wounds.

Microarchitecture

The porous collagen–chondroitin sponge has a void volume of 95%. Pore diameters are typically 5–150 μm, averaging 80–100 μm. The septae of the sponge are several micrometers thick, comparable to the size of individual cells which will invade and populate the sponge. These microdimensions of the matrix were deliberately engineered because geometry, space, and surface all have effects on cell behavior. If the pores are too small, histogenetic cells cannot invade or occupy the matrix. Too large and potential histogenetic cells would "see" a nonstimulatory flat surface. At the chosen size, histogenetic cells "feel at home" and are induced to proliferate (Fig. 16–2).

Macroarchitecture

During manufacture, the spongy Integra material is formed into a sheet about 1–2 mm thick, comparable to the average thickness of human dermis. Liquid silicone (polysiloxane) elastomer is poured as a second layer. The silicone barely penetrates the sponge, but enough to bond the two lamina. The final composite of spongy matrix overlayered with transparent silicone rubber is about 3–3.5 mm thick. The composite material is pliable and conformable to gross anatomical contours. The silicone serves as an effective epidermis—airtight and water tight as long as it is undamaged. The matrix in contact with the host has the important job of regulating reactions and inducing histogenesis. Nonspecific chemistry loosely adheres the sponge to healthy tissue within a few days, but histogenesis is a delayed event and there is no formal histologic connection between the material and the host for approximately 10 days.

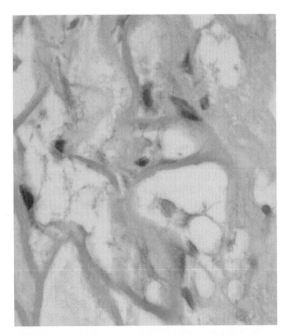

Fig. 16-2. This micrograph, 17 days after placement, shows the sizes and relationships of cells and matrix. The smallest dark round. Lymphoid cells are the pioneer cells. The larger flatter cells are the transitional cells.

Acute Physiologic Effects

When Integra is applied to a wound, all of the normal physiologic responses to injury cease. Recognition of injury is so severely attenuated that inflammation and its derivative events never emerge. Integra, therefore, favorably influences clinical outcomes immediately upon placement. As the entire process evolves in time, from nonliving matrix to autogenous tissue, each of its important biologic properties is relevant to one or more of its clinical indications, such as preventing scarring or closing exposed bones and joints. At the front end, its abilities to immediately close a wound, to be recognized as normal tissue, to suppress inflammation, and to control acute wound failure, are especially important. These are the properties that make Integra dependable for critical coverage where life and limb are threatened and for closure of pathologic wounds.

Immediate Closure of Wound and Recognition as Normal Tissue

The composite Integra implant, matrix with silicone, is an effective artificial skin. The silicone pseudoepidermis has an obvious function because it is a thorough barrier against environmental exposure. However, it is the bio-compatible sponge, looking to the body like aminoglycan ground substance, which has the less intuitive but more potent beneficial effect on the wound. When Integra is applied to a wound, the wound immediately stops being a wound. It may still be an injury or defect, but from a physiologic point of view, all of the events which define the usual response to injury cease. The sponge is accepted by local cells as "self." To lymphoid patrol cells, which eventually find the matrix, the chondroitin lattice appears to be an acellular but otherwise normal tissue. The only response triggered is a regenerative one. This means that inflammation and other defensive responses do not occur.

Inflammation: Suppression of Effects

Inflammation is the normal protective response to injury. Depending on its cause, injury is recognized by platelets or leukocytes. They trigger an autoamplifying cascade of cells and chemicals, which is meant to defend the host and stabilize the injury, recognized clinically by custom-ary signs, such as redness, swelling, and pain. Wound repair is the latter response, which makes scar and restores the host. Repair is an integrated sequential consequence of inflammation, appearing as injury and inflammation subside. Inflammation is an inherently destructive process. While inflammation begins the sequence leading to wound repair, repair processes are suppressed by acute inflammation. Acute inflammation can also dismantle early products of repair. Collagenolysis and other prote-olysis during inflammation will lyse scar, commonly seen clinically when an abscess drains through a recently healed wound. These are the reasons that inflammation is the enemy of the wound physician. When inflammation occurs reactively for identifiable reasons, such as an infec-tion or a fracture pseudarthrosis, the physician must con-trol the cause of the inflammation. When inflammation arises for erroneous reasons, such as rheumatoid disease, then inflammation per se must be stopped. Until then, physiologic wound repair will remain suppressed and sur-gical wound repair is prone to fail.

When Integra is applied to a wound, inflammation ceases. It is not only recognized as self, but it also seems to be "invisible" to platelets and inflammatory leukocytes. Observed histologically, at no time are there inflammatory cell infiltrates in the matrix. At no time do inflammatory cell exudates or even intravascular leukocyte margination appear in the adjacent tissues (Fig. 16–3). Clinical signs of inflammation are suppressed or eliminated. Pain is often conspicuously absent after Integra application, and any preoperative periwound erythema and edema rapidly abate (Fig. 16–4). At least three characteristics of Integra explain this phenomenon. (1) Because of masked binding sites, platelets cannot recognize the collagen, and platelet adhesion is absent. This prevents the thrombotic cascade to inflammation from being triggered (Fig. 16–5). (2) The

artificial epidermis sequesters the wound, eliminating ambient exposure, desiccation, bioburden, and their injurious effects. (3) The chondroitin matrix looks sufficiently like normal tissue that blood-borne leukocytes and lymphoid cells that might find their way into the matrix do not recognize anything abnormal that would trigger a defensive response.[7a]

Pathergy Is Preempted

"Pathergy" has the general meaning of an abnormal or exaggerated response to an injury or challenge. Originally applied to allergens, it has taken on broader meanings, such as the intense inflammatory response to minor trauma in Behcet's syndrome (Fig. 16–6). Lately, it has come to signify an unexpected or disproportionate adverse response of a wound to accident, disease, or deliberate injury (débridement and surgery). The injury-induced necrosis of pyoderma gangrenosum is a paradigm. In this chapter, "pathergy" will be synonymous with "unexpected acute wound failure." It is a tokenized way to describe pro-gressive inflammation, necrosis, tissue lysis, wound bursi-tis, dehiscence, and other undesirable wound complica-tions not due to obvious causes, such as infection or excess mechanical load, especially if they are unanticipated, exag-gerated, or a consequence of treatment or injury-triggered flare-up of underlying disease.

Wound pathergy is most prone to occur with any disorder that causes severe ischemia or severe inflamma-tion. This includes athero-and other macro-occlusive arterial diseases, hypercoagulable, microthrombotic, and microocclusive disorders, autoimmune vasculitis and angiopathies, and the various active immuno-pathies, including connective tissue disorders, panniculopathies, inflammatory dermatoses, and any similar disease of immunity and inflammation. In these disorders, every surgical procedure, from simple débride-ments and biopsies to amputations and complex wound closures, is at risk for necrosis, lysis, dehiscence, and ulceration. These undesirable responses are mediated in many ways, including acute neutrophilic inflammation, complement and lymphocyte activation, abnormal cytokine profiles, protease activation, thrombosis, and ischemic infarction, to name a few that are most under-stood. A robustly healthy wound and host weather injury and inflammation and they easily get on with repair when the acute events subside. Sick wounds and hosts do not have the same degrees of freedom to accommodate the secondary injury that inflammation creates. Anything that mitigates inflammation lessens the chances of wound failure.

Regardless of the disease and the pathogenetic path-way to wound failure, almost anytime that Integra is applied to such wounds or patients, these risks are controlled and adverse wound behaviors are eliminated. By sequestering mesenchyme and creating a closed

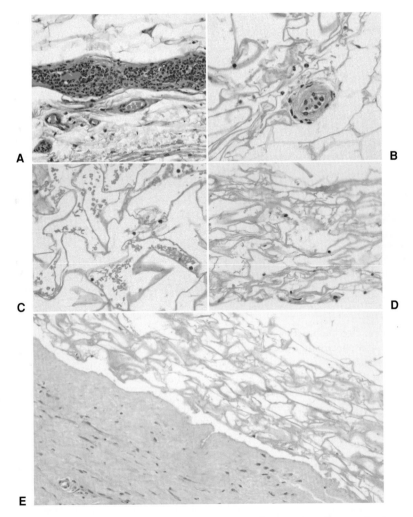

Fig. 16-3. Integra suppresses or eliminates inflammation. Figures 3a, b, c were taken from a patient having lower extremity dermatofasciectomy for Milroy's primary lymphedema. **A.** Biopsy taken 4 hours after a fasciectomy for lymphedema, just prior to Integra. Neutrophils have congregated in blood vessels on the wound surface, the normal response to injury, the start of inflammation. **B.** Biopsy 4 hours later. Between Integra matrix (top and left) and normal adipose (bottom and right), a blood vessel has some, but reduced, leukocyte margination. **C.** At 24 hours, neutrophils are few, in proportion to red cells that bled into the matrix. **D.** At 5 days (from another patient), there are only early histogenetic cells. There are no neutrophils, plasma cells, eosinophils, lymphocytes, nor monocyte-macrophages. A defensive response never appears in the matrix. **E.** At 11 days, the matrix remains mostly empty. The host wound is also normal, devoid of any of the normal histological response to injury, but with early entrainment of cells starting to migrate toward the matrix. (Note: unless otherwise stated or obvious, all histological images presented throughout the chapter are oriented with the outer superficial surface, silicone or epidermis, at the top.)

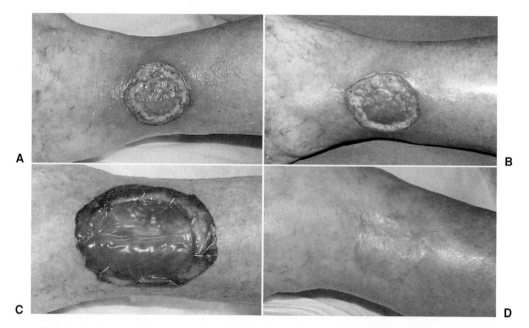

Fig. 16-4. Chronic ulceration in a 61 year old woman due to protein-S deficient hypercoagulability, with histology-confirmed periwound microthrombosis. Inflammation, necrosis, and ulceration were refractory to topical care. **A.** Prior to consistent topical care, periwound inflammation is intense. **B.** With strict care and increased warfarin, the wound and periwound are improved, but inflammation and active necrosis-ulceration still persist. **C.** Six days after wound excision and Integra, periwound inflammation, erythema, and edema, have completely subsided. **D.** Healed. This is a typical example of a chronic refractory ulcer, due to active pathology, which failed multiple prior care but healed promptly with Integra.

wound, by mimicking normal autogenous tissue, and by suppressing inflammation, the various deleterious effects of injury and inflammation, which lead to acute wound failure, are arrested. Because Integra should never be applied to a natural wound surface, but rather to an acutely, fully, surgically excised surface which is histologically normal, these various factors are stopped before they ever start.

Subacute Physiologic Effects

Subacute Integra effects are those related to its regeneration phase. From the patient's perspective, this is a busy time, with clinic visits, dressing changes, anticipation of skin grafts, and anxiety over outcome. From a general physiologic point of view though, Integra's abilities to suppress acute inflammation mean that this period of several weeks is very benign and uneventful. From the point of view of the wound, this is a crucial but orderly, controlled, and productive time in which normal wound repair is suppressed and an embryonic form of histogenesis grows the neodermis.

Suppression of Normal Inflammatory Wound Repair

Inflammation begets normal wound repair. This process, in which the wound contracts and is cemented together by fibrous scar, is known as the "wound module".[7b] It is the body's standard mode of repair after injury. It begins as blood-borne monocytes in the inflammatory zone of the wound are transformed to macrophages. As mobile phagocytes, macrophages have an afferent function to recognize debris and remove it, resulting in eschar separation. Their efferent role is to make cytokines, which stimulate local vascular and perivascular histoprogenitor cells. Stimulated cells migrate to the wound and establish new blood vessels, recognized as "granulation tissue." Behind them come myofibroblasts, which contract the wound, and regular fibroblasts, which make the collagenized scar. As the proliferative wound module covers the original defect, epithelial cells migrate across it. The wound is "closed" when epithelialization is complete, when mesenchyme underneath is fully sequestered from the ambient world. Chronic wounds are all due to some component of this

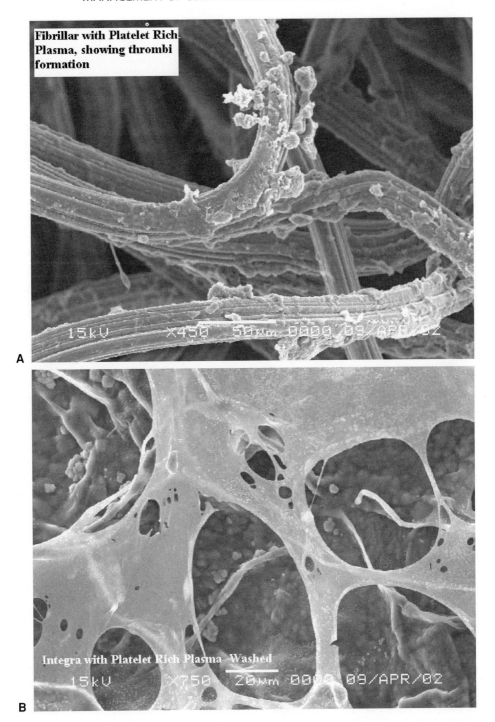

Fig. 16-5. Electron micrographs of matrices incubated with platelet rich plasma: **A.** Platelets adhere as expected to a collagen-cellulose matrix. **B.** Platelets do not adhere to the Integra collagen-GAG matrix. The chondroitin has rendered the collagen invisible to platelets. (Photos on file, Ethicon, somerville, New Jersey, USA)

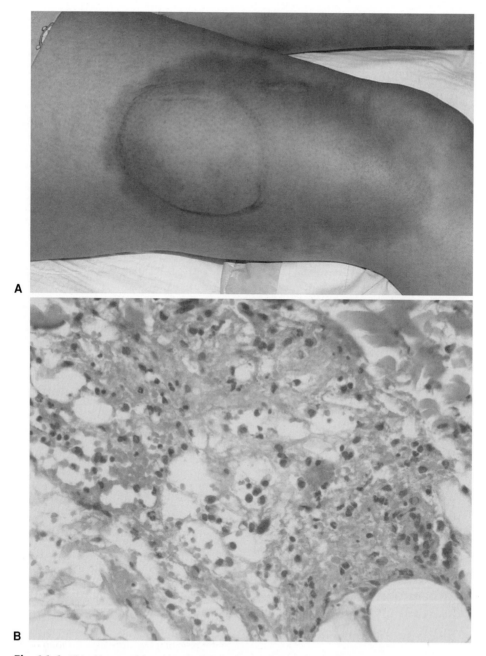

A

B

Fig. 16-6. This 43 year old woman had previously undiagnosed Behçet's syndrome, now with multiple acute manifestations. Illustrated is the standard "pathergy test", the response to a needle prick. **A.** This is the result 12 hours after a single prick to the thigh with an 18 gauge needle. **B.** There is hemorrhage and complex mixed inflammation at the dermis-hypodermis boundary. This is one of the classic but more parochial definitions of pathergy. In this chapter, the contemporary more liberal meaning of "pathergy" is used: acute, unexpected wound and soft tissue complications, disproportionate to the injury. Although not an Integra case, this illustrates the type of immunopathic events that often lead to refractory ulcers that Integra can heal.

process failing. However, even in healthy subjects, normal inflammatory wound repair can be the proverbial "double-edged sword," ensuring the immediate health of the subject, but leading to undesirable late effects due to scar and contracture. By turning off inflammation, Integra turns off the master switch that triggers this entire series of events. Fibroplasia never occurs, meaning that contractures, keloids, and other reactive or pathologic scars and their clinical effects also never occur.

Induction Of Embryonic Histogenesis

If Integra did nothing other than control inflammation and pathergy, and thereby stabilize a sick wound, it would still be a valuable device. However, it would then be just another biologic dressing ultimately needing replacement by autogenous grafts. What makes Integra unique among all other surgical grafts and implants is its ability to regenerate an embryogenic tissue. The surgeon who uses Integra is incubating an engineered tissue devoid of scar and having the characteristics of dermis. The aminoglycans and the geometry of the matrix are presumed to be the key triggers and regulators of this phenomenon. It is easy enough to observe Integra regeneration histologically and observe that the process is completely different from ordinary wound module fibroplasia. Understanding that the process is comparable to embryonic histogenesis comes by inference and cross–correlation with available information on that subject. Notable parallels include the lack of inflammation in fetal wound repair, the lack of fibroplasia and the prompt regeneration of tissues in fetal wound repair, the predominant role of aminoglycan ground substance in embryonic histogenesis and fetal wound repair, the comparable development and morphology of dermatocytes during embryogenesis and Integra histogenesis,[8] and the biophysics of tissue growth and vasculogenesis.[9–11]

Histogenetic Process

As Integra histogenesis proceeds, several distinctive events or phases occur. The following images are taken from among 11 different individuals with extensive histologic documentation of their Integra reconstruction (unless explicitly stated, sequential images are not necessarily from the same patient):

Wound closure and suppression of inflammation— The most immediate effects of Integra are to sequester mesenchyme from the ambient environment and to suppress inflammation (Fig. 16–3 and 16–4).

Recognition of the matrix, pioneer cells—Small lymphoid-looking cells enter the matrix in small numbers. Integra was engineered to be nonsoluble. There is no evidence that Integra has any diffusible moieties or any cytotactic properties. These lymphoid "pioneer cells"

seem to be patrol cells, either blood-borne or resident in normal tissues, which find the matrix by happenstance. They do not recruit other cells. They migrate or diffuse freely through the matrix, and, when they do react, they simply adhere to the matrix (Fig. 16–7a).

Transition—Adherent pioneer cells undergo a transformation. They elongate along the septae of the matrix, then enlarge as cytoplasm and nucleoplasm accumulate in preparation for proteogenesis and mitosis. These behaviors are characteristic of cell–aminoglycan interactions. These transitional cells mark the beginning of active histogenesis (Fig. 16–7b).

Syncytial transformation and clusters—The transitional cells develop into "syncytial fibroblasts." These are large cells. Under light microscopy, their boundaries are indistinct, hence, the designation "syncytial." They are proteogenic, with large pseudopods surrounding foci of young amorphous collagen. They are also mitotic and eventuate in small clusters of cells (approximately 1–12) occupying a domain or pore of the matrix. The clusters are evenly scattered throughout the matrix, wherever there was a pioneer cell (Figs. 16–7c and d). These events usually occur between 5 and 15 days (all event times are expressed as days or weeks after Integra placement; the time frame of Integra events has wide variability, from person to person and within different locales in the same person, and the given values are very rough approximations; events tend to be quicker in healthier people, on upper parts of the body, and in children). There are two notable observations about these cells: (1) as characterized by light microscopy, appearance and behavior of these cells are identical to the syncytial fibroblasts characteristic of embryonic dermatogenesis,[8] (2) there is nothing like this that ever occurs in normal inflammatory wound repair. Syncytial fibroblast transformation is the keystone event in Integra histogenesis. It occurs because the collagen–chondroitin matrix is directing cells to do something that mature cells ordinarily will not do.

Stimulation and entrainment of perivascular cells—The syncytial clusters are metabolically active, and the diffusibility of gases from the host wound and competition between clusters are limiting factors. As demand outpaces supply, angiogenic factors are made in order to summon new blood vessels. At the heart of embryonic biophysics, this closed-loop demand–supply interaction regulates vasculogenesis and substrate-dependent histogenesis, which depends on vascular endothelial growth factor (VEGF) and other angiogenic growth factors. New blood vessels must come from pre-existing blood vessels, and stimulation causes nearby angiocytes, both endothelial and perivascular cells, to enlarge, multiply, and migrate (Figs. 16–7e, f, and g).

Vasculogenesis—Migrating angiocytes aim for the sources of stimulation, each syncytial cluster, then

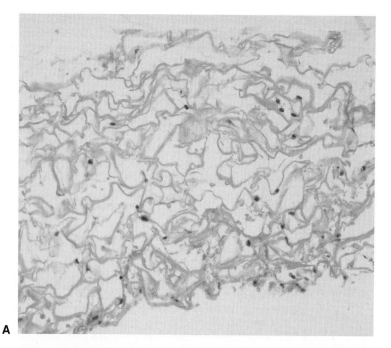

A

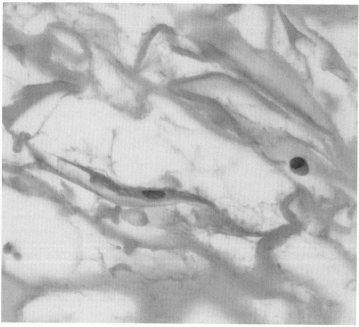

B

Fig. 16-7. A. Recognition of the matrix, pioneer cells. Integra 5 days after placement. Sparsely scattered in the matrix are small lymphoid-looking cells with dark nuclei. These are the pioneer cells. There is neither hemorrhage nor inflammation in the matrix, neither of the usual mechanisms which would transport cells. These pioneers have randomly found the matrix. Some are still free and round, and some are adhering to the matrix and starting to flatten. **B. Transition.** A closer view. One cell is still a round unattached pioneer. The other cell has transitioned, attached to the matrix, flattened and elongated. Attachment with morphological transformation is a characteristic cell-glycosaminoglycan interaction.

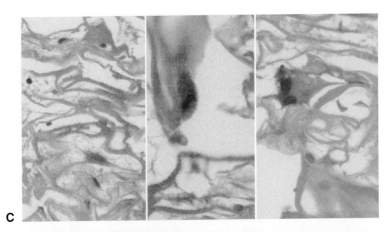

C

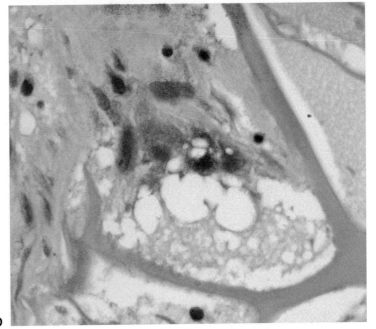

Fig. 16-7. **C. Syncytial transformation.** (left) The adherent elongated transitional cells again transform, becoming syncytial fibroblasts, large cells with large nuclei, long pseudopods, and indistinct boundaries. Pioneer, transitional, and syncytial cells are all seen here. (middle) This transition is the keystone event in Integra regeneration. These cells are the first to be histogenetically active, generating new tissue by mitotic cell replication and by production of connective proteins. (right) Doubled by mitosis, these large stellate cells seem confluent, hence "syncytial." Pale young fibrillar collagen is present in the cells. (The separation between cells and matrix is a fixation-dehydration artifact.) **D. Syncytial clusters.** A 17 day view of a syncytial cluster, indistinct large embryonoid cells interspersed with young collagen. It is an insular cluster without gross organization, not yet a tissue. Substrate supply depends on diffusion of nutrients and gases from the host. Having about a dozen cells, this cluster can grow no more until pending revascularization fulfills the metabolic needs of this and competing clusters.

D

reassemble themselves into luminal vessels that can conduct blood. As further histogenesis proceeds to fill the matrix, the vascular network continues to branch and expand as required. An anatomical connection between host and Integra is now starting to form (Fig. 16–7h; 5–15 days for the initiation of this process).

Second-set histogenesis—Now that new blood vessels directly supply the early clusters, more robust histogenesis can proceed. There is empty space to be filled and it is filled both by mitotic new cells (which can proliferate until loss of contact is corrected), and by the more voluminous and more mature collagen which they can now make. As the widely dispersed syncytial clusters

grow larger, they grow to confluence, and the matrix fills with tissue (Fig. 16–7i; 10–20 days for the initiation of this process).

Matrix filling—The first round of histogenesis could occur anywhere in the matrix, deep or superficial, wherever there were pioneer cells and syncytial clusters. However, second-set histogenesis must start at the base, because this is where new blood vessels must enter. It develops layer by layer, a broad tangential front rising through the matrix like a tide, from base up to silicone, as progressive vascularization allows the process to occur at ever higher levels. The events are qualitatively identical at all levels, but the surface lags behind the base by

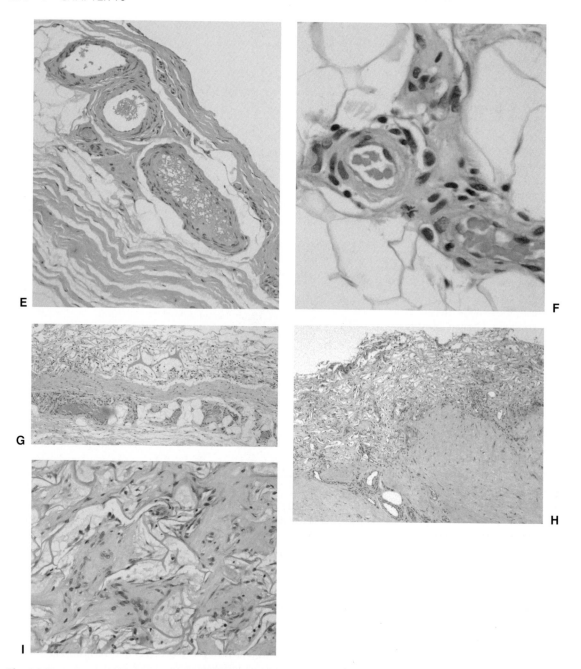

Fig. 16-7. **E. Normal angiocytes prior to Integra.** Figures 7e, 7f, 7g are from the same patient. The first is normal tissue prior to Integra. Among blood vessels large and small, the angiocytes, both endothelial and medial, are small and uniform in size. Many are flattened due to intraluminal blood shearing and mural tension and geometry. These are normal blood vessels. **F. Stimulation of perivascular cells.** At 10 days after Integra, syncytial clusters are starting to demand revascularization, mediated by the diffusion of angiogenic cytokines. Angiocytes in subjacent host blood vessels respond to these transforming, mitogenic, cytotactic peptides. Nuclei enlarge, with stippled chromatin. Cell sizes and shapes are enlarged and variable. Cells are breaking away from their native positions as they begin migration toward the source of angiogenic stimulus. Some undergo mitosis, seen in anaphase near the center.

1–2 weeks (Fig. 16–7j; onset at 3–6 weeks, depending on many factors).

Consolidation—Because the top levels lag behind the base, there is a period in which the base is both maturing and also serving as the source of migratory angioblasts and histioblasts needed at still developing higher strata. As histogenesis completes itself, the entire matrix consolidates to a uniform final appearance, domains filled, and all mitosis, migration, and reorganization ceased. Skin grafts are usually ready to be placed before this process is complete (Fig. 16–7k; 3–16 weeks).

Domain maturation—Pores that are newly filled with cells and connective proteins typically have loosely organized collagen bundles, still immature fibroblasts, and vessels not yet fully coalesced. There is a maturation period in which these structures assume their final histologic structure. Only a few weeks long, this maturation period is very brief by the standards of normal inflammatory scar maturation. This is when the tissue settles down to become typical mature mesenchyme. The cells that generated the new tissue need never again replicate unless injury or embryonic events once again recruit them to do so (Fig. 16–7l).

Epidermal events—Epithelium is usually restored surgically. Transplanted cells reestablish a basement membrane, then engineer the formation of a lamina propria to supply their metabolic needs. Papillation of the epidermis, formation of the papillary dermis, and proliferation of the subepidermal vascular plexus are events governed by the new epidermis. They are entirely independent of the substrate, and these events are identical for scars, ordinary skin grafts, Integra, or reepithelialization of any other wound or tissue (Fig. 16–7m and n).

The Histogenetic Process Compared to Normal Inflammatory Repair

The wound module of inflammatory repair was epitomized in a preceding paragraph, the anatomy of which is depicted in Fig. 16–8. To fully understand the advantages of Integra, the histology of these two systems must be directly compared. Key distinctions between the two are listed below.

Wound module versus histogenesis—Normal repair is triggered by and is contingent on inflammation, resulting in the wound module of inflammatory repair. Inflammation is antithetical to histogenesis, and Integra suppresses inflammation while undergoing a developmental rather than a reactive process (Fig. 16–9).

Timing—Inflammation is rapid, the entire process from onset to a nominally healed wound being measured in hours to days. Normal fibrous repair is sufficiently mature at 5–15 days to permit suture removal. Yet, at 5–15 days with Integra, the process of histogenesis is just barely underway. Integra is a more controlled and more paced process.

Cellular controllers—The "hornet's nest" of acute inflammation is stirred up by blood-borne neutrophils, monocytes, and lymphocytes. These cells are transient and extrinsic to the tissue, disappearing when injury is

---

Fig. 16–7. **Continued**

G. Entrainment of perivascular cells. A wide view of the 10 day events in figure 7f. The matrix, lying on the sural fascia of the leg, has numerous syncytial clusters. Metabolically active but without circulation, these clusters are signaling the need for angiogenesis. Diffusion of angiogenic factors into the subfascial areolar adipose has caused marked hyperplasia of host vessels. Subsequent migration of activated angioblasts across the fascia and into the matrix is obvious. This entrainment of angiogenic cells is the inception of true histogenesis, the formation of a multicellular structure with a tissue level of organization. **H. Vasculogenesis.** At 17 days, vascular hypertrophy and cell streaming toward the matrix are very active. A few blood vessels crossing into the matrix are well established. From these, newer vessels branch wider and deeper into the matrix, with erythrocytes in young vascular lumina. As vasculogenesis establishes circulation, cells and their products can proliferate. This allows the early syncytial clusters to begin a second set of more robust histogenesis. Note that the lower strata of the sponge, where vessels have entered, are filling with tissue, but the upper layers are still largely a void, awaiting the arrival of blood vessels. **I. Second set histogenesis.** A 17 day view of histogenesis after blood vessels arrive. The upper left corner, toward silicone, is unvascularized matrix, containing scattered syncytial cells making pale fibrillar collagen. The rest of the image is a zone of active angio-organization, with vessels seen in cross section and as longitudinal chords of clustered angioblasts. Some of the vessels have enlarged to a higher order to supply capillaries downstream. Angioblasts are still migratory or transformational, with large ovoid nuclei, stippled chromatin, and a loose intercellular organization, active in three processes: coalescence into blood conducting vessels, enlargement of diameter and mural thickness to serve as arterioles, and sourcing new angioblasts for more distal vessels. Wherever a pore has been infiltrated or traversed by a vessel, the pore has become filled with fibrous tissue, dense fibrous collagen trapping original syncytial cells, which are now beginning to have the classic fibroblast appearance. As vasculogenesis pushes upward toward the silicone or tangentially across non-vascular substrate, more and more of the matrix will become filled in this way.

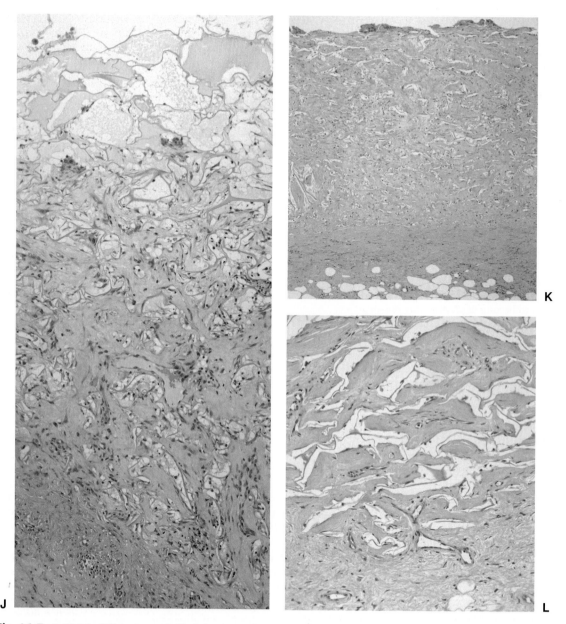

Fig. 16-7. J. Matrix filling. Latter half of the regeneration. At top, serum filled pores have pioneer and transitional cells. In the stratum below, syncytial clusters wait for nutrient capillaries. At center level are migratory angioblasts and erythrocyte-conducting vessels. Fibrous collagen is present, but this central layer is still more cellular than proteinized. Toward the base, large conducting vessels carry blood locally and to developing strata above, surrounded by dense fibrous collagen which is now predominant. At the lowest level, mature fibroblasts are trapped in maturing collagen bundles. A firm physical connection of collagen and vessels unites matrix and host. As active histogenesis and angiogenesis rise to higher strata, established vessels within the matrix become the angiogenic source, and vessels in the host substrate are returning to a normal non-proliferative state. The process will continue shifting upward. **K. Consolidation.** At 6 weeks, the matrix is consolidated, all pores and domains filled with regenerated tissue. Collagen in the newer upper strata is still young and amorphous, but the lower strata are assuming their final mature structure, and the matrix will become uniform over the next few weeks. (Note the large accumulation of foreign body giant cells at the

controlled. These cells never appear in healthy Integra. The pioneer cells, which find the Integra matrix, while lymphoid in appearance, are not lymphocytes. A defensive response is never initiated and these cells become intrinsic, the sires of the new tissue.

Control dynamics—As an engineering control system, inflammation and early repair is an open-loop process. The outputs of the system, angiogenesis and fibroplasia, have no direct inhibitory feedback on the system controllers, the leukocytes and macrophages, who answer to an independent set of triggers. New vessels reaching the inflammatory cells do not inhibit further production of angiogenic factors. Repair cells, under the uninhibited control of inflammatory cells, accumulate in supernormal numbers, leading to the excessive density of blood vessels and disorganized solid fibrosis that characterize young scar. The Integra control system has closed-loop feedback. Syncytial cells and angiocytes have a mutual cooperative regulation without the need for a third extrinsic party. New vessels are summoned only by legitimate metabolic need and the relief of ischemia by the arrival of new vessels turns off further production of angiogenic factors. The resulting vascular density is exactly what it needs to be to supply the needs of the tissue—no more, no less. Closed-loop control means that histogenesis more accurately targets a model of normal embryonically developed tissue, without excesses.

Order of events—In normal inflammatory repair, angiogenesis precedes any other reparative event. Angioblasts migrate from underlying source vessels toward the source of angiogenic stimulation, which is the inflammatory cell layer on the surface of the wound. Dense angioplasia is always present just below the wound surface, the vessels organizing in a layer of acute inflammatory glycosaminoglycans devoid of fibroblasts or proteins. Fibroblasts only appear deep to this, after vessels are well organized, conducting blood, and maintaining an environment where inflammatory cells are no longer needed. Angiogenesis leads. Fibroplasia follows. In Integra, fibroplasia leads and angiogenesis follows,

just as in normal embryogenesis. There is a second wave of fibroplasia, but this is due to the cooperative facilitation between the two sets of cells.

Fibroblasts—The reparative cells of inflammatory healing, angioblasts and fibroblasts, both originate from underlying vascular cells. Newly generated fibroblasts are typically round with large active nuclei. With time, they become denser and more compact, first filling their strata of the wound with cells, then becoming flattened by the collagen they produce. Whether first populating the revascularized aminoglycan ground substance or later entrapped in collagen, they are, at all times, distinct from each other, individually identifiable, never contiguous or entangled with each other. In Integra, syncytial fibroblasts are so-called because they are large, entangled, and indistinct. They look like embryonic dermatoblasts, not like ordinary reparative fibroblasts. Later cells appearing during second-set histogenesis are more like typical fibroblasts, but appear concurrently with collagen; they do not become dense and space filling themselves.

Vascular density—In inflammatory repair, new vessels are abundant, far in excess of normal vascular density and far in excess of what is needed for normal blood supply. Vessels are attracted to a broad tangential extrinsic boundary of stimulation (the macrophage zone), which is unconcerned about the normal vascular needs of the tissue. Because of the open-loop state of the system, angiogenesis just keeps going. This is recognized clinically as the robust red color of hypervascular granulation tissue. As the healed wound matures, excess vessels slowly involute and vascular density returns to normal over months or years. In Integra, vascular density remains accurate—exactly what is needed to meet the metabolic requirements of the tissue. This is because vasculogenesis is under the control of distributed attracting points (syncytial clusters), each intrinsic to the developing tissue, each having its own closed-loop interaction with arriving vessels. Having normal vascular density, regenerated Integra remains white, looking like dermis or fascia. Vascular density does not change much with

---

***Fig. 16–7.* Continued**
top, a response to the silicone rubber which can appear within a week of Integra's placement. This can cause some turbid blistering of the silicone, but it is not accompanied by inflammation. This is benign, and gentle curettage of the surface allows skin grafts to take without problem.) **L. Domain maturation.** At 8 weeks, histogenesis has ceased, and regeneration is complete. Collagen bundles are large and lamellated. Fibrocytes are flat, mature, and normal size. Blood vessels, both in the matrix and in the base, are of normal size and histology. The fibrous bond between host and matrix is completely natural. There is not an inflammatory cell in sight. This the final output of the histogenetic process, a compliant fibrous tissue, histologically and mechanically comparable to normal dermis, and distinct from scar. From this point forward, slow remodeling will occur, measurable only in months and years, just as native dermal collagen turns over. Note that the collagen-GAG matrix itself is entirely unaltered, neither resorbed by cellular nor chemical processes, nor in any way distorted by fibrous contraction or compression.

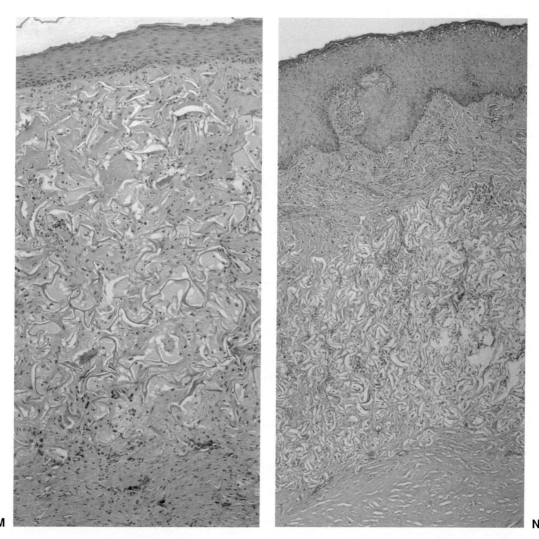

M

N

Fig. 16-7. **M. Epidermal events, early.** This is consolidated maturing. Integra a few weeks after skin grafting. The graft is still young, not yet mature enough to thicken and develop papillae, but all strata of the epidermis (germinativum, spinosum, granulosum, lucidum, corneum) are reorganized and functioning to expectations. As a metabolically active cellular tissue, the epidermis needs a robust circulation, and its effects on the Integra are already evident: numerous new capillaries have formed in the subepithelial zone. This is the beginning of a papillary dermis. **N. Epidermal events, late.** Mature, skin grafted Integra at one year. Loosely collagenized, the intrinsic matrix is nearly unaltered. There is no evidence whatsoever of matrix distortion due to fibrous contracture. What is new, compared to the preceding figure, is the papillary dermis. As the lamina propria of the epidermis, the epidermis, governs its formation, regardless of the original substrate. Characterized by a structural layer of thick collagen, a dense vascular plexus, and papillary rete ridges, it is, in all respects, a normal papillary dermis.

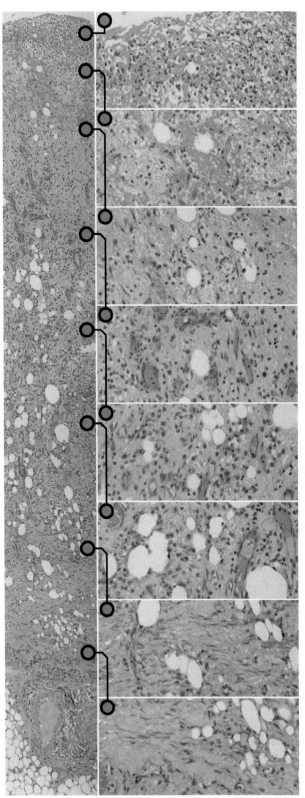

Fig. 16-8. This is a healthy wound, covered with typical "granulation tissue". This biopsy demonstrates the normal process of inflammatory repair, the "wound module". Inflammation, which triggers the events, always occurs at the surface. Strata develop, each layer down representing events from earlier days; looking deeper is to see the entire history of the wound. The wound is 2 weeks old, the specimen 6–8 millimeters thick. On the right are high resolution views of the strata.

Level 1, inflammatory zone. Fibrin and plasma cover the surface, heavily infiltrated with acute inflammatory cells (neutrophils, lymphocytes, monocytes). Platelet and leukocyte cytokines are transforming monocytes to macrophages, seen as occasional enlarged mononuclear cells.

Level 2, macrophage zone. Inflammatory cells are fewer, mixed with large transformed macrophages. They operate in a pale, acellular, non-proteinized "ground substance". This glycosaminoglycan "ether", made by inflammatory and transformed cells, has a different composition and structure than Integra GAG'S, and thus different effects. Macrophages have the keystone role of making pro-proliferative cytokines which will transform and attract histogenetic cells from underlying blood vessels.

Level 3, angioblast streaming. Stimulated angioblasts (migratory spindle cells), arisen from deeper source vessels, are streaming through the ground substance toward the stimulus macrophages. Arriving angioblasts start to reform tubular vessels.

Level 4, vessel organization zone. Organized tubular vessels are conducting blood, providing crucial support for the next major cell line, the fibroblasts. Neutrophils are still present, exiting vessels here to make their way to the top. A few young round fibroblasts and faint eosinophilia attest to the onset of connective protein formation.

Level 5, non-inflammatory transition zone. At this level, the incipient tissue is sequestered from inflammatory stimuli. There are no inflammatory cells (except a few in-transit neutrophils). Small round cells between vessels are young fibroblasts. Young collagen is still amorphous, but more abundant.

Level 6, fibroblast accumulation zone. Young round histogenetic cells fill the space between vessels with some early clustering and orientation. Collagen shows some fibrous structure, the first level at which things are becoming more "tissue" than "granulation".

Level 7, fibroblast maturation zone. Inflammatory cells have long since disappeared. Nearby large vessels conduct blood to proliferating capillaries above. Entrapped in the abundant collagen they are making, cells are flattened, oriented, and clustered, looking like classic fibroblasts.

Level 8, fibrous consolidation zone. The tissue is now more protein than cell. Collagen is in long thick bundles. Tensile strength is developing. As time continues, this collagen will become clinical scar, thicker, denser, and more non-compliant (Figure 16-11).

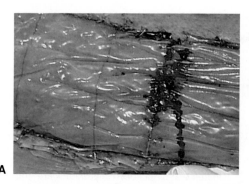
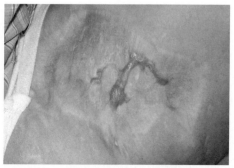

A   B

Fig. 16-9. **A.** Integra is fully regenerated, ready for skin grafts. In a seam between pieces, an open area has caused some normal wound healing, resulting in granulation pieces, an open area has caused some normal wound healing, resulting in granulation tissue. The side-by-side difference between normal repair and Integra is as obvious grossly as it is histologically, and this will result in different types of healed tissue, as shown next. **B.** Healed Integra at 24 months. Discounting the depression due to absence of subcutaneous adipose, it looks mostly like normal skin, soft, pliable, free of erythema and fibrosis. The only exception is the red scar in the center, a typical hypertrophic scar that occured where granulation tissue developed in a seam. The clinical differences between hypertrophic scar and mature Integra reflect the significant biological differences between wound module repair and Integra histogenesis.

maturation because it is already what it should be. Integra's vascular biophysics are identical to normal closed-loop embryonic vasculogenesis (Fig. 16–10).

Collagen density and organization—Inflammatory repair results in fibrous collagen, dense to the point of complete filling, with little lymph or ground substance. Large collagen bundles are arranged arbitrarily, but they develop tropic–anisotropic directionality if the scar is subjected to tensile loads (Wolf–Davis Law). The dense packing of collagen means that fibers have no tertiary or three-dimensional form (wavy, springy, or coiled), which would confer extensibility. The scar is therefore inelastic, noncompliant, and poorly deformable, leading to its many complications. Absent significant mechanical load, scar collagen slowly remodels, returning after months or years to an architecture akin to dermis or fascia. Integra collagen is less fibrous. It has no overall directionality. The matrix septae partition the space so that large-scale collagen organization is incoherent, unable to form long bundles. Rather, collagen forms casts of the matrix pores, following the contours of the bounding septae. This creates both a highly partitioned architecture and tertiary structure, which permits tensile strains. To the extent that a domain is fully bounded and tends to form closed "onion skin" loops of collagen, net local tension at rest tends toward zero. Collagen density can be no greater than 95% (matrix is 5% of volume), and the matrix serves as a percolation network of empty space between collagen bundles, giving it some fluidity. The regenerated material remains highly pliable and deformable (Fig. 16–11 and 16–12).

Contraction—Normal scar contracts, the natural means of closing a wound, but also the other reason for a scar's many complications. Integra does not contract. In addition to the properties discussed in the preceding paragraph, the appearance of the matrix remains unaltered. If Integra collagen did contract, one would expect to see the matrix material become stretched, distended, ruptured, folded, pinched, compressed, compacted, or any other conceivable deformation due to the force of contracting scar. None of this happens. Developing collagen respects and conforms to the material, and the native morphology of the matrix is unaltered during histogenesis (review any of the Integra histology images). Septal architecture also remains unaltered for as long as the matrix persists, which is years (Fig. 16–13)

Maturation—Normal inflammatory wound healing follows a pattern of "overshoot-then-involute." The acute inflammatory repair phase is rapid, aggressive, and open loop. Instead of the wound creating a model of normal tissue, it "overshoots," quickly resulting in an excessive density and quantity of new blood vessels and immature connective proteins. These early events are measured in days to weeks. Once the wound is epithelialized and proliferation ceases, the scar undergoes a maturation process in which excessive elements of repair involute. Erythema fades, scar becomes more compliant, and scar histology gradually transforms back toward normal dermis. Scar maturation is measured in months and years, and, in the interval, scar complications can cause all manner of troubles. Integra does not have this overshoot–involute pattern. Instead, Integra

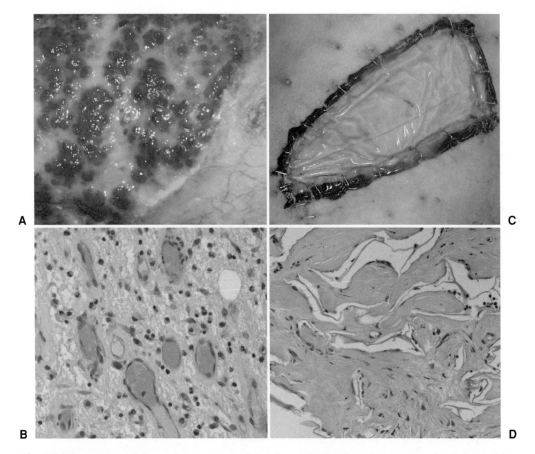

Fig. 16-10. **A, B.** In this normal wound, vascularized granulation tissue is a saturated red, due to high density of voluminous vessels. It contrasts sharply with pale surrounding skin. Histology corroborates the gross appearance. Hypervascularity, in excess of physiologic vessel density, results from an unregulated open loop process forced by cells (macrophages) extrinsic to the developing tissue. **C, D.** Integra neo-dermis is regenerated, ready for skin grafts. Histology shows just a few vessels, their number and volume much lower than in granulation tissue. Color (hue and saturation) matches the adjacent skin because they have equal vascular density. Precise, efficient network formation results from embryonic vasculo-genesis, a tightly regulated closed loop process controlled by cells (syncytial fibroblasts and embryonic dermatoblasts) that are intrinsic to the developing tissue.

undergoes an orderly targeted evolution, which leads to a dermal analog without any oscillatory behavior. Regenerated Integra is a nearly mature, mechanically compliant, esthetically acceptable tissue by the time that skin grafts are healed. This behavior is a conse-quence of closed-loop controls on cell migration and proliferation, which are typical of both Integra and embryonic histogenesis. Integra histogenesis is mea-sured in weeks to months, in a middle zone between inflammatory repair and scar maturation. The matrix itself disappears slowly by passive hydrolysis, preserving much of its original architecture for as long as 4 years. (Fig. 16–14).

Figures 16–15 and 16–16 highlight all of these dif-ferences. They show Integra juxtaposed directly against inflammatory repair and scar. In these images, the two processes operate concurrently, side by side within micrometers of each other. Yet the processes remain distinct, each preserving its own distinctive anatomy. The microanatomic differences correlate directly with differences in clinical behavior, potential morbidity and sequelae, and ability to have a well-behaved properly heal-ing wound. It must be understood that Integra does not alter basic biologic systems. The body has genetic processes that allow it to respond to different conditions. Injury is recognized as such, and the body responds accordingly,

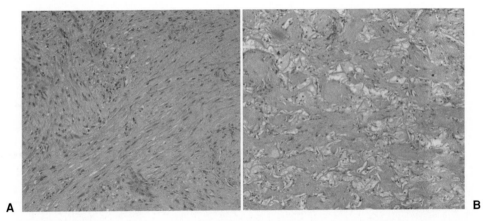

A **B**

Fig. 16-11. **A.** Fibroplasia in a normal wound. In the zone of fibrous consolidation, densely packed fibroblasts make thick chords of collagenized scar. Increasing connective proteins make the scar progressively less compliant or deformable. Initially omnidirectional, these chords will remodel themselves to resist applied tensile loads, thereby distorting features and obstructing motion. **B.** Integra collagenization. Cellularity is low. Collagen conforms to the matrix, forming discrete packets molded within the pores of the sponge. "Incoherence", spaces and interruptions between collagen clusters, mean that the material remains more fluid and deformable, more like normal tissue, less like scar.

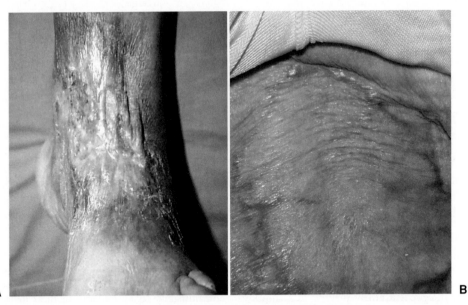

A **B**

Fig. 16-12. **A.** Scar contracture. Scar contraction and non-compliance causes the common clinical problem of joint contractures. In this dorsal ankle burn scar, motion puts tension on the scar, inducing tendinous metaplasia, further decreasing compliance. Motion also fractures the scar causing ulceration, begetting more scar. This is precisely the kind of case which is reconstructable with Integra. **B.** Compliant Integra. Integra was used here to close a large back wound. Just a few months later, while other normal scars are still young, red, and stiff, the new Integra skin is very deformable, wrinkling and folding normally in response to any motion or force. This property allows joints, the face, and other mobile parts to be reconstructed without contractures.

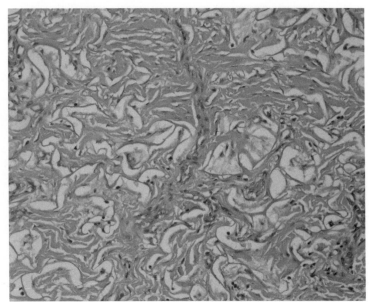

Fig. 16-13. Integra at one year. With time, normal physiologic collagen dynamics make the neodermis slowly look more like natural dermis, seen here as the formation of discrete loose parallel wavy collagen bundles. However, most of the matrix still persists, and whatever collagen remodeling is taking place, it continues to respect the boundaries imposed by the matrix. The neodermis conforms to the matrix, rather than distorting it, in contradistinction to the way that contracting scar distorts or obliterates anything.

with inflammatory repair. If other conditions are met, the body can respond by embryonic histogenesis. It is, therefore, not surprising that Integra does what it does, but without an artificial device to create the necessary stimulus, this histogenetic process has no natural triggers in adult life. It is erroneous to think of Integra as just another ordinary graft or repair. It invokes an entirely different biologic response than any other form of injury, surgery, or other treatment, accounting for its favorable properties (Table 16–1).

Related Therapeutic Effects

Semibiologic Non-Living Material

"Biologic dressings" are used to protect wounds, control inflammation, prevent pathergy and complications, and promote wound repair prior to definitive closure. Cadaver allograft, porcine xenograft, allogeneic amnion, and nonbiologic materials (eg, Biobrane, Bertek Pharmaceuticals, Inc., West Virginia) are commonly used in lieu of using (wasting) autogenous skin grafts simply for interim wound control. Integra is semibiologic. It is composed of biologic materials that identify itself to a wound as compatible. Aminoglycan biocompatibility, sequestration of the wound, and suppression of inflammation make Integra a comparable or superior biological dressing. Its key advantage, though, is that it is not alive. Other biologic dressings will die, degenerate, be rejected, or otherwise require periodic replacement. Integra does not die. It does not degenerate. Assuming that the wound has been properly prepared, it just sits on the wound, providing

biologic coverage without jeopardy to itself. It can serve its purpose as a biologic dressing for a prolonged interval (weeks to months) and it need not be replaced. It is available in limitless quantities without procurement issues.

Biologic Superdressing

As a nonliving semibiologic material, Integra is an excellent biologic dressing, but it has an added advantage. As the Integra-covered wound becomes healthy and competent to proliferate new tissue, the Integra then acts as the matrix for new tissue growth. Thus, Integra does double duty, first as a nonliving biologic dressing, which cannot die nor degenerate, and then as the agent of skin regeneration and reconstruction. As such, it is much more than just a simple or passive biologic dressing, and the term "biologic superdressing" designates its ability to automatically transition into the mode of active histogenesis and skin regeneration.

Histoconduction and Bridging

The Integra sponge is a trellis that guides the ingrowth of new tissue. When Integra is placed on a healthy wound, histogenetic cells and new blood vessels migrate into the material. It is customary to think of this ingrowth as an orthogonal function, the direction of growth being vertical through the matrix, at right angles to the wound surface, the same process taking place concurrently at each infinitesimal area of the wound. There is nothing that prevents histioblasts from migrating tangentially. If there is a gap or void in the wound, which cannot source cells into the overlying Integra, cells will migrate in from

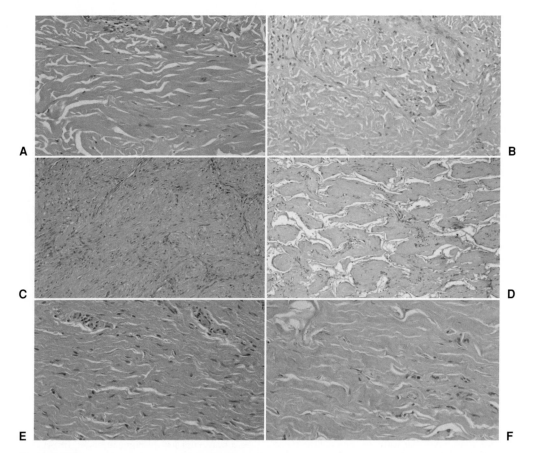

Fig. 16-14. **A.** Normal reticular dermis. Large, parallel, mostly horizontal collagen bundles are separated by interstitial spaces. Typical fibroblasts in typical densities are dispersed throughout. **B.** Normal reticular dermis from another subject, orthogonal view. Mechanical skin anisotropies (Langer's lines) mean that collagen might be seen tangentially or crosscut. Either way, collagen bundles are large, distinct, and coiled, wavy, or springy, with interstitial gaps. These properties confer elastic compliance, permitting normal motion of body parts. **C.** Young scar, normal repair at peak fibroplasia. The scar is highly cellular, to be heavily collagenized in ensuing weeks. Dense packing of fibers means no fluidity of the material. Lack of folding or waviness means that there can be no distensibility. This is basis of contractures, strictures, stenoses, stiffness, and other typical adverse effects of scar. **D.** Young Integra has a completely different histology, morphology, and biomechanics. The matrix partitions the collagen, creating interstitial spaces. It has many of the structural properties of normal dermis, explaining their mechanical and clinical similarities. **E.** Matured scar at 2 years. It is still cellular compared to normal dermis, but not by much. The scar collagen has undergone a gradual transformation. It is now bundled and springy, looking mostly like normal dermis. **F.** Old Integra at 4 years. Some of the original matrix is now gone, but for septae that do remain, their morphology is still unaltered. As with scar, physiological collagen remodeling is slowly making this specimen look like normal dermis. However, in sharp contrast to scar, Integra has, from the outset, a structure and properties that are always very close to dermis, thereby avoiding scar complications.

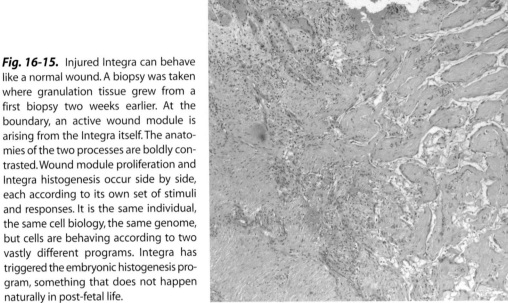

Fig. 16-15. Injured Integra can behave like a normal wound. A biopsy was taken where granulation tissue grew from a first biopsy two weeks earlier. At the boundary, an active wound module is arising from the Integra itself. The anatomies of the two processes are boldly contrasted. Wound module proliferation and Integra histogenesis occur side by side, each according to its own set of stimuli and responses. It is the same individual, the same cell biology, the same genome, but cells are behaving according to two vastly different programs. Integra has triggered the embryonic histogenesis program, something that does not happen naturally in post-fetal life.

surrounding healthy regeneration-competent areas. This property is analogous to other histoconductive matrices such as bone grafts. Tangential histoconduction means that Integra regeneration can "bridge" over surfaces that cannot heal. Objects that customarily need flaps for closure can instead be healed with Integra. This includes bone, tendons, open joints, cartilage, and even alloplastic hardware.

Suppression of Scar and Avoidance of Scar Sequelae

Scar is the consequence of inflammatory wound healing, a disorganized deposition of collagen distinctly different than normal dermis and fascias. An indiscriminate glue that binds injured tissues together, scar ensures the health of subjects after injury and surgery. For all the good that it does though, scar has its dark

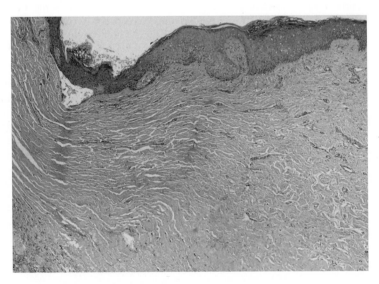

Fig. 16-16. The right half of this image is normal Integra at one year, the neodermis looking very much like normal dermis (Fig. 16-14). Epidermis and papillary dermis are normal. The Integra skin converges on an area of normal wound healing and ordinary contracted scar (the left half). As a mature scar, it is beginning to look somewhat like dermis, but juxtaposed against the Integra, one can appreciate why Integra behaves so much more like normal skin.

Table 16–1. Repair and histogenesis

Condition	Inflammatory repair	Integra histogenesis	Embryonic dermatogenesis and fetal wound repair
Inflammation	Inflammation triggers the process	Inflammation is suppressed	No inflammation
Cell controllers	Chemotactically summoned marrow-derived cells	Resident local mesenchyme (or possibly marrow derived patrol cells)	Locally developing mesenchyme
Type of cell response	Defensive	Nondefensive, histogenetic	Nondefensive, histogenetic
Type of healing	Wound module inflammatory repair	Generative (embryonic) histogenesis	Generative and regenerative histogenesis
Dynamical control system	Open-loop, controllers extrinsic to tissue	Closed-loop, controllers intrinsic to tissue	Closed-loop, controllers intrinsic to tissue
Order of histogenesis	Angiogenesis leads, fibroblasts follow	Fibroblasts lead, angiogenesis follows	Dermatoblasts lead, angiogenesis follows
Vasculogenic dynamics	Target or gradient angiogenesis	Distributed field angiogenesis	Distributed field angiogenesis
Vascular density	Hyperdensity angiogenesis	Correct density angiogenesis	Correct density angiogenesis
Type of histogenetic cell	Classic fibroblasts	Syncytial fibroblasts	Syncytial fibroblasts (dermatoblasts)
Collagen architecture	Dense, noncompliant	Percolated, distensible	Percolated, distensible
Scar contraction	Prominent	Absent	Absent
Star chemical	Collagen (structural)	Glycosaminoglycans (process regulator)	Glycosaminoglycans (process and structure)

side. Prior to maturation, scars and their sequelae can become foremost clinical issues. From skin deformities after burns and dermatoses, to joint contractures and tendon entrapment after all types of extremity injury, to strictures, stenoses, and obstructions of tubular viscera, restriction of lungs, dyskinesias of the heart and valves, and sclerosis and dystrophy of tissues everywhere, scar can be a potent troublemaker. Throughout all of medicine, it is one of the most prevalent causes of long-term morbidity and dysfunction and the need for corrective surgery, physical therapy, and other clinical care. Because Integra stops inflammation and normal repair, it stops scar formation. No scar means none of its complications. It can control fibroplasia where old scars once were, it can prevent the formation of new scars, and it can correct the adverse consequences of scar, such as contractures and stenoses. It even suppresses or prevents pathologic types of scar, such as keloids.

Similarity to Normal Dermis and Favorable Mechanics

More than just taming scar, regenerated Integra has properties comparable to normal dermis. This can be inferred

from its histology and histogenesis. Mechanical testing of these materials has provided documentary confirmation.[12] The real proof though is "in the pudding." Clinical observations of its texture and quality, its suppleness, and pliability readily confirm its distinction from scar and similarity to normal skin. This means that mechanical compliance is good (more elastic, lower Young's modulus), that scars are not apt to contract, and that the resulting sequelae of scar contracture do not occur.

Control of Local Soft–Tissue Pathology

Integra does not cure nor have any direct active therapeutic effect on any of the diseases that create pathologic wounds and chronic ulcers. However, Integra does have the ability to control the local effects of disease. Injury, disease, inflammation, ulceration, wound closure, and various therapies are all part of a complex nonlinear dynamical multicontrol system, just like any complex system in physiology and pathology. Normal tissue, active but stable disease, rampant disease, a normal healthy healing wound, a stalled wound, and an actively ulcerating wound are all basins of attraction or local stability on the chaotic attractor of the system's state space. In the chronic pathologic wound, sick controllers and impaired degrees of freedom in the system cannot easily keep the host in a desirable state. Any perturbation of the system, by disease, trauma, or therapy, can have no effect or dramatic effects, expected results or contrary results. How a therapeutic intervention might effect the system cannot be predicted, even when the linear one-to-one relationships between particular components of the system are well characterized. The body has various systems for fighting, controlling, and eliminating disease, but in the chaotic pathologic wound, these systems cannot prevail. While Integra does not directly cure any diseases, its ability to control the wound is profound enough to permit normal physiologic systems to recover, regain the upper hand, and eliminate residual pathology. Thus, via complex nonlinear interactions, Integra controls local soft-tissue pathology and keeps it controlled. Active inflammation and ulceration cease, and reconstructed areas seem resistant to recurrent disease.

Resistance to Recurrent Disease

Continued management of underlying diseases and risks is mandatory for any wound in any patient, before, during, and after acute phases of healing and reconstruction. This is for both the general health of the patient and the continued health of the closed wound. Reality is though that some patients will have flare-ups of disease or unexpected injury or they will lapse in their follow-up and preventive care. Like anything else, Integra can be damaged by trauma such as lacerations or pressure. However, it seems to be relatively resistant to the effects of recurrent inflammatory and lytic disorders, such as venous or rheumatoid ulceration.

INDICATIONS AND USES OF INTEGRA

Integra General Indications

Integra's use can be classified or conceptualized in several ways. It is both an acute *artificial skin* and a *skin regenerant*, and it can be used to serve either or both of these functions. Most Integra cases can be classified into four general modes of use. (1) *Critical coverage* for salvage of life and limb. As an artificial skin, Integra blocks recognition of injury, quenches inflammation, and controls pain, pathergy, edema, and fluid fluxes. These properties help stabilize general metabolism with large injuries, significantly reduce nursing requirements, and accelerate recovery and rehabilitation. Integra can be life saving for large wounds, such as burns, deglovings, and fasciitis.[13–18] (2) Integra provides *essential coverage*, closing exposed visceral, skeletal, and other structures. As artificial skin, it provides interim protection for these structures, and as an agent of regeneration, it creates the final skin coverage, often supplanting the flaps or complex repairs usually required for their closure. (3) As a

skin regenerant, Integra is valuable for any soft-tissue *reconstruction* where quality of the skin and avoidance of scars and contractures is desirable. (4) Integra's dual nature also allows it to act as a *"biologic superdressing."* Like any acute biologic dressing, Integra, can have a true therapeutic role, controlling inflammation, environmental exposure, and other risks, which threaten wound healing and surgical repair. However, unlike ordinary biologic dressings, Integra need not be removed, and it automatically assumes the role of skin regenerant.

For many wounds, acute and chronic, traumatic and pathologic, Integra's ability to fulfill these roles easily and at low risk makes it equivalent to or superior to conventional methods of wound closure. For example, its ability to conduct tissue tangentially allows it to bridge gaps, such as open joints, and cover structures, such as large tendons. This means that a simple safe procedure can supplant a traditional large operation, with equivalent and, sometimes, better results. Choosing among various options for wound closure is based on many factors related to the wound, the disease and risks, and the patient. To understand Integra's indications and advantages, it is first necessary to understand the general principles of reconstructive plastic surgery and operative wound closure.

Overview of Wound Repair Surgery

Therapeutic wound repair, as opposed to physiologic wound repair, means surgical closure. Many wounds do not need surgery to close. They simply need good hygienic care in support of natural contraction and epithelialization. However, some wounds do need surgery for closure, either for the sake of timeliness and efficiency, or for the sake of safety and preservation of parts and function, or because they will not heal otherwise. When surgery is required or desirable, the methods generally fall into three categories: repair, grafts, and flaps.

General Issues and Topical Care

In discussing the methods of wound management and closure, there are several important concepts that must be remembered in every case, every patient, and every wound. These are: (1) Wounds heal. It is nature's way. In a healthy patient, operative repair is not necessary for many wounds. (2) However, operative repair of simple wounds is done for many good reasons, such as symptomatic and psychologic relief, convenience, expediting the end result and minimizing costs, and controlling the functional and cosmetic outcome. (3) Healthy wounds heal, and while good care supports this, all too often bad care impedes what nature can already do on its own. Do not mistake poor care for a pathologic wound. (4) Pathologic wounds do not heal on their own. In order to plan treatment an accurate diagnosis and understanding the pathophysiology is necessary. (5) Nonoperative topical care in support of contraction and epithelialization is always a good choice in healthy simple wounds. (6) When a wound is not capable of healing by normal contraction, or when a wound must not be allowed to heal that way, by reason of disease, anatomical complexity, altered function, or threat to the patient, this is when choices must be made about surgical closure. (7) Wounds that are not properly prepared and do not meet criteria of suitability-for-closure cannot be closed. This is true from the repair of simple lacerations to managing major trauma to doing elective surgery to placing implants like Integra. Premature closure of an unprepared wound will result in abscess or dehiscence. Wounds that are not ready to close, must not be closed. Proper preparation means complete control or correction of disease, elimination of injury, removal of debris and eschar, alleviation of adverse mechanics, and thorough control of edema and inflammation. Throughout this chapter, any discussion of operative wound closure, by Integra or by any conventional method, is hereby explicitly understood to be a wound that has had the necessary preoperative evaluation and preparation appropriate for the circumstances of the wound, and that the wound is as fully controlled and prepared as the current state of the art, the efforts of physician and patient, and the nature of the underlying disease permit.

Wound Repair

"Wound repair" in its most liberal definition refers to (1) the physiological process of wound healing, (2) any type of wound-closure surgery, and (3) certain tactical methods of wound closure. In the latter sense, repair refers to the simple methods of directly approximating wound margins. These basic techniques are used when injured anatomy can or must be reduced, significant amounts of skin are not missing, and additional incisions and advancement of tissue are not needed. Any procedure, which requires the replacement of missing anatomy or the elaborate design and rearrangement of skin, is considered reconstruction. Repairs are generally done for acute benign wounds following trauma and surgery.

Grafts

Grafts are pieces of tissue that come from a variety of sources and which are sutured into the recipient wound (in this chapter, "suture" implies any suitable form of surgical fixation, including sutures, staples, tapes, and glues). A graft is a graft by virtue of the fact that it has no anatomical attachment to the host, no circulation of its own, and it is not capable of living independently away from a recipient wound. Any type of tissue can be grafted for many reasons. Some grafts are alive and some

need not be. For example, cadaveric fascia, tendon, and bone are everyday surgical implants because even though dead, their desirable biomechanical and bone regenerative properties persist. However, for skin grafts and wound repair purposes, grafts must be alive. This puts certain constraints on a successful graft: (1) Grafts, even living grafts, depend on the host or recipient wound to do the healing. (2) They will neither survive nor heal if the host wound is incompetent to heal. (3) Because a graft is completely dependent on the health of the recipient wound, the wound must be properly prepared, nonpathologic, and adequately vascularized. (4) The graft must be in firm direct contact with the wound. Failure to have a mechanically stable graft means no adhesion, no revascularization, and no healing. Improper application, seromas, hematomas, and motion are categorically intolerable. All manner of dressings and splints are used to avoid these. (5) The graft must be suitably thin to stay alive. Too many cells, too thick, and their metabolic needs outstrip the diffusibility of gases and nutrients from the host wound, and it dies. (6) Skin grafts do not carry with them the cellular machinery of repair. Therefore, the recipient wound, which does all of the healing for the whole system, must be healthy. (7) A healed skin graft is epidermis on scar, and like any scar, it is subject to hypertrophy, contracture, and related problems. (8) Grafts are technically simple and clinically convenient, but, biologically, are very complex. In short, a skin graft is a way to put skin someplace that it is needed, but the recipient wound must be healthy, wound healing competent, independently capable of healing, and have no special needs other than the need to restore missing epithelium; the mechanics and appearance of the healed wound must not be an issue. Excision of a large nevus on the back or closure of a large burn at mid-thigh in a healthy person are examples of ideal suitability for a skin graft. Chronic irradiated wounds of mobile tissues around the mouth or perineum are the worst conceivable circumstances to use a skin graft, and poor appearance and function of the grafts will be moot because they will not heal in the first place.

There are three main reasons that grafts are used. (1) Convenient wound closure. When rapid or extensive closure is desirable in a healthy wound, and when scars and function are not foremost concerns, skin grafts are the most pragmatic method to close a wound that cannot be repaired by simple suture or minor flaps. (2) Biologic dressing. Dressings made of compatible biologic materials provide high-quality short-term protection for wounds under those circumstances where autogenous skin is in short supply, minor inflammation or injury persist despite care, or the wound or patient are not yet ready for final closure. Biologic dressings are temporary by design. Skin grafts are a suitable way to do this. However, since loss of the grafts is also likely, the method is best managed with disposable materials, such as cadaver allograft, porcine xenografts, and alloplastic materials such as Biobrane. (3) Specialized reconstruction. Special grafts are used for specific reconstructive needs—functional and cosmetic. A variety of tissues are valuable as reconstructive grafts, including bone, fascia, tendon, cartilage, mucosas, and full-thickness skin. Skin grafts are of two varieties. Those used for convenient wound closure are usually "split thickness," tangential shaves of epidermis, which allow the donor site to re-epithelialize. They are very convenient, utilitarian, and the best option for covering large areas. However they also heal with scar and contract. "Full-thickness" grafts transport both dermis and epidermis. They are limited in availability, and they require deliberate operative repair of the donor site, but they are similar to native skin when healed, so they are used when high-quality skin reconstruction is needed in relatively small areas, especially around joints, face, and mobile structures, which cannot afford to contract.

Flaps

Flaps, like grafts, are pieces of tissue transferred from one place to another for the sake of reconstruction or wound closure, but with crucial differences. A flap is a flap by virtue of the fact that it does maintain an anatomic attachment to the host (the pedicle), carrying its own circulation, and being perfectly capable of living independent of any other anatomy other than its own pedicle. While skin flaps are the most common, flaps come from all variety of tissues for the sake of myriad types of reconstruction. They are all typically thick, complete structures, such as a whole muscle, or composite structures of skin and fascia or skin, fascia, and muscle. Unlike certain grafts which can be nonliving, flaps are categorically alive, and any necrosis of a flap due to inadequate circulation is a failure. The biology, techniques, and indications for flaps are completely different than those of grafts: (1) Healthy properly made flaps are independently capable of healing and do not depend on any substrate or recipient area. (2) Flaps will live and heal even when the recipient wound is incompetent to heal. (3) Any target wound to be closed with a flap must meet basic closure criteria of hygiene, débridement, and control of disease and inflammation, but need not be fully vascularized or inherently healthy. (4) The technical deficiencies, which can kill a graft (mechanical dehiscence or impaired adhesion) do not kill flaps; they can be advanced and inset again. (5) Whereas grafts depend on diffusion of gases and nutrients from the host wound, flaps get these via the circulation through their pedicles, and flap failure is usually due to poor design, poor technique, or vascular disease, all of which can result in inadequate perfusion. (6) Because flaps are

normal, vascularized, independently viable composite tissues, they carry with them all of the machinery of wound repair, and can heal when the recipient wound is ill and cannot heal. (7) Flaps retain their original normal characteristics and mechanics as they heal and thus avoid problems due to tangential scarring. (8) Flaps can be technically elaborate, but properly designed, they are biologically very simple, simply healing a circumferential "cut" by ordinary means. Some flaps are small and technically trivial, such as for minor trauma repair, small scar revisions, and reconstruction after the excision of small skin lesions. Some flaps require substantial technique with significant possible risk to the patient, including the risks of any prolonged and elaborate operation, and the sacrifice of donor structures (done for the greater good, but still a sacrifice). While some small flaps are done simply for convenience, major flaps are done because the wound cannot be directly repaired, simple grafts will not heal, essential structures must be protected, problematic scars must be avoided, or various other site-specific reconstructive criteria must be met.

The main caveat of flaps is that the circulation through the pedicle may be inadequate to meet the perfusion needs of the entire mass of the flap. Unlike split-thickness skin grafts (STSG), flaps are not a renewable resource, so proper design and execution are of paramount importance so that they remain viable. Some flaps are "random," meaning that they are designed based on local geometry, tissue mechanics, and the desirability of a particular piece of skin for a particular purpose, but not designed with regard to the vascular anatomy of the tissue. There are general design rules that govern how to create a successful random flap. Many factors can interfere, such as anisotropic skin elasticity which can keep a flap from reaching the target, or a poorly placed suture that creates a line of tension across a flap which will kill it. In the interest of having flaps reach their targets successfully, they are sometimes raised and advanced in incremental stages known as "delays," each delay allowing the flap's vascular network a chance to adapt. Large random flaps may be tricky to pull off, but they often provide the best functional and cosmetic results by restoring precisely the type of tissue needed. When safety, a healed wound, and preservation of life and limb are of paramount importance, the most dependable flaps are "anatomical" flaps, flaps that are designed explicitly around the vascular anatomy of the tissue to be used. Skin and fascia are supplied, in part, by direct fasciocutaneous vessels arising from the major distributing vessels and are supplied, in part, by perforators arising in underlying muscles. The circulatory anatomy of skin, fascias, and muscles is well mapped, and it is easy to design flaps where the incorporation of these vessels or muscles ensures a fully perfused flap. Many standard flaps (such as the rectus abdominis or the latissimus dorsi muscles) are based on a single vascular pedicle, allowing those flaps to be transplanted to remote locations where the pedicle vessels can be anastomosed to vessels at the recipient site (a "free flap"). These flaps may sacrifice useful muscles and can be bulky and require later revisions, but they reliably get wounds healed. As such, they are used when large amounts of tissue are needed, or when open important structures demand dependable coverage. In short, flaps can be technically elaborate and laborious, but they bring inherently healthy, wound-healing competent tissues to the problem area. When the stakes are high for successful wound closure, good flaps get the job done.

There are four main reasons to use flaps. (1) Convenient wound closure—Typically for small traumatic or surgical defects where simple direct repair is not possible, the simplest, most efficient, and most dependable way to close a wound is a small nearby flap. (2) Essential coverage—The conventional arts of repair dictate that exposed visceral and skeletal structures should be closed with flaps. This is because skin grafts cannot take or cannot perform properly in this role. The reasons are many. Grafts cannot take over moving skeletal parts, such as joints and tendons. They cannot take over voids such as joint spaces and serous cavities or over alloplastic non-living materials, such as hernia mesh and metal joint prostheses. Even if grafts could theoretically be coaxed to heal over some of these structures, the noncompliant scar will rupture with subsequent movement, or scarring in the grafts will inhibit movement. Skin grafts over rigid materials (bone) are subject to shear ulceration with only minor force. Pathologic conditions in exposed structures, such as a bowel fistula, may destroy skin grafts or lyse any direct repair under tension. Exposed vital organs like heart, lung, and brain may require ample protection from injury and exposure. In these situations, skin grafts and similar materials can have a role as biologic dressings for acute, short-term protection. However, definitive closure of these essential structures requires thick, durable, mechanically compliant, anatomically normal tissues that ensure healing and do not depend for their survival on the wound or the structures that are being closed. (3) Reconstruction—Flaps are often used when reconstructive requirements are foremost considerations. Reconstruction means restoring tissues or entire structures, the reconstitution of form and function to avoid or correct disabilities or cosmetic defects. Such functional problems may be acute and wound related, or they may be chronic, elective, and associated with disease, birth defects, or remote healed trauma. The restoration of injured or missing complex structures can be for any reason on any part of the body. Situations are as diverse as medicine and pathology themselves; from the release and reconstruction of burn and scar contractures to the replacement of missing facial features after cancer surgery, from ears to eyelids, abdominal wall defects to anal strictures, pharynx to fingers. Anything that needs form or function or must move or look correct needs to be reconstructed. Flaps fulfill the reconstructive requirements of specific tissue types for specific tasks without excessive scarring. (4) Wound healing incompetence—This is essentially synonymous with chronic and pathologic wounds. Wounds that can heal do so. When a wound or injury cannot heal, it becomes a chronic ulcer. Radiation, venous disease, arterial disease, immunopathies, and so on all create circumstances in which the inherent machinery of repair, the local progenitor cells and the derivative wound module, are impaired, inhibited, or dysfunctional, to one degree or another. All operative wound closures involve the juxtaposition of one wound surface against another. While it is nice when a wound is completely healthy and both surfaces can heal, nevertheless, it is only necessary for one of the two surfaces to be wound-healing competent. If both surfaces are wound-healing incompetent, nothing heals. This is why skin grafts usually fail over chronic wounds, because neither the wound nor the graft are independently capable of healing. When operative wound closure demands that competent tissues be juxtaposed against the incompetent ones, flaps provide this service. Obviously, the flap itself must be fully healthy. For instance, a radiation ulcer cannot be closed by the mobilization and advancement of adjacent irradiated skin, so a flap from a farther region is needed.

Good flaps are the romantic heroes of reconstructive plastic surgery. However, as good as they are, they have their limitations. Certain areas of the body, notably around the ankle and foot, often do not have enough skin to close the defects that occur there. Local soft-tissue mechanics may prevent a flap from reaching its target. Certain areas do not have any direct anatomical flaps. Flaps can die, either in whole, or, more commonly, the distal end of the flap which is, of course, the part being stretched into service to cover the target defect. Underlying vascular disease may kill a flap. Atherosclerotic vessels may prevent anastomosis of a free flap. Potential local flaps may be within the zone of injury. Occult hematological disorders can kill a flap. Active inflammatory or other disorders may threaten the flap as much as they have caused the primary problem, either by necrosis or by dehiscence and failure to heal. Whatever illnesses and comorbidities have created the wound may make the patient too ill or high risk for an elaborate operation. Flaps can sacrifice useful parts and create secondary disabilities. Flap donor sites can have complications and make the whole problem larger. Failed flaps take away anatomy and limit further options. A core skill of plastic surgery is knowing how to make a good flap and avoid these problems and pitfalls. In patients who have chronic and pathologic wounds, these problems and pitfalls may not be avoidable. Flaps play a pivotal role in the closure of complex wounds, but there are times when flaps simply cannot be done or will not survive. Integra is the new alternate option that often works where flaps cannot. Understanding when a flap should be but cannot be used is to understand when Integra should be used.

Integra and Conventional Wound Surgery

By now, it should be clear that, when dealing with chronic and pathologic wounds, especially those that have exposure of bones, tendons, joints, and other essential structures, conventional simple direct closure and skin grafts, the technically simple options, are usually doomed to fail. Deliberate conscientious open wound care is usually superior, safer, and more successful. If surgery is indicated, conventional principles of plastic surgery, prior to Integra, required flaps for dependable closure. This principle has always been, and always will be, valid, but as just discussed, the same problems that create pathologic wounds also create problems for flaps. Problem wounds have a well deserved bad reputation, and conventional principles of operative plastic surgery, which succeed in healthy wounds, have their limitations in problem wounds.

Integra is a new paradigm of wound closure. Its technical use is nearly identical to ordinary skin grafts, but the similarities end there. It is an implant, it is not living, it suppresses repair, it induces histogenesis, it has histoconductive properties, all unique among ordinary wound closure materials and methods. Integra is not meant to be used for every wound. The entire art of surgical wound repair and reconstructive plastic surgery offers many options to get good results in simple, effective, dependable ways. Most problems can be solved by usual methods. Integra is used for two important reasons. First, in certain situations, it gives superior results compared to conventional methods, either a better biological result, or improved safety, convenience, or economy. Second, it solves problems which are not remediable by conventional means. The following sections will explain Integra's general indications and uses, after which its role in chronic wounds will be detailed.

Integra for Acute Wounds and Critical Coverage

Integra functions as a high-quality artificial skin. Whether for burns, fasciitis, degloving injuries, or any trauma or surgery resulting in large loss of skin, it has proven itself a superior tool to minimize morbidity, accelerate recovery, and avoid residual sequelae. Its

effects on an acute wound can be dramatic, and on large acute wounds, life saving. Control of extensive platelet and leukocyte activation and subsequent inflammation have a potent beneficial effect on general posttrauma physiology. Fluid fluxes, evaporative cooling, environmental exposure, and microbial bioburden are immediately eliminated. No donor sites are created, which would enlarge the wound and compound these problems. Dressing changes are infrequent and nursing requirements for the wounds are nil. Its dependability as an acute skin replacement has even extended the range of surgical procedures, allowing elective excision of huge areas of skin for problems such as lymphedema.[19]

Integra for Essential Coverage

Integra can cover and close those internal structures that convention says should be managed with flaps. As a high-grade skin substitute, it can protect those structures. Because it is not alive, it cannot degenerate and disappear simply because it is overlying a nonvascular structure which cannot support an ordinary skin graft. Because it regenerates new tissue, it eventually builds its own final living coverage. Because it can conduct tissue tangentially, it can bridge, building new tissue across gaps that ordinarily mandate closure with flaps. Because of its superior mechanics compared to skin grafts, it often functions as effectively as flaps over mechanical structures. It has these properties without creating donor wounds or sacrificing other autogenous tissues. It permits closure and salvage of injured extremities that might otherwise be amputated for lack of a good flap.

Integra for Reconstruction

If a wound or injury crosses joints or mobile structures, contractures may occur. Integra can be used for initial wound closure in order to avoid contactures from occurring. Integra can also be used as a later procedure to correct already stiff or contracted joints. Many circumstances will affect whether Integra or any other surgical method is used either sooner or later for these purposes, but if the goal is to avoid scar-related morbidity, disability, and disfigurement, Integra can solve the problem. Its crucial property in this regard is its ability to arrest normal fibroplasia and instead create a more normal embryonic type of tissue which has favorable mechanics. Flaps are conventional and they may often be superior, but Integra has some preferential properties, such as control of scar, lack of donor sites, formation of a thin tissue, and no need for later "debulking" procedures. Practical clinical uses of this property of Integra include the correction or elimination of keloids, the prevention or correction of contractures, the restoration of features to face, breast, genitalia, and other soft structures, and restoration of a more normal skin surface to areas of older scar tissue and skin graft.

INTEGRA FOR CHRONIC AND PATHOLOGIC WOUNDS

The overall success rate in completely healing chronic wounds with Integra is nearly 90% in properly selected patients. This is exceptionally good when one considers that Integra is used for the extreme situations of refractory pathology, extensive ulceration, exposed vital structures, and other risk factors for which conventional repair and reconstruction are apt to fail or have already failed. All of the foregoing discussion about the general use of Integra is fundamental to understanding how to use Integra for chronic wounds. The difference is that chronic and pathologic ulcers are hard to treat and are prone to complications and failure. For these wounds, Integra not only fulfills its nominal roles as artificial skin and skin regenerant, but it is therapeutic, helping to tame inflammation and residual pathology, thereby giving an advantage to the wound and its treatment that few other therapies, if any, can match. Throughout this section, quantitative and outcome-oriented statements will be made, such as "most common risk factor," "20% incidence," "length of treatment averages 5 months," "95% success." These valuations are based on the author's cumulative experience and compiled data, as well as other sources. This data is summarized in the "Review of Experience" section that follows.

The Problem of the Chronic Problem Wound

The book *Wound Repair*, 2nd edition, by Peacock and VanWinkle, 1976, is a milestone publication, being the first contemporary textbook widely circulated devoted to this subject.[20] However, textbooks reflect the problems and perspectives of their times and, in 1976, the issues of the day were precytokine wound-healing physiology, surgical technique, burns, trauma, surgical wounds, and repair of tendons and other special structures. The foremost basic science topics were collagen biology and scar. Only 14 of 699 pages are devoted to a rudimentary discussion of venous and pressure ulcers, with treatment emphasis on skin grafts. Published just a few years later, the small book *Chronic Problem Wounds* by Rudolph and Noe, 1983, reflects the awakening appreciation that these problems are distinct from ordinary surgical wounds, that there must be some diagnosis-oriented formality in the approach to pathologic ulcers, and that their good care requires a different frame of mind.[21] Contemporary wound research and practice is now centered on problem wounds, in no small part, because we have been so successful in learning how to manage and resolve acute healthy traumatic wounds. One might hope that in decades to come, that chronic pathologic wounds will become equally easy to manage; for now, the designation "problematic" is well earned.

Some chronic and pathologic ulcers are due to diseases such as lupus or hemoglobinopathies that are persistent and difficult to treat. Some, such as pressure ulcers, are due to repetitive unrelieved injuries that arise from complex physical and psychosocial problems that cannot easily be corrected. The problem is made more complex because there are always two sets of issues to diagnose and treat, what caused the injury or tissue loss, and what is inhibiting healing. Sometimes these are the same and sometimes they are distinct. Trivial assumptions about successfully repairing healthy wounds, as ordinarily practiced for everyday trauma and surgery, are invalidated because some of these chronic wounds simply cannot heal. Many of these problems are in older patients where there are multiple concurrent risk factors that compound the severity and refractoriness of the ulcer. These are chronic problems, which heal slowly, and whose care requires the diligent and extended participation of patient, family, and professional providers. However, many patients cannot cooperate with the prescribed care, due to disease, physical disabilities, and psychological, social, and economic factors. An older patient with rheumatoid ankle ulcers or diabetic foot ulcers who might be blind, obese, crippled in the hands, stiff in the back or hips, has no companions at home, and has inadequate economic resources to afford help, simply cannot perform the seemingly simple tasks of wound bathing and bandaging. These wounds are chronic problems with a chronic risk of recurrence if the underlying disease is not managed. The problem is compounded by huge gaps in our knowledge of the biophysics and pathology of these problems. The number of rational, scientific, and thoughtfully invented therapeutic products is still limited, and the subject is an invisible orphan in the undergraduate curriculum of medical education. Thus, problem wounds will be a problem for a long time.

Effective management of problem wounds follows the same models of clinical care that are applied to any issue in medicine. This means proper history and examination, a differential diagnosis of the causes, and a refined diagnosis based, as needed, on laboratory and imaging studies. Unlike most other medical problems, thorough wound diagnosis also depends on a period of observation to ascertain the behavior of the wound, its dynamics, and its response to nonspecific introductory wound care. It must be concluded whether a wound is being sustained by ongoing trauma or if it is failing due to persistent disease. It must be determined if wound healing physiology is inherently competent, responding but losing to repetitive injury, or if wound healing per se is failing. If the problem is repetitive injury, is it due to some pathologic or physical condition inherent to the patient, or is it the result of inept injurious care? If the wound is failing, incompetent to heal, is it due to correctable extrinsic factors, such as arterial insufficiency, or is the intrinsic machinery of repair inhibited or damaged, such as by antimetabolite chemotherapy or radiation? Once these questions are answered, then a diagnosis-specific treatment plan must be implemented. Some therapies will be obvious, rational, and effective. Some will be favorite nostrums and "shot in the dark" choices from the often irrational supply depot of wound care products. Some patients need pharmaceuticals, some need physical modalities, some need surgery, and some just need good nursing. Progress must be monitored and measured and the treatment changed as needed if the wound is not responding as expected to prescribed care. It is not the purpose of this chapter to discuss the general biology of the problem wound and its overall clinical management. It is presumed that every clinician treating these problems understands the basic structure of medical diagnosis and treatment and how they apply to this particular subject, regardless of the specific diagnoses or what the treatment plan and choices are for any individual patient and wound.

The preceding discussion of conventional wound repair represents the current common art of reconstructive plastic surgery. While customary repair, grafts, and flaps are eminently successful in curing acute wounds in healthy people, they cannot be trusted in chronic wounds. The new quest to cure chronic pathologic wounds is, therefore, fostering many novel approaches to all aspects of wound therapeutics, both surgical and nonsurgical. Integra is one of the new thoughtfully invented products that works well. It is versatile, effective, and safe, and like anything else, it must be selected and used properly in order to succeed.

RATIONALE AND INDICATIONS FOR INTEGRA ON CHRONIC WOUNDS

Surgical closure of chronic and pathologic wounds is difficult and unreliable for the same reasons that they are difficult to manage without surgery. Underlying disease perpetuates the ulcer or inhibits healing. Control of underlying disease is mandatory, in principle, but it can be impossible to eliminate adverse factors such as autoimmune inflammation, arterial insufficiency, and the effects of radiation. These disorders can also cause anatomical complications or caveats, such as rheumatoid synovitis exposing ankle tendons or severe atherosclerosis eliminating the usual flaps used to cover those tendons. These are the wounds subject to pathergy and wound healing failure, leading to prolonged care, multiple failed procedures, risk of amputation, and prolonged frustration and expense. For unwary surgeons, autogenous materials are prone to be wasted and donor

site complications may enlarge the original wound. Even when a standard flap is available, underlying illness and risks may cause complications or make the patient too ill for major surgery. These are the problems of trying to do surgery for chronic pathological wounds. Integra's properties solve most of these problems and it is often the only option which will succeed. The art of efficient, expeditious, effective wound repair or reconstruction is in knowing when to apply each of the tools. Integra should be used preferentially for the circumstances listed below.

High-Risk History and Susceptible Disorders

If the patient has a history of failed surgery for the ulcer or related conditions. If the patient has a history of failed surgery for other reasons, or wound and soft-tissue complications of prior surgery or trauma (pathergy). If prior reconstruction or wound closure has become reulcerated. If the patient has arterial disease, immunopathies, longstanding or severe venous disease, or hypercoagulable and micro-occlusive disorders, especially if severe, difficult to manage, or actively flared up.

High-Risk Ulcer Profile

If the current ulcer has failed or progressed in spite of reasonable prior care. If examination shows persistent inflammation, necrosis, lysis, and progressive ulceration. If there is pathergy and progressive necrosis or ulceration after débridement and other supervised care. If pain is difficult to control. If skeletal or visceral structures are exposed or exposure can be anticipated after débridement. If periwound transcutaneous oxygen levels or other regional measures of blood flow are diminished. If the ulcer or location would ordinarily be considered at high risk for complications or amputation.

Inflammation and Disease Persist

If the physician has done everything that current art and science permit to treat the disease and control the wound, but inflammation or active ulceration persist, then conventional repair or grafts with living materials are apt to fail, and Integra should be used. Integra is not only preferred because it is not alive, but its ability to control inflammation is also therapeutic, and rapid subsidence of pain, drainage, ulceration, and pathologic wound dynamics can be expected.

Unsuccessful Topical Care

It is necessary with any chronic wound to have a preliminary treatment phase in which diagnosis is made, risk factors are corrected, and basic wound care is initiated. By the time these activities are concluded, a few weeks of hygienic treatment and observation will have revealed if the wound is wound healing competent, beginning to proliferate an active wound module. If not, if the wound is incompetent to heal under ordinary circumstances, Integra ought to be used in lieu of conventional surgery.

Control of Symptoms

In a problem wound, severe pain may be present due to persistent pathologic inflammation (ie, the inappropriate inflammation of immunopathic or similar disorders, as opposed to the reactive inflammation of controllable factors, such as trauma and bioburden). The patient may have constitutional symptoms of malaise and tiredness. In these cases, wound excision and closure with Integra can immediately cure the pain and relieve other symptoms; it should be done for humane symptomatic relief.

Surgical Complications or Anticipated Wound Failure

If residual pathology, inflammation, or ischemia threaten complications of conventional flaps, grafts, and repairs. If prior attempts to do surgery for the same condition did, in fact, fail. If the established diagnoses or confirmed ischemia carry a high risk of pathergy and surgical complications.

Ineligible Skin Grafts

Skin grafts are technically convenient, but biologically complex, being completely dependent on a healthy and wound-healing competent host wound. Conditions such as ischemia, devascularized structures, and minor residual inflammation nullify the use of skin grafts because the grafts will die or not adhere. Not being alive, Integra does well in these circumstances.

Ineligible or High-Risk Flaps

Flaps ordinarily solve what grafts cannot, because they are normal vascularized tissues, which are independently capable of and responsible for healing the wound. Integra can be used safely and dependably when flaps cannot or should not be used: if location and local anatomy have limited flaps (such as the distal leg and ankle); eligible flaps are in the zone of risk and will probably fail; active inflammatory diseases threaten wound complications along all new incisions; vascular disease and ischemia threaten flap necrosis; atherosclerosis or hypercoagulability or general patient condition preclude free flaps.

Exposed Essential Structures

One of the preeminent indications for flaps is the closure of visceral, skeletal, and alloplastic structures. If flaps are ineligible for any of the above reasons, Integra is a highly dependable substitute, because of tangential histoconduction and its ability to bridge a nonliving hiatus.

Biologic Coverage Is Desirable

Integra should be used wherever a conventional biological dressing might be used for interim wound closure, including persistent mild inflammation or interval protection of a wound in preparation for later closure. It will eliminate intermediate steps, because it serves both purposes, short-term biologic coverage and definitive reconstruction or wound closure.

High-Risk Patient

Integra placement is quick and safe, the only "cut and bleed" risk to the patient being the wound excision. Subsequent skin grafts have no risk other than the graft donor site. Integra should be used in lieu of conventional repairs for any patient who is sick or a poor risk for surgery and anesthesia. If disabilities and psychosocial circumstances warrant minimum surgery-induced disruption of daily affairs, Integra can be the simplest, yet most dependable, approach to wound closure. Integra is the ultimate "play it safe" wound closure option.

Large Surface Areas

For large wounds, skin graft needs will be correspondingly large, but creating donor wounds concurrent with the primary wound can complicate postoperative care. Inflammation, physiologic challenge, pain, drainage, soiled dressings, septic risk, nursing requirements, and various functional inhibitions will all increase. In a sick or disabled person, a large wound excision with simultaneous large donor sites can sometimes be overwhelming. Integra requires two procedures, but as with much of reconstructive surgery, multiple small operations are safer and yield better outcomes than performing one big heroic operation fraught with pitfalls. Using Integra, net physiologic load on the body is significantly reduced. During the first procedure, the primary defect immediately ceases to be a wound, physiologically speaking, and the latter skin grafts done by themselves are simpler to cope with. Whenever it is desirable to limit collateral injury, minimize wound surfaces, minimize acute physiologic stress, or simplify postoperative symptoms and nursing care, Integra serves this function.

High-Risk Donor Sites

Flap and graft donor sites can be at risk because of disease, location, ischemia, inflammation, and any other factor discussed above. Arterial insufficiency is probably the most common risk that jeopardizes a donor site. The high incidence of necrosis and ulceration after saphenous vein donation for heart and vascular surgery is common evidence of this risk. Even if a donor site can be harvested without wound complications, there can be functional contraindications. For example, the latissimus dorsi muscle is crucial to be able to use crutches, walkers, and wheelchairs, those orthotics necessary for many chronic wound patients. Yet a latissimus free flap is one of the first choices for many plastic surgeons wanting to cover a complex lower extremity wound. Preservation of health, function, and lifestyle are the real goals, not simply wound closure for its own sake. If it is desirable to avoid donor sites, Integra eliminates this risk while giving equivalent or superior coverage of the target wound.

High Risk for Recurrent Disease

Patients with chronic wounds have chronic disorders. Recurrent ulceration of skin, scars, and skin grafts is a risk, especially for immunopathic, venous, lymphatic, and hematologic disorders. Integra reconstructed skin seems to be somewhat resistant to recurrent disease and, therefore, more durable and less prone to ulceration. These disorders also risk new wounds in areas not yet ulcerated, meaning that Integra can have a role for prophylactic skin reconstruction. If there are extensive trophic changes of skin, if there is obliterative liposclerosis, if there is chronic dermatitis or recurrent transient erosions of skin, or if there is any other irreparable pathology of skin and fascias, then this risk is real. Preemptive excision and reconstruction absent any ulcers may or may not be justified. However, if there is already an ulcer which has failed other care and is scheduled for surgery, then strong consideration should be given to excising the entire affected area (usually the distal leg and ankle) and reconstructing skin with Integra.

Avoiding Scar and Improving Reconstruction

Regardless of why it is used, Integra controls scarring. Unlike split-thickness skin grafts, an Integra reconstruction is unlikely to contract and require late revision. It is, therefore, useful both for the prevention of contractures and for the correction of established contractures. The value for burn closure and similar acute wound repair is obvious. For chronic wounds, if the area involves joints, hands, face, neck, breasts, genitalia, skin folds, or any other mobile anatomy, then Integra should be given primary consideration unless some suitable flap or direct repair can do an equivalent or quicker job.

Simplifying Care and Preserving Function

Upon placement of Integra, the wound is immediately closed. Pain, drainage, and other symptoms cease. Nursing requirements are nil, permitting almost all care to be as an outpatient, requiring only infrequent dressing changes. For patients with obligations at work or home, who must preserve function and lifestyle, who must travel, who live remotely and cannot come for frequent medical visits, or in whom other illnesses take precedence, Integra can be used because of its ability to simplify care.

Absent Risk Factors—A Superior Reconstruction

Integra's ability to heal wounds, to succeed where flaps would ordinarily be used, to achieve superior results in some cases (avoiding scars, graft contractures, revisions, and flap debulkings), and to do so with no risk, no donor sites, and little to no inpatient care are valuable properties in their own right. For situations where flaps or grafts would be conventional, easy, safe, and successful, Integra might sometimes be preferred because of these advantageous properties.

Integra and Chronic Wound, Surgical Planning, Compared to Conventional Methods

The above discussion of Integra indications does not imply that Integra replaces conventional methods of wound surgery. All methods are important and reconstructive plastic surgery and wound surgery are, at their core, a doctor's "black bag" of principles and techniques that are selected and applied based on individual circumstances. When conventional repair, grafts, and flaps are likely to give the fastest, surest, most dependable, least complicated or disabling way to resolve a problem, that is what should be done. Since the majority of all surgery is done in people in whom physiologic wound repair is intrinsically healthy, conventional methods will always be the most common. However, Integra is an important new tool in that "black bag", because it can simplify care, make it safer, and succeed where conventional modalities fail. This is especially true in problem wounds where normal wound healing is damaged or inhibited. The best way to appreciate circumstances in which Integra is superior to conventional surgery for chronic wounds is to look at some case studies.

Case Study A1. Indications and Surgical Planning

Male patient, 73 years old with an embolic foot necrosis; leg salvage with Integra. The patient had embolization and distal foot necrosis following femoral catheterization for coronary angioplasty. Amputation through the distal tarsal row removed all necrosis. This is a functionally good amputation because all major ankle stabilizers, including tibialis anterior and peroneus longus, are still inserted. The dilemma is that there is insufficient skin to close the wound (Fig. 16–17a). If more bone is removed for the sake of skin closure, the tendons will be disinserted, ankle control lost, and a below-knee amputation (BKA) would be warranted. There are no local flaps to cover the defect. Skin grafts are contraindicated over the open joints. The patient has atherosclerotic arteries making a free flap risky.

Most surgeons would have opted for a BKA. By placing Integra over the open osteotomies, these problems evaporate. Integra keeps the wound safe, tolerates arterial insufficiency, heals over bone, and bridges the joints. Skin grafts were placed at 6 weeks. They were completely healed and mature several months later. The patient wears a customized shoe and is fully ambulatory (Fig. 16–17b–e).

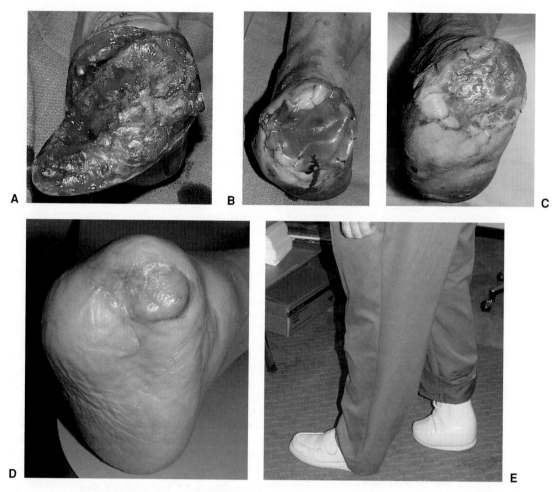

Fig. 16-17. **Case Study 1. A.** Amputation through the distal tarsus. Cuboid and cuneiform osteotomies and intertarsal joints are open without sufficient skin to close them. **B.** Some lateral skin was sutured, and everything else was covered with Integra, shown here stapled in place before fixation dressings. **C.** The regenerated Integra a few days after placing skin grafts. **D.** The healed result. Note that the Integra is become smaller. Diminution in size, with dilation or advancement of adjacent normal skin, occurs occasionally. This is normal accommodation to mechanical load and anatomical geometry, often seen in the atrophy of bulky flaps and surgical "dog ears". It is different than scar contracture because it remains compliant and not stiff, without tendinous banding or limitations of motion. **E.** At 5 months, the patient is walking normally in a custom fitted shoe.

Case Study A2. Indications and Surgical Planning

Female patient, 74 years old; mixed pathologic ulceration into the ankle; closed with Integra. The patient presented with a 30-year history of recurrent ankle ulcers, old skin grafts, and a nominal history of venous disease. Figure 16–18a demonstrates the frequent inflammatory papules and ulcers. Absence of venous stigmata such as edema, liposclerosis, and pigment changes, pertinent features such as history, distribution, and appearance of the lesions, and her ultimate response to antimetabolic chemotherapy confirm this as an immunopathy. The patient was already being treated with anticoagulants for a thrombotic history. Seronegative rheumatoid arthritis, Sweet's neutrophilic dermatitis, and an antiphospholipid antibody syndrome are the most probable diagnoses. The lesions as seen were intermittently controlled with various treatments, but during an intense flare-up, all of the old skin grafts lysed. Ulceration was into the major underlying tendons and into the ankle mortise. The author treated this by excision and closure with a scapular free flap. At 9 and 10 days after surgery, gastrointestinal bleeding forced discontinuation of anticoagulants. The flap promptly began dying from its margins inward (the vascular anastomoses were patent at the time of débridement 4 days later, a characteristic history with hypercoagulable disorders). The ankle now requires closure. Further free flaps are contraindicated. Local flaps are not large enough and they risk necrosis because of disease. Skin grafts cannot cover the open tendons and joint. Amputation would be considered by many surgeons. Interim biologic dressings are suitable, but the closure dilemma cannot be avoided indefinitely. This was the author's third Integra case. Integra was not used in the anticipation that it would work, it was used as a temporization, a biological dressing to buy time while alternate options were considered. It healed and stayed healed through 4 years of follow-up (Fig. 16–18b). It was one of the seminal cases that led to the writing of this chapter. Similar cases would now be managed preemptively with Integra rather than by any other method.

Case Study A3. Indications and Surgical Planning

Female patient, 44 years old; hypercoagulable disorder and chronic achilles ulceration; healed with Integra. The patient had a spontaneous achilles tendon rupture. Tendon repair was followed by multiple complications and necrosis of the tendon. The ankle was ultimately closed with a rectus abdominis muscle free flap and skin grafts. The patient presented to the author for consultation because of villous dysplasia of the skin grafts, chronic recurring ulceration, and pain and dysfunction (Fig. 16–19a). The plan was to do serial excisions of excess old flap and advancement of surrounding skin. The first such procedure caused prompt dehiscence and necrosis of the wound. These events and a history of retinal artery thrombosis pinpoint a hypercoagulable disorder, confirmed by multiple postacute elevations of fibrinogen and anticardiolipins. Any further effort to close and revise this wound has these challenges and requirements: any incision risks more necrosis and complications, a free flap already failed to give a desirable result and more donor sites are unwarranted, more skin grafts will have the same problem of mechanical dystrophy and ulceration, the reconstruction must be mechanically compliant and thin enough to accommodate normal footwear. Wound débridement and warfarin anticoagulation were followed by Integra. There were no further adverse events. A second piece of Integra was placed after the first one regenerated in order to obtain a thicker neodermis in this area of significant stress and strain (Fig. 16–19b). The area healed without any of the pathologic changes that affected the original skin grafts (Fig. 16–19c).

Case Study A4. Indications and Surgical Planning

Male patient, 58 years old; vascular infarction of hand; preservation of length with Integra. The problem resulted from accidental brachial artey drug injection (Fig. 16–20a). Initial débridement preserved metacarpophalangeal joints and proximal phalangeal bone, intending to use them as grafts under a hypogastric flap that would preserve some length and mobility. An abdominal pedicle transfer is an inherently difficult reconstruction, made more difficult here because of prior above-knee amputation (AKA), an obese abdominal panniculus, cardiovascular disease, and depression. The patient opted out of this flap after 1 week and all nonviable bone and joint was removed, just below the metacarpal heads. The margins of skin viability were a centimeter or two proximal to the osteotomies, creating a problem for closure. One option is to shorten bone, leaving him without metacarpals, but a mobile carpus. Aside from the general disabilities that this causes, it takes away this patient's ability to hold a cane, crutch, or walker that he needs because of the ipsilateral thigh amputation. To preserve length, soft tissues are needed. A flap from the trunk was already a failed bad idea. A radial forearm flap is disqualified by the vascular injection injury and so is a free flap. Skin grafts will either not take on the open bone or will be prone to recurrent ulceration. The solution was to create a first web space by wrap-around of a dorsal skin flap over the thumb metacarpal and then closure of all wounds and osteotomies with Integra (Fig. 16–20b). After it was healed, tendon transfers and osteotomies in

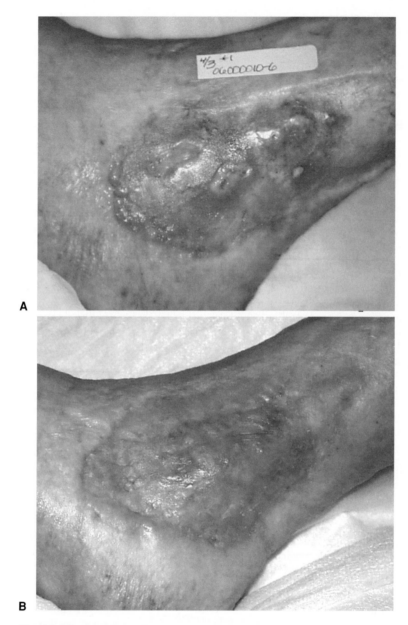

Fig. 16-18. **Case Study 2. A.** A view of the chronic lateral ankle pathology. Acute and chronic inflammation of decades duration are affecting old skin grafts. A few months later, intense inflammation lysed all of the skin in this area, leading to the failed free flap and then Integra. **B.** Integra was placed over the fibula, the open ankle joint just anterior to the fibula, and the surrounding soft tissues. The image shown is two years later. The Integra has been problem free, and inflammation and ulceration no longer affect the area.

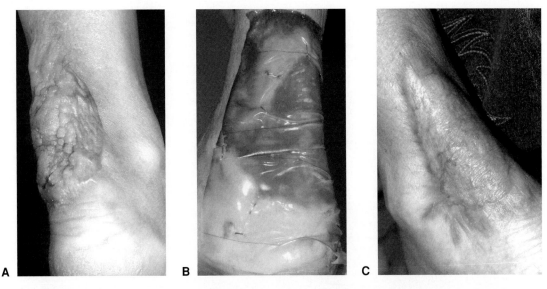

Fig. 16-19. **Case Study 3. A.** Skin grafts over muscle flap over missing achilles tendon. Villous dysplasia of skin grafts is common in areas of repetitive mechanical strain, and the scar remains juvenile, hyperemic, pathologically active. There are multiple skin ulcers near the distal end. **B.** Integra in place. It is fully regenerated and silicone is separating. It is desirable to place grafts before this happens, but this does happen and is manageable as discussed in the text. **C.** The reconstruction at one year. In contrast to what had happened with the original ordinary skin grafts, notice how this skin in thin, soft, compliant, with normal texture, that it has even developed the normal transverse dermal creases that occur in this area.

select areas were able to restore some mobility and pinch (Fig. 16–20b, c). In the author's practice, Integra would now be opted as primary reconstruction for any such situation, abandoning the radial forearm flap and other traditional options just listed.

Case Study A5. Indications and Surgical Planning

Male patient, 60 years old; severe arterial disease with heel necrosis; leg salvage with Integra. The patient has diabetes, end-stage renal disease, and severe atherosclerosis. Left foot ulceration resulted in septic gangrene, necessitating BKA. While recuperating, a large heel pressure ulcer formed. Toes on the right foot were already missing from previous vascular events. The patient was sent for consultation after refusing right-leg amputation. The problem was how to close the large heel wound and preserve function. Severe arterial disease and deficient local resources precluded any type of local or free flap. Skin grafts were sure to fail over a calcaneal osteotomy accompanied by advanced vasculopathy. Integra easily solves the problem. It succeeds without donor sites or other risk to the patient. He was managed as an outpatient and has maintained function and lifestyle (Figure 16–21).

Use of Integra and Discussion by Diagnosis and Pathology

The diagnosis which underlies a chronic pathologic ulcer has significant implications for type, length, and success of treatment, resource utilization, collateral morbidity, and stability of result. While Integra is useful for a variety of chronic wounds, its relative indications, contraindications, and details of use vary with the cause of the ulcer. This section describes the use of Integra based on underlying diagnosis.

Macroarterial

Ulceration associated with arterial insufficiency, usually atherosclerotic, is one of the most common reasons to use Integra. The degree of arterial insufficiency governs the ease or difficulty, success or failure, of wound repair and reconstruction. This is true for Integra or any other surgery, and if technically possible, arterial insufficiency should be corrected prior to any wound-closure surgery. To the extent that revascularization succeeds and restores wound-healing competence, an ulcer might close by topical care only or by customary one-stage grafts and flaps. In patients with more severe or uncorrectable disease,

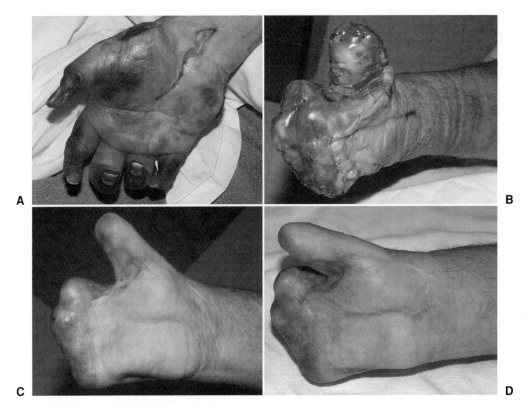

***Fig. 16-20.* Case Study 4. A.** The infarcted hand, prior to debridements. Various ischemic areas can be coaxed to survive with good wound care, pharmacological intervention, and patience. **B.** There is more salvageable hand than might at first be appreciated. The problem is that soft tissues are insufficient to cover remaining bone. The first web space has been reconstructed with a dorsal skin flap. Integra covers the bones (osteotomies just below the metacarpal heads), and parts of the web space, shown at two weeks. **C.** The healed hand. Thumb carpometacarpal extension is preserved. **D.** In this image at one year, the reconstruction is matured. Skin is durable. Tendon and muscle transfers have restored some flexion and pinch at the thumb base. The skin is healed and trouble free, and the hand is functional for the patient.

Integra is valuable for two reasons. The first is its ability to control wound conditions, averting the pathergy that ordinarily complicates severe arterial insufficiency. As a nonliving material it will not fail the way that grafts and flaps might and it is ideally suited to the retarded or delayed healing typical of arterial insufficiency. The second reason is its ability to bridge essential structures, performing well in lieu of conventional flaps, which might be unavailable or too risky. In these conditions, Integra is very successful in closing wounds and salvaging limbs when conventional surgery would fail. Salvaging complicated stumps, such as coaxing a dehisced or partially necrotic BKA wound to heal rather than conversion to an AKA is a particularly valuable capability.

Integra will fail when arterial insufficiency is severe (easy to recognize, because the matrix turns black). For mild insufficiency, ankle–brachial indices (ABIs) of 0.7 to 0.8, conventional repair, grafts, and flaps are permissible and are likely to heal. In these circumstances, Integra might often be preferable for the closure of tendons, bones, and joints in lieu of higher risk flaps, but it is not essential. ABIs below 0.2–0.3 are likely to result in failure regardless of method. In these extreme circumstances, if Integra was used, it would be safe, losing nothing but time if it fails, but at these low ABIs, failure is mostly assured. Alternately, transcutaneous oxygen pressure measurements (TcPO$_2$) can be used to assess risk, and values of 10 torr or lower without improvement when breathing is 100% oxygen is another marker of extreme arterial insufficiency likely to fail surgery, including Integra. It is in the middle zone, where conventional surgery is likely to fail or carry substantial risk,

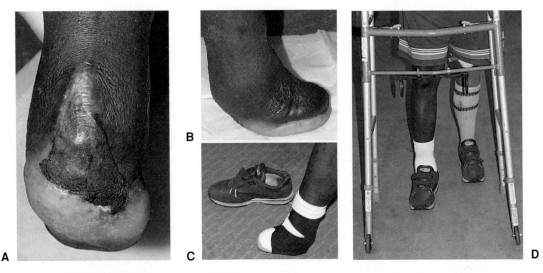

Fig. 16-21. Case Study 5. A. This is a face on view of the reconstruction, healed Integra over a large posterior calcanectomy and the achilles insertion. **B.** The patient is in full weight bearing on his healed foot. The oblique calcanectomy merely followed the contours of skin necrosis; the toes are missing from previous vascular complications. **C.** For stability, the patient uses a space filling orthotic wrapped around his ankle. **D.** Using his sneaker, his left leg prosthesis, and a walker, he is independent and ambulatory.

that Integra can be successful. Hyperbaric oxygen therapy can be a worthwhile adjunct treatment, typically started at the time of Integra placement or up to a few weeks in advance, with courses of treatment typically 20–40 sessions.

Atherosclerotic macroarteriopathy is distinctive in that it is an anatomical condition of blood vessels, which impedes, but does not damage wound repair. It is not a soft tissue disease, and it does not cause pathologic ulceration. Wound physiology remains intrinsically healthy, and length of treatment (from placement of Integra to healed skin grafts) for arterial ulcers is one of the most rapid compared to other diagnoses. Simply stated, for arterial ulcers, Integra heals wounds and salvages limbs, which could not have been managed by any other means, and it does so with no added risk to the patient. The only caveat is that if ischemia is too severe, Integra will not help, and extreme degrees of arterial insufficiency with significant morbidity or complications are still best managed by amputation.

Microarterial

Microangiopathies include thromboangiitis obliterans and other arteritides, vasculitides associated with systemic immunopathies (lupus, calcinosis cutis, Raynaud phenomenon, sclerodactyly, and telangiectasia [CRST], scleroderma, etc.), and metabolic disorders, such as certain calcium dystrophies. Unlike atherosclerosis,

the upper extremities are frequently involved with disease and ulceration, and often young people are affected. Compared to the macroangiopathies, general patient management differs in many ways, with the focus being more on managing the underlying diseases rather than reestablishing circulation. When ulcers develop, their clinical pathology and management share features of both arterial insufficiency, proportional to the degree of ischemia, and the underlying immunopathy. Nonangiopathic calcium disorders are discussed below, but special note should be made of ulcers due to systemic calcinosis-calciphylaxis. This is due to secondary and tertiary hyperparathyroidism and its various causes, usually end-stage renal disease. Histologically, it is characterized by diffuse medial arteriosclerosis in small and micro vessels. It is sometimes accompanied by hypercoagulability and microvascular thrombosis. The problem causes ischemic infarction and ulceration of skin and subcutaneous fascias. The problem can occur anywhere, but it has a predilection for central areas, usually abdomen, pelvis, and thighs. The disorder is problematic enough by itself, but, in some patients, it is compounded by macroatherosclerosis due to the diabetes or hypertension that caused the renal disease. Characteristic of any severe vascular insufficiency, transcutaneous oxygen pressures are low, pain is severe, and the wounds heal exceedingly slowly with topical care alone. Pathergy is the rule, with attempts to débride such wounds usually rewarded with more to débride. Integra is remarkably successful in these patients. Areas of necrosis and ulceration are completely excised, and Integra is placed immediately to cover the wounds. Relief of pain is instantaneous, pathergy is prevented, and the wounds heal. Integra regeneration proceeds at relatively normal rates, ready for skin grafts in 5 to 6 weeks. Hyperbaric oxygen therapy can be a useful adjunct during early phases of the reconstruction.

Hypercoagulable and Other Micro-Occlusive

These are a wide range of metabolic and hematologic disorders which cause microvascular occlusion, but no other active injurious pathology. They include hemato-pathologies (hemoglobinopathies, polycythemias, red cell and platelet disorders, and dys- and cryopro-teinemias) and hypercoagulopathies (prethrombotic disorders, antiphospholipid antibodies, homocysteine-mias). Clinical symptoms, wound pathophysiology, and wound natural history are comparable to atherosclerotic or other arterial ulcers, including severe ischemic pain, pathergy, refractoriness and multiple treatment failures, and threatened or prior amputations. However, there is an important difference: Most of these conditions are easier to manage. They tend to occur in younger other-wise healthier patients and the problems or their effects are usually correctable or more easily managed, such as treating hypercoagulable patients with anticoagulants. The consequence is that patients in this category have high Integra success rates with few failures or complica-tions. As with any ulcer of any diagnosis, initial treat-ment phases involve basic topical hygienic wound care, diagnosis, and initiation of disease specific therapies. Many such ulcers are small and heal with anticoagula-tion and topical care alone, and larger ones can improve to the point of successful skin grafting. However, these are "chronic problem wounds," and some remain refrac-tory to care, exhibiting continued ischemia and wound misbehavior in the form of pain, pathergy, delayed heal-ing, and defiance of conventional surgery. When ischemia and delayed wound healing persist, Integra controls symptoms and pathergy, tolerates the ischemia without consequence, and gradually heals the wound. Periwound ischemia helps confirm the diagnosis and may indicate hyperbaric oxygen as short-term adjunct therapy (as with the other ischemic ulcers, transcuta-neous oxygen pressures are a useful tool to assist diagno-sis, assess risk, and plan treatment; Doppler pressures, photoplethysmography, pulse volume measurements, and similar measures of bulk macroarterial flow will not be helpful in these disorders).

Diabetes

Diabetes does not cause any unique ulcerative pathology nor does it intrinsically retard wound repair. Three categories of ulceration in diabetic patients should be con-sidered. The first are ulcers due to any other diagnosis which incidentally occur in a diabetic person. In these patients, the diabetes per se is generally not relevant to the wound and its management. Diabetes is, of course, associated with accelerated and distal-acral atherosclero-sis, and it is the arterial disease, not the diabetes, which can make these wounds problematic. Wound and Inte-gra management are typically the same as for other arterial ulcers. The second type of ulcer is necrobiosis lipoidica. This occurs in nondiabetic patients as well, but it has a well-characterized association with diabetes. It is a chronic necrotizing inflammation of subcutaneous adipose fascias having a somewhat distinctive distribu-tion over the pretibial region. It is most comparable to an immunopathic panniculitis (discussed below). Like other such disorders, aggressive excision and skin recon-struction with Integra is very successful, not only healing the wounds, but eliminating the inflammatory phlegmon, which makes these patients chronically ill, minimizing the risks of future ulceration.

The third category is the characteristic "diabetic ulcer." This is really a neuropathic ulcer, often com-pounded by associated arterial disease and noncompliant patient behaviors. The paradigms are the mal perforans and the Charcot ulcers on plantar surfaces. Results with Integra are mostly poor. Even when arterial insufficiency is not a contributing factor, patient compliance and loca-tion in weight-bearing areas can be insurmountable problems. Integra's biologic performance will be correct, undergoing thorough regeneration and partial or com-plete take of skin grafts as long as patients are kept non-ambulatory or nonweight bearing. However, lack of patient compliance and participation may keep the skin grafts from ever being applied; reulceration is likely. Note that Integra performs well on the foot for other prob-lems. It does well in diabetics on nonweight-bearing sur-faces and it does well on the plantar in other patients who are sensate and responsible about activities and orthotics. Opting Integra or any other form of reconstructive foot surgery in these patients must be tempered by two prin-ciples. (1) If a patient cannot be compliant during a plan-tar reconstruction, it might be best not to begin at all (true for any type of diabetic foot surgery or reconstruc-tion). (2) Healed Integra under the calcaneus or other plantar weight-bearing surfaces is subject to reulceration. Integra reconstruction on weight-bearing plantar sur-faces is probably best avoided in diabetic foot patients.

As long as the problem is not a plantar "diabetic ulcer," Integra salvages many necrotic and ulcerated feet in dia-betic patients. When arterial insufficiency causes prob-lematic wound behavior, Integra can control pathergy and stabilize the wound. When vascular disease precludes grafts and flaps, Integra is a dependable way to heal the wound and restore new skin over tendons, ligaments, and other structures. When open bones and joints, after foot débridement, threaten high-level amputation, Integra's ability to regenerate over these structures heals them with minimum risk and disability.

Venous Disease

Venous ulcers are the most common lower-extremity ulcers. Key features of the disease and its management are venous hemodynamics, venous vasculitis, venous thrombosis (and hypercoagulability in some patients), acute dermatitis, chronic trophic tissue changes and liposclerosis, and the paramount necessity of good control of edema and venous hypertension. For many patients, the problem is not the disease but the lack of competent care. Once a good program of systematic sustained care and compression is initiated, many of these patients and ulcers will heal and stay healed without surgery. If an ulcer persists after that, vein excision or interruption can be the simple trick that works next and, for those with larger ulcers that need skin replacement, complete excision and ordinary skin grafts usually then succeed. However, some patients have more difficult situations due to advanced, refractory, complicated disease: (1) extensive circumferential ulceration, (2) long duration with prior failed skin grafts, (3) refractory inflammation (venous vasculitis and dermatitis), (4) advanced liposclerosis and scarification of the sural fascias which, after excision, leave bare muscle, tendon, and synovium upon which to place grafts, (5) preexcisional ulceration into skeletal structures such as tibialis and peroneus tendons, the bony malleoli and malleolar bursas, and the ankle joint, and (6) concomitant unrelated diseases such as atherosclerotic arterial insufficiency or a connective tissue disorder. In these patients, Integra successfully reconstructs stable skin, regardless of how many prior skin grafts failed. Good preparation is essential, including good wound hygiene, topical or systemic steroids if needed to control refractory venous vasculitis and dermatitis, anticoagulation for that subpopulation in whom the problem is due to hypercoagulability, strict compression to control edema and venous hypertension, and complete wound excision and venous interruption at the time of surgery. Integra's abilities to control inflammation and bridge essential structures ensure that the wounds heal and that disease stays quiet in reconstructed areas. In the patient who is responsible about compression and edema management, these goals are easily achieved, and the success rate of Integra is one of the highest for all diagnoses.

Lymphatic

Dermatitis and ulcers due to lymph stasis and postural edema are quite different than venous stasis in many ways, but they also have features in common. Similarities include late-stage soft-tissue pathology, frustrations over failed treatments and recurrent problems, and the general concepts and methods of management. While wound, skin, and edema treatment principles are largely the same as those for venous disease, most surgeons learn to stay away from lymphatic conditions. If surgery is done for any reason, either minor wound surgery and skin grafts, or regional panniculectomies and skin grafts, or even just incisions through the edema for musculoskeletal surgery underneath, the operative wounds can be harder to manage than the original ulcers; they often do not heal. Integra is effective. It can greatly simplify excision and closure of such wounds and it can reliably heal. Its role as a high-grade artificial skin allows for complete elective dermatofasciectomy of an entire limb for lymphedema and the resulting reconstructed skin tends to stay edema-free.

Immunopathic

The immunopathies are a broad category of autoimmune and inflammatory pathologies. They include the classic collagen-vascular and connective tissue disorders (rheumatoid, lupus, scleroderma, polymyositis, ankylosing spondylitis, Behçet's, Sjögren's, Wegener's, and so on), the arteritides (polyarteritis nodosum, giant cell arteritis, thromboangiitis, etc.), the inflammatory dermatoses and panniculopathies (pyoderma gangrenosum, erythema nodosum, neutrophilic dermatitis, Weber-Christian, etc.), and various other illnesses such as sarcoidosis, Crohn's, and other inflammatory bowel diseases. Immunopathies are active diseases with protean manifestations. They are double trouble: they cause soft-tissue injury and ulceration and they also impair the healing of that damage. Progressive necrosis and lysis of skin and fascias can occur, causing chronic ulceration, most commonly on leg and ankle, but also in many other locations. When these diseases are active, pathergy and wound failure are ever present demons waiting to complicate trauma and surgery. (Fortunately, rheumatoid and similar patients have many elective operations, including prosthetic arthroplasties, without any complications, but active phases of leg ulceration or recent surgical complications are tip-offs to potential trouble.) Immunopathic ulcers are often misdiagnosed and mistreated. Even when diagnosis and care are properly instituted, these diseases consistently stymie attempts to treat and resolution of these wounds can be difficult and prolonged. Histories of many years or decades duration and many failed prior wound operations are common.

The prospects for successful ulcer surgery using simple repair, skin grafts, and nearby small flaps are very small. Active refractory ulcerative pathology is problematic enough by itself, but many of these patients, being older, also have concurrent venous or arterial disease of varying degrees. Issues of essential coverage further compound the problem because the pathologic lysis of skin and subcutaneous fascias commonly expose muscles, tendons, retinacular ligaments, bones, and joints. Multiple and multifocal ulceration is characteristic. Many immunopathic ulcers remain small, but this combination of factors tends to produce the largest and most complex chronic leg ulcers that occur across all diagnoses. Effective management begins with control of the underlying disease to the extent that it is possible. It is not always possible though, and residual dermatitis, panniculitis, positive serologies, and systemic symptoms may prevail in spite of aggressive antiinflammatory, antimetabolic, and anti-immune therapies. It is in these circumstances, where aggressive treatment has improved, but not eliminated, pathologic inflammation, that the concept of a biologic superdressing is particularly applicable. Integra's ability to subside the residual inflammation, then reconstruct skin and cover exposed essential structures has consistently shown good results in these patients, with complete or partial healing in 90% of patients. As with generic length-of-care data for these patients, the length of Integra reconstruction is one of the longest, averaging 10 months for complete final epithelialization. However, this statistic belies the fact that most of these patients have a nearly instantaneous improvement in symptoms, a rapid return to meaningful lifestyle, and that late residual healing is only in small areas that remain uninflammed and asymptomatic. If there are subsequent flare-ups of disease with new wounds, the Integra reconstructed skin tends to be spared from disease and reulceration.

Mechanical, Anatomical, Trauma, and Surgery

There are some chronic ulcers that result from mechanical, traumatic, and anatomic conditions rather than from disease. This is a diverse group of problems including pressure ulcers, congenital, traumatic, and surgical defects of chest, spine, and abdominal wall, persistent ulcers due to mechanical gliding of joints and tendons or due to fracture pseudarthroses, and many other incidental conditions. Within the broad scope of wounds and surgery, only a tiny fraction of these problems qualify for Integra. Many of them are acute or occur in otherwise young and perfectly healthy people where customary wound care and surgery easily succeed. Many are due to skeletal injury where appropriate bone and joint stabilization will correct the problems. Integra ought to be avoided for pressure ulcers in the neurologically impaired because it will fail for the same reasons that it fails diabetic plantar reconstruction (ie, the typical sacral, coccygeal, ischial, and trochanteric ulcers). There are ulcers due to illicit drug abuse, psychoneurotic "neurodermatoses," and other problems that result from complex psychosocial factors that are not easily correctable. Most of these are inherently healthy wounds

for which no wound surgery other than débridement is ever indicated, at least not until the underlying problems are managed and injury is relieved, and after which they will probably heal by natural contraction supported with basic hygienic care. When surgery is needed, ordinary repairs, grafts, and flaps, the basic stuff of textbook surgery in healthy people, almost always suffice.

However, Integra might be selectively preferred for some of these situations. Essential coverage of exposed structures in areas impoverished of good flaps, or the desire to avoid donor sites or late revisions might be compelling reasons to use Integra. There might be deliberate reconstructive goals, such as restoring the dorsum of the hand, where thin compliant tissue is needed and Integra is superior to legacy options such as groin flaps. There are those ulcers, due to anatomic, traumatic, and mechanical conditions, which become chronic and nonhealing in spite of responsible compliant care. A typical example is ulceration in a contracted tendinous scar crossing a joint where repetitive stress–strain continually fractures the scar, liable to occur at any joint, but especially common on the dorsal ankle and the popliteal. Even when such scars are not ulcerated, the contractures themselves are still disabling problems. Another common example is laceration or ulceration into the tendon sheath of the tibialis anterior or other large tendon, where constant shearing induces serosal or synovial metaplasia and inhibits fibrous repair and wound closure. Minor ankle trauma causing erosion into a malleolar bursa will not heal for the same reasons, especially in a person with concurrent vascular or autoimmune disease. Injury due to toxic chemicals and chemotherapy drugs can quickly become pathologic ulcers devoid of reparative potential. It is in these patients, where an ordinarily simple acute problem has become refractory and chronic, that Integra is valuable. It can relieve adverse mechanics, cover essential structures, control unstable wounds, and prevail under the burden of concurrent risk factors, such as arterial insufficiency. Whatever the original cause of a problem, when it becomes a chronic ulcer, Integra is indicated for any of the criteria discussed in the "Rationale and Indications" section above.

Radiation and Malignancy

There is only limited experience with Integra and malignant ulcers. Cancer should be managed by wide excision, but not all tumors are resectable or operable. If a satisfactory wide excision results in a large defect with specific needs for closure or reconstruction, Integra can be used for the same indications that apply after any trauma or surgery. Unresectable tumor and wide micrometastasis always present a challenge. Some type of closure and symptomatic control is theoretically desirable, but using large flaps is often unnecessary risk for no advantage, and skin grafts quickly reulcerate. Nevertheless, it has been an historic practice to at least try to ameliorate a malignant wound with skin grafts, typically for extensive skin and breast cancers. The grafts may take transiently, but they are quickly replaced by tumor. While there are no satisfactory choices for unresectable tumors, Integra can be no worse than flaps and grafts. It has a tangible advantage in that the silicone is an impenetrable barrier that can at least block exposure and drainage, maintain some hygiene, and afford some symptomatic palliation. It has a theoretical advantage in that the aminoglycan in the Integra may have some effect to tame or regulate the malignant behavior of tumor cells. While strictly anecdotal, cases support the possibility of this hypothesis. While Integra will not cure the problem, its ability to provide some symptomatic relief and simplify care without additional morbidity, donor sites, pain, disability, or significant intrusion on life style are desirable properties, and Integra ought to be considered for these unfortunate situations.

Integra over radiated tissues is also of limited experience. Radiation damage to deoxyribonucleic acid (DNA) induces latent cell kill, manifest when cells try to replicate. Wounds cannot heal because the local progenitor cells of wound repair cannot proliferate. For the same reasons, Integra regeneration over a radiated wound might fail. However, to the extent that lower radiation doses or better contemporary radiation therapy practices leave residual wound healing potential, Integra provides such good protection to the wound that this potential has a chance to be expressed. Recall, too, that the early histogenetic pioneer cells may be blood borne, so Integra may be hosting remote cells that are not influenced by the damaged wound. Histoconductive bridging from surrounding healthy areas also applies. Among the author's few cases, this category had one of the lower success rates, as might be expected, but it was also better than might be expected. There are other reports of success.[22] Flaps remain the preferred method of closing radiation wounds, but when circumstances preclude flaps, Integra remains the next best method, possibly succeeding, and at least serving as an effective artificial skin to protect the wound and manage life style.

Granulomatous and Infectious

Closure of any infected wound by any means is categorically contraindicated, but there are different kinds of infections with different principles of care. Physicians are generally very familiar with ordinary suppurative infections due to pyogenic bacteria. These infections are acute. Either they are there or they are not and they do not become chronic ulcers or panniculitis. Integra has a role in their surgery only to the extent that drainage and débridement leave large defects that meet the indications for Integra closure. However, there are also atypical infections that cause skin and fascial ulcers—those due to fungi, mycobacteria, actinomycetes, and protozoa. These infections often present as a chronic ulcerative panniculitis. They may be small and focal or quite extensive. They may be acute and fulminant or relatively indolent and chronic. They are all comparable in that they must be treated by aggressive total excision, by either surgery alone (such as Buruli ulcer due to *Mycobacterium ulcerans*), or by surgery and antimicrobials (such as panniculitis and ulceration due to *Mycobacterium fortuitum* or *marinum* or complex wounds due to actinomycosis or mucormycosis). Once the wound is completely excised, it can be closed. Because the disease and the required surgery can be extensive or destructive, the defects will often meet the criteria for Integra closure. A particular benefit of Integra is that it closes the wound without any additional incisions or dissection for the sake of moving flaps or grafts. This is a crucial issue, because with these unusual pathogens, secondary surgical fields are always at risk for infection due to inoculation from the primary wound. There are also the occasional ulcers with granulomatous pathology of uncertain origin. After wound excision, Integra can help control residual inflammation, leading to a healed wound.

Miscellaneous Other Disorders

Some ulcers are due to uncommon causes in minor categories. An example are the metabolic ulcers due to calcium disorders. Systemic calcinosis or calciphylaxis was discussed above as a microangiopathic entity, but there are also the calcium dystrophies. These include calcinosis cutis, calcifying panniculitis, pannicular ossification, and myositis ossificans, which, once they become ulcerated, are impossible to heal without complete excision. Integra is applicable because excision of these lesions is apt to result in large wounds with exposed musculoskeletal structures requiring deliberate closure. There are also a small number of chronic ulcers that defy accurate diagnosis. In a certain sense, the specific diagnosis does not matter. If underlying disease and risks can be identified, each needs to be treated or managed. Beyond that, the wound must be cared for according to principles of good wound management. Integra serves a vital role for the resolution of many of the more persistent, refractory, problematic chronic wounds, and its use is guided by the criteria in the "Rationale and Indications" section.

Adjunct

Integra is useful as a supporting modality for conventional surgery. A flap might be unequivocally the best thing for a given situation, but flaps can create secondary dilemmas which need their own solution. (1) A flap donor site might be large or mechanically noncompliant, impossible to repair directly. It then requires its own deliberate closure and Integra can be used instead of traditional flaps and grafts. (2) A flap in intermediate stages of transfer has a bare underside. This needs its own care, since it risks contraction and loss of flap extensibility as it heals, and it risks necrosis if it is improperly "tubed" under tension. The distal working part of the flap can also be an "unsatisfied end" that risks necrosis if, while under the vascular stress of a delay, it is left exposed and not inset. Integra is a very simple and effective way to close these open surfaces. It protects the flap from exposure and physiological stress, it halts scar and contraction, and it eliminates the typically cumbersome wound care that is required, all without any tension or additional insult to the flap. (3) One method of delaying a flap is to elevate it and then replace it *in situ*, waiting a few weeks for its circulation to adapt before trying to move it to the target. However, back in its original position, the deep surface starts to heal, and in so doing, scar and revascularization restore circulation to the way it was. This negates the delay, nullifying the hoped for vascular adaptation and jeopardizing the flap during subsequent transfer. By intercalating a barrier between the flap and its donor base, the two surfaces are kept separate. This allows the delay effect to occur, and it makes the second-stage dissection and transfer much easier. Integra is ideal for this job. The silicone is the immediate barrier. Then, at the time of transfer, since flap delay and Integra regeneration times are roughly equal, the donor surface is ready to accept skin grafts and requires little other care. (4) Some reconstructions are necessarily complex due to local anatomy and mechanics, lack of adequately large flaps, or a need to minimize the amount of dissection. Integra is an ideal companion to flaps. A small, safe, dependable flap can be used where it is most crucially needed, allowing Integra to close the remaining areas of a complex wound. All of these four scenarios are regular events in plastic surgery, conventionally managed by secondary flaps, skin grafts, biological dressings, and topical care. Integra will often be better, simpler, safer, more effective, cause fewer complications and be better tolerated by the patient. It should be used for these purposes whenever there is a need to simplify a complex reconstruction, protect an open or delayed flap, make the flap donor site easier to manage, or avoid secondary donor sites.

Use of Integra and Discussion by Anatomy

Head, Trunk, and Upper Extremity

The number of chronic wounds on upper parts of the body is small compared to the lower extremity, and wounds here typically have far fewer problems. Integra is more likely to be used in these areas for trauma and reconstruction. Pathologic wound-healing impairments are less of a concern. Issues of exposed essential structures,

biomechanics and scar, lack of suitable local flaps, the desire to limit donor sites, and simplification of care are more likely to be the motivations to use Integra. Results are dependably good. It even works well in vasculopathic hands associated with immune disorders or atherosclerosis. For certain select problems, such as the scalp and dorsum of the hand, Integra ought to be opted as the preferred reconstruction (discussed below).

Lower Extremity

Most chronic wounds are on the lower extremity. Special circumstances and caveats apply when doing any reconstruction on the lower extremity, Integra or otherwise. Integra tends to mitigate pathology and inflammation, which is why it is effective when other treatments have failed. However, the following issues must always be considered. Never overlook the possibility of concurrent arterial or venous disease, or any other combination of multiple risks, and treat each risk accordingly. Regeneration times may be prolonged, sometimes 6–7 weeks. Edema control and graft fixation are essential. Use splints or boots to control motion of joints or major tendons that are covered with Integra. Avoid pressure injury due to tight bandaging around the foot and ankle. Do whatever is required to protect the reconstruction, but do allow ambulation and preserve function as long as mechanical loads and strains on the graft are completely eliminated in responsible patients. Concurrent treatment of the underlying disorder must continue, depending on the status of the disease and complications of treatment.

Exposed Structures

Conventional plastic surgery principles dictate that open bones, joints and bursa, tendons, viscera, and alloplastic materials all be covered with flaps, and that skin grafts and other materials can be, at best, only temporary biologic dressings. As a skin substitute, Integra provides superior acute coverage of these structures. Then, by its ability to conduct histogenesis tangentially, it readily bridges these structures, even when they cannot support a conventional skin graft. Integra can close most instances of exposed structures (See Table 16–6c). It does so when flaps are not possible, without donor sites and donor morbidity, and without late revision. Since exposure of these structures is what prompts many surgeons to suggest amputation, Integra results in saved limbs. Notable points are the following.

Integra does well on living bone, cortical or cancellous, because healthy bone is capable of sourcing cells and circulation into the graft. If Integra over bone (or any other structure) turns black, it means that the subjacent bone is dead. Further tangential bone débridement and reapplication of Integra will succeed. Integra performs well over open joints, especially small joints of the hand and foot. Until healed, control of motion by splints or orthotics is essential. Integra performs well over tendons, doing especially well over small extensor tendons. Tendon diameter itself does not seem to be important, but the combination of size and length of excursion is—along with viability and adequacy of débridement. The peroneus tendons just above the malleolus and the tibialis anterior tendon across the ankle are most likely to require secondary coverage by flaps or new Integra. If Integra can control and heal a large complex wound to the point that only a small residual tendon exposure needs to be covered with a small safe flap, this is a clinical success for Integra. One of Integra's values is that it buys time for the surgeon and patient. It can protect a wound or structure while ancillary matters are stabilized or while a final flap is being delayed. If, while being used as an interim skin substitute, it regenerates and heals the wound, then any parallel plan of closure can be curtailed.

The following paragraphs detail the use of Integra for some select areas and anatomical problems. This is not a comprehensive list of clinical problems that Integra can solve. Rather, these items were selected because they arise frequently enough in practice, they are a natural fit for Integra, and various investigators have reported comparable good results. These are also all situations in which Integra outperforms the usual approaches to care and should be considered a preferred method of closure.

Scalp

Large scalp defects, with or without calvarial exposure, occur from disease, trauma, and surgery. Small defects, even up to 10–15 cm, are often best managed by simple topical care as the scalp contracts. For larger defects, conventional methods of closure are skin grafts, scalp flaps, shoulder and neck flaps, and free flaps. These all have drawbacks in terms of durability, donor sites, or risks and costs of the reconstruction. Many surgeons have reported on the exceptional ease, safety, dependability, and good results of using Integra on the scalp. Remember, Integra buys time. Even if later surgery is to be done for esthetic restoration of forehead or hairline, it can be done electively when all else is healed and healthy. The healed Integra will even accept hair transplant plugs. Integra should be considered a preferred choice when operative closure is required for large scalp defects.

Dorsum of Hand

Integra was particularly effective for closing the dorsum of the hand. Large defects in this area are conventionally closed with groin, abdominal, and radial forearm flaps, free flaps, and skin grafts. These all have disadvantages related to: staged flap transfers temporary disabilities, difficulties with the aftercare, problematic donor sites, risk to the forearm and hand, contractures and deformities, and bulky flaps requiring staged reduction once healed. Full-thickness skin grafts give outstanding results in this location, but donor skin may be limited, or exposed bones, joints, and tendons may limit their applicability. Integra results in a thin and compliant tissue comparable to normal dorsal hand skin. It does so with neither donor sites, nursing and functional problems, risk of flap necrosis, nor late revisions. Whether for trauma, chronic wounds, or elective reconstruction, Integra and full-thickness skin grafts should both be considered the options of choice for restoring skin on the dorsum of the hand and wrist. Full-thickness grafts are best suited for elective planned reconstructions (eg, excision of a giant hairy nevus covering the entire dorsal hand and wrist), and Integra is best suited for trauma, burns, chronic wounds, or any situation where donor sites are insufficient or anatomy is complex.

Visceral and Alloplastic Coverage

Visceral organs and alloplastic hardware are best closed by flaps, but when flaps are unavailable or patient risk contradicts their use, Integra does a remarkably good job of closing and protecting them and restoring new skin over them. Even if the intent is to eventually use a flap, Integra serves as high-quality interim coverage, allowing the wound and patient time to stabilize and allowing the surgeon time to plan the definitive reconstruction and delay flaps. Any organ can, in principle, be closed with Integra. On an open thorax, it is a competent gas barrier which maintains an expanded lung as long as the silicone is undamaged. Its most common reported use, along these lines, is for closure of an open abdomen. It can be used after trauma, compartment syndrome, congenital abdominal wall defects, tumor resection, and even fasciitis and peritonitis after adequate débridement and control of infection. In the author's one case of Integra over orthopedic hardware, the patient had had multiple wound complications which precluded major surgery until after diagnostic workup and related care. Integra was used as interim coverage, the plan being to use it either until other attempts could be made to close the wound, or until the fracture was sufficiently healed to permit removal of the hardware. The key to any management of this type is to stay ahead of separating silicone. To prevent premature exposure of the underlying structures, removal of old silicone and placement of a new sheet of Integra should be planned for every 4 weeks. In this one case, after placement of three pieces of Integra, a lamina of new skin had formed tangentially, completely covering the plate and fracture, allowing the fracture to heal, thereby obviating any other surgery of any kind.

Achilles Tendon

Achilles tendon exposure is common, due to chronic venous or rheumatoid ulceration, arterial ulcers, pressure ulceration (usually with underlying arterial insufficiency), and complications of Achilles rupture and surgery. Achilles ulcers are all manageable, with or without Integra. However, there is a general (mis)perception that they are difficult and refractory. It is true that wounds, flaps, and grafts do have real problems in this area. The ulcers often accompany vascular diseases and other high-risk illnesses, and surgery may fail due to those comorbidities. Failed surgery, contractures, and reulceration can also result from motion. Large flaps can require late revision to accommodate activity and footwear. Skin grafts usually fail. However, the common notion that grafts categorically cannot heal over the Achilles is erroneous. Failed grafts result from three manageable factors. Two are surgical errors, (1) exposed tendon surfaces may be dry and dead but they are not properly decorticated, and (2) motion is not adequately controlled. The third reason is physiologic. Vascular density in this largely collagenous hypocellular structure is just what it needs to be for its own circumstances, but it may or may not be insufficient to support a skin graft. The value of Integra is that it is not alive, so it will not die while waiting for revascularization. Once the process begins, the biophysics of vasculogenesis ensure that sufficient vascularity develops. In the interim, Integra artificial skin protects the tendon and keeps it completely viable. Assuming that good wound preparation and débridement have been done, Integra will succeed where a skin graft might die. After it heals, the final result is thin, like normal Achilles skin, and it is more tolerant of local mechanics, avoiding later ulcers, contractures, and skin dystrophy. As a genuinely different paradigm of surgery, Integra circumvents, prevents, preempts, solves, and resolves the many factors that make Achilles closure problematic. Barring extreme degrees of arterial insufficiency, Integra can be expected to do well over properly débrided Achilles tendon. Along with small local reliable flaps that can be done in one stage when circumstances are good, Integra ought to be considered as the primary modality of Achilles closure.

Heel

Every comment just made about the Achilles is equally true for the heel and the two often occur simultaneously. Calcaneal ulceration is almost always due to pressure in patients with arterial disease. Among "old school" surgeons whose first choice of care for any lower-extremity wound in a diabetic or elderly patient is pre-emptive amputation, heel ulceration is one of the common inciting conditions. However, as with the Achilles, heel ulcers are almost all manageable. Smaller ulcers, up to 4–5 cm diameter, in patients with sufficient arterial circulation will heal by contraction with topical care alone. Sometimes, small local flaps are useful. Larger ulcers and lesser circulation make the problem more challenging, the wounds more prone to stall or fail and flaps harder to find or more likely to die. If skin loss is large enough that the calcaneus projects posteriorly beyond the skin margins, closure by contraction is unlikely. Integra is used in these latter situations, where topical care only or simple one-stage procedures cannot be done. Placing it over a calcaneal ostectomy is easy, safe, and uniformly effective (barring extreme arterial disease). In cases where topical care alone will not work, Integra ought to be considered the primary option of surgical closure of the posterior heel.

Amputation and Limb Salvage

Integra can prevent amputations because it can solve difficult limb salvage problems where grafts and flaps will fail. Three general scenarios occur. (Scenario 1) Preventing peremptory amputation. Injury, infarction, or ulceration of an extremity are often automatically amputated by surgeons who do not know how to manage complex wounds and limb salvage. Rather than lose the entire extremity, these wounds can instead be managed and healed, with Integra having a central place in the schema of débridement and reconstruction. (Scenario 2) Preventing unnecessarily high amputation. When amputation is required, it can be kept at a low level, near the zone of débridement. Just because an otherwise satisfactory amputation results in insufficient skin and exposed structures, or the wound cannot support ordinary skin grafts, or there are no nearby flaps to close the wound, none of these justify carrying the amputation to a higher level. The wounds can be closed easily with Integra, preserving joints and limb segments. Preserving a midfoot rather than a BKA or keeping the knee rather than doing an AKA are the typical situations. (Scenario 3) Avoiding progressive amputation. An amputation already performed may have complications (necrosis, ulceration, dehiscence, and abscess) prompting the surgeon to do a higher level amputation. Conversion of a below knee to an above knee amputation is the typical event. As long as the problem is just a local wound complication, as opposed to complete necrosis of a limb segment, the wound can be managed like any other risky wound: débridement, good preparatory care, followed by closure with Integra. Amputation scenarios generally imply arterial disease rather than an inflammatory pathology, meaning that Integra will have a high success rate in these situations (except with extreme ischemia). In all of these situations, due to arterial disease, other components of care are equally mandatory: operative or endovascular revascularization, hyperbaric oxygen therapy for defined criteria, pressure relief, and general care of the patient.

There are also the few patients who are not salvageable, or who would suffer more by prolonged care, and amputation should be done when it is clear that a patient meets these criteria.

TECHNIQUE AND MANAGEMENT

Technique and Management

Good outcomes with Integra are contingent on technique and details of management. The nominal methods of use are described in prior literature and in the package insert. This section discusses additional details especially relevant to its use in chronic wounds.

Control Disease and Prepare Wound

All chronic wound patients must have accurate diagnosis and treatment of underlying disease and risks. There must be thorough preoperative management of inflammation, ulceration, edema, debris, and bioburden, controlled as thoroughly as the disease and available treatments permit. Integra can control some residual pathological inflammation, but to ignore proper wound preparation invites abscess and loss of the material. The most common preparatory treatment profile for patients in the author's practice is twice daily hygiene and silver sulfadiazine dressings, edema control by elastic or multilayer bandaging, periodic examination and minor débridement, and incidental therapies related to individual diagnoses.

Wound Excision

Regardless of how well the wound has been prepared and how healthy it looks, Integra must not be placed on an existing wound surface. Not only does this risk infection, but if Integra is placed on a proliferative wound module of cells already committed to conventional inflammatory fibrous repair, the full late-phase benefits of a compliant scarless tissue will not be realized. At the time of surgery, the entire existing wound must be completely excised. If anatomical circumstances preclude safe excision (eg, the wound is on open internal organs), then thorough curettage should be done to remove all "granulation tissue." Integra is a surgical implant, not a wound dressing, and it must be accorded due respect.

Forms and Availability

The original product, packaged in isopropyl alcohol, is available in three rectangular size, 4×5, 4×10, and 8×10 inches. As much as is needed can be opened and applied to cover the prepared wound after first rinsing out the alcohol. Recently available is a new package using only electrolyte buffer. If needed, the Integra sponge can be gently scraped from the silicone and used by itself for extra thickness or bulk filling in small bursas or cavities.

Table 16–2. Antibiotic usage[1]

	Vancomycin	Gentamicin
Patient A		
Vancomycin 3,000 mg		
Gentamicin 720 mg		
5 Hours	<2	0.90
14 Hours	<2	0.43
Patient B		
Vancomycin 8,000 mg		
Gentamicin 1,920 mg		
15 hours	4	1.07
Patient C		
Vancomycin 4,000 mg		
Gentamicin 960 mg		
4 hours	11.8	0.96
Normal values		
Peak	15–35	4–8
Trough	<10	<2

[1]All values in μg/ml.

Antibiotics

Infections are a potential complication, but if Integra is properly managed, they are avoidable. Prophylactic antibiotics are used by many surgeons, either as part of the preliminary rinse or impregnated into the sponge after the rinses are complete (Table 16–2), supplemented by several days of oral antibiotics. Low, nearly zero infection rates are due predominantly to good preoperative preparation, complete excision of the wound, and good fixation and compression of the graft. Whether antibiotics are useful or not is a matter of faith, but they are a cheap and safe hedge against an undesirable complication.

Application to Wound

The Integra must conform to and contact the wound surface. Tension within the material will shear the sponge from the silicone, so the material must not be stretched. The material as is is sufficiently deformable to let it conform to most wound surfaces, but it can be folded, pleated, darted, and mosaicized in any way desired so that unstrained material is everywhere in contact with the wound. It can be affixed with sutures, staples, or any suitable alternative. Some surgeons have reported good success using fibrin glues to cement the product on the wound.

Fixation and Compression

Fixation and compression are of paramount importance. The principles and art are no different than for affixing any skin graft. The goal is to ensure that the material adheres to the wound without shear and that hematomas and seromas do not accumulate. Depending on circumstances, the common methods of graft fixation and compression are elastic bandages, padded "tie-over" dressings, and vacuum devices. Joint immobilization and mechanical offloading are achieved with splints, boots, various other orthotics, and even interphalangeal pins or other hardware fixation as needed. Activities and life style are permitted to the extent that splinting and edema control can be maintained.

Interim Management and Observation

If disease has been controlled, the wound properly prepared and excised, and the graft properly fixated, then postoperative care and concerns are minimal. Because histogenesis is observable through the silicone, it is necessary to periodically examine the graft. Examinations are typically done at 1–week intervals, consisting of unwrapping and then rewrapping new compression bandages. If there are no problems with the graft or the dressings, intervals of 2 to 3 weeks suffice. When the graft is fully opacified with new tissue, skin grafts are ready to be placed. The time from placement of Integra until placement of skin grafts averages 3 weeks for upper-body trauma reconstructions in young healthy people. For chronic pathologic ulcers of the lower extremity in older patients, Integra-to-skin graft intervals average 5–6 weeks, depending on severity of illness (see Table 16–7a).

Separated Silicone

When Integra is regenerated, tissue filling the sponge dislodges the silicone overlayer. The nominal usage of Integra is to place skin grafts when histogenesis is complete, but before the silicone separates. If silicone does separate before grafts are placed, this is almost always of no adverse consequence. Blistering of the silicone is irrelevant, but if it opens onto an edge, then some minor inflammation and benign sub-silicone abscess can result. Simply removing the silicone and instituting regular daily hygienic topical care will keep the regenerated Integra healthy and ready for the skin grafts. This will not affect whether the wound heals, although it does risk some inflammatory wound module and scar. What is more common is ejection due to benign foreign-body reaction against the silicone, which should not be confused with acute inflammation or infection, and which will not jeopardize the skin grafts (Fig. 16–7k).

Overgrafts

When dermatogenesis is complete, the silicone is lifted, and thin epidermal autografts are placed on the "neodermis." These skin grafts are managed as any other, but thin grafts are typically used (3–8 thousandths of an inch), trying to minimize the amount of mature dermis which is transplanted and minimizing donor site problems in these at-risk patients. Customary skin graft care is practiced. Small remaining bare areas will epithelialize naturally and, in healthy wounds and patients, grafts are usually healed within 2–8 weeks of placement. For chronic problem wounds, epithelium is sometimes difficult to cultivate on top of otherwise healthy Integra, and complete epidermal healing times can be several months (Table 16–7a). This can be a frustration, but it is usually an acceptable one because much of the skin graft has taken, residual open areas tend to be small, and the patients are already much improved. If the Integra is open by circumstances of premature silicone separation or failure of the skin grafts, then one must choose between continued topical care, adjuvant therapies, such as platelet-derived growth factor, or new skin grafts. Regenerated Integra is inherently healthy, a "naked dermis," which is effectively closing native tissues underneath. With some basic hygienic care, it can remain open like any other wound. An oft asked question is whether the initial skin grafts need to be placed at all. They are a qualified necessity. Left ungrafted, regenerated Integra will either epithelialize from the margins, or it will not. In healthy wounds and patients, epithelial ingrowth can and does happen; for smaller wounds and this can be opted in lieu of operative skin grafts.[23] For large wounds, anything more than a few centimeters, and for complex or pathologic wounds, operative skin grafting is required if results are to be best and the duration of care optimized. Whatever choices are made, it must be remembered that regenerated Integra is a mesodermal structure and, until epithelialized, some kind of active care will always be required.

Planned Second Integra

If an Integra reconstruction does mostly well, but there are some unhealed areas, a secondary procedure can be done—usually small flaps or another piece of Integra. However, there are also circumstances in which using multiple sequential pieces of Integra is part of the *a priori* treatment plan. Situations warranting this include: using Integra as a long duration artificial skin, replacing a fresh piece before silicone separates on the first piece; maintaining uninterrupted coverage while waiting for tangential histogenesis to bridge a gap; needing a thicker (multiple) layer of regenerated tissue.

Secondary Procedures

With any skin graft, it is common for there to be small scattered open areas, which require further topical care as the wounds fully reepithelialize. Typically just a tiny fraction of the total reconstructed surface, these areas heal within a few weeks in healthy patients and wounds, and Integra skin grafts are no different than ordinary skin grafts in this regard. However, for chronic wounds, although Integra fully succeeds in 90–95% of properly selected patients, the nominal pathway of "Integra–skin graft–quickly healed" occurs in only 20–25% of these patients. The other patients require some additional care, either prolonged topical care of several months duration, a second set of skin grafts, or some new Integra or local flaps to close focal small areas. Nearly all of this secondary care is supplemental to the original reconstruction in patients mostly healed and doing well, rather than a bailout from the original plan in patients doing poorly. There are no hard rules about when to do another procedure. Whenever it becomes clear that the current situation will not improve further with topical care only, then a follow-up procedure should be done.

Ancillary Therapies

When more prolonged care is required to get the skin overgrafts completely healed, this is just mostly ordinary topical care with hygienic products. However, several therapies with wound stimulatory effects can be opted to promote or accelerate complete healing in these delayed wounds. Platelet-derived growth factor (PDGF, recombinant human PDGF-BB, becaplermin, Regranex, Ortho-McNeil, Raritan, NJ) seems to be particularly effective at forcing complete re-epithelialization of otherwise healthy regenerated Integra (however, it must be used cautiously in patients with immunopathic disorders, because it can have a contrary ulcerative effect). Apligraf (neonatal living skin equivalent, Organogenesis, Canton, MA) and comparable living devices can have a similar effect. Hyperbaric oxygen therapy may be worthwhile for a very limited set of indications, namely, those patients with severe macro- or microarterial insufficiency and, in particular, those who have low transcutaneous oxygen tensions, which increase while breathing 1-atm 100% oxygen. Custom orthotics for control of motion and edema may be required in select situations and all other ordinary modalities of postoperative care and wound care must be maintained. Management of the underlying diseases must continue unabated.

Long Term Management

Integra maturation is that period of a few months in which the regenerated matrix is consolidating to uniform histology and full tensile strength is developing. Until then, minor trauma can cause tangential avulsion lacerations of the reconstructed tissue. Simple protective wraps and continued edema control are desirable until the new skin is no longer fragile. Underlying diseases and disabilities require continuing management, regardless of whether Integra or any other method was used to heal the wound.

Logistics

Integra and skin grafts are formal procedures conducted in the operating room, Unless a patient's underlying disease or the complexity of a particular problem or operation warrants inpatient care, all management can and should be done as an outpatient. Skin graft timing is judged by how thoroughly regenerated the matrix appears. However, actual intervals are influenced as much by the realities of outpatient services and surgery scheduling, but there is sufficient latitude in the timing of the grafts to accommodate reality. Most patients are not significantly disabled by the required dressings, splints, and aftercare, and most can carry on with ordinary activities of daily living at home. It is most important to realize that the cumulative time required to complete an Integra reconstruction is anything but trivial. None of the methods of using Integra are difficult or arcane and 4–6 weeks of intrinsic matrix regeneration time may not seem very long, yet until that last little square centimeter is epithelialized, active care must continue. Not surprisingly, time-to-completion is much less for trauma wounds in young healthy people. However, for chronic and pathologic wounds, treatment averages 5 to 6 months for most diagnoses, and as much as 10 months for radiation and immunopathic disorders. Physicians who do not regularly treat chronic wounds must appreciate these times and not become anxious or lose interest. The logistics of an Integra reconstruction, compared to conventional surgery, are really just mirroring the biology of its regeneration. Recall that normal inflammatory wound healing works quickly, over days to weeks, but it leaves a wake of scar-related complications that may require months or years of disability or future care. Integra occupies the middle ground, regenerating and healing, and requiring care, over weeks to months. However, once it is healed, it rarely needs further attention or late revision. Fortunately, although these treatment intervals may seem long to physicians who are anxious to see good results, they are accepted by most patients because (1) the ulcer itself has been present for months or years, (2) they are already used to the idea of needing daily care, (3) once Integra is placed, symptoms, progressive disease, and various disabilities resolve, so function, lifestyle, and peace of mind are improved for most patients, (4) most of the prolonged care is for small unepithelialized but otherwise stable areas, and the patients have long since returned to otherwise normal healthy activities, and (5) Integra is succeeding where all else had failed.

Complications and Problems

With proper wound preparation, excision of the wound, and graft fixation, complication rates should be low. Acute hematomas and loss of adhesion due to motion are avoidable and can be easily managed by evacuation, better fixation, and a new piece of Integra if needed. If regenerated Integra ejects the silicone before skin grafts are placed, it is managed topically (as already discussed). In these circumstances, the original wound is healed under the Integra, and what happens on the superficial surface is of no great concern. If silicone separates prematurely before the sponge is regenerated, this too is managed by customary daily hygiene and wound care until skin grafts can be placed. In these situations, as long as the Integra sponge remains healthy, primary disease and inflammation are kept under control, and good daily care of the wound is maintained, the Integra will continue to regenerate. Occasionally, silicone separates in limited areas, with tubid milky exudates in the resulting blisters. Whatever the cause of these seemingly sterile abscesses (foreign-body giant cell reaction under the silicone is the cause, in some cases), they are usually not accompanied by pain erythema, or destruction of the regenerated matrix. Local silicone removal and good daily care preserves the matrix and skin grafts typically do take in these areas. True infection, manifested as intense inflammation, pain, suppuration, and loss of the material, should be very infrequent if the wound is properly prepared and excised, edema controlled, and the graft effectively fixated. The management of lost or delayed skin grafts is discussed above.

Open Integra

It should be clear that, while loss of silicone or epithelium is not the preferred pathway, it is no catastrophe, and the reconstructed new dermis can be safely managed without the silicone. A consistent observation is that even when regenerated Integra remains unepithelialized, the wound and periwound tissues remain free of inflammation, pain, further necrosis and ulceration, and all evidence of the original problem (as long as the underlying diseases are also adequately treated). Thus, even unepithelialized "naked dermis" Integra is therapeutic and it is far more tolerable to patients than the original wound was, sometimes even perfectly acceptable.

Failed Integra

A core concept about Integra is that it works well for pathologic wounds where conventional repairs are likely to fail. This means that Integra is regularly being challenged by proverbial "poor protoplasm." Assuming that patients are correctly diagnosed, thoroughly treated, that the wound is properly prepared, and that good care continues after surgery, Integra usually succeeds. However, there are the few times when it simply fails. Failure comes in several forms. (1) "Gangrene" of the matrix. When Integra covers nonviable tissues it turns black, a sure sign of residual undébrided eschar or of extreme artial insufficiency. (2) Failure to regenerate. Areas of the matrix can persist as is, without evidence of histogenesis. Usually just patchy, this seems to correlate with general debility or advanced illness. (3) Early lysis or ulceration. Matrix which appears to have regenerated can suddenly ulcerate or involute, either before or soon after skin

grafting. This is a dependable marker of underlying disease flaring up, typically immunopathic or hematologic disorders, and it may be accompanied by new ulcers in previously uninvolved skin. While Integra can help control or resist active disease and may be more resilient than native local tissues, it is not a cure for these diseases and it is not invulnerable. If the flare is severe, matrix regenerated tissue can reulcerate. (4) Failure to accept or support skin grafts. Many practitioners have observed the "disappearing skin graft" phenomenon in which a first set of skin grafts adheres and then dissolves. Second skin grafts usually succeed. The problem is when Integra remains persistently open after several grafts. Surprisingly, in the author's practice, this has occurred almost exclusively in a few younger patients (less than 40 years old), on the lower extremity, where status of the wound waxed and waned with activity. Patient compliance with restricted activities, leg elevation, and good compression seem to favorably influence this problem. (5) Conversion to a conventional wound with inflammatory healing. This is a combination of the above situations. If grafts do not adhere and disease takes over, the open Integra eventually reverts to an ordinary wound. (6) Late ulceration. Integra, which has completely healed, might reulcerate if disease or maintenance care get out of control. If it already healed once, it should be easy to get an incipient new lesion rehealed with good hygiene, compression, antiinflammatory control, and other basic care. In all of these situations, the problem is not inherent to the matrix, but reflects problems with disease, patient, and their management. When these events do occur, the following should be done: reestablish good daily wound care; reassess patient and disease status; intensify treatment of underlying disease if needed; check to make sure that arterial vascular status has not changed during the course of treatment; perform further débridement as needed; rethink the overall treatment plan; when wound and disease are again under control, try again for closure, with new Integra or by other means, depending on the new plans.

Caveats and Contraindications

There are no formal contraindications to Integra. Used correctly, it is categorically safe and does not jeopardize tissue, limb, or life. Even if treatment plans change along the way, it is always a good interim artificial skin in advance of any other reconstruction. The main reason not to use it is that a problem can be solved more expeditiously by conventional means. Relative indications for Integra are presented above. The inverse is true, if those conditions do not exist, Integra is not necessary. If underlying structures are not exposed, if disease and risks are easily or fully controlled, if dependable flaps are present, if prior conventional procedures were uncomplicated, if a preliminary period of observation and topical care show that the wound is wound-healing competent, then conventional management and surgery should be done. All decisions should be predicated on the goals of controlling disease and symptoms, healing the wound, doing so as quickly and efficiently as possible with minimized costs and resource utilization, all while preserving function and lifestyle. Whatever treatment can be anticipated to best fulfill these goals should be selected. The great majority of wounds are best managed by ordinary means. Integra is used for those large, life-threatening, complex, pathologic, or refractory problems for which customary methods of care have not or will not work.

REVIEW OF EXPERIENCE

In the preceding sections, many of the statements about outcomes, incidence, duration, and other quantitative information were based on data compiled from the author's own practice. This section will summarize some of that data for a clearer understanding of the patients and problems suitable for treatment with Integra and a realistic picture of management and outcomes.

The data summarized here reflect a 72–month study interval in which Integra was used in a total of 132 patients.[24] It was used for chronic wounds in 111 patients, the subjects of the tables and discussion below. In 107 of those patients having 158 individual ulcers, Integra was used to directly close the wounds. In the other 4 patients with 7 lesions, Integra was an adjunct to chronic wound surgery, used mainly to close donor sites when flaps were used for the primary closure. Among the 111 patients with 165 ulcers, there were 173 instances of exposed skeletal or visceral structures which, under the conventional rules of plastic surgery, would have required flaps for closure. The first set of tables profiles all 111 patients with 165 ulcers and 173 exposed structures. The second set of tables presents outcomes, limited to the 103 patients with 151 ulcers and 166 exposed structures who concluded care and had complete data.

Patients and Ulcers

Table 16–3, Data: Patient Profiles and Ulcer History

These are the profiles of the 111 chronic wound patients and their ulcer history, stratified by diagnostic category. Many patients had multiple risks or diagnoses. Typically one diagnosis predominated as the most immediate or problematic factor, designated the "primary diagnosis." There were 90 instances of secondary diagnoses (for example, some of the rheumatoid and all of the diabetic patients also had artherosclerotic arterial insufficiency, and some venous patients had a hypercoagulable disorder responsible for their original

venous thrombosis). Individual diagnoses within categories were diverse (immunopathic: rheumatoid, lupus, Sjögren's, polymyalgia rheumatica, Wegener's granulomatosis, pyoderma gangrenosum, calcinosis cutis, Raynaud phenomenon, esophageal motility disorder, sclerodactyly, and telangiectasia [CREST]; hypercoagulable: protein C, protein S, antithrombin III, fibrinogen, anticardiolipin, plasminogen, homocysteine; micro-occlusive: polycythemia vera, hyperparathyroidism-calciphylaxis). The diagnostic categories are ranked in order of incidence; sex and age distributions are given for each. Histories of less than 2 years duration are listed in months, longer histories are given in years. Also listed is the percentage of patients who had one or more failed prior procedures for those ulcers.

Table 16–3, Analysis

These 111 are a small fraction of all patients in the author's practice during 6 years, reflecting that Integra was not used indiscriminately, neither for its novelty nor any other unconsidered reason. All patients were treated according to some disciplined schema for the evaluation and treatment of chronic wounds, with Integra opted based upon certain consistent criteria. For example, for each venous patient treated with Integra, many more were treated by compression, topical modalities, skin grafts, venous interruption, and other conventional care. Integra was used only for selective reasons, as detailed in the indications sections above. These 111 patients represent the extreme of multiple risk factors, prolonged refractory disease, failed procedures, and anatomical complexities. The ranking of the data portrays the frequency with which certain diagnoses will create problems manageable with Integra, with arterial, immunopathic, venous, and hypercoagulable disorders predominating. This should be no surprise, because these are the diagnoses most likely to fail topical care and defy conventional surgery. The low incidence of prior procedures for atherosclerotic macroarterial ulcers is also no surprise, because failed prior surgery in these patients implies a subsequent amputation, and most such patients never have the chance for limb salvage consultation and care.

Table 16–4, Data: Ulcer Anatomy—Site

This table details ulcer location. The left side panels correlate general location with primary diagnosis. Values for each are stated as percentage of all ulcers. The right side of the table is not correlated with diagnosis, but rather gives a more detailed profile of ulcer location, instances listed as percentage of all 165 ulcers.

Table 16–5, Data: Ulcer Anatomy—Complications

This table details "anatomical complications," referring to exposure of internal structures. The 173

Table 16–3. Patient profiles and ulcer history

Diagnostic category	Primary diagnosis % of all 111 patients	Male :: Female (%)	Age Range years	Age Mean years	Duration of ulcers, less than 2 years (months) % of all Pts	Mean ± std	Range	Duration of ulcers, greater than 2 years (years) % of all Pts	Mean ± std	Range	Prior failed procedures % of patients per category
Macroarterial	24	67::33	42–83	68	14	4	1–11	2	2	—	11
Immunopathic	19	19::81	29–86	65	15	6	3–8	3	22	3–40	19
Venous/lymphatic	16	72::28	32–86	67	10	9	3–14	10	16 ± 13	2–40	44
Hypercoagulable	8	11::89	34–80	58	7	6	3–11	3	7	2–12	33
Mechanical/ anatomical	7	37::63	16–90	59	3	5	2–7	3	23	2–44	38
Radiation/ malignancy	6	0::100	21–93	67	3	16	14–18	—	—	—	43
Diabetes/ neuropathy	5	100::0	51–67	56	3	12	3–21	—	—	—	40
Unknown	4	0::100	36–76	54	7	7	1–11	—	2	—	80
Micro-occlusive	3	0::100	45–72	62	2	15	—	2	3	—	33
Trauma and surgery	2	50::50	39–66	53	2	2	—	—	—	—	0
Granulomatous/ infectious	2	50::50	37–56	47	—	—	—	2	19	—	50
Total, chronic (107 patients, 158 ulcers)	**96**	**43::57**	**16–93**	**64**	**66**	**7 ± 5**	**1–21**	**27**	**14 ± 15**	**2–44**	**30**
Adjunct to chronic wound surgery	4	50::50	6–66	33	7	1	0–4	—	—	—	25
Total patients in study (111 Patients, 165 ulcers)	**100**	**43::57**	**6–93**	**63**	**73**	**6 ± 5**	**0–21**	**27**	**14 ± 15**	**2–44**	**30**

Table 16–4. Ulcer anatomy, site

Diagnostic category	Primary diagnosis % of all 111 patients	Location and number of ulcers			Location of ulcers, detailed	Instances, % of all 165 ulcers
		Head & trunk % of all 165 ulcers	Upper extremity % of all 165 ulcers	Lower extremity % of all 165 ulcers		
Macroarterial	24	—	1	19	**Total, head & trunk**	**8**
Immunopathic	19	—	—	25	Head	1
Venous/lymphatic	16	—	—	13	Back	5
Hypercoagulable	8	—	1	10	Abdomen	1
Mechanical/anatomical	7	1	1	7	Chest	1
Radiation/malignancy	6	3	—	1	**Total, upper extremity**	**6**
Diabetes/neuropathy	5	—	—	3	Hand/wrist	4
Unknown	4	—	1	2	Forearm	1
Micro-occlusive	3	—	1	2	**Total, lower extremity**	**86**
Trauma and surgery	2	—	1	1	Thigh	6
Granulomatous/infectious	2	1	—	2	Leg	34
Total, chronic	**96**	**5**	**6**	**85**	Ankle	26
Adjunct to chronic wound surgery	4	3	—	1	Foot	20
Total patients in study	**100**	**8**	**6**	**86**	**Total ulcers**	**100**

279

Table 16–5. Ulcer anatomy, complications

Diagnostic category	Primary diagnosis % of all 111 patients	Anatomical complications		Instances % of all 173 ulcers	Structures exposed
		% of Patients per category	Detailed		
Macroarterial	24	74	**Total open bone**	**36**	
Immunopathic	19	76	Cortical	16	Sternum, ribs, tibia, fibula, malleoli, calcaneus, tarsals, metatarsals, phalanges
Venous/lymphatic	16	72	Cancellous	20	Sacrum, tibia, fibula, malleoli, calcaneus, tarsal, metatarsals, phalanges (hand & foot)
Hypercoagulable	8	56	**Total open joints**	**14**	
Mechanical/anatomical	7	88	Major	5	Tibiotalar, talofibular
Radiation/malignancy	6	100	Minor	9	Metacarpophalangeal, intertarsal, tarsometatarsal, metatarso-phalangeal, interphalangeal
Diabetes/neuropathy	5	100	**Total open tendons**	**48**	
Unknown	4	40	Major	42	Finger & wrist extensors, Achilles, tibialis anterior, tibialis posterior, peroneus longus & brevis, extrinsic toe extensors
Micro-occlusive	3	33	Minor	6	Extensor digitorum brevis, intrinsic & distal toe flexors
Trauma and surgery	2	100	**Total others**	**2**	
Granulomatous/Infectious	2	50	Internal organs	1	Lung, kidney
Total, chronic	**96**	**74**	Alloplastic materials	1	Metal plate (distal tibia fracture)
Adjunct to chronic wound surgery	4	0			
Total patients in study	**100**	**71**	**Total exposed structures**	**100**	

instances of exposure occurred in 111 individual ulcers (67% of all ulcers) in 78 patients (71% of all patients). The left-side panels list incidence as percentage of the patients in each diagnostic category who had such complications. The right-side panels (not correlated with diagnosis) give a detailed profile of the exposed structures, incidence listed as percentage of the 173 structures exposed. Exposed bone is partitioned by cortical bone only versus cancellous bone exposed by disease, débridement, or ostectomy. "Open joint" refers explicitly to joints having an arthrotomy, loss of joint capsule and synovium, and exposure of the joint space, due to either disease or debridement. Major/minor tendons are classed based on physical size or functional significance. Grouped tendons, such as finger and toe extensors, are counted only once for each instance, even when multiple individual tendons were exposed. Many instances of exposed minor tendons, joint capsules, and retinacular ligaments were not tabulated, because while flaps are often used for their closure, flaps would not have been considered categorically necessary. Many pieces of Integra were applied directly to large areas of muscle where the results are dependably good. Coverage of viscera and hardware are presented in the case studies.

Tables 16–4 and 16–5, Analysis

The anatomical distribution of these lesions is as one would expect, with the major ulcerative pathologies (arterial, immunopathic, venous, and hypercoagulable disorders) causing mostly leg and foot ulcers, and other diagnoses having more generalized distributions. The incidence of exposed skeletal and visceral structures is high, reflecting, in part, the destructive effects of these underlying disorders on skin and fascias. However, these values are exaggerated compared to the natural incidence of these situations. This is because the patients in this study were selected for Integra precisely because of these anatomical conditions. These are the situations where closure by conventional means is unreliable and where Integra is dependably effective and of low risk.

Outcomes

Table 16–6, Data: Outcomes— Outcome Category

Outcomes in 103 patients are divided into three groups. Group 1 "healed" patients were completely healed by Integra, subdivided into four categories: 1a, the nominal uncomplicated reconstruction (excise wound, place Integra, place skin grafts when regenerated, healed); 1b, the nominal reconstruction, but persistent open areas after the epidermal overgrafts required more than 6 weeks of care, including additional topical modalities, such as platelet derived growth factor; 1c, incomplete take or delayed re-epithelialization of the first skin grafts prompted a second skin graft over the original Integra; 1d, residual open areas or lost Integra were successfully closed with a second application of Integra and subsequent skin grafts. Group 2 "incomplete" patients all had successful Integra-dependent outcomes, but Integra alone did not fully heal the wound: 2a, conventional flaps or skin grafts were used to complete closure of small areas where Integra did not heal; 2b, Integra created a healthy stable wound, free of active pathology and ulceration, permitting the wound to be healed with subsequent flaps or grafts that replaced areas of unepithelialized Integra; 2c, same circumstances as 2b, but remaining open. Integra, stable and asymptomatic, was left open for chronic topical wound

Table 16–6. Outcomes, by category

	Outcomes, detailed	1 Healed % of all 103 patients	2 Incomplete % of all 103 patients	3 Failed % of all 103 patients
1a	Prescribed reconstruction, nominal, healed	22		
1b	Topical care to complete epithelialization	10		
1c	Second skin grafts	25		
1d	Second Integra	14		
2a	Secondary flaps or grafts		14	
2b	Pathology controlled		3	
2c	Persistent open Integra		3	
3a	Loss or failure of Integra			3
3b	Persistence of wound or continued pathology			1
3c	Amputation			5
	Totals	**71**	**20**	**9**

Table 16–7. Outcomes, by diagnosis

Diagnostic category	1 Fully healed % of patients per category	2M Mostly healed (>2/3) % of patients per category	2P Partly healed (<2/3) % of patients per category	3 Failed % of patients per category
Macroarterial	58	8	16	18
Immunopathic	74	16	5	5
Venous/lymphedema	88	—	6	6
Hypercoagulable	86	—	14	0
Mechanical/anatomical	88	12	—	0
Radiation/malignancy	72	28	—	0
Diabetes/neuropathy	0	20	40	40
Unknown	60	20	20	0
Micro-occlusive	100	—	—	0
Trauma/surgery	100	—	—	0
G anulomatous/infectious	50	50	—	0
Adjunct	100	—	—	0
Total	**71**	**10**	**10**	**9**

care. Group 3 were failures: 3a, loss or failure of the Integra with a persistent wound; 3b, persistent or progressive ulcerative wound pathology; 3c, failure of the reconstruction leading to amputation.

Table 16–6, Analysis

Integra successfully closed all wounds in 71% of the patients. In 20% of patients, Integra contributed to a successful outcome, supplemented by other operations. Integra failed to close the wound or resolve the clinical problem in 9% of patients. Integra actually performed properly in nearly 100% of patients. There were a few patients with extreme degrees of arterial insufficiency in whom Integra failed to adhere or regenerate to any degree whatsoever. In all other "incomplete" or "failure" patients, adherence and regeneration of the matrix occurred, but with patchy loss or failure due to conditions of disease and patient compliance. Even in some of the "failure" patients, there was nearly complete healing of the Integra and skin grafts. These cases were designated "failures" because there was an eventual amputation and Integra ultimately contributed nothing to the final outcome. This was notably in the diabetics with plantar ulceration, where failure was due to noncompliance with prescribed care rather than any deficiency of the Integra. Integra is safe, and potential minor complications, as detailed in the "Techniques and Management" section, are no different than the nuisance issues that arise with all chronic wound care. Miscellaneous events of this nature did occur, but were all managed in the daily course of care; they did not significantly influence outcomes. The only notable adverse event was one infection under one sheet of Integra (pain, fever, suppuration, periwound erythema, lysis of the Integra), in a patient with high-grade arterial insufficiency and active rheumatoid arthritis.

Table 16–7, Data: Outcomes—Diagnosis

In this table, the three general outcome categories (healed, incomplete, failed) are stratified by diagnosis. It was obvious in the review of data that among the Group 2 "incomplete" patients, there were two subpopulations. Some did extremely well, qualifying as incomplete only on minor technicalities and healing after some accessory surgery, whereas some had deficiencies, which remained unhealed or required a different strategy for subsequent care. Within this group, this partition of better or worse outcomes correlated with the degree to which the original skin grafts healed, greater than or less than two thirds of the original wound area. In this and the next table, the "incomplete" Group 2 is subdivided into "mostly healed" and "partly healed" based on this discriminator. In this and the next two tables, data are presented as percent age of patients per category, so that on each row, all values sum to 100%.

Table 16–8, Data: Outcomes—Site

This table is comparable to the preceding one, with general outcomes correlated against anatomical location rather than underlying diagnosis. All instances of multiple ulcers (151 ulcers in 103 patients) were on the lower extremity (eg, leg and ankle, or leg and foot). Because this table describes outcomes by patient rather than

Table 16–8. Outcomes, by site

Location	1 Fully healed % of patients per category	2M Mostly healed (>2/3) % of patients per category	2P Partly healed (<2/3) % of patients per category	3 Failed % of patients per category
Upper extremity	60	20	20	—
Head and trunk	80	20	—	—
Thigh	25	25	—	50
Leg	72	4	16	8
Ankle	82	5	5	8
Foot	42	17	24	17
Lower extremity, multiple	80	12	4	4
Total	**71**	**10**	**10**	**9**

outcomes by ulcer, a new "multiple" entry refers to patients that had ulcers at more than just one of the sites listed in the other rows.

Tables 16-7 and 16–8—Analysis

Outcomes based on diagnosis were meaningful. The lowest success rates and the highest failure rates were among patients with arterial insufficiency and diabetic neuropathy. Outcomes by site show that the foot was a poor performer compared to most other locations. However, data from Tables 16-3 and 16-4a remind that there were many arterial and foot ulcers treated. The implications of this experience are very clear. As already discussed in the "Uses of Integra" section, Integra not only performs well when arterial insufficiency is mild to moderate, it can be the only practical modality that can ensure success in these circumstances. However, when arterial insufficiency is extreme, as it was in some of these patients, Integra will fail. Proper patient selection is, therefore, important if unnecessary failed procedures are to be avoided in advance of inevitable amputation. Ankle–brachial indices of 0.2 to 0.3, and a $TcPO_2$ below 10 torr without a response to oxygen challenge are criteria by which these judgments can be made. Integra likewise performs very nicely on the foot, salvaging many extremities that all too often are peremptorily and unnecessarily amputated. The foot is a challenge, but it is not per se the problem. Noncompliant middle-aged ambulatory neuropathic diabetic patients are the problem and a lesson learned is that it is best not to waste resources attempting to use Integra to resolve diabetic plantar ulcers.

F. Table 16–9, Data: Outcomes—Closure of Internal Structures

This table documents outcomes for the closure of 166 exposed structures. The three columns are simply the three outcome categories retitled to reflect the means of resolution: closure of the structure by healed Integra (healed), closure by a secondary flap or graft (incomplete), or unresolved, including amputation (failed).

G. Table 16–9, Analysis

Of the 166 instances of exposed structures, 90% were successfully closed by Integra. For 6%, secondary surgery was required for eventual closure, but Integra functioned as a competent artificial skin, keeping those structures safe, thereby permitting late closure and salvage. Only 4% of these structures were not closed by Integra and were eliminated by later débridement or amputation. Each one of these salvaged structures would have required flaps according to the usual principles of plastic surgery. This is one of the benefits of Integra, that it can perform as well as flaps, but without morbidity and donor sites, especially in circumstances where there are no flaps to give away.

H. Table 16–10, Data: Utilization and Length of Treatment

Direct costs of care were not tabulated, but lifestyle impact was assessed by looking at the length of time to complete a reconstruction, and economic impact was estimated by analyzing venues of care, inpatient versus outpatient. For length of treatment, "Integra-to-skin grafts" is the regeneration time in weeks, the mean time between placing Integra and placing the first set of skin grafts (counted in days, then converted to weeks), stratified by diagnosis. This parameter was controlled by surgical scheduling and by the basic physiology of Integra as much as by anything else. Therefore, values are relatively uniform, with not even a weeks difference between more benign and more pathologic diagnoses. The exception is the radiation category, where, as might be expected, radiation caused a high-end second mode. "Integra-to-healed" is the interval, in months, between

Table 16–9. Outcomes, closure of internal structures

	Closure by Integra % of patients per category	Closure by secondary surgery	
Circumstance		**Flaps or grafts % of patients per category**	**Amputation or unresolved % of patients per category**
Open bone			
Cortical	89	4	7
Cancellous	94	3	3
Open joints			
Major	74	13	13
Minor	87	13	—
Open tendons			
Major	93	5	2
Minor	80	20	—
Open internal organs	100	—	—
Open hardware	100	—	—
Totals	**90**	**6**	**4**

placing Integra and when the wound was fully epithelialized. This data also includes patients in the Group 2 partial success category, their intervals measured when secondary grafts or flaps were healed. In four groups, there is a clear outlier (the parenthetical values under "range"), which is excluded from the averages.

Table 16–11, Data: Utilization—Inpatient Versus Outpatient

This table assesses inpatient hospitalization versus care that was entirely outpatient (clinic and outpatient surgery). The first column is the number of patients each year (data available for 107 patients, because the study covered only 6 months of 1996 and 2002, the numbers in parentheses are pro rata annualizations that make all rows comparable). The second column is the number of patients who had an inpatient admission at any time related to their Integra reconstruction, either for the primary excision and Integra or for the skin grafts. "Inpatient admission" is defined as a formal hospitalization of greater than 24 hours duration subject to the legal and administrative criteria of inpatient

Table 16–10. Utilization and length of treatment

	Integra-to-skin grafts (weeks)		Integra-to-healed (months)		
Primary diagnosis	**Mean**	**Std**	**Mean**	**Std**	**Range**
Macroarterial	5.3	1.2	5.0	2.5	1–9 (19)
Immunopathic	5.4	1.6	9.6	5.3	2–18
Venous/lymphatic	4.6	1.3	6.2	3.2	2–11
Hypercoagulable	5.3	2.0	5.8	2.1	4–9 (19)
Mechanical/anatomical	5.0	1.3	5.2	1.5	3–7 (12)
Radiation/malignancy	7.4	3.9	9.8	4.3	5–15
Diabetes/neuropathy	4.3	1.1	6.5	2.1	5–8 (15)
Unknown	4.1	1.4	7.0	0.8	6–8
Micro-occlusive	6.0	—	4	—	—
Trauma and surgery	4.6	—	3	—	—
Granulomatous/infectious	4.1	—	2	—	—
Total, chronic	**5.3**	**2.0**	**7.2**	**4.3**	**1–19**
Adjunct	4.1	0.7	3.8	1.7	2–6
Total	**5.3**	**1.9**	**7.0**	**4.3**	**1–19**

Table 16–11. Utilization—inpatient versus outpatient

Year	Total Integra patients	Number of inpatients	Percentage inpatients
1996	4 (8)	3	75
1997	18	11	61
1998	10	5	50
1999	19	9	47
2000	16	4	25
2001	28	6	21
2002	12 (24)	0	0
Total	**107**	**38**	**36**

reimbursement, and does not include overnight stays of less than 24 hours. The last column is the percentage inpatients— the ratio of the first two columns.

Tables 16–10 and 16–11—Analysis

The logistics of an Integra reconstruction were explained in the "Techniques and Management" section and should now be reread. That discussion is based on this data. An Integra reconstruction is not a trivial affair. It is a staged reconstruction that requires the commitment of the patient and dedicated persistence of the surgeon and allied health staff. Length of care is relative. For most surgeons, who take care of people with acute injuries without wound-healing problems, any chronic wound reconstruction can be a tedious affair not suited to the surgeon's manner of practice. For patients who have endured the ulcer and its diseases for months or years, Integra control of a problem wound usually means dramatic improvement, and most patients are far more understanding about the time required than the physician is. Patient acceptance is even greater because most of it can be done as an outpatient. The inpatient rate declined to zero over 6 years. The problems and the severity of the patients being treated did not change during this interval. What did change was: (1) increasing familiarity of the author with Integra and its capabilities; (2) increasing infrastructure of wound services through outpatient clinics and home health agencies; (3) concurrent socioeconomic changes in the delivery and payment of medical services (in the United States) which have steered care away from hospitals. Integra is a product very well suited to taking care of complex problems as an outpatient. While costs were not explicitly analyzed, Integra's ability to keep patients out of the hospital and free of numerous failed procedures would seem to make Integra reconstruction for chronic or pathological wounds economically favorable.

Summary of Author's Data

Tables 16–7 to 16–9 show that 81% of patients had excellent outcomes, either complete success with Integra itself (71%, outcome group 1) or after some minor subsidiary surgery (10%, outcome Group 2M). However, the way in which data was tallied, good results are somewhat underestimated. For example, Case E3 was assigned to Group 2 because she died before the final skin graft healed, but Integra had performed well with dramatic improvements in the patient and her wounds. Case F1 was likewise classified a partial success because a small secondary procedure was needed, but the ability of Integra to close a flexor tendon and salvage a finger in an atherosclerotic hand is a truly great success. The category 3 failures were, indeed, failures, but in retrospect, seven patients with extreme arterial insufficiency or diabetic plantar ulcers should be considered poorly selected. The remaining 96 patients had a realistic potential for success and, among these patients, the good results were 88% (76% Group 1, 12% Group 2M).

The 10% of patients with neither a good result or outright failure still benefited from Integra, either in partial closure of the wounds, control of further ulceration, or sufficient stability of the wound to permit reconstruction by other means. Lesser results were largely on the lower extremity associated with severe arterial insufficiency and diabetic neuropathy. It was learned that Integra and time ought not to be wasted on extreme patients of these types. However, for most of the other arterial patients, including diabetics, Integra not only performed well, but it was often the only salvation for a threatened extremity. Integra also closed and healed 90% of the exposed bones, joints, tendons, and other structures that it was applied to, and protected another 6% leading to closure with flaps. This demonstrates Integra's ability to supplant flaps, oftentimes in situations were flaps are needed but are not available, getting the same job done, sometimes a better job, without donor sites or risk to the patient. While many acute conditions best treated with Integra, such as burns and degloving injuries, must be treated in the hospital, Integra reconstruction for chronic wounds can be managed almost entirely as an outpatient, with preservation of activity and lifestyle.

Other Sources

Integra was released for general use in 1996, after 2 decades of development and then various clinical trials for burns. There is now a full decade of clinical experience, and numerous investigators and clinicians from around the world have reported favorable experiences, in peer-reviewed publications and at burn and wound symposia. Many of the exciting cases and extended indications are the subject of case reports presented at conferences for which there is no public citation. References 25 to 54 are some of the published resources. They discuss a wide spectrum of clinical scenarios, including acute and chronic wounds, large trauma cases, and carefully planned elective operations, both in adults and in children. In reading them, certain themes recur and certain common conclusions are drawn, all of which echo what has been discussed in this chapter. Notable points include: Integra is useful for a broad range of acute, large, critical wounds and a variety of reconstructive problems;[25–31] it is very useful for managing acute, severe, and chronic illness in children;[32–35] Integra has a beneficial effect on posttraumatic wound and patient physiology;[36] it simplifies care, shortens recovery, and shortens length of care;[29,32,34,37,38] it minimizes morbidity and saves lives;[17,37,38] it is good for a wide range of anatomically and pathologically specific problems such as scalp, breast, upper extremity, limb and stump salvage;[33–35,39–46] it can solve chronic wound problems;[35] it covers essential structures and alloplastic materials;[18,47,48] there is value in eliminating concurrent donor sites;[32,43] the healed material is comparable to normal skin and much better than skin grafts;[28,42,43,49,50] tissue mechanics, lack of scar and contractures, and physical properties of the healed material are comparable to skin and superior to skin grafts, yielding good or superior functional results and improved range of motion;[18,28,29,32,42–45,51–53] cosmetic appearance is likewise very good, and much better than ordinary skin grafts;[22,25,26,28,39,40,43–45,47,51,54] sequential layers of Integra can produce desirable effects and it works well as a composite or adjunct with flaps.[28,47,54] The general impressions are that for select problems of critical wound care and reconstruction, that Integra outperforms conventional methods of care, simplifying complex care, minimizing morbidity and utilization, and yielding superior results.

Other Indications

While the focus of this chapter is on wounds and, especially, chronic wounds, the properties of Integra's collagen–chondroitin matrix make it suitable for other problems in surgery. Most interest is in using the matrix itself, without the silicone, for implantation purposes. The general areas of interest and investigation are listed below.

Bulk Filling

Bursas or wound "dead space" are usually controlled by negative-pressure suction drainage, positive-pressure compression bandaging, or filling with flaps (not controlling the space risks abscess and dehiscence). Integra matrix can be used instead, eventually turning into buried tissue. This can simplify closure of a complex wound in the same way as it simplifies closure of surface wounds.

Contour Correction

This may be for cosmetic or reconstructive purposes, large contour depressions, or fine wrinkles. The attraction of using the matrix is that it and the regenerated tissue are durable and long lasting. Along with its other properties, this makes it safer and simpler than many flaps, more durable and less prone to complication than large tissue grafts, and superior to reabsorbing injectable filler materials in current practice, such as bovine collagen.

Control of Inflammation and Scar Contracture

In principle, the matrix could be used as a liner along any type of serosal or mesenchymal surface to inhibit inflammatory changes and scar. Theoretical advantages run a gamut from controlling capsular contracture around breast implants to minimizing strictures and obstructions of tubular viscera to controlling serositis, effusions, and adhesions in the thorax, pericardium, peritoneum, around joints and tendons, and anywhere else where scar must be eliminated to preserve function. These are speculative uses, but presumably they will get attention as the material becomes more familiar to more surgeons.

Peripheral Nerve Management

The matrix has been shown to be superior to other methods of controlling epineurial fibrosis and guiding the regeneration of nerve axons.[55] The author has twice used the sponge by itself for the buffering or sequestration of an entrapped nerve with chronic severe neuralgia. In both instances, the nerve was the posterior tibial or common plantar nerve at the ankle. Both patients had a history of failed operations and other care. Integra matrix allowed the nerves to be completely decompressed and lysed and then closed with nonscarring tissue, without needing elaborate flaps. Both patients were entirely relieved of pain. What is important is that the principles of care were those of all good peripheral nerve surgery. Integra is simply a very good tool that allows a surgeon to effectively fulfill those principles of care. The matrix seems like a natural fit for problems related to nerve entrapment, nerve injury, and plexitis.

New Product Forms

In order to support these extended indications, there has been developmental work on a bulk implantable form of the sponge and on a micronized injectable form.[56] They were not available for general use by the time that this chapter was written. This is a matter of living history, these circumstances reflecting the ongoing evolution of a new, but very important, product.

Keratinocytes

The possibility of completing the entire reconstruction with just one operation has received much attention. There are two approaches to this problem. One is to use laboratory-cultured autografts derived from a skin biopsy. While the mesenchymal matrix is regenerating *in situ*, the epithelial grafts are growing in the laboratory, ready for application by the time the matrix is regenerated. This concept is limited by the availability and expense of this service, and it is not appropriate for small wounds. However, the concept has been proved and, for large burns, it can be a valuable strategy.[17, 38, 57, 58] The second approach is to seed the matrix with keratinocytes, and allow them to grow as the matrix is regenerating. While maintaining the viability of these explanted cells might seem to be problematic, this concept, too, has been proved.[59, 60] There is not yet any readily adaptable clinical technique that all surgeons might use, but development in this area continues.

Tissue Engineering

As discussed earlier the nominal technique of applying Integra is a form of *in situ* tissue engineering. However, it is somewhat passive, presenting the scaffold to the wound, then allowing cells to find it and do what they will. Adding keratinocytes to the matrix is a more active intervention, taking some control over which cells appear and when. The matrix permits this type of engineering. It is a highly biocompatible environment with a critical attachment chemical (the chondroitin) that affords superlative protection and organizational guidance to cells that find themselves there. In principle, any type of cell could be seeded and, in theory, one can foresee the possibility of using a matrix of this sort for the regeneration of hepatic cells, renal cells, pancreatic islet cells, or cells of any other visceral organ, epithelium, or gland. In 2003, bioengineering new tissues and organs has become a forefront academic research issue, and Integra-like matrices can be anticipated to be important in decades to come.

REFERENCES

1. Yannas IV, Burke JF. Design of an artificial skin. I. Basic design principles. *J Biomed Mater Res.* 1980;14:65–81.

2. Yannas IV, Burke JF, Gordon PL, et al. Design of an artificial skin. II. Control of chemical composition. *J Biomed Mater Res.* 1980;14:107–131.

3. Yannas IV. Studies on the biological activity of the dermal regeneration template. *Wound Repair Regen.* 1998;6:518–523.

4. Dostal GH, Gamelli RL. Fetal wound healing. *Surg Gynecol Obstet* 1993;176:299–306.

5. Bullard KM, Longaker MT, Lorenz HP. Fetal wound healing: current biology. *World J Surg.* 2003;27:54–61.

6. Bertolami CN. Glycosaminoglycan interactions in early wound repair. In: Hunt TK, Heppenstall RB, Pines E, et al. eds. *Soft and hard tissue repair: biological and clinical aspects.* New York, Praeger, 1984:67–97.

7a. Ronca F, Palmieri L, Panicucci P, et al. Antiinflammatory activity of chondroitin sulfate. *Osteoarthr Cartil.* 6 (Suppl A) 1998;14–21.

7b. Hunt TK, Knighton DR, Thakral KK, et al. Cellular control of repair. In: Hunt TK, Heppenstall RB, Pines E, et al. eds. *Soft and hard tissue repair: biological and clinical aspects.* New York, Praeger, 1984:3–19.

8. Holbrook KA, Smith LT. Ultrastructural aspects of human skin during the embryonic, fetal, premature, neonatal, and adult periods of life. *Birth Defects.* 1981;17:9–38.

9. Gottlieb ME. Modeling blood vessels: a deterministic method with fractal structure based on physiological rules. *Proc 12th Int Meet IEEE Eng Med, Biol Soc.* 1990.

10. Gottlieb, ME. The VT model: a deterministic model of angiogenesis and biofractals based on physiological rules. *Proc 17th Annu Northeast Bioeng Conf.* 1991.

11. Gottlieb, ME. Vascular networks: fractal anatomies from nonlinear physiologies. *Proc 13th Int Meet IEEE Eng Med Biol Soc.* 1991.

12. Mozingo DW, Ben-David K, Perrin KJ, et al. Comparison of the biomechanical properties of burns grafted with conventional split thickness skin vs. Integra artificial skin. *Boswick Burn Wound Symp,* Maui, 2001. Data on file Surgical Research Laboratory, Inc., Nashville, TN.

13. Burke JF, Yannas IV, Quinby WC, Jr., et al. Successful use of a physiologically acceptable artificial skin in the treatment of extensive burn injury. *Ann Surg.* 1981;194:413–428.

14. Heimbach D, Luterman A, Burke J, et al. Artificial dermis for major burns: a multicenter randomized clinical trial. *Ann Surg.* 1988;208:313–320.

15. Heimbach DM, Warden GD, Luterman A, et al. Multicenter postapproval clinical trial of Integra dermal regeneration template for burn treatment. *J Burn Care Rehabil.* 2003;24:42–48.

16. Sheridan RL, Hegarty M, Tompkins RG, et al. Artificial skin in massive burns—results to ten years. *Eur J Plast Surg.* 1994;17:91–93.

17. Loss M, Wedler V, Kunzi W, et al. Artificial skin, split-thickness autograft and cultured autologous keratinocytes combined to treat a severe burn injury of 93% of TBSA *Burns.* 2000;26:644–652.

18. Dabney A, Voigt D, Metz P, et al. The use of Integra in traumatic degloving and soft tissue injuries. *Boswick Burn Wound Symp.* Maui, 2003 [in *J Burns Surg Wound Care,* Feb, 2003].

19. Gottlieb ME. Lower extremity lymphedema-management by total dermatofasciectomy and skin reconstruction with Integra. *Boswick Burn Wound Symp.* Maui, 2003 [in *J Burns Surg Wound Care,* Mar. 2003].

20. Peacock EE, Van Winkle W. *Wound Repair.* 2nd ed. Philadelphia, W. B. Saunders, 1976.

21. Rudolph R, Noe JM. *Chronic problem wounds.* Boston, Little, Brown, 1983.

22. Gonyon DL, Zenn MR. Simple approach to the radiated scalp wound using Integra skin substitute. *Ann Plast Surg.* 2003; 50:315–320.

23. Prystowsky JH, Siegel DM, Ascherman JA. Artificial skin for closure and healing of wounds created by skin cancer excisions. *Dermatol Surg.* 2001;27:648–653.

24. Gottlieb ME, Furman J. Successful management and surgical closure of chronic and pathological wounds using Integra. *J Burns Surg Wound Care,* Feb, 2004.

25. Dantzer E, Braye FM. Reconstructive surgery using an artificial dermis (Integra): results with 39 grafts. *Br J Plas Surg.* 2001;54:659–664.

26. Dantzer E, Queruel P, Salinier L, et al. Integra, a new surgical alternative for the treatment of massive burns. Clinical evaluation of acute and reconstructive surgery: 39 cases. *Ann Chir Plast Aesthe.* 2001;46:173–189.

27. Demarest GB, Resurrecion R, Lu S, et al. Experience with bilaminate bioartificial skin substitute and ultrathin skin grafting in non-burn soft-tissue wound defects. *Wounds.* 2003;15: 250–256.

28. Orgill DP, Straus FH, II, Lee RC. The use of collagen-GAG membranes in reconstructive surgery. *Ann NY Acad Sci.* 1999;888:233–248.

29. Wiley DE, Kowal-Vern A, Latenser BA. Successful application of Integra in a polytrauma case. *Boswick Burn Wound Symp.* Maui, 2003 [in *J Burns Surg Wound Care,* Mar, 2003].

30. Suzuki S, Matsuda K, Isshiki N, et al. Clinical evaluation of a new bilayer "artificial skin" composed of collagen sponge and silicone layer. *Br J Plast Surg.* 1990;43:47–54.

31. Larson KW. Treatment of necrotizing fasciitis wounds with Integra dermal regeneration template. *Boswick Burn Wound Symp.* Maui, 2003 [in *J Burns Surg Wound Care,* Mar, 2003].

32. Lorenz C, Petracic A, Hohl HP, et al. Early wound closure and early reconstruction. Experience with a dermal substitute in a child with 60 percent surface area burn. *Burns.* 1997; 23:505–508.

33. Vazquez Rueda F, Ayala Montoro J, Blanco Lopez F, et al. First results with Integra artificial skin in the management of severe tissue defects in children. *Cir Pediat.* 2001;14:91–94.

34. Besner GE, Klamar JE. Integra artificial skin as a useful adjunct in the treatment of purpura fulminans. *J Burn Care Rehabil.* 1998; 19: 324–329.

35. Greenberg JE, Falabella AF, Bello YM, et al. Tissue-engineered skin in the healing of wound stumps from limb amputations secondary to purpura fulminans. *Pediatr Dermatol.* 2003; 20:169–172.

36. King P. Artificial skin reduces nutritional requirements in a severely burned child. *Burns.* 2000;26:501–503.

37. Ryan CM, Schoenfeld DA, Malloy M, et al. Use of Integra artificial skin is associated with decreased length of stay for severely injured adult burn survivors. *J Burn Care Rehabil.* 2002;23:311–317.

38. Boyce ST, Kagan RJ, Meyer NA, et al. The 1999 clinical research award. Cultured skin substitutes combined with Integra artificial skin to replace native skin autograft and allograft for the closure of excised full-thickness burns. *J Burn Care Rehabil.* 1991;20:453–461.

39. Wang JCY, To EWH. Application of dermal substitute (Integra) to donor site defect of forehead flap. *Br J Plast Surg.* 2000;53:70–72.

40. Hunt JA, Moisidis É, Haertsch P. Initial experience of Integra in the treatment of postburn anterior cervical neck contracture. *Br J Plast Surg.* 2000;53:652–658.

41. Soejima K, Nozaki M, Sasaki K, et al. Treatment of giant pigmented nerus using artificial dermis and a secondary skin graft from the scalp. *Ann Plast Surg.* 1997;39:489–494.

42. Chou TD, Chen SL, Lee TW, et al. Reconstruction of burn scar of the upper extremities with artificial skin. *Plast Reconstr Surg.* 2001;108:378–384.

43. Dantzer E, Queruel P, Salinier L, et al. Dermal regeneration template for deep hand burns: clinical utility for both early grafting and reconstructive surgery. *Br J Plast Surg.* 2003; 56:764–774.

44. Palao R, Gomez P, Huguet P. Burned breast reconstructive surgery with Integra dermal regeneration template. *Br J Plast Surg.* 2003;56:252–259.

45. Kopp J, Magnus NE, Rubben A, et al. Radical resection of giant congenital melanocytic nevus and reconstruction with meek-graft covered integra dermal template. *Dermatol Surg.* 2003;29:653–657.

46. Thomas WO, Rayburn S, Leblanc RT, et al. Artificial skin in the treatment of a large congenital nevus. *South Med J* 2001;94:325–328.

47. Giovannini UM, Teot L. Aesthetic complex reconstruction of the lower leg: application of a dermal substitute (Integra) to an adipofascial flap. *Br J Plast Surg.* 2002;55:171–172.

48. Shermak MA, Wong L, Inoue N, et al. Reconstruction of complex cranial wounds with demineralized bone matrix and bilayer artificial skin. *J Craniofac Surg.* 2000;11: 224–231.

49. Moiemen NS, Staiano JJ, Ojeh NO, et al. Reconstructive surgery with a dermal regeneration template: clinical and histologic study. *Plast Reconstr Surg.* 2001;108:93–103.

50. Stem R, McPherson M, Longaker MT. Histologic study of artificial skin used in the treatment of full-thickness thermal injury. *J Burn Care Rehabil.* 1990;11:7–13.

51. Berger A, Tanzella U, Machens HG, et al. Administration of Integra on primary burn wounds and unstable secondary scars. *Chirurg* 2000;71:558–563.

52. Fitton AR, Drew P, Dickson WA. The use of a bilaminate artificial skin substitute (Integra) in acute resurfacing of burns: an early experience. *Br J Plast Surg.* 2001;54: 208–212.

53. Soejima K, Nozaki M, Sasaki K, et al. Reconstruction of burn deformity using artificial dermis combined with thin split-skin grafting. *Burns* 1997;23:501–504.

54. Moore C, Lee S, Hart A, et al. Use of Integra to resurface a latissimus dorsi free flap. *Br J Plast Surg.* 2003;56:66–69.

55. Lut BS, Ma SF, Chuang DC, et al. Specificity of reinnervation and motor recovery after interposition of an artificial barrier between transected and repaired nerves in adjacency- an experimental study in the rat. *Acta Neurochir (Wien).* 2001;143: 393–399.

56. Research on file, Ethicon, Somerville, New Jersey.

57. Pandya AN, Woodward B, Parkhouse N. The use of cultured autologous keratinocytes with Integra in the resurfacing of acute burns. *Plast Reconstr Surg.* 1998;102:825–828.

58. Wisser D, Steffes J. Skin replacement with a collagen based dermal substitute, autologous keratinocytes and fibroblasts in burn trauma. *Burns.* 2003;29:375–380.

59. Jones I, James SE, Rubin P, et al. Upward migration of cultured autologous keratinocytes in Integra artificial skin: a preliminary report. *Wound Repair Regen* 2003;11:132–138.

60. Kremmer M, Lang E, Berger AC. Evaluation of dermal-epidenmal skin equivalents ('composite-skin') of human keratinocytes in a collagen-glycosaminoglycan matrix (Integra artificial skin). *Br J Plast Surg.* 2000;53:459–465.

17 Biomaterial Wound Matrix from Small Intestine Submucosa: Review and Efficacy in Diabetic Wound Healing

Robert G. Frykberg and Jason P. Hodde

Introduction
    Background
    SIS: A New Biomaterial Wound Matrix
    Preclinical Evaluation of SIS in Wound
    Healing
    Clinical Evaluation of SIS in Wound
    Healing

SIS Wound Matrix to Treat Diabetic Ulcers
    Case 1
    Case 2
Discussion
Conclusion
Acknowledgment
References

INTRODUCTION

Wound healing is a complex process of tissue restoration that is often refractory to currently available treatments. Modern wound-care techniques too often only offer palliative care, failing to address underlying mechanisms of disease, leading to wound closure through the deposition of suboptimal fibrotic tissue. Recently developed wound-care products derived from natural tissue sources may tilt the healing response toward the restoration of functional tissues and away from fibrosis. A biomaterial derived from porcine small intestinal submucosa (SIS) has been developed into a new biologic wound-care product. This review describes the origin of the biomaterial, its compositional properties, and its transformation into a clinical product that has been proved effective in diabetic wound management. The wound matrix developed from this unique biomaterial has previously been evaluated in a preclinical full-thickness wound-healing study in rats. This manuscript extends the utility of the SIS wound matrix to humans in a pilot study of chronic human diabetic ulcers. Results indicate the effectiveness of the SIS biomaterial to cause rapid tissue restoration and epithelialization in clinically treat hard-to-heal full-thickness diabetic ulcers.

Background

Wound healing is a complex process of tissue restoration[1,2] that can either lead to fibrotic tissue replacement (scarring) with limited functional restoration or to the restoration of natural tissue with normal structure and function. An accepted goal of modern wound care includes facilitating the healing response toward the restoration of functional tissues. This goal is accomplished by providing a conducive environment for wound healing through the means of maintaining wound hydration,[3] offering thermal insulation, and providing protection from infection.

Very few current wound-care products have the capacity to direct the healing process toward functional tissue restoration; most only offer palliative care. The spectrum of available products can be broadly divided into two categories: synthetic (including biosynthetic) and biologic (tissue origin). Synthetic wound products are typically inexpensive, have long shelf life, induce minimal inflammatory reaction, and lack the risk of disease transmission.

Such synthetics and biosynthetics include polyurethane films and foams, hydrogels, textiles, hydrocolloids, and collagen/alginate combinations. All of these products function well as short-term moisture barriers, but are insufficient in promoting regenerative wound healing.[4]

Biomaterials have recently become critical components in the development of effective new medical therapies for wound care. They are able to more effectively promote granulation and epithelialization of dermal wounds than synthetic materials.[5] In addition, biologic wound products effectively regulate evaporation and exudation and effectively protect the wound site from bacterial infection. Biologic-derived wound dressings are not new, but their effectiveness has greatly increased with recent innovative developments.

Biologic wound dressings have been used in clinical medicine since 1973, when the use of a porcine skin dressing was first reported.[6] Sheets of collagen harvested from sheep intestine have also been used.[7] Specialized biologic dressings have been developed more recently and include products derived from human cadaver skin (Alloderm, Lifecell Inc., Branchburg, NJ); a product prepared by seeding dermal fibroblasts on a biodegradable matrix (Dermagraft, Smith & Nephew Inc., Largo, FL); and a tissue-engineered human skin equivalent (HSE) made by layering a sheet of stratified human epithelium onto a bovine collagen matrix impregnated with human foreskin fibroblasts (Apligraf, Novartis Pharmaceuticals Corp., East Hanover, NJ). Such technologically advanced products are approaching the equivalent of human skin replacement, but are still limited by the extensive preparation time, high cost of manufacture, and short shelf life.[8,9]

Other biologic alternatives for wound care include autologous skin grafts and living, cellular xenografts. Autologous skin grafts probably represent an optimal wound dressing when considered in terms of healing, but morbidity associated with the additional tissue harvest site and limited supply compromise the benefits of this alternative and eliminates it completely as a viable option in the severely diseased or injured patient. Cellular xenografts (ie, biologic products derived from animals, which contain cells) remain immunologically incompatible for human use.

An ideal wound dressing would be one made from a readily available biomaterial that requires minimal processing and, after sterilization and storage, retains the biologic characteristics that promote wound healing. Such a biologic dressing would incorporate both the advantages typical of synthetic dressings (low cost, long shelf life, and low risk of immunologic reaction) and those typical of biologic dressings (regulated fluid flow, increased resistance to bacterial contamination, enhanced granulation tissue formation, and more rapid epithelialization).

SIS: A New Biomaterial Wound Matrix

A biomaterial derived from the pig small intestine submucosa (SIS) has been extensively evaluated in preclinical models and in clinical settings since its unique properties were first reported in 1989.[10] This novel material, a thin, translucent layer of the intestine, is approximately 0.15 mm thick and consists primarily of a collagen-based extracellular matrix (ECM) (Fig. 17–1). In its native state, this intestinal layer contains relatively few resident connective tissue cells and provides structural support, stability, and biochemical signals to the rapidly regenerating mucosal cell layer. The naturally cross-linked collagen network of the submucosal layer also gives strength to the intestine.

In preparation for clinical use, SIS is harvested from the pig and is gently processed to lyse all resident cells, remove cellular debris, and reduce the risk of disease transmission.[11] It is then sterilized using proprietary methods that include treatment with ethylene oxide gas.

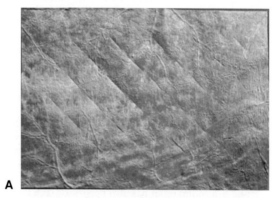

A

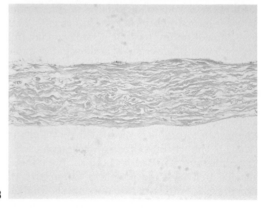

B

Fig. 17–1. SIS-wound matrix. The prepared SIS is an acellular collagen-based wound care product approximately 0.15 mm thick. **A.** Gross image; **B.** H&E. Original magnification, 100×.

This preparation technique retains not only the collagen component of the ECM, but has also been shown to retain other components of the matrix, such as glycosaminoglycans (ie, hyaluronic acid),[12] proteoglycans, fibronectin,[13] and other matrix-associated factors.[14] The sequential processing methods utilized in the transformation of SIS into a clinical product allows long-term storage of the acellular sheet of ECM without destroying its natural architecture and ability to support wound healing and tissue repair.

Preclinical Evaluation of SIS in Wound Healing

Since the initial report of its preclinical use as a vascular conduit in 1989,[10] the SIS biomaterial has been evaluated successfully in numerous species and organ systems. Induction of host tissue proliferation and replacement following SIS implant has been demonstrated in many tissues, including blood vessels,[15–18] lower urinary tract,[19,20] body wall[21,22] tendon,[23,24] ligament,[25] dura,[26,27] and cartilage.[28] Over time, the biomaterial is gradually incorporated and replaced by new host tissues, acting as a support for tissue growth and maturation that leads to a lasting repair. The new tissue generated by the host in response to SIS implantation is specific to the site of implantation; generalized fibrosis does not occur.

An early study to evaluate SIS as a blood conduit showed, for example, that when SIS was implanted in place of an artery, new tissue invaded the SIS biomaterial within 4 weeks; the graft site appeared nearly identical to the original vessel after as little as 8 weeks.[29] Even though the conduit had been formed from a single layer of the thin SIS biomaterial, a multilayered vessel resembling the native tissue structure of artery was formed.

The SIS biomaterial has also been used as a covering for dermal wounds in rats following the creation of an experimental full-thickness skin defect.[30] Wounds were allowed to heal for time periods ranging from 3 days to 8 weeks. The extent of healing and wound contraction was measured against a control group that was treated with OpSite dressing. Results showed that wound contraction was 33% in the SIS-treated group, but that contraction accounted for 56% of reduction in wound size in the control group. In the SIS-treated wounds, histopathology revealed that wounds completely re-epithelialized over a 6-week period and that the epithelium resumed its normal appearance and blended well with the peripheral connective tissue after 8 weeks. Further *in vitro* work has shown that SIS supports the differentiation of primary human epidermal cells, as well as the synthesis of basement membrane proteins (Fig. 17–2).[31]

Preclinical studies such as these and others have repeatedly demonstrated the ability of SIS to regenerate

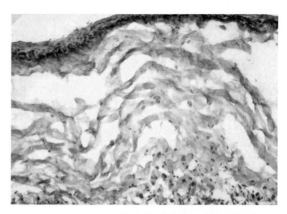

Fig. 17–2. Collagen VII immunostaining following the cultivation of human primary epidermal cells on SIS for 10 days shows the presence of collagen VII at the cell–SIS interface; collagen VII is absent in the SIS biomaterial when evaluated prior to cell conditioning. See Lindberg (Ref. 31) for methods. 200×

as host tissue, induce rapid capillary ingrowth,[24,29] be resistant to infection,[32,33] and to induce little or no immunologic reaction. Specific studies to examine the SIS biomaterial in wound models have indicated that SIS supports rapid epithelialization and differentiation of resident tissue cells and allows the deposition of basement membrane proteins appropriate to dermal and epidermal tissues.[31] All of these characteristics are desirable to effect wound healing with the restoration of functional tissue instead of scar tissue formation.

Clinical Evaluation of SIS in Wound Healing

The SIS biomaterial has been available for clinical use to treat diabetic ulcers, venous stasis ulcers, pressure sores, and other chronic, nonhealing wounds since 2000. More recently, SIS has been approved as a device to repair the rotator cuff (Restore Orthobiologic, DePuy Inc., Warsaw, IN), as a treatment for incontinence (Stratasis, Cook Biotech Incorporated, West Lafayette, IN), and as a surgical graft for soft tissue reinforcement (Surgisis, Cook Biotech Incorporated, West Lafayette, IN).

The first clinical report of the use of SIS to treat partial-thickness skin wounds was published in 2001.[34] A total of 14 patients were evaluated for wound healing using two different SIS preparations. Patients were divided into equal groups and treated with either moist SIS or with a lyophilized form of the biomaterial. Time to complete epithelialization was measured and the results were reported. Results indicated that the lyophilized form of the SIS wound matrix was superior to the wet form of the product. All 7 patients treated with the lyophilized form of the biomaterial healed completely within 10 weeks; 6 of the wounds had completely epithelialized in less than 8 weeks. It was reported that in none of the 14 patients did the SIS biomaterial show signs of toxicity, clinical signs of rejection, or cause subepithelial seroma formation as the wounds progressed to full healing. All wounds epithelialized with minimal or no scar tissue formation.

SIS WOUND MATRIX TO TREAT DIABETIC ULCERS

As part of an ongoing open-label clinical trial, SIS (Oasis) was provided by Cook Biotech Incorporated (West Lafayette, IN) as an acellular, lyophilized, and sterilized sheet of ECM. This material has been shown to retain the three-dimensional architecture, structural collagen composition, and matrix-associated component structure of the submucosal ECM. Patients were randomized to receive either the SIS wound matrix or becaplermin (PDGF) gel (Regranex, Ortho-McNeil Pharmaceuticals, Raritan, NJ) for diabetic foot ulcers with a minimum size of 1 cm^2 and present for at least 1 month. Patients with severe ischemia, renal failure, and clinical infection were excluded from enrollment.

For all patients, the chronic ulcers were routinely debrided, evaluated, measured, and photographed prior to application of either the SIS wound matrix or becaplermin gel. The latter subjects were typically treated with twice daily saline-moistened gauze pads after cleansing with saline. The growth factor gel was applied to the wound only once per day at the time of one of these moistened dressing changes. Those patients randomized to the SIS group followed a different dressing protocol, although weekly wound care and evaluation was standard for both groups. The sterile SIS was cut to size slightly larger than the ulcer, placed upon the wound bed, and moistened with sterile saline for rehydration. If the wound was moist, this was not necessary, since the tissue fluids would rehydrate the wound matrix. Secondary absorbent film dressing, foam, or hydrocolloid was applied after placement of the SIS to provide a moist healing environment and to maintain direct contact of the SIS with the wound bed. Early in the study, patients applied a moist saline gauze over the SIS matrix twice daily. Repeat applications of the SIS were applied only as needed prior to the next weekly visit. In most instances, dressings remained intact for the entire week and were, therefore, changed by the investigator at the study visit. SIS was reapplied according to the amount of dressing observed on the surface of the wound and the extent of epithelialization at each change of the secondary dressing. Usually, the wound matrix was hydrated at the center of the wound and developed

a caramel appearance, with overlapping portions on intact skin retaining the lyophilized (dry) characteristic. Off-loading was accomplished through the use of wedged postoperative shoes, fixed-ankle walking brace, or a surgical shoe with removable plugs under the ulcer site. Patients were instructed to limit weight-bearing activities as much as possible despite their ambulatory status and to use crutches or a walker when feasible.

Two patients randomized to the SIS arm of the study are presented as case studies to highlight the clinical utility of a wound-matrix dressing as incorporated into a comprehensive wound-healing protocol.

Case 1

DH was a 77-year old type 2 diabetic man with a several month history of a chronic neuropathic ulceration on his left medial heel. Prior dressings consisted only of daily moist saline dressings. His medical history was also significant for coronary artery disease and previous coronary artery bypass graft, previous stroke, and a history of critical ischemia of his left foot and leg requiring femoral-tibial bypass graft and first ray amputation several months previously. All surgical wounds on the right leg were healed on presentation with the index ulcer on his left heel. Pulses were palpable in his left foot and neuropathy was documented by an inability to sense a 10-g monofilament at several sites on his foot.

After meeting the enrollment criteria and obtaining informed consent, the patient was randomized to receive treatment with the SIS matrix dressing on October 30, 2001. Figure 17–3 shows his wound at baseline prior to SIS application. At this time, the greatest dimensions

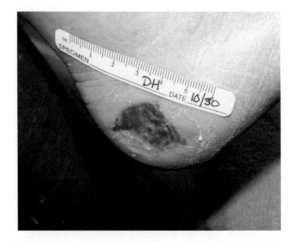

Fig. 17–3. Case 1. DH. Neuropathic ulcer of left heel at baseline and initiation of SIS wound matrix treatment (October 30, 2001).

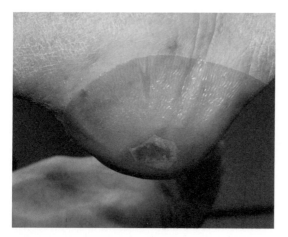

Fig. 17–4. Hydrocolloid used as the secondary dressing over the SIS matrix dressing.

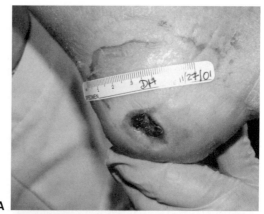

A

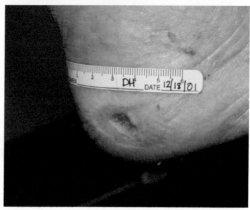

B

Fig. 17–5. A. At 4 weeks (November 27, 2001), there were notable signs of healing. **B.** By week 7 (December 18, 2001) the wound had decreased to 1.0 × 0.4 cm diameter.

were 2.1 × 1.9 cm with the wound having a fairly granular base. There were no signs of clinical infection. The secondary dressings consisted only of hydrocolloid over the moistened SIS matrix and were changed on a weekly basis during his study visits (Fig. 17–4). The patient was seen weekly and by November 27, 2001 his wound had decreased in size to 1.0 × 1.8 cm diameter and retained its healthy appearance. Three weeks later the wound measured 1.0 × 0.4 cm with obvious epithelialization on the periphery (Fig. 17–5A and B). His wound was completely epithelialized at week 10 with only a small area of overlying hyperkeratosis remaining (Fig. 17–6). During subsequent followup over the next year there was no recurrence of this lesion or did any new lesions develop.

Case 2

EC is a 34-year-old man with a 15-year history of type 1 diabetes and recurrent neuropathic ulcers on both feet. On December 16, 2002, he presented to our Wound Healing Center with a 4-month history of a nonhealing neuropathic ulcer on the plantar aspect of his right heel measuring 1.2 × 1.0 cm in diameter. There was an abundance of callus on the periphery, which was debrided prior to taking measurements (Fig. 17–7A). The wound had a granular base and did not demonstrate any signs of clinical infection. After meeting all inclusion criteria and providing his informed consent, he was randomized to receive the wound matrix dressing. In his case, the secondary dressing consisted of a two-layered foam dressing with the inner portion cut as an aperture to provide further off-loading from the plantar heel ulcer. He was also prescribed a pressure-relieving

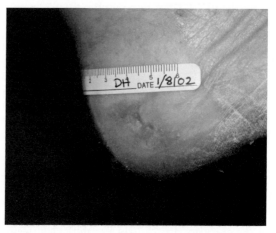

Fig. 17–6. Healed on January 8, 2002 at week 10

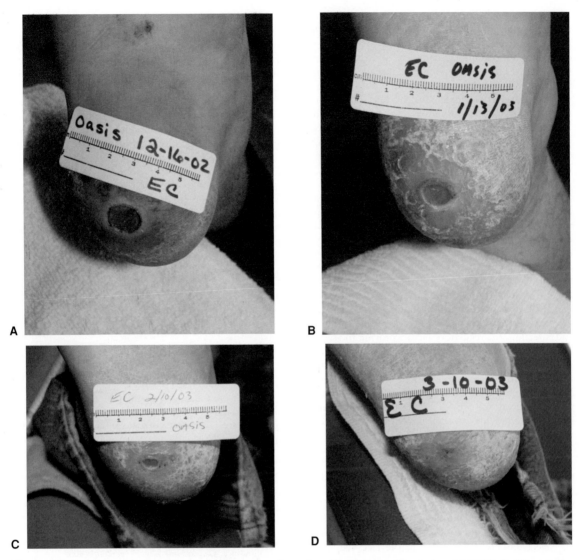

Figure 17–7. Case 2. EC. **A.** Right heel ulcer at baseline after débridement (December 16, 2002). **B.** Ulcer at the 4-week visit with minimal improvement. **C.** By week 9 (February 10, 2003) the ulcer had decreased in size to 0.4 × 0.7 cm. **D.** Ulcer healed by week 14 despite noncompliance with off-loading footwear.

surgical shoe designed to off-load the heel. He was noncompliant in this regard, however, due to imbalance from his neuropathy and retinopathy. Therefore, a well-cushioned postoperative shoe was provided instead.

He was followed weekly according to the protocol. At visit 4, he had made minimal progress with the wound measuring 1.0 × 0.8 cm (Fig. 17–7*B–D*). This was attributed to his noncompliance with off-loading and excessive activity. However, by week 9, his wound had reduced to a diameter of 0.4 × 0.7 cm and was showing a reduction in

surrounding hyperkeratosis. He remained free of infection and was healed by week 14 despite his failure to fully comply with the use of the appropriate off-loading shoe. After several months of followup, no recurrence was noted.

DISCUSSION

This report on the use of the SIS biomaterial to treat diabetic ulcers demonstrates that the wound matrix is easy to apply, is nontoxic, and does not induce an adverse immunologic reaction, even in patients given repeated applications. The results also demonstrate that placement of the SIS wound matrix on diabetic ulcers can result in initiation and complete epithelialization of the wounds. These observations and initial clinical findings are consistent with the known properties of the biomaterial, support the preclinical findings, and extend the preclinical observations to a human population. Results indicate that the SIS wound matrix can be used to successfully manage chronic diabetic ulcers due to its excellent protective properties and ability to act as a natural template for tissue regrowth.

Wound care products derived from acellular ECM tissues provide optimal environments for wound repair. Further, the three-dimensional architecture and composition of the SIS biomaterial appears to be an ideal environment for diabetic wound healing. The complex composition of collagens, proteoglycans, glycosaminoglycans, and other ECM-associated factors found in the SIS wound matrix provides the structural integrity, flexibility, and elasticity appropriate for dermal wound covering and subsequent epithelialization. The structural integrity of the matrix provides a barrier to dehydration and infection, the regulatory factors provide the signals necessary for the propagation of new and healthy tissue, and the native tissue architecture provides a stable structure for cell attachment, proliferation, and differentiation. Unlike most materials available to treat chronic wounds, the SIS biomaterial provides more than just palliative treatment; it provides an environment that is conducive to, and effective for, wound healing.

Advances in biomedical engineering and in techniques for matrix procurement have allowed the fabrication of a collagen-based wound matrix material that is effective in healing human wounds. Even though the source material is porcine derived, extensive preclinical research and human clinical experience[35–38] has indicated that the xenograft is accepted by the host and is not rejected. This is likely due to the fact that ECM components, including collagen, are highly conserved across mammalian species. Processing steps are minimal, yet have been shown to provide a virus-safe biomaterial for human use while retaining bioactive factors that may play important roles in the host response to implantation of the SIS biomaterial.

CONCLUSION

Biomaterials have recently become critical components in the development of effective new medical therapies for wound care because they are able to more effectively promote granulation and epithelialization of dermal wounds than synthetic materials. They are able to lead to the restoration of natural tissue with normal structure and function, and facilitate rapid, pain-free, regenerative healing. Advances in the procurement and processing of natural materials for wound healing have largely overcome the complications of immunologic rejection, risk of disease transfer, and issues of insufficient structural integrity that have historically limited their utility in human medicine.

A new biomaterial derived from the submucosal portion of porcine small intestine has been used successfully in preclinical studies of wound healing and in other surgical procedures where soft-tissue reinforcement is indicated. This SIS biomaterial has now been developed into a wound-care product that successfully manages human partial-thickness wounds and chronic diabetic ulcers. While we await the completion of the ongoing clinical trial for diabetic foot ulcers, these promising results justify further evaluation of this biologic matrix for its effectiveness in the treatment of chronic wounds of all types.

ACKNOWLEDGMENT

This study was supported by a grant from Cook Biotech Incorporated, West Lafayette, Indiana.

REFERENCES

1. Brown-Etris M. Measuring healing in wounds. *Adv Wound Care.* 1995;8:53–58.

2. Calvin M. Cutaneous wound repair. *WOUNDS.* 1998;10: 12–32.

3. Winter GD. Formation of scab and the rate of epithelialization of superficial wounds in the skin of the domestic pig. *Nature.* 1962;200:377–378.

4. Leipziger LS, Glushko V, DiBernardo B, et al. Dermal wound repair: Role of collagen matrix implants and synthetic polymer dressings. *J Am Acad Dermatol.* 1985;12:409–419.

5. Gao ZR, Hao ZQ, Li Y, et al. Porcine dermal collagen as a wound dressing for skin donor sites and deep partial skin thickness burns. *Burns.* 1992;18:492–496.

6. Elliot R, Hoehn J. Use of commercial porcine skin for wound dressings. *Plast Reconstr Surg.* 1973;52:401–405.

7. Shettigar UG, Jagannathan R, Natarajan R. Collagen film for burn wound dressings reconstituted from animal intestines. *Artif Organs.* 1982;6:256–260.

8. Greenfield E, Jordan B. Advances in burn wound care. *Crit Care Nurs Clin North Am.* 1996;8:203–215.

9. Eaglstein WH, Falanga V. Tissue engineering and the development of Apligraf, a human skin equivalent. *Adv Wound Care.* 1998;11(4 Suppl):1–8.

10. Badylak SF, Lantz GC, Coffey A, et al. Small intestinal submucosa as a large diameter vascular graft in the dog. *J Surg Res.* 1989;47:74–80.

11. Hodde JP, Hiles MC. Virus safety of a porcine-derived medical device: evaluation of a viral inactivation method. *Biotechnol Bioeng.* 2002;79:211–216.

12. Hodde JP, Badylak SF, Brightman AO, Voytik-Harbin SL. Glycosaminoglycan content of small intestinal submucosa: a bioscaffold for tissue replacement *Tissue Eng.* 1996;2:209–217.

13. McPherson TB, Badylak SF. Characterization of fibronectin derived from porcine small intestinal submucosa. *Tissue Eng.* 1998;4:75–83.

14. Hodde JP, Hiles MC. Bioactive FGF-2 in sterilized extracellular matrix. *WOUNDS.* 2001;13:195–201.

15. Lantz GC, Badylak SF, Coffey AC, et al. Small intestinal submucosa as a small diameter arterial graft in the dog. *J Invest Surg.* 1990;3:217–227.

16. Lantz GC, Badylak SF, Coffey AC, et al. Small intestinal submucosa as a superior vena cava graft in the dog. *J Surg Res.* 1992;53:175–181.

17. Sandusky GE, Badylak SF, Morff RJ, et al. Histologic findings after *in vivo* placement of small intestinal submucosal vascular grafts and saphenous vein grafts in the carotid artery in dogs. *Am J Pathol.* 1992;140:317–324.

18. Sandusky GE, Lantz GC, Badylak SF. Healing comparison of small intestine submucosa and ePTFE grafts in the canine carotid artery. *J Surg Res.* 1995;58:415–420.

19. Vaught JD, Kropp BP, Sawyer BD, et al. Detrusor regeneration in the rat using porcine small intestinal submucosal grafts: functional innervation and receptor expression. *J Urol.* 1996; 155:374–378.

20. Kropp BP, Ludlow JK, Spicer D, et al. Rabbit urethral regeneration using small intestinal submucosa onlay grafts. *Urology.* 1998;52:138–142.

21. Clarke KM, Lantz GC, Salisbury SK, et al. Intestine submucosa and polypropylene mesh for abdominal wall repair in dogs. *J Surg Res.* 1996;60:107–114.

22. Badylak S, Kokini K, Tullius B, Simmons-Byrd A, Morff R. Morphologic study of small intestinal submucosa as a body wall repair device. *J Surg Res.* 2002;103:190–202.

23. Badylak SF, Tullius R, Kokini K, et al. The use of xenogeneic small intestinal submucosa as a biomaterial for Achilles tendon repair in a dog model. *J Biomed Mater Res.* 1995;29: 977–985.

24. Hodde JP, Badylak SF, Shelbourne KD. The effect of range of motion on remodeling of small intestinal submucosa (SIS) when used as an Achilles tendon repair material in the rabbit. *Tissue Eng* 1997;3:27–37.

25. Aiken SW, Badylak SF, Toombs JP, et al. Small intestinal submucosa as an intra-articular ligamentous graft material: a pilot study in dogs. *Vet Comp Orthopedics Traumatol.* 1994;7: 124–128.

26. Cobb MA, Badylak SF, Janas W, Boop FA. Histology after dural grafting with small intestinal submucosa. *Surg Neurol.* 1996; 46:389–394.

27. Cobb MA, Badylak SF, Janas W, et al. Porcine small intestinal submucosa as a dural substitute. *Surg Neurol.* 1999;51: 99–104.

28. Welch JA, Montgomery RD, Lenz SD, et al. Evaluation of small intestinal submucosa implants for repair of meniscal defects in dogs. *Am J Vet Res.* 2002;63:427–431.

29. Lantz GC, Badylak SF, Hiles MC, et al. Small intestinal submucosa as a vascular graft: a review. *J Invest Surg.* 1993;6: 297–310.

30. Prevel CD, Eppley BL, Summerlin DJ, et al. Small intestinal submucosa: utilization as a wound dressing in full-thickness rodent wounds. *Ann Plast Surg.* 1995;35:381–388.

31. Lindberg K, Badylak SF. Porcine small intestinal submucosa (SIS): a bioscaffold supporting *in vitro* primary human epidermal cell differentiation and synthesis of basement membrane proteins. *Burns.* 2001;27:254–266.

32. Badylak SF, Coffey AC, Lantz GC, Tacker WA, Geddes LA. Comparison of the resistance to infection of intestinal submucosa arterial autografts versus polytetrafluoroethylene arterial prostheses in a dog model. *J Vasc Surg.* 1994;19: 465–472.

33. Badylak SF, Wu CC, Bible M, McPherson E. Host protection against deliberate bacterial contamination of an extracellular matrix bioscaffold versus DacronTM mesh in a dog model of orthopedic soft tissue repair. J Biomed Mater Res 2003;67B: 648-654.

34. Brown-Etris M, Cutshall WD, Hiles MC. A new biomaterial derived from small intestine submucosa and developed into a wound matrix device. *WOUNDS.* 2002;14:150–166.

35. Franklin ME, Gonzalez JJ, Michaelson RP, Glass JL, Chock DA. Preliminary experience with new bioactive prosthetic material for repair of hernias in infected fields. *Hernia.* 2002; 6:171–174.

36. Knoll LD. Use of porcine small intestinal submucosal graft in the surgical management of tunical deficiencies with penile prosthetic surgery. *Urology.* 2002;59:758–761.

37. O'Connor RC, Harding JN, Steinberg GD. Novel modification of partial nephrectomy technique using porcine small intestine submucosa. *Urology.* 2002;60:906–909.

38. Rutner AB, Levine SR, Schmaelzle JF. Processed porcine small intestine submucosa as a graft material for pubovaginal slings: durability and results. *Urology* 2003;62:805-809.

18 | Skin Substitutes in Acute and Chronic Wounds

Kevin G. Donohue and Vincent Falanga

Introduction
  Basis for Skin Substitutes
  Defining Skin Substitutes
History of Skin Substitutes
  Excisional Grafts
  Autologous Keratinocyte Sheets
  Allogeneic Keratinocyte Sheets
  Dermal Constructs
  Bilayered Constructs
Skin Substitutes in Acute and Chronic Wounds
  Acute Wounds Treated Electively
  Acute Wounds Treated Urgently
  Chronic Wounds Treated Electively
Ideal Properties of Skin Substitutes
  Adherence
  Elasticity, Flexibility, and Pliability
  Barrier to Microbial Invasion
  Aid in Fluid Balance
  Nontoxic/Nonantigenic

  Biodegradable
  Long Shelf Life, Minimal Storage
    Requirements, and Low Cost
Overview of Current Skin Substitutes
  Keratinocyte Sheets
  Dermal Constructs
  Bilayered Constructs
Wound-Bed Preparation
  Débridement
  Control of Exudate
  Control of Bacterial Burden
Mechanism of Action
  Keratinocyte Sheets
  Dermal Constructs
  Skin Equivalents
Economics of Skin Substitutes
Acknowledgment
References

Skin substitutes are either acellular or composed of nonviable or living cells. Examples of these therapeutic agents are keratinocyte sheets, dermal constructs, or skin equivalents consisting of both epidermal and dermal components. Skin substitutes have been made possible by advances in tissue culture and our ability to manipulate matrix components. They have now been used in a variety of clinical applications, including burns, excisional wounds, and chronic wounds. Some skin substitutes are already commercially available and have received official regulatory approval for the treatment of venous and diabetic foot ulcers. Certain skin substitutes have been shown to synthesize a number of matrix materials and growth factors and appear to respond to injury in a manner consistent with the normal process of

wound healing. However, their mode of action *in vivo* remains unclear. As demonstrated in clinical trials, the benefits of skin substitutes include decreased healing time, reduced wound pain, and avoidance of a donor site for graft harvesting. However, skin substitutes should not be regarded as being the same as autografts. Using biochemical markers and deoxyribonucleic acid (DNA) evidence, it has been found that at least some of these skin substitutes do not remain in chronic wounds for more than a few weeks. There is also evidence that allogeneic constructs elicit an inflammatory reaction by the host, although that does not seem to interfere with their effectiveness. As with any advanced therapeutic product, wound-bed preparation is instrumental to maximizing the benefit of skin substitutes.

INTRODUCTION

Basis for Skin Substitutes

Skin is made up of two layers. The outer layer, the epidermis, is densely cellular and comprised primarily of keratinocytes, arranged in layers that become denser and more impermeable as they progress from the innermost basal layer to the outermost corneal layer. One of the main functions of the epidermis is that of a barrier for sealing in moisture and keeping out microbes and toxins. Epidermal loss leaves the body susceptible to microbial invasion and to fluid and electrolyte imbalance. The epidermis is avascular and bound to the lower layer, the dermis, by a basement membrane. The epidermis receives nutrients by diffusion from a capillary bed just below the basement membrane, within the dermis. Epidermal appendages like hair follicles and sweat glands traverse the two layers but serve nonvital roles.[1] The appendages, being downward projections of the epidermal layer into the dermis, provide an important reservoir of epithelial cells. When the epidermis is lost, the appendages serve as islands of replacement epithelial cells throughout the injured area. They allow re-epithelialization to occur quickly with cells provided from both these and from the wound edges. Skin injury severe enough to destroy these appendages requires more time to replace the epithelial layer because it grows solely from the edges inward.

The dermis, the lower layer, is less cellular and made up primarily of connective tissue components like collagen, fibronectin, and elastin; these matrix proteins supply pliability and elasticity that allow the skin to be form-fitting, yet nonconstraining in relation to underlying structures. The dermis also contains blood vessels and sensory components. These structures help nourish and sustain the skin, function in temperature regulation, and provide warning against outside insults. When the dermis is destroyed, repair is imperfect and is accompanied by scar formation and contraction. True regeneration does not occur.

To deal with both partial and full-thickness loss of skin, a wide variety of skin substitutes have been developed. Various living, nonviable, or acellular autologous and allogeneic skin substitutes have been used alone or in combinations. We will review their history, development, and clinical use.

Defining Skin Substitutes

A universal definition of a skin substitute has not been made. Many synthetic skin substitutes were produced in the 1950s, 1960s, and 1970s and are discussed in detail elsewhere.[2] Currently, skin substitutes derive much of their effectiveness from their biologic components. We will focus only on those constructs containing biologic components.

HISTORY OF SKIN SUBSTITUTES

The history of skin substitutes is not a clear stepwise journey ending with the single most advanced product to date. Rather, it is a number of different, but related, ventures each seeking to replicate one or more functions of skin and in some way collectively progressing toward a human skin equivalent. We will discuss their history by focusing on human split- and full-thickness allografts and autografts (grouped under "excisional grafts"), cultured autologous keratinocyte constructs, cultured allogeneic keratinocyte constructs, dermal constructs, and, finally, bilayered constructs. The latter containing both living epidermal and dermal components.

Excisional Grafts

Although full-thickness skin grafts were used several thousand years ago in the Far East, skin grafts do not appear to have entered medical practice in the West until much more recently.[1,3] Use of autologous split-thickness grafts in Europe was reported in the latter half of the 19th century.[1,4] From the late 19th into the 20th century, autografts were the main treatment for open wounds, so long as adequate donor sites were available.[1] The major problem with autologous skin grafts was the creation of a second wound in the form of a donor site. Allografts were used when donor sites were not available, but were noted to serve only as temporary coverage; adhering well to the wound and even becoming vascularized, they protected against water loss and bacterial invasion but eventually were rejected.[1] In addition, allografts decrease the bacterial count of granulation tissue, providing a cleaner wound for autografting.[5] Attempts were made to extend allograft lifespan with systemic immunosuppression but not many cases were reported and it is unclear if they had a significant impact.[1] Investigation of immunosuppression with allografts appeared to fall by the wayside when cell culture techniques improved.

Autologous Keratinocyte Sheets

The success of many of today's skin substitutes is due to key discoveries in cell culture techniques made over the last few decades. The major advance marking the beginning of this period was the ability to culture human keratinocytes.[6] In 1975, Rheinwald and Green[6] reported large-scale production of human keratinocytes from serial culture techniques that allowed for exponential growth. In time, their techniques were refined with advances that included supplementation of the culture media with growth factors.[1] Eventually sheets of autologous keratinocytes suitable for wound coverage were created, with the first clinical successes reported in burn patients in 1981.[7,8] The process involved taking a biopsy of the patient's skin and enzymatically processing it to yield keratinocytes, which were serially cultured to create sheets of the patient's own cells. The advantages of this process included the small size of donor tissue, and its autologous nature, which avoided the infectious and antigenic concerns of allogeneic grafts. This process, although a great advance, still held drawbacks. Lag time was a major problem from biopsy to patient application, which, under optimal conditions, still required 3 weeks. Other limitations included construct fragility due to lack of a dermal component, as well as a short shelf life.

Allogeneic Keratinocyte Sheets

Attention then shifted to culturing allogeneic grafts. Keratinocytes from neonatal foreskin were grown the same as were the autologous grafts. An advantage of foreskin cells is their greater proliferative potential.[6] For support, keratinocytes sheets were placed on gauze. If not immediately applied, they could be cryopreserved. Freezing allowed for large quantities of ready available grafts. A significant concern though, as with any allogeneic transplant, was the possibility of rejection. Fortunately, Langerhans cells, a primary source of antigenicity in the epidermis, are removed in the processing of the tissue.[9] In addition, keratinocytes stop expressing major histocompatibility complex (MHC) class II antigens after about 7 days of culture.[10] The immunologically less inert nature of the allogeneic grafts allowed them to take without obvious rejection.[11] These grafts proved rather successful with numerous patients being treated.[12] Interestingly, the allogeneic constructs persisted only for a limited period, eventually being replaced by host cells.[13] Even in leg ulcers when the graft did not persist, the allogeneic keratinocyte grafts promoted healing, particularly from the edges, suggesting a mechanism beyond just replacement of cells.[14–16] Lack of a dermis continued to cause problems of wound contracture, instability, and poor cosmesis.

Dermal Constructs

It was known over 100 years ago that a successful dermal graft would decrease wound contracture and scar formation while increasing healing time and overall functionality of repaired skin.[1] Early methods used full-thickness cadaveric grafts. These were left on for several days to facilitate take before the epidermis, being more antigenic than the dermis, was stripped away and replaced with a split-thickness graft or, more recently, cultured autologous keratinocytes.[4] However, problems with fragility of the replaced epidermis persisted and revascularization of the graft was unreliable.[17] In an effort to improve on this, a bilayered artificial skin involving a dermal construct and a synthetic epidermis was developed.[18] This involved a thin Silastic (Dow-Corning Corp. Midland, Michigan) membrane as an epidermal analog, which was bonded to a dermis of bovine collagen and shark condroitin cross-linked with glutaraldehyde. Following graft take, the Silastic would be removed and replaced by keratinocyte sheets. Although this resulted in functional tissue covering the wound more quickly than did keratinocyte sheets, it still held some drawbacks. The impermeability of the Silastic-inhibited drainage of exudates, increasing seroma formation and premature separation.[4] Further improvements led to the Silastic being replaced with cultured autologous human keratinocytes and a dermis of autologous fibroblasts incorporated into a collagen–glycosaminoglycan base.[19] This worked well in stimulating the ingrowth of fibrovascular tissue but, unfortunately, showed a particular predisposition for infection and enzymatic breakdown.[19] Eventually this work led to the development of a human dermal equivalent, namely Dermagraft (Advanced Tissue Sciences, La Jolla, CA; now marketed by Smith and Nephew). Dermagraft is a living dermal replacement constructed by growing neonatal fibroblasts within a bioabsorbable mesh of polyglactin or polyglycolic acid. As the fibroblasts proliferate, they produce their own dermal matrix by secreting collagen, growth factors, and other extracellular proteins. Dermagraft will be discussed in more detail later.

Bilayered Constructs

About the same time Dermagraft was being produced, a bilayered human skin construct with both living dermal and epidermal layers (Apligraf, Organogenesis, Canton, MA) was also being developed. To date, Apligraf is the most complex human skin equivalent, containing human fibroblasts and keratinocytes in respective dermal and epidermal layers. These cells are harvested from neonatal foreskin. The fibroblasts are seeded into a bovine collagen gel and, over time, produce their own extracellular matrix. The keratinocytes are cultured separately and once confluent are exposed to air, facilitating the formation of a stratified epithelium. The keratinocyte sheet is then placed on top of the neodermis and further cultured to allow adherence. Apligraf will be discussed later in greater detail.

SKIN SUBSTITUTES IN ACUTE AND CHRONIC WOUNDS

Wounds being treated with skin substitutes can be grouped into three main categories: acute wounds being treated electively, or urgently, and chronic wounds treated electively.[20,21]

Acute Wounds Treated Electively

Surgical wounds that would otherwise be allowed to heal by second intention are a prime example of an acute wound that could be treated with a skin substitute. For the most part, these wounds are free of pathologic roadblocks to healing. With standard of care, these surgical wounds should heal readily. However, any wound is best healed as quickly as possible since each represents a threat of infection and a drain on medical resources and quality of life. Similarly important, is the need to maximize cosmetic outcome to benefit the patient's emotional well-being. Since skin substitutes, particularly skin equivalents, have resulted in shortened healing times and apparent improved cosmetic outcome in chronic wounds, it was felt that they could do the same for acute nonemergent wounds. Studies of dermatologic surgical wounds treated with a skin equivalent (Apligraf) have shown it to be safe and effective.[22–25] However, conclusive benefits of decreased healing and superior cosmetic outcome in comparison to second-intention healing have only been subjective. Acute wounds are distinctly different from chronic wounds, with the latter having clear pathologic abnormalities to healing. It is likely that the mechanisms through which skin substitutes are suspected to promote healing, such as supplying growth factors and cytokines, are not lacking in acute wounds and thus skin substitutes do not impart a benefit. A clear benefit may be realized in surgical defects requiring an autologous graft; use of Apligraf in place of an autograft will allow avoidance of a second wound from graft harvesting.[25,26]

Acute Wounds Treated Urgently

Acute wounds treated urgently with skin substitutes include burns and toxic epidermal necrolysis. These conditions have unique, often life-threatening reasons for wanting to restore skin function and expedite their healing, such as maintaining homeostasis of water and electrolytes and preventing infection and sepsis. Skin substitutes, similar to moisture-retentive dressings, help decrease pain, a complication these wounds are well-known for. There is no clear algorithm to use in deciding which wounds will benefit most from one or another of the different skin substitutes. Superficial wounds with damage primarily to the epidermal layer basically need wound coverage. These wounds may do well with keratinocyte grafts, Biobrane coupled with a split-thickness graft, or Apligraf. Each of these modalities supplies a neoepidermis.

The destruction and loss of the dermal layer and the subsequent contraction and scar formation extend the morbidity of burns and other deep wounds. Skin substitutes that are intended for use in full-thickness wounds, like Integra and Alloderm, seek to provide a dermal matrix. They are thought to decrease contraction and scar formation.

Chronic Wounds Treated Electively

The greatest experience with skin substitutes has likely been with chronic wounds. Although burns are a great focus for the development and use of skin substitutes, chronic wounds affect a far greater number of patients. Diabetic foot ulcers and venous ulcers are the chronic wounds for which skin substitutes have received regulatory approval. These chronic wounds have pathologic abnormalities preventing their healing. It is not known what prevents these wounds from healing. It is suspected that they are stuck at some point in the healing process. Skin substitutes, particularly those with living cells, like Dermagraft and Apligraf, have been shown to improve their healing. Their possible mechanisms of action in healing will be discussed in detail later.

IDEAL PROPERTIES OF SKIN SUBSTITUTES

In general, the ideal properties for a skin substitute will simulate the functions of normal skin, facilitate healing, and make the product easily available and economically viable. Ideal properties of skin substitutes were reviewed by Burke et al. in 1981 and have been further elaborated on in several reviews since then.[2,10,17,18,20] Below is a list of the properties which these reviews all touch on in one way or another.

Adherence

Immediate and sustained adherence of the substitute to the wound surface preserves the viability of graft cells through diffusion of nutrients. These properties also facilitate ingrowth of native tissues. Continued adherence is strongly dependent on the inner surface of the substitute, which should be a material that facilitates this ingrowth. Cell migration into the substitute is dependent on many factors. The presence of living fibroblasts may be critical. These constructs have already been producing a dermal-like extracellular matrix. Their growth factors and other peptides may lend chemotactant properties while structural proteins, like collagen, facilitate migration of cells. Pore size is important; if too small it will not allow access; if too large, it may compromise construct handling.[20] An optimal pore size has been estimated at 200–300 μm.[20] A well-prepared wound bed is vital to adherence. It needs to have fibrinous and necrotic debris removed and bacterial colonization and exudate production reduced to a minimum.

Elasticity, Flexibility, and Pliability

As properties of the construct, these allow it to conform to the wound bed, aiding adherence. They should also disperse stresses on the substitute that might cause it to tear or shear. The morbidity of full thickness wounds extends far beyond the healing process due, in part, to contracture and scar tissue formation. Skin substitutes that decrease contracture and create the least scar tissue and the most mobility are preferred.

Barrier to Microbial Invasion

In normal skin the cornified layer of the stratified epithelium acts as the main barrier to microbial invasion. In addition, there are immune cells within the dermis and a few in the epidermis, which serve to control bacterial invasion. Skin substitutes do not contain immune mediated cells but they should preferably act as barriers to infectious organisms.

Aid in Fluid Balance

Skin substitutes should reduce fluid loss from the wound to prevent dehydration and electrolyte imbalance, prevent desiccation of the wound, and allow for moist healing. However, complete occlusion predisposes to trapping of exudate. This can result in seroma formation, precluding adequate adherence. These conflicting needs can be difficult to achieve with bilayer constructs that contain a synthetic epidermal analog.[20] With autografts and Apligraf a stratified epithelium is already there and these can be meshed or lightly fenestrated to allow for exudate flow to the surface, reducing the chance of a seroma forming. With synthetic components, such as the silastic neoepidermis, micropores are created to allow for limited evaporation. Although the optimal rate of water flux through the construct is not known, based on studies of occlusive and semipermeable dressings some have suggested 5 mg/cm^2/hr as ideal.[20]

Nontoxic/Nonantigenic

A skin substitute should not elicit an allergic or irritant reaction that would compromise its benefit. It should be immunocompatible with the host tissue. Autologous grafts of any sort, being from the patient, are nonantigenic. Although Apligraf has been shown in a number of studies to elicit no clinical rejection at the treated site or in systemic cellular and humoral analyses, one study did unexpectedly observe a foreign body-like granulomatous response in 4 of 11 patients.[24,27–29] Multinucleated giant cells were observed at the interface between the Apligraf and the patient's dermis.[29] These findings showed no correlation with either poor clinical outcome or prior exposure to Apligraf. This response was thought to represent an innate reaction to the foreign substance and it supports the hypothesis that allogeneic grafts are slowly replaced by host tissue.

Biodegradable

Nonbiologic component materials should be biodegradable, like polyglactin. This is to prevent possible foreign-body reactions and facilitate the remodeling by native cells of the construct into true native tissue. Nonbiodegradeable materials also require removal, which predisposes to complications.

Long Shelf Life, Minimal Storage Requirements, and Low Cost

In general, these properties make skin substitutes readily available and economically viable for all wounds that can benefit from a skin substitute. In addition, ideal properties of skin substitutes include easy handling, reduced pain, and improved cosmetic outcome.

OVERVIEW OF CURRENT SKIN SUBSTITUTES

Here we will review current skin substitutes, covering many of the available commercial products in the United States. We have grouped them into keratinocyte sheets, dermal constructs (those with biologic components only in the dermal layer), and bilayered constructs. We will begin with a review of some of their general properties.

Introduction of infectious disease is a concern for all of these products, but particularly for allografts and xenografts because organisms, like human immunodeficiency virus (HIV), can originate from the donor. Autografts, because they come from the patient, are not tested for diseases like HIV. Cultured cells, including autologous cells, are grown under aseptic conditions. With the use of nonautologous tissues, governmental regulations require testing to safeguard against infectious organisms, particularly viruses like HIV and hepatitis. Likewise, xenografts are tested for organisms appropriate to their source. For allogeneic cultured cells the use of neonatal foreskin is particularly useful. They have great expansive potential in culture. This allows for a smaller number of donors, making the testing for infectious organisms more cost-effective and decreasing the chance of a contaminated product.

Dermal constructs with or without cells supply a scaffold for the regeneration of native tissues. They are thought to stimulate and guide the migration of native cells. Collagen, especially type I collagen, has been shown to provide contact guidance, providing superior cell migration and orientation.[30] Materials, such as polyglycolic acid, can serve as a template, but they are best when engineered to particular filament and pore sizes. Dermal constructs that are seeded with human fibroblasts are allowed to grow for some time as part of the manufacturing process. This allows them to begin producing human extracellular matrix including collagen, glycosaminoglycans, cytokines, and growth factors, which are thought to play a part in the healing properties of these products. In general, the living cells used in skin substitutes do not persist for more than a few weeks after application and are replaced with native cells.[31]

Dermal constructs with or without a synthetic epidermal analog, such as a silicone membrane, are often used in conjunction with split-thickness autografts or cultured keratinocyte sheets. Upon adequate vascularization of the dermal construct and availability of donor autograft tissue, the temporary silicone layer is removed, if present, and an autograft is placed over the neodermis. If a split-thickness graft is required, these dermal constructs allow a thinner graft than would otherwise have been performed.

Keratinocyte Sheets

Epicel (Genzyme Corp., Cambridge, MA)[31]

Epicel is a cultured autologous keratinocyte sheet. Using a small piece of the patient's own skin (about 2 cm^2), the keratinocytes are enzymatically separated and cocultured on top of irradiated murine cells (feeder layer) to produce epidermal autografts. Within weeks, enough keratinocyte sheets can be grown to cover the patient's entire body. For support in transporting and application, keratinocyte sheets of approximately 50 cm^2 are placed onto petrolatum gauze. It is recommended that on initial patient presentation, the wounds be débrided and a dermal substitute be applied to keep the wound clean and encourage revascularization until the keratinocytes grafts can be applied. Epicel is indicated for deep dermal and full-thickness burns comprising a total body surface area of greater than or equal to 30% and for grafting after congenital nevus removal. The final product has a shelf life of 24 hours under proper refrigeration and so should be used the day of its delivery.[32]

VivoDerm (ER Squibb and Co., Princeton, NJ)[33]

This product is not yet available in the United States, but has been used in several European countries under the trade name Laserskin. It is comprised of a hyaluronic acid membrane, containing laser-induced micropores, onto which autologous keratinocytes are seeded and grown. When applied to a wound, the pores facilitate migration of cells onto the wound surface.[10] This product has shown success in treating burns and chronic venous ulcers.[33]

Inverted Keratinocyte Delivery System

A recently reported, unnamed delivery system for allogeneic keratinocyte sheets involved an upside down human-porcine skin substitute. Originally planned as a skin equivalent with human keratinocytes cultured on acellular pig dermis, it failed to take when grafted onto burn patients.[34] When placed in an inverted position, with keratinocytes down, it significantly improved healing of graft donor sites, suggesting the dermal component protected the keratinocyte layer. It did not prove useful on full-thickness burns, healing only one of five sites and, then, only after repeated attempts.[34]

Dermal Constructs

Biobrane (Bertek Pharmaceuticals, Morgantown, WV)[35]

Biobrane is a trilayered, acellular, composite skin substitute. It is made with a specially knitted nylon fabric. Porcine dermal collagen is applied on one side and a permeable silicone membrane is bonded to the other. The porcine collagen side is placed against the wound bed to facilitate adherence. Biobrane is intended as a temporary dressing. It should be removed approximately 7–14 days after application, once the wound has re-epithelialized or when a skin graft is planned. Biobrane is indicated for use on superficial partial-thickness burns and graft donor sites. Biobrane has a shelf life of 3 years when stored at room temperature.[30,35]

Early reports of patients treated with Biobrane suggested it increased infection rates.[36] However, several studies with many more patients have since concluded Biobrane to be safe and effective in treating superficial partial-thickness burns in pediatric patients.[37–39] In these studies, when compared to standard treatment with 1% silver sulfadiazine, Biobrane decreased healing time, length of hospital stay, pain, and use of pain medication. It was determined that the infection rate increased when patients with deeper thickness burns were treated.[39] In a series of 8 patients with toxic epidermolysis bullosa involving an average of 80% of body surface, Biobrane appeared to reduce pain and infection, improve fluid and electrolyte balance, and better control heat loss.[40]

Oasis (Cook Biotech, Lafayette, Indiana; marketed by Healthpoint, Ltd. Fort Worth, TX)

Oasis is an acellular xenograft derived from porcine small intestinal submucosa (SIS). The SIS is processed to remove all cells, leaving the extracellular matrix, including structural components and growth factors. It is supplied as a dry sheet and is rehydrated immediately prior to placement. It is intended for temporary coverage of partial-thickness skin loss injuries such as burns, abrasions, pressure and chronic vascular ulcers, and autograft donor sites. Oasis has a shelf life of one year.[41] Little is known of the capacity of Oasis to stimulate wound healing.

AlloDerm (LifeCell Corp., Branchburg, NJ)

Alloderm is an acellular, dermal allograft. Cadaveric human skin is processed to first remove the entire epidermis and then the dermal cells, leaving the dermal extracellular matrix. The product is then freeze dried, through a patented process, preserving the structure of the matrix. Alloderm is approved for use in burns, alone or in conjunction with an autograft, and may also be used as an implant for cosmetic and reconstructive purposes. AlloDerm is stored at 1–10°C and has a 2-year shelf life.[42]

In side-by-side comparison, the use of Alloderm as a dermal transplant in conjunction with a thin split-thickness autograft was equivalent in its 14-day take rate as that of a thicker split-thickness graft.[21] There were no statistical differences in scarring, elasticity, contracture, or patient and physician assessment of final cosmetic result. With the Alloderm-treated wounds, split-thickness autografts ranged from 0.005 to 0.009 inches thick. Within this group, the thinnest autografts had the best take rate. It was hypothesized that the porosity of the Alloderm and the thinness of the graft allowed better nutrient diffusion.

Integra (Integra LifeSciences Corp., Plainsboro, NJ; distributed by Ethicon, Inc.)

Integra is a composite, acellular, dermal substitute. Constructed as a bilayer, it has a bovine collagen and chondroitin-6-sulfate matrix overlaid with a silicone membrane. Approximately 1–2 weeks after its application, the silicone component is removed and replaced with a split-thickness graft. Integra is approved for use in burns and in burn scar revision. Integra is stored in 70% isopropyl alcohol and has a shelf life of 2 years.[30,43,44]

Integra has been shown to markedly decrease length of hospital stay in severely burned adults.[45] Average stay in the Integra group was 63 days compared to 107 days in the control group. Integra has also shown promising results in reducing contracture in reconstruction of burn scars. Five patients with burn scars of the anterior cervical neck underwent reconstruction with Integra and each experienced reduced contracture and an improved cosmetic result, particularly in the bearded area.[46] However, recurrence of contracture of >50% occurred in all cases.

TransCyte (Smith and Nephew, Inc. Largo, FL)

TransCyte is a trilayered composite, dermal substitute with nonviable human cells. Manufacturing begins similarly to Biobrane with a nylon mesh that is coated on one side with porcine collagen and bonded to a silicone membrane on the other. Human fibroblasts from neonatal foreskin are seeded into the nylon mesh and allowed to proliferate. When adequately mature, this is preserved by freezing. The freezing process kills the cells but, upon thawing, the matrix contains active growth factors. TransCyte is indicated for use as a temporary wound covering for full- and partial-thickness burns prior to autograft placement. It must be kept frozen until use.[30,47]

Extensive partial-thickness burns treated with TransCyte, in comparison to a standard topical antibiotic regimen (silver sulfadiazine, repetitive wound débridement, and dressing changes), had significantly shorter healing time and less hypertrophic scar formation.[48] TransCyte has also been shown to significantly reduce length of stay in pediatric scald burn patients.[49] The TransCyte group averaged 5.9 +/− 0.9 days in the hospital as opposed to 13.8 +/− 2.2 days for those receiving standard therapy. In the treatment of partial thickness facial burns, Transcyte was significantly better than standard topical antibiotic therapy, requiring less wound care time and less time to re-epithelialize.[50]

Dermagraft (Smith and Nephew, Inc. Largo, FL)

Dermagraft is a living human dermal substitute produced by seeding human fibroblasts from neonatal foreskin onto a bioabsorbable scaffold. The scaffold is a mesh made of polyglactin or polyglycolic acid, the same materials used to make absorbable sutures. The fibroblasts proliferate, creating extracellular matrix proteins like collagen and growth factors; this, coupled with the breakdown of the scaffold, remodels the construct making it more like human dermis. Dermagraft is approved for use in full-thickness neuropathic diabetic foot ulcers. Dermagraft has a 6-month shelf life, but needs to be kept at or below −70°C. It requires a rapid time-sensitive thawing procedure and should be applied within 30 minutes after thawing.

In a pivotal study of diabetic foot ulcers, wounds treated with Dermagraft and standard treatment (débridement, moist dressings, and pressure relief) in comparison to wounds treated with standard treatment alone were more likely to be completely healed by week 12 (50.8 vs. 31.7%, $p = 0.006$) and week 32 (57.7 vs. 42.4%, $p = 0.04$).[51] Dermagraft-treated wounds also had a shorter median time to complete healing (13 vs. 28 weeks, $p = 0.01$). The wounds treated with Dermagraft received weekly applications of the dermal substitute for up to 8 weeks unless completely healed. These findings were comparable to the pilot study and later confirmed in a supplemental trial.[52,53]

Bilayered Constructs

OrCel (Ortec Int'l., NY)[54]

OrCel is a bilayered, living, cellular substitute. It is comprised of human keratinocytes and fibroblasts derived from neonatal foreskin. The fibroblasts are seeded into and on one side of a bovine collagen matrix. The other side is coated with a nonporous collagen gel to which the keratinocytes are applied. OrCel is indicated for treating donor site wounds in burn victims. Under the Humanitarian Device Exemption it is also indicated for use in epidermolysis bullosa, specifically for reconstructive hand surgery and donor site wounds. Trials are underway for assessing OrCel use in venous leg ulcers and diabetic foot ulcers. OrCel is shipped in a cooled package (11–19°C) where it remains viable for 72 hours. It should remain in the shipping package until use.[54]

Apligraf (Organogenesis, Inc. Canton, MA)

Apligraf is a bilayered, living, cellular substitute. It is made with fibroblasts and keratinocytes derived from human neonatal foreskin. The fibroblasts are grown in a bovine type I collagen gel to form a dermal substitute. Keratinocytes are grown separately into a stratified epithelium and then placed on top of the neodermis. The construct is allowed to grow a few more days before shipping. Apligraf has been Food and Drug Administration (FDA) approved for use in diabetic foot ulcers and venous ulcers. It has a 5-day shelf life and can be stored at room temperature until use.

Apligraf has been shown to significantly reduce the time to complete wound closure in venous and diabetic ulcers.[27,55] It has also been shown to be especially helpful in healing hard-to-heal venous ulcers of long duration.[28,56,57] Additional reports suggest that Apligraf is safe and effective in a variety of acute and chronic wounds including epidermolysis bullosa, pyoderma gangrenosum, and postsurgical wounds.[24,58,59]

WOUND-BED PREPARATION

Wound-bed preparation is vital to achieving maximal benefit from skin substitutes. These constructs will fail if placed on wounds that are heavily colonized by microbes, not thoroughly cleared of necrotic and fibrinous debris, or heavily exudative.

Débridement

Necrotic tissue, fibrinous debris, and eschar physically interfere with adherence and act as foci of bacterial colonization and proliferation. Acute and chronic wounds should be surgically cleared of necrotic debris. A regimen of maintenance débridement may be necessary in some chronic wounds to deal with reoccurring fibrinous debris and the likely associated bacterial load.

Control of Exudate

Exudate should be reduced as much as possible. Exudate of chronic wounds has been shown to hinder prolifera-

tion and is thought to bind or break down growth factors.[60,61] In chronic lower-extremity wounds, exudate is often due to dependent edema, as in venous ulcers. In this case, compression dressings and lower-extremity elevation will help reduce exudate. Reduction in bacterial burden also reduces exudate.

Control of Bacterial Burden

Bacteria hinder wound healing on several levels. They cause inflammation that drives exudate production, compete with the host for vital nutrients, and produce toxic substances that can further break down tissue. There are a number of methods to control bacterial burden, some of which act on different levels. Removal of necrotic and fibrinous debris will reduce the bacterial load and, at the same time, remove areas for bacteria to proliferate. In these types of chronic wounds, the use of slow-release antiseptics containing silver or iodine can be particularly helpful. For the deeply infected wound, systemic antibiotics should be instituted.

Vacuum-assisted closure devices offer benefits in all three of these areas and are quite good at preparing wounds for skin substitutes. Comprised of a pump with an airtight dressing, it supplies constant negative pressure throughout the wound bed. This removes exudate as it forms. In so doing, it also carries away superficial bacteria and fibrin and other proteins within exudate.[62]

MECHANISM OF ACTION

Skin substitutes clearly act as a protection against infection and dessication and help provide a moist wound environment. It is highly suspected that skin substitutes also stimulate the endogenous healing process in biochemical and biologic ways that are still poorly understood.

Keratinocyte Sheets

Autologous keratinocyte sheets act by cell replacement. They are also thought to act through stimulation of endogenous cells.[31] Autologous full-thickness punch grafts that were prewounded 3 days prior to harvesting demonstrated greater wound edge stimulation in treating chronic wounds than grafts that were not prewounded.[63]

Although allogeneic keratinocyte sheets may appear to take and are not associated with acute rejection, persistence of their cells only ranges from 1 to 6 weeks.[10,11] The graft cells are progressively replaced by native cells.[64] The improved healing that occurs after their placement is thought, in part, to result from the growth factors and other proteins they secrete.[15,65] Chronic wounds are characterized by inactive wound edges, with keratinocytes that have hightened proliferation, but do not migrate. Allogeneic keratinocyte sheets are known to stimulate epithelial migration, likely from the growth factors and cytokines they secrete.[15,65]

Dermal Constructs

Dermal constructs have been reported to decrease healing time and to reduce the necessary thickness of skin grafts used.[20,66–68] Dermal constructs are intended to speed wound closure by more quickly supplying a surface for epithelial migration. They do this by providing an existing structure, often made up of dermal matrix components like collagen. By using the same matrix components found in human dermis, like collagen, they encourage more rapid in-growth of fibroblasts and endothelial cells due to interactions with the cells.

Dermal constructs are also hypothesized to reduce scarring and contracture. Normal dermis has a sophisticated structure of collagen intimately associated with other connective tissues, like elastin, whereas scars consist primarily of less complex, denser bundles of collagen with no associated elastin.[66] Dermal constructs, with or without living cells, are thought to decrease scar formation by providing a scaffold or template to facilitate a more organized formation of neodermis. Although there have been subjective and nonsignificant objective reports of dermal grafts and skin equivalents reducing scar formation and wound contracture, there is no conclusive evidence for this. It is possible that in the short term a more pliable scar is obtained, but as the scar remodels over time much of this benefit is lost. This is consistent with Integra use in reconstruction of burn scars; as previously mentioned, there was initial improvement with reduced contraction, but much of this improvement was lost over time as the new scar with the dermal construct matured.[46] Autografts retain their original dermal architecture, even though the graft cells and collagen are nearly completely replaced by 6 months.[1] Allografts are eventually replaced with scar after complete healing and an early good cosmetic result.[1]

Skin Equivalents

Skin equivalents provide a combination of keratinocyte sheets and dermal constructs and, therefore, act through a combination of the above-mentioned mechanisms. Apligraf, in particular, has had considerable research aimed at its mechanism of action. Graft cells in venous ulcers treated with Apligraf do not persist for more than a few weeks. Therefore, its benefit must be other than cell replacement.[31] When Apligraf was wounded *in vitro* and examined at histological and molecular levels for characteristics of healing, it demonstrated the ability to re-epithelialize itself and to heal in a sequential response method similar to *in vivo* healing of skin.[69] In particular, there was appropriately sequenced secretion of cytokines and growth factors consistent with the first (inflammatory)

and second (proliferation) phases of healing. In addition, the re-epithelialization was associated with a shift in the keratinocytes from proliferation to migration. This is consistent with skin's normal response to wounding and supports the hypotheses that bioengineered skin acts in dynamic biologic ways on multiple levels.

ECONOMICS OF SKIN SUBSTITUTES

There have been several studies showing the cost-effectiveness of skin substitutes. The cost benefit comes from decreasing healing time and the subsequent savings in direct costs, dressings, hospital days, and office and nursing visits.

As mentioned earlier, acute surgical wounds do not appear to heal any faster with skin substitutes than by second intention healing. Therefore skin substitutes may not offer cost savings in acute wounds. Severe burns require intensive specialty care costing thousands of dollars per hospital day. Decreasing the number of hospital days has a great potential savings. As previously mentioned, TransCyte use in pediatric scald burns reduced length of hospital stay by as much as half.[49] Although it has not been reported, there is a good chance this would show a cost benefit. In superficial outpatient burns treatment with Biobrane was shown to cost less than treatment with a standard topical antibiotic regimen.[70]

Several studies have demonstrated the cost-effectiveness of some of the more expensive skin substitutes in treating chronic wounds. A prospective, multicenter, randomized study involving 240 participants examined the direct medical cost in treating hard-to-heal venous ulcers with Apligraf versus Unna's boot over a 12-month period.[71] The assessment included the cost of primary therapeutic intervention, additional compression dressings, physician office visits, laboratory tests and procedures, management of adverse events, and hospitalizations. The annual average cost per patient came out to $20,041 for the Apligraf group and $27,493 for the Unna's boot group. The strongest factor in this difference was that Apligraf patients experienced approximately 3 months more in the healed state than did their control group.

Even with multiple applications Dermagraft offers a cost benefit. In a French study, Allenet et al. used a Markov model to assess the cost-effectiveness of Dermagraft in comparison to standard therapy. Using a 100-person cohort followed for 52 weeks they determined a 6% long-term cost savings with Dermagraft.[72]

ACKNOWLEDGMENT

Work supported by National Institutes of Health (NIH) Grants AR42936 and AR46557.

REFERENCES

1. Galico GG. Biologic skin substitutes. *Clin Plast Surg.* 1990; 17:519–526.

2. Pruitt BA, Levine NS. Characteristics and uses of biologic dressings and skin substitutes. *Arch Surg.* 1984;119: 312–322.

3. Limova M, Grekin RC. Synthetic membranes and cultured keratinocytes grafts. *J Am Acad Dermatol.* 1990;23:713–719.

4. Eaglestein WH, Falanga V. Tissue engineering and the development of Apligraf a human skin equivalent. *Clin Therap.* 1997;19(5):894–905.

5. Morris PJ, Bondoc CC, Burke JE. The use of frequently changed skin allografts to promote healing in the non-healing infected ulcer. *Surgery.* 1966;60:30.

6. Rheinwald JG, Green H. Serial cultivation of human epidermal keratinocytes: the formation of keratinizing colonies from single cells. *Cell.* 1975;6:331–334.

7. Green H, Kehinde O, Thomas J. Growth of cultured human epidermal cells into multiple epithelia suitable for grafting. *Proc Natl Acad Sci USA.* 1979;76:5665–5668.

8. O'Connor NE, Mulliken JB. Banks-Schlegal, et al. Grafting of burns with cultured epithelium prepared from autologous epidermal cells. *Lancet.* 1981;10:75–78.

9. Hefton JM, Ambershon JB, Bizes DG, et al. Loss of HLADR expression by human epidermal cells after growth in culture. *J Invest Dermatol.* 1984;83:48–50.

10. Jones I, Currie L, Martin R. A guide to biological skin substitutes. *Brit J Plast Surg.* 2002;55:185–193.

11. Thiovolet J, Faure M, Demidem A, et al. Long term survival and immunologic tolerance of human epidermal allografts produced in culture. *Transplantation.* 1986;42:274–280.

12. Arons JA, Wainwright DJ, Jordan RE. The surgical applications and implications of cultured human epidermis: a comprehensive review. *Surgery.* 1992;111:4–11.

13. Burt Am, Pallet CD, Sloane JP, et al. Survival of cultured allografts in patients with burns assessed with a probe specific for Y chromosome. *BMJ.* 1989;298:915–917.

14. Leigh IM, Purkis PE, Navsaria HA, et al. Treatment of chronic venous ulcers with sheets of cultured allogeneic keratinocytes. *Br J Dermatol.* 1987;17:591–597.

15. Shehade S, Clancy J, Blight A, et al. Cultured epithelial allografting of leg ulcers. *J Dermatol Treatment.* 1989;1:79–82.

16. Phillips TJ, Kehinde O, Green H, et al. Treatment of skin ulcers with cultured epidermal allografts. *J Am Acad Dermatol.* 1989;21:191–199.

17. Phillips TJ Biologic skin substitutes. *J Dermatol Surg Oncol.* 1993;19:794–800.

18. Burke JF, Yannas IV, Quinby WC, et al. Successful use of physiologically acceptable artificial skin in treatment of extensive burn injury. *Ann Surg.* 1981;194:413–428.

19. Hansbrough JF, Boyce ST, Cooper ML, et al. Burn wound closure with cultured autologous keratinocytes and fibroblasts attached to a collagen glycosaminoglycan substrate. *JAMA.* 1989;262:2125–2130.

20. Sefton MV, Woodhouse KA. Tissue Engineering. *J Cutaneous Med Surg.* 1998;3:S1–S18.

21. Wainwright D, Madden M, Luterman A, et al. Clinical evaluation of an acellular allograft dermal matrix in full-thickness burns. *J Burn Care Rehab.* 1996;17:124–136.

22. Eaglestein WH, Iriondo M, Laszlo K. A composite skin substitute (Graftskin) for surgical wounds. *Dermatol Surg.* 1995;21:839–843.

23. Gohari S, Gambla C, Healey M, et al. Evaluation of tissue-engineered skin (Human skin substitute) and secondary intention healing in the treatment of full thickness wounds after Mohs micrographic or excisional surgery. *Dermatol Surg.* 2002;28:1107–1114.

24. Eaglestein WH, Alvarez OM, Auletta M, et al. Acute excisional wounds treated with a tissue-engineered skin (Apligraf). *Dermatol Surg.* 1999;25:195–201.

25. Tarlow MM, Nossa, R, Spencer JM. Effective management of difficult surgical defects using tissue-engineered skin. *Dermatol Surg.* 2001;27:71–74.

26. Kirsner RS. The use of Apligraf in acute wounds. *J Dermatol* 1998;25:805–811.

27. Falanga V, Margolis D, Alvarez O, et al. Rapid healing of venous ulcers and lack of clinical rejection with an allogeneic cultured human skin equivalent. *Arch Dermatol.* 1998; 134:293–300.

28. Falanga V, Sabolinski M. A bilayered living skin construct (Apligraf) accelerates complete closure of hard-to-heal venous ulcers. *Wound Rep Reg.* 1999;7:201–207.

29. Badiavas EV, Paquette D, Carson P, et al. Human chronic wounds treated with bioengineered skin: histologic evidence host-graft interactions. *J Am Acad Dermatol.* 2002;46:524–530.

30. www.burnsurgery. org/Modules/skinsubstitutes/sec4.htm

31. Phillips TJ, Manzoor J, Rojas A, et al. The longevity of a bilayered skin substitute after application to venous ulcers. *Arch Dermatol.* 2002;138:1079–1081.

32. www.genzyme.com

33. biomed.brown.edu/Courses/BI108/BI108_2001_Groups/Tissue_Engineered_Skin/Alternatives.htm

34. Matouskova E, Bucek S, Vogtova D, et al. Treatment of burns and donor sites with human allogeneic keratinocytes grown on acellular dermis. *Br J Dermatol.* 1997;136:901–907.

35. Smith DJ. Use of Biobrane in wound management. Proceedings of a conference held on September 17, 1994, in Houston, Texas. *J Burn Care Rehab.* 1995;16:317–320.

36. Feldman DL, Rogers A, Karpinski RH. A prospective trial comparing Biobrane, Duoderm, and xeroform for skin graft donor sites. *Surg, Gyn & Obstet.* 1991;173:1–5.

37. Barret JP, Dziewulski P, Ramzy, PI, et al. Biobrane verses 1% silver sulfiadiazine in second degree pediatric burns. *Plast Reconstr Surg.* 2000;105:62–65.

38. Lal S, Barrow RE, Wolf SE, et al. Biobrane improves wound healing in burned children without increased risk of infection. *Shock* 2000;14:318–319.

39. Ou LF, Lee SY, chen YC, et al. Use of Biobrane in pediatric scald burns—experience in 106 children. *Burns.* 1998;24:49–53.

40. Arevalo JM, Lorente JA. Skin coverage with Biobrane biomaterial for the treatment of patients with toxic epidermal necrolysis. *J Burn Care Rehab.* 1999;20:406–410.

41. www.woundcare.org/newsvol5nl/pr3.htm

42. www.lifecell.com/healthcare/products/alloderm/index.cfm (LifeCell Corp website). Last accessed May 2003.

43. www.integra-ls.com/bus-skin_mstr.htm?bus-skin_main.htm (Integra website, Life Sciences Holdings Corporation). Last accessed May 2003.

44. www.skinhealing.com. Last accessed May 2003.

45. Ryan CM, Schoenfeld DA, Malloy M, et al. Use of Integra artificial skin is associated with deceased length of stay for severely injured adult burn survivors. *J Burn Care Rehab.* 2002;23:311–317.

46. Hunt JA, Moisidis E, Haertsch P. Initial experience of Integra in the treatment of post-burn anterior cervical neck contracture. *Br J Plast Surg.* 2000;53:652–658.

47. www.smith-nephew.com/businesses/W_TransCyte.html (TransCyte webpage, Smith and Nephew, Inc). Last accessed May 2003.

48. Noordenbos J, Dore C, Hansborough JF. Safety and efficacy of TransCyte for the treatment of partial-thickness burns. *J Burn Care Rehab.* 1999;20:275–281.

49. Lukesh JR, Eichelberger MR, Newman KD, et al. The use of a bioactive skin substitute reduces length of stay for pediatric burn patients. *J Ped Surg.* 2001;36:1118–1121.

50. Demler RH, DeSanti L. Management of partial thickness facial burns (comparison of topical antibiotics and bio-engineered skin substitutes). *Burns.* 1999;25:256–261.

51. Pollack RA, Edington H, Jensen JL, et al. A human dermal replacement for the treatment of diabetic foot ulcers. *Wounds.* 1997;9:175–183.

52. Gentzkow GD, Iwasaki SD, Hershon KS, et al. Use of Dermagraft, a cultured human dermis, to treat diabetic foot ulcers. *Diabetes Care.* 1997;4:350–354.

53. Gentzkow GD, Jensen JL, Pollak RA, et al. Improved healing of diabetic foot ulcers after grafting with a living human dermal replacement. *Wounds.* 1999;11:77–84.

54. www.ortecinternational.com (Ortec Int'l website). Last accessed May 2003.

55. Veves A, Falanga V, Armstrong D, et al. Graftskin, a human skin equivalent, is effective in the management of noninfected neuropathic diabetic foot ulcers. *Diabetes Care.* 2001;24:290–295.

56. Brem H, Balledux J, Sukkarieh, et al. Healing of venous ulcers of long duration with a bilayered living skin substitute: results from a general surgery and dermatology department. *Dermatol Surg.* 2001;27:915–919.

57. Long RE, Falabella AF, Valencia I, et al. Treatment of refractory, atypical lower extremity ulcers with tissue engineered skin (Apligraf). *Arch Dermatol.* 2001; 137:1660–1661.

58. Falabella AF, Valencia IC, Eaglestein WH, et al. Tissue engineered skin (Apligraf) in the healing of patients with epidermolysis bullosa wounds. *Arch Dermatol.* 2000;136: 1225–1230.

59. de Imus G, Golumb C, Wilkel C, et al. Accelerated healing of pyoderma gangrenosum treated with bioengineered skin and concomitant immunosuppression. *J Am Acad Dermatol.* 2001 44:61–66.

60. Bucalo B, Eaglestein WH, Falanga V. Inhibition of cell proliferation by chronic wound fluid. *Wound Rep Reg.* 1993;1:181–186.

61. Falanga V, Eaglestein WH. The "trap" hypothesis for venous ulceration. *Lancet.* 1993;341:1006–1008.

62. Argenta LC, Morykwas MJ. Vacuum-assisted closure: a new method for wound control and treatment: clinical experience. *Ann Plast Surg.* 1997;38:563–577.

63. Kirsner RS, Falanga V, Kerdel FA, et al. Skin grafts as pharmacological agents: pre-wounding of the donor site. *Br J Dermatol.* 1996;135:292–296.

64. Gielen V, Faure M, Mauduit G, et al. Progressive replacement of human cultured epithelial autografts by recipient cells as evidenced by HLA class I antigen expression. *Dermatologica.* 1987;175:166–170.

65. Phillips TJ, Gilchrest BA. Cultured epidermal allografts as biological wound dressings. *Prog Clin Biol Res.* 1991;365:77–94.

66. Wainwright DJ. Use of an acellular allograft dermal matrix (Alloderm) in the management of full-thickness burns. *Burns.* 1995;21:243–248.

67. Fitton AR, Drew P, Dickson WA. The use of a bilaminate artificial skin substitute (Integra) in acute resurfacing of burns: an early experience. *Br J Plast Surg.* 2001;54:208–212.

68. Sheridan RL, Hegarty M, Tompkins RG, et al. Artificial skin in massive burns – results to ten years. *Eur J Plast Surg.* 1994; 17:91–93.

69. Falanga V, Isaacs C, Paquette D, et al. Wounding of bioengineered skin: cellular and molecular aspects after injury. *J Invest Dermatol.* 2002;119:653–660.

70. Gerding RI, Emerman CL, Effron D, et al. Outpatient management of partial thickness burns. Biobrane versus 1% silver sulfadiazine. *Ann Emerg Med.* 1990;19:121–124.

71. Schonfeld WH, Villa KF, Fastenau JM, et al. An economic assessment of Apligraf (Graftskin) for the treatment of hard-to-heal venous leg ulcers. *Wound Rep Reg.* 2000;8:251–257.

72. Allenet B, Paree F, Lebrun T, et al. Cost-effectiveness modeling of Dermagraft for the treatment of diabetic foot ulcers in the French context. *Diabetes Metab.* 2000;26:125–132.

19

Wound Closure by External Tissue Expansion

Ralph Ger and Eli S. Schessel

Introduction
Wound Closure by External Constant
 Tension Approximation
Wound Management
General Principles of Wound
 Closure
 Technique
 Pain Management
Lesions of the Lower Extremity
 Thigh
 Knee Joint
 Leg
 Foot and Ankle
Pressure Sores

Sacral Pressure Sores
Ischial Pressure Sores
Trochanteric Pressure Sores
Heel Ulcers
Abdominal Wall Wounds
Thoracic Wounds
Breast Surgery
Head and Neck Lesions
Discussion
 Special Considerations for
  Elderly Patients
 Contraindications
 Economic Considerations
References

INTRODUCTION

The frustration accompanying efforts to improve methods of wound healing has a long history. In the 4th century, Hippocrates declared; "Healing is a matter of time, but it is also sometimes a matter of opportunity." The earlier history of wound therapy consisted mostly of attempts to stimulate the rate of natural healing by stimulating epithelialization using local wound therapy. The resulting thin fragile scar, although prone to break down, was often gratefully accepted. Attempts to improve the quality of the healed wound led to the introduction of surgical interventions. The latter approaches were rewarded by more expeditious healing, and, more importantly, by a wound covered by full-thickness skin. The price paid for these benefits were operative procedures that became, *pari passu*, progressively more complicated. Most recently, intense investigation into the biochemical factors associated with the healing process are taking place; as yet, the translation into beneficial results have been less rewarding than had

been hoped. The ultimate aim of the various therapeutic measures is the replacement of lost skin by local site full-thickness skin and, in certain sites, it is underlying subcutaneous tissue. In other words, replaced skin should resemble the quality of the lost skin as much as possible.

Surgical interventions, such as various forms of flaps, are relatively major procedures. In an attempt to avoid the latter, Neumann[1] in 1957, investigated the stretching of skin by the subcutaneous placement of an inflatable balloon that is intermittently distended. The skin that is eventually gained was then transposed to close the wound defect. It is somewhat surprising that this principle was not explored earlier in the search for more rapid wound closure by better quality skin. The enlarging breasts and abdominal walls of pregnant women and, unnaturally, the enlarged lower lips and ears of some tribal Africans that followed the implantation of large plates in those parts did not appear to arouse much curiosity in the medical establishment. Various other techniques of skin expansion followed Neuman's work and continue to be introduced.

WOUND CLOSURE BY EXTERNAL CONSTANT TENSION APPROXIMATION

This presentation is concerned with a method of treatment that converts a nonhealing wound into a fresh clean wound by a combination of minimally invasive sharp débridement and regular or pulsed irrigation, following which the wound is closed by delayed primary wound closure. All skin is expandable, the degree and rate of expansion being related to the interstices between the cells, the amount of elastic tissue present, and the degree of fixation to the underlying tissues. The closure is achieved by approximating local tissues that have been expanded by the use of a device named the Proxiderm (Progressive Surgical Products, Westbury, NY).[2] The Proxiderm is an external tissue expansion device (Fig. 19–1A, B) that consists of a pair of tissue hooks that are inserted through healthy skin into subcutaneous tissue approximately 2 cm from the opposing wound margins into the subcutaneous tissue. The Proxiderm automatically applies a constant, sustained, low-grade force of no more than 460 g to the margins of the wound and gradually stretches the nearby skin to close the wound with full-thickness skin and the cavity with subcutaneous tissue. The devices are typically left in place for periods of 2 to 3 days. During this time period, the wound edges gradually approach other. (Fig. 19–1 C) Significantly contaminated wounds are evaluated once

or more daily. Large wounds may require multiple applications of the devices until the wound can be closed by sutures in a tension-free environment. The devices vary in number, size, and shape, depending on the size and site of the lesion and the contour of the surrounding surface. For the latter situation, the devices are shaped from slightly curved to that of a right angle.

Constant long-term stretching of the skin by this method leads to the approximation of the skin edges and to physiologic changes that induce angiogenesis and increased mitotic activity of the epithelial cells.[3] Approximation is a well known and rapid method of closing defects and has long been used in recent wounds when tissues are pliable and able to be moved. However, in tissues fixed by chronic inflammatory states, such as occurs in older wounds or in skin deficient wounds, current methods of approximation have limitations.

WOUND MANAGEMENT

Local conditions that preclude closure include the presence of a persistent discharge, which usually indicates the presence of nonviable tissues and signs of active inflammation, such as edema, erythema, and increased heat. These situations require resolution before treatment is commenced. Currently, this is carried out by a variety of methods that usually include sharp débridement of necrotic tissues, the systematic administration

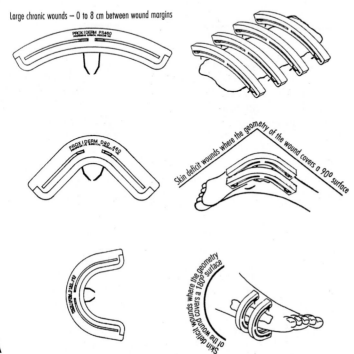

Large chronic wounds — 0 to 8 cm between wound margins

Skin deficit wounds where the geometry of the wound covers a 90° surface

Skin deficit wounds where the geometry of the wound covers a 180° surface

A

Fig. 19–1. **A.** Diagrammatic illustrations of different sizes and shapes of the Proxiderm devices. **B.** Photographic rendering of different sizes and shapes of the Proxiderm devices. **C.** Diagrammatic illustration of gradual approximation of wound margins.

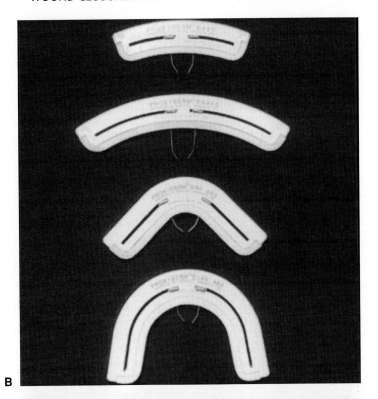

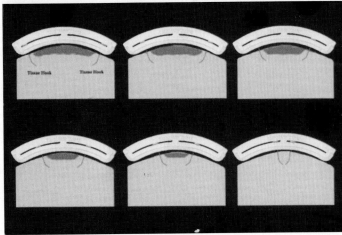

Fig. 19–1. Continued **C**

of antimicrobial agents, and intensive local toilette. Cultures, preferably using excised tissues, maybe be helpful, in that a dominant organism, sensitive only to a specific medication, may be identified, requiring the administration of a specific medication. The prevention of cross-contamination during wound toilette is important, especially in many of the elderly and/or diabetic patients, who may be immunocompromised.

GENERAL PRINCIPLES OF WOUND CLOSURE

The closure of wounds that are skin deficient and contaminated require preparation for conversion into clean wounds that are closed in a tension-free environment. The contamination needs to be eliminated by a combination of intensive wound toilette, including the removal of necrotic and marginal tissue, antimicrobial therapy, general and/or local, and frequent irrigation, with or without the addition of specific medications. The tension-free environment is mediated by the application of the Proxiderm devices, leading to delayed primary closure of the healing wound. When the wound is finally closed by suture, an irrigating catheter may be placed in the deeper parts of the wound to prevent the collection of possible remaining anaerobic collections. The final result should be a vascular, tension-free closure with local site skin.

Technique

After the wound has been prepared for closure, the patient is sedated by analgesic and/or sedative drugs and, if necessary, anesthetic agents are infiltrated locally. The wound margins are sharply excised and, if necessary, gently undermined, usually by finger dissection at a fascial level. In chronic wounds that are adherent to the underlying tissue, this step is required so as to allow the skin and subcutaneous tissue to slide without inverting the margins. Subacute wounds are not usually adherent and, in these circumstances, the underminings maneuver may be unnecessary. A series of 2/0 nylon paired sutures are placed 2–3 cm from the wound margin and 2 cm apart. One suture of each pair is tied with modest tension and the ends are left long (Fig. 19–2A); these long ends will be looped around the devices and tied at a later stage. The adjacent suture is left untied and secured by Steristrips (Fig. 19–2B). The use of rubber booties to reduce pressure on the skin is optional. The purposes of the tied sutures are threefold: the surface area of the wound is decreased, the security of the devices is increased by the looped long ends, and the obliteration of any dead space is enhanced. The untied sutures are used in the same manner as the tied sutures at the first dressing change; at this time, their initial placement simplifies this procedure. Devices are now placed between the previously tied sutures and additionally secured by the long ends of the tied sutures. Well-padded occlusive dressings are placed under the ends of the Proxiderms to prevent pressure on the skin, on the sides and between the Proxiderms to prevent movement of the devices (Fig. 19–2C), and over the top of the devices where it is secured to the patient by Elastoplast and/or adhesive tape to prevent dislodgement of the devices and wound contamination (Fig. 19–2D). Dressing changes are carried out approximately every 2–3 days. In contaminated wounds and in all sacral lesions, dressings are changed once or more daily; under these conditions, contamination of the devices is possible. Dislodgement, soiling, or the expenditure of tension of the devices requires the latter's replacement. If clean and in good position with tension still present, as judged by the position of the knobs, the devices are left in place until the next dressing change. After final approximation of the skin and subcutaneous tissue, the wound is sutured. Patients in good general condition undergo healing. In debilitated and hypoproteinemic patients, it is wise to retain the sutures until sound healing of the wound takes place; in these same patients an additional application of the Proxiderms is recommended so as to allow the wound to heal in a tension-free environment. At times, during the course of the treatment, edema, inflammation or a purulent discharge may occur; these conditions require the temporary discontinuation of the devices and attention to the cause(s) of the onset of the sepsis. Once these conditions have been dealt with, the expansion can be recommended.

The clinical experience in early 2003 covers over 2,000 patients. Lesions in most areas of the body have been treated. The illustrative material presented can be supplemented by referring to the www.Proxiderm.com, where some 150 cases are graphically described. While the principles of management enunciated above apply generally, mention is made of particular deviations and modifications that may apply to specific sites or lesions.

Pain Management

In general, as in intravenous catheters, indwelling needles, and orthopedic pins, tissue hook insertion of the Proxiderms may be uncomfortable and require local anesthesia/sedation. Thereafter some patients may experience a slight pulling sensation and analgesics may be necessary. The above does not apply to insensate patients such as those with diabetic neuropathy or paraplegia.

LESIONS OF THE LOWER EXTREMITY[4,5]

Thigh

Lesions of the thigh lend themselves to relatively easy closure because of the good blood supply and the substantial subcutaneous layer that moves easily over the strong fascia lata (Fig. 19–3).

Knee Joint

Traumatic and postoperative lesions that expose the knee joint and/or hardware associated with joint replacement present difficult situations that demand timely closure of the joint, together with preservation of joint mobility (Fig. 19–4). It is possible for the patient to undergo active supervised physiotherapy during the wound closure and thereby avoid limitation of movement.

Leg

The upper and lower halves of the leg have different anatomic features that impact on the healing of lesions. The muscles of the upper leg are large and become tendinous in the lower leg; the muscles of the lower leg, smaller than those in the upper leg, become tendinous in

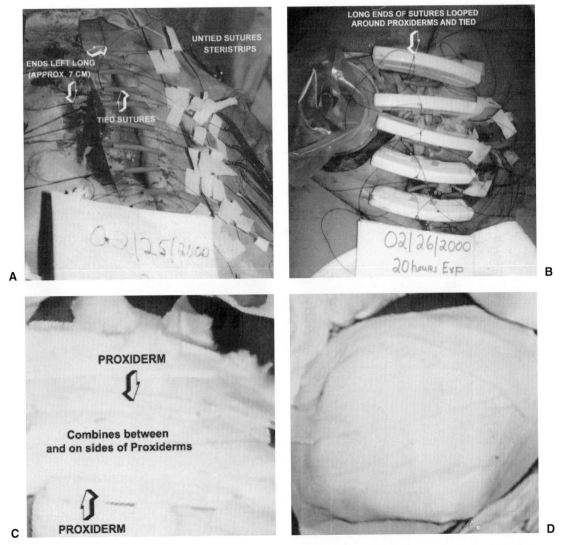

Fig. 19–2. **A.** Long ends of tied sutures left approx. 7 cm long. Long ends of untied sutures secured by Steristrips. **B.** Long ends of adjacent paired suture looped around Proxiderm and tied firmly. **C.** To prevent movement of Proxiderms, padded occlusive dressings are placed between the Proxiderms. **D.** Padded occlusive dressings placed on top of Proxiderms; Proxiderms and dressings secured to patient by Elastoplast and/or adhesive tape.

the foot. It follows that, in the upper leg, the arterial supply is superior and the muscle pump, on which the venous and lymphatic drainage are partly dependent, is more efficient. In addition, the subcutaneous position of the tibia renders it liable to open fractures that are more difficult to close in the lower leg.

Traumatic Lesions

Open tibial fractures are common lesions that require closure. Currently managed by muscle or myocutaneous flaps, local or free, certain cases can be managed by constant-tension skin approximation thereby avoiding major surgery (Fig. 19–5). Postoperative wounds may also expose the large tendons of the leg. Like bone, tendons require early coverage to prevent the onset of infection and/or necrosis. This situation is liable to occur in wounds resulting from extensive débridement (Fig. 19–6) and the common operation of decompression of the leg in cases of compartment syndrome (Fig. 19–7). In the latter situation, the closure of operative wounds

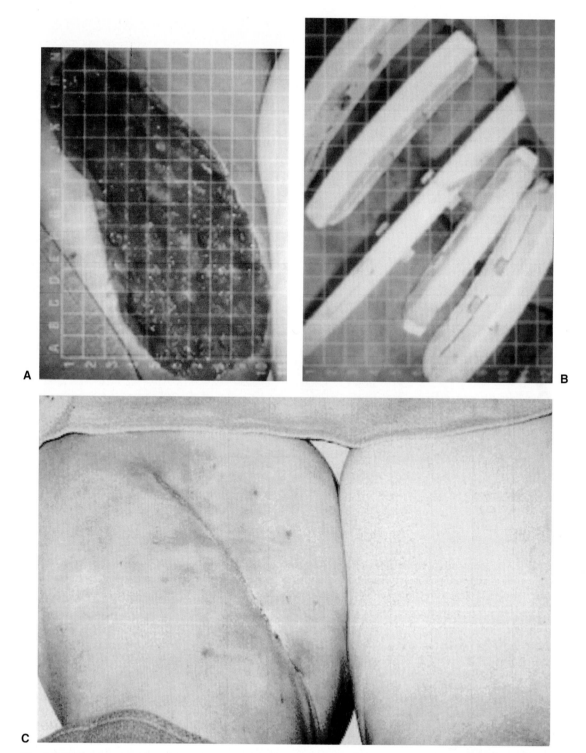

Fig. 19–3. **A.** A 60-year-old patient developed a large hematoma on the right thigh, which resulted in necrotizing fasciitis. Postdébridement, the wound measured 20.5 × 7.8 cm; appearance 4 days later. **B.** Proxiderms seen applied to wound. **C.** Two applications of Proxiderms; wound closed by suture on day 7; appearance at 18 days.

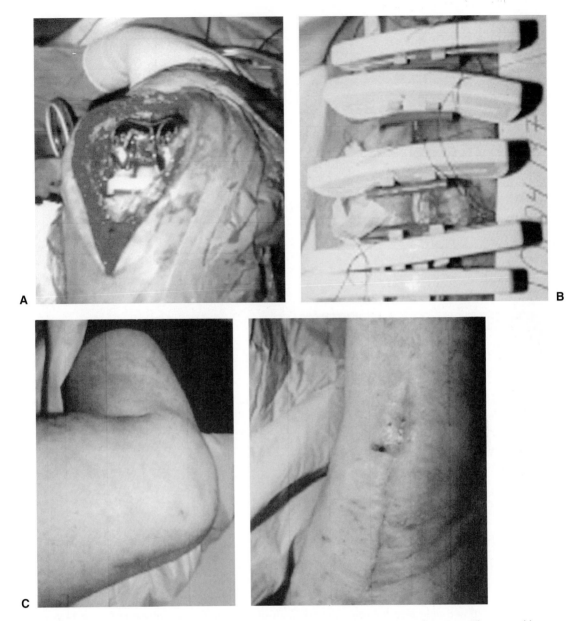

Fig. 19–4. **A.** A 71-year-old diabetic arthritic patient underwent a knee joint replacement. The wound became infected and dehisced, exposing the prostheses. **B.** Appearance following application of Proxiderms. Supervised physiotherapy was carried out during the healing process. **C.** Appearance at 1 month shows full flexion and a well-healed wound.

may result in disfiguring scars that require further treatment (Fig. 19–8).

Foot and Ankle

The foot and ankle are common sites for wounds that are generally difficult to close because of the deleterious effects of peripheral neuropathy, vascular disorders, and diabetes. In addition, with the feet being vital to weight bearing and ambulation, the healing of lesions by full-thickness skin and subcutaneous padding is mandatory; healing by secondary intention commonly results in scars that fail to stand up to the pressure of ambulation. The status of the peripheral circulation assumes great

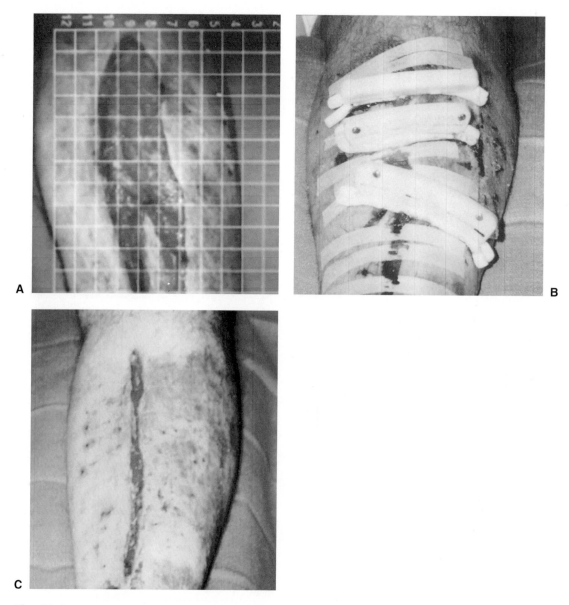

Fig. 19–5. **A.** Exposed tibia seen following débridement of an open fracture of the tibia in a 34-year-old patient caused by an avulsion injury as a result of a motor vehicle accident. **B.** Proxiderms seen applied to wound. **C.** Three applications of Proxiderms over 13 days; patient discharged.

importance in lesions below the level of the knee joint. The absence of peripheral pulses and/or the signs of ischemia, such as color and temperature changes and absent hair growth on the toes, demands further investigation. Positive Doppler auscultation is encouraging and the ankle/brachial indices (ABI) may be helpful. The latter test maybe questionable in the presence of calcified, incompressible vessels. It has been our experience that in patients with an ABI above 0.7 and with satisfactory signs of skin nutrition, the use of the Proxiderm devices has not caused untoward complications. Difficulties may arise with the application of the devices to lesions around the malleoli. Lesions on the borders of the foot and posterior heel will require right-angled devices. Wounds on the dorsum of the foot (an uncommon site) in thin patients may constitute a

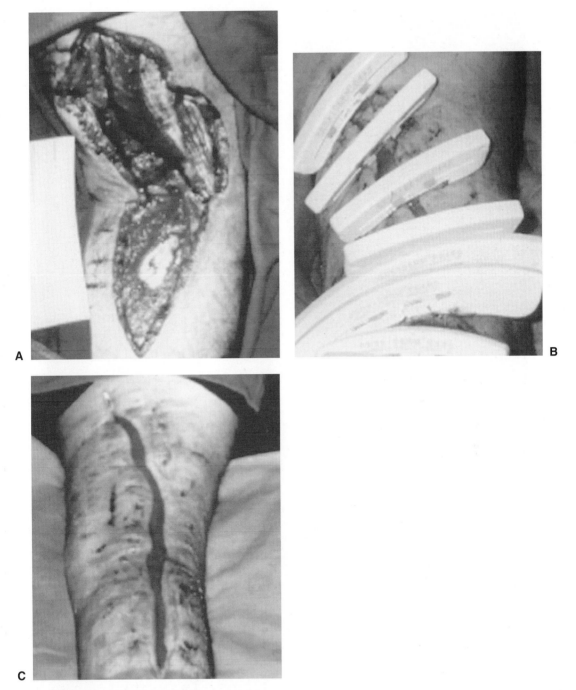

Fig. 19–6. **A.** Appearance of leg following extensive débridement of necrotic tissues as a result of an extension of Fournier's gangrene due to an inadequately drained perianal abscess in a 34-year-old patient. **B.** Application of Proxiderm devices. **C.** Appearance prior to discharge on 16th day. Reproduced with permission from, Wound closure by external tissue Expansion, *Annals of Plastic Surg.,* 1997; 38(4): 352–357.

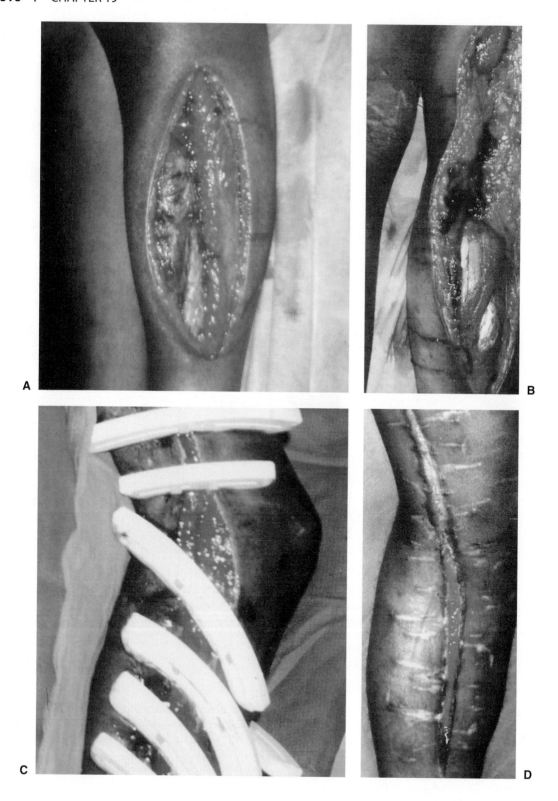

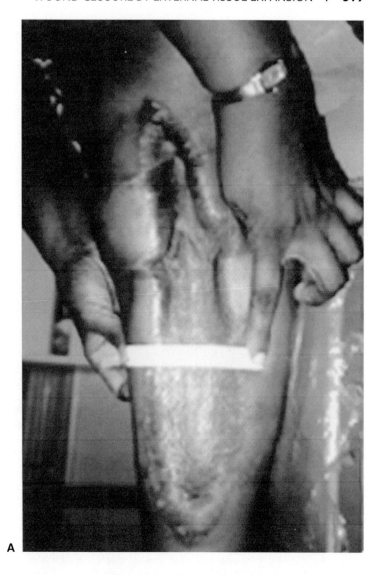

Fig. 19–8. **A.** A 53-year-old patient showing a poor cosmetic result following skin grafting procedures for closure of two postfasciotomy wounds of the same leg for decompression of a compartment syndrome 3 years previously. **B.** Proxiderms were applied anteriorly and laterally after excision of both skin grafts. **C.** Appearance at 6 weeks. **A**

contraindication to the use of the devices because of possible ensnaring of the tendons. Ambulation with weight-bearing devices attached to the foot is ill-advised and is a major problem with noncompliant patients. On the other hand, it is possible to treat certain cases on an outpatient basis; for example, a compliant patient who is to receive home care and can remain confined to bed for a week, can be satisfactorily managed. In all

circumstances, off-loading weight for 2 weeks after closure is advisable. In general, the most rapid healing will take place by off-loading weight and preventing edema by modest elevation of the limb. In favorable cases with relatively clean wounds and minimal discharge, patients have had their legs encased in an Unna boot. This compression bandage not only acts as a dressing that does not require changing, but also assists in the stabilization

Fig. 19–7. **A.** Appearance of leg following erroneous decompression of lateral compartment of the leg (seen on the right part of the wound) in a 21-year-old patient with an anterior compartment syndrome (seen on the left part of the wound). **B.** Postdébridement of necrotic anterior compartment structures. **C.** Wound with application of Proxiderm devices. **D.** Appearance on discharge at 16 days after several applications of Proxiderms. Patient is prone to the development of keloid wounds.

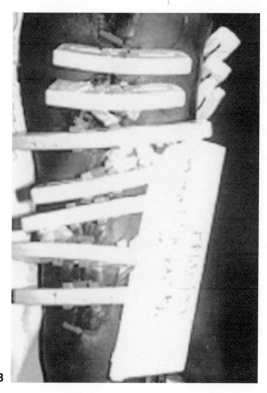

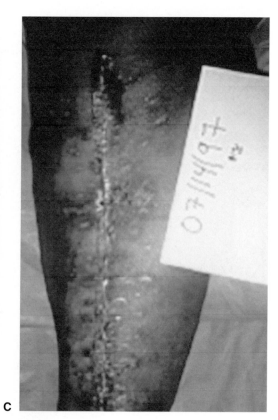

B **C**

Fig. 19–8. Continued

of the devices. In compliant and fitter patients, crutch walking is acceptable with or without a wheelchair. Debilitated and/or noncompliant patients need to be institutionalized, which can be at a reduced level of care.

The most common lesions treated were diabetic ulcers (Fig. 19–9), posttraumatic and postoperative defects, neuropathic ulcers, and pressure sores. Venous (stasis, postphlebitic) ulcers were not treated; the fibrosis and calcification/ossification of the skin and subcutaneous tissues prevent both approximation of the tissues, as well as angiogenesis and epithelial proliferation.

Experience has led to the adoption of certain practices. Suture of the margins of a small wound, for example,

under 2 cm, encapsulates contamination and can lead to wound breakdown and infection. Such a small wound should be converted into a fresh clean wound as described above and approximated by the Proxiderm devices only. Sutures can be used to complete the final-healing process when the skin approximation is well advanced.

The orientation of the devices is usually such that the devices are at a right angle to the long axis of the wound. This should be kept in mind when a wound is excised. For example, when closing a transmetatarsal or midtarsal amputation, the fashioning of a fish-mouth wound, rather than a long plantar flap, facilitates the application of the Proxiderm device (Fig. 19–10). In a heel ulcer

---

Fig. 19–9. **A.** A 68-year-old diabetic patient with a recalcitrant plantar ulcer of 4 months duration. Previous tissue flap procedure failed. **B.** Appearance after sharp débridement. Wound measured 3.8 × 5 cm. **C.** Wound margins sutured by number 2/0 nylon passed through rubber booties, other sutures left untied. **D.** Application of Proxiderms. **E.** Appearance at 2 days. Untied sutures tied. **F.** Appearance 7th postexpansion day. Proxiderm applied for an additional 2 days to allow wound healing in a tension-free environment. **G.** Appearance at 3 years. Reproduced with permission from Schessel E, Ger R, Wound Closure by External Tissue Expansion, *J. of Foot and Ankle Surg.*, 2000; 39(5).

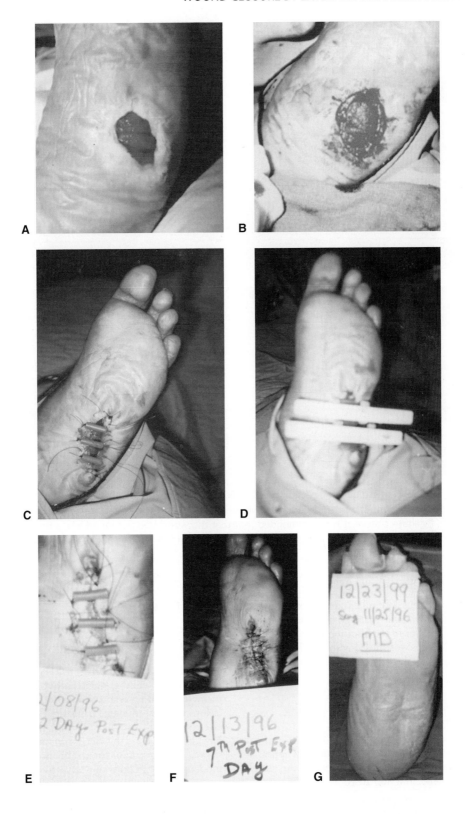

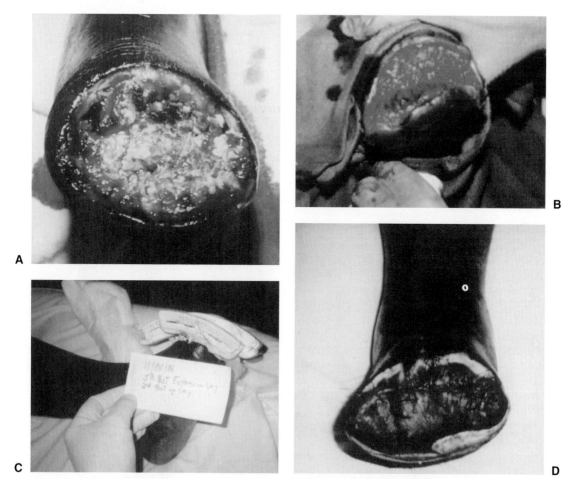

Fig. 19–10. A. A 62-year-old diabetic patient on dialysis with a marginal blood supply (ABI less than 0.7) underwent a transmetatarsal amputation. Appearance 2 weeks postamputation; below-knee amputation (BKA) recommended. **B.** To facilitate closure, it is recommended that that the wound be fashioned into a fish-mouth appearance, as seen in this photo of another patient. **C.** Application of Proxiderms in the above patient. **D.** Appearance at 7 days.

involving the calcaneus, wound closure is fascilitated by resection of the nonweight-bearing part of the tuberosity of the bone inferior to the insertion of the tendo calcaneus. Most wounds were closed within 7–10 days, but strict observance to the principles of wound healing need to be followed to achieve a well-healed stable wound.

PRESSURE SORES

Pressure sores are very common lesions whose treatment demands appear to be on the rise. Lesions can appear at any area, but the most common sites are the sacral, ischial, trochanteric, and heel areas.

Sacral Pressure Sores (Fig. 19–11)

These lesions are the most difficult to close because this area bears weight in the immobile patient and is commonly contaminated by bladder and rectal contents. Efforts to control the bowel so as to avoid postoperative fecal soiling are necessary; in this regard supplemental feeding is a common cause of diarrhea and lesions abutting the anal canal are especially problematic. In a small number of cases, the rectal contents have been diverted by the insertion of an intrarectal sleeve.[7] It is common for treatment in this area to be interrupted by periods of dedicated cleansing and irrigation. In some patients, especially the obese, the

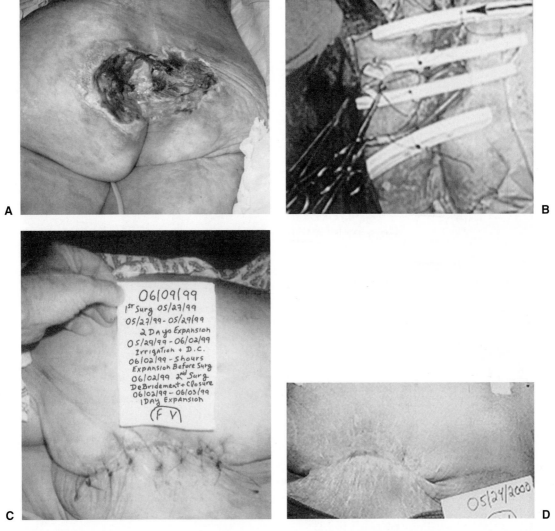

Fig. 19–11. **A.** Sacral pressure sore, 14.2 × 11.9 × 4.5 cm in size, in a 77-year-old patient. **B.** Excised wound 4 days after initial débridement. Four Proxiderms are seen, between which lie rubber booties containing 2/0 nylon sutures, whose long ends are looped around the devices for additional security (arrow). **C.** Appearance on 13th postoperative day showing intact 2/0 nylon sutures. **D.** Well-healed wound seen 1 year later. No recurrence. Reprinted from *British journal of Plastic Surgery*, **54**; Schessel ES. Ger R, The management of pressure sores by constant tension, approximation, 439–446, © 2001 with permission from Elsevier Ltd.

lesion may be quite deep; in these circumstances, a layered closure using 2/0 nylon sutures will assist in the obliteration of a dead space.

Ischial Pressure Sores (Fig. 19–12)

These lesions are somewhat easier to manage than sacral ulcers, as they are less likely to be soiled by the patient's effluents.

Trochanteric Pressure Sores (Fig. 19–13)

These lesions are the easiest pressure sores to manage because fecal contamination is uncommon. This situation may allow tissue expansion prior to definitive débridement and closure, a factor that may reduce the period of institutionalization (see later under prestretching). Undermining is usually necessary and extends for about 2–3 cm; wound evaluation may only be necessary every 2–3 days.

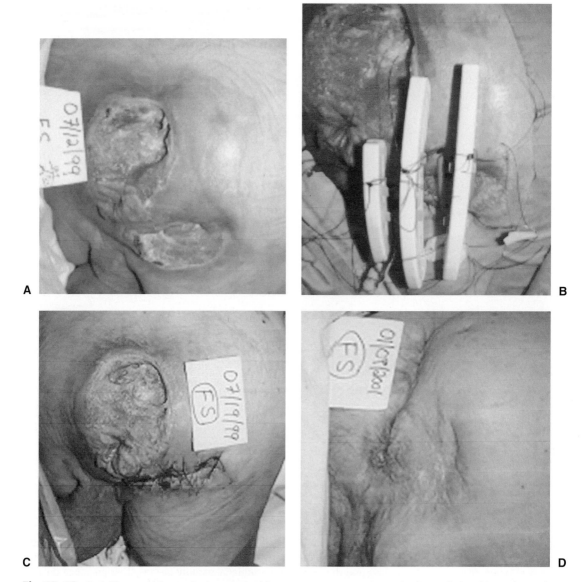

Fig. 19–12. **A.** A 62-year-old paraplegic patient with concurrent pressure sores in close relationship to the anal orifice; ischial measuring 5.3 × 10.9 cm and sacral measuring 9.4 × 10.5 cm **B.** Application of Proxiderms. The wounds were closed sequentially; the ischial being closed first. **C.** After 3 applications of Proxiderms the ischial pressure sore was closed by suture. Appearance 4 days postclosure. **D.** Appearance at 16 months: no recurrence.

Heel Ulcers (Fig. 19–14)

Local conditions often dictate the therapeutic approach. The skin at the margins of the ulcer is often fibrous, inverted, and adherent to the underlying structures, in which case the margins are sharply excised and undermined at a suprafascial level for about 10 mm. The wound is then approximated by sutures and Proxiderm devices are applied, using devices that best fit the local conditions and contour. An Unna boot supplants the Elastoplast dressing. The wound is evaluated at 2- to 3-day intervals, except in cases where a major amputation is being considered because of a marginal vascular supply, in which case daily inspections are necessary. In the event of the lesion involving the underlying bone, a common event, partial excision of the nonweight-bearing

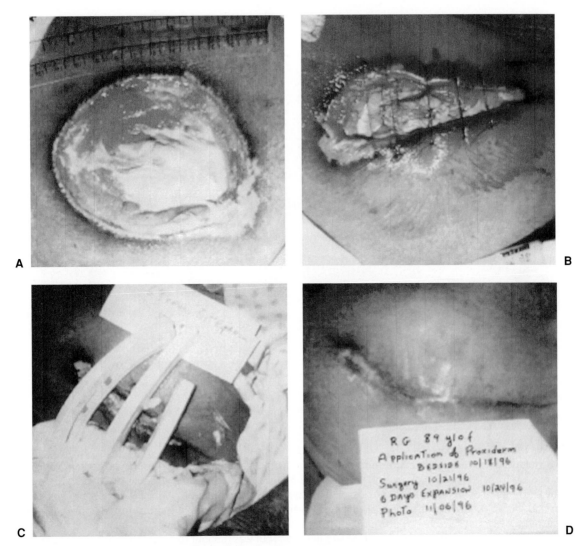

Fig. 19–13. A. A bone-based trochanteric lesion in an 89-year-old patient, measuring 12.5 × 9.2 cm. **B.** Proxiderm expansion for 63 hours has resulted in considerable approximation. **C.** Application of Proxiderms. A catheter has been placed in the wound for irrigation purposes. **D.** At 19 days satisfactory healing is present. The patient died 18 months later with a healed wound.

part of the tuberosity is performed. The latter maneuver, in any event, facilitates closure of the defect and is advisable in the larger pressure sore.

ABDOMINAL WALL WOUNDS[8]

Dehisced abdominal wall wounds are common and usually follow laparotomies that are associated with contamination (Fig. 19–15) and/or necrosis (Fig. 19–16). A five-

fold increase in the incidence of incisional hernias can be expected when postoperative wound infections complicate intra-abdominal operations.[9] It has been shown that delayed closure of skin and subcutaneous tissue in the infected abdominal walls of experimental animals, result in a stronger fascial closure than that obtained in primary wound closure.[10] Similarly, in a literature review of abdominal wall dehiscences over a 35-year period, it was concluded that delayed primary closure is preferable in

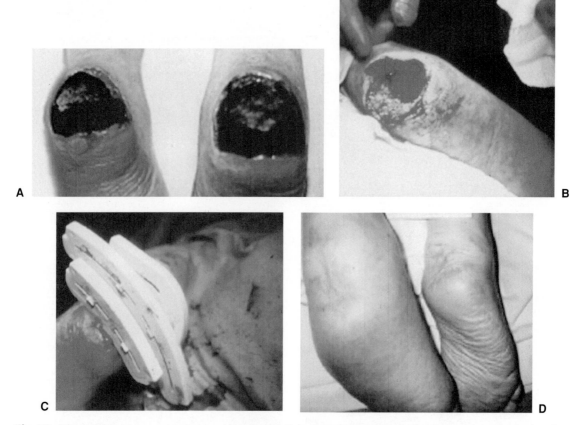

Fig. 19–14. **A.** Bilateral pressure sores in a 59-year-old diabetic patient, in poor general condition, who had undergone multiple unsuccessful procedures, including skin grafts, flaps, and muscle-transposition procedures over a 4-year period. The peripheral vascular supply was marginal. **B.** Appearance after surgical débridement of necrotic soft tissue and removal of nonweight-bearing portion of posterior calcaneus. **C.** Application of 3 Proxiderms of different sizes and shapes. **D.** Proxiderms were applied 4 times over a 6 week period, at which time the wound was healed. Appearance 2 years later. The heels remained healed for a further 2 years, at which time the patient succumbed from medical causes. The cause of the left leg edema was unknown, but was thought to be due to venous thrombosis.

cases where contamination has occurred as a result of surgery.[11] Furthermore, undue delay of approximation of the anterior aponeuroses appears to result in a higher incidence of herniations. Primary closure of a contaminated wound is an ideal that cannot currently be achieved. This importance of obtaining rapid wound closure is a tenet to which not all subscribe; some professionals in the field prefer to close the wound only when vents and fistulae are operatively sealed.[12]

Currently dehiscences are managed by control of the infection by systemic medications together with local wound toilette until local conditions allow delayed primary closure by a variety of methods or, if the latter are not possible, by secondary healing.

Because delayed healing carries significant disadvantages, a method of accelerating the delayed closure by full-thickness skin and subcutaneous tissue by external expansion is advantageous. The presence of fistulae has not delayed closure in our experience where fistulae lay lateral to the skin margins of the wound, only one being placed in the center of the wound. The method of closure follows the general principles described previously. In a series of 16 cases,[12] comorbid conditions were notably severe, the most common being cardiovascular disease. The ages

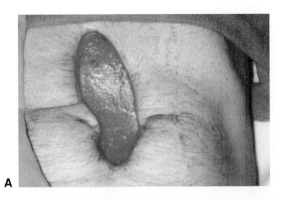

A

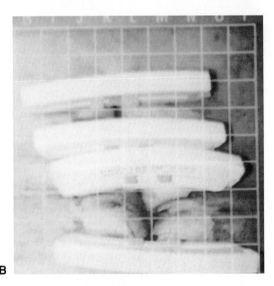

B

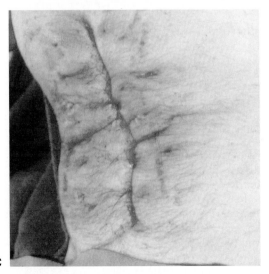

C

varied between 21 and 83 years, with an average of 55 years. The wounds tended to be large, measuring 29×24 cm to 10.5×5 cm, with the remainder falling between these parameters, except for the smallest wound that measured 7×4 cm, but 7.5 cm deep. Ten patients had one or more intestinal stomas, namely three colostomies, three ileostomies, and four bowel fistulae. Wound closure was achieved in an average time of 7.5 days with a maximum of 18 days and a minimum of 2 days. Contraindications are as described previously, with deep lesions in obese patients constituting a special problem.

THORACIC WOUNDS

Experience with these wounds are mostly in patients who undergo sternal splitting to gain access to the coronary arteries. While generally healing well, these incisions sometimes dehisce. Because these operations tend to occur in older and sicker patients, the morbidity and mortality from these complications are often of major significance and wound management is often complicated. Some of these cases had been unsuccessfully treated by pectoralis muscle flap operations (Fig. 19–17). All patients had serious pre- and postoperative morbid conditions and a technique that is simplistic and avoids major operative procedures is desirable. The principles of treatment were no different from those previously described.

BREAST SURGERY

Operations on the breast often require skin expansion in order to accommodate implanted prostheses. Current techniques using muscle and free flaps require extensive surgery, general anesthesia, a donor defect, a high degree of surgical skill, and are associated with complications—at times serious. External skin expansion is a simple rapid method, which requires a short stay in a ambulatory facility, minimal anesthesia, and modest surgical skill. The insertion of a 250- to 300-cc prosthesis requires 2–3 months of internal tissue expansion before a satisfactory breast mound is created. In contrast, external expansion can attain the same result in 4–6 days, the rate being approximately 60 cc per 24-hour period. The reconstruction can be carried out on an immediate or delayed basis.

Fig. 19–15. **A.** Abdominal wall, postcolectomy, in a 42-year-old patient; healing by secondary intention. **B.** Application of Proxiderms. **C.** Final result at 10 days following accelerated healing with the use of Proxiderm devices. Reproduced with permission from, The use of external tissue expansion in the management of wounds and ulcers, *Annals of Plastic Surg.*, 1997;**38**(4): 352–357.

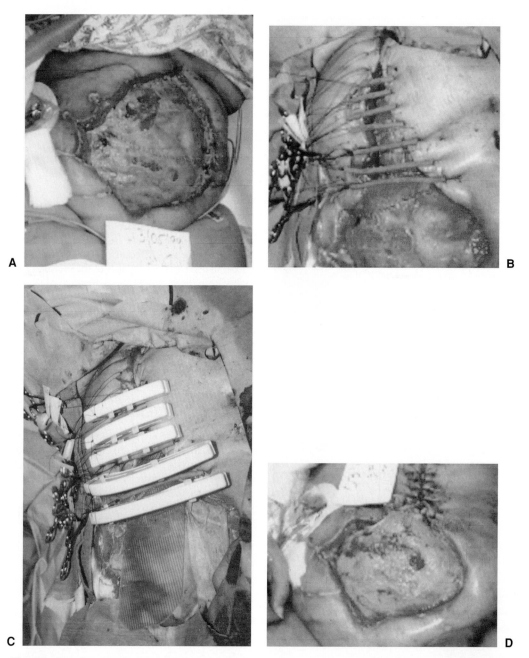

Fig. 19–16. **A.** Contaminated abdominal wall wound measuring 29 × 24 cm, with an ileostomy bag seen on the right, in a 73-year-old diabetic patient. A suture securing an implanted mesh is visible; both were removed. **B.** Nylon sutures are passed through rubber booties in the superior and cleaner part of the wound and tied; the ends are left long and secured by Steristrips. **C.** Proxiderms are seen in place and additionally secured by encirclement with the long sutures. **D.** The upper half of the wound closed by suture on the 3rd day. **E.** The same procedure as above was repeated in the lower half of the wound after a period of vigorous wound toilette. Appearance on 14th day with devices in place. **F.** The wound was closed by the 18th day; photograph taken 3 days later. Reprinted from American Journal of Surgery, V184, Schessel ES, Ger R, et al. The management of the postoperative disruptive abdominal wall, pp. 263–268, © 2002 with permission from Excerpta Medica.

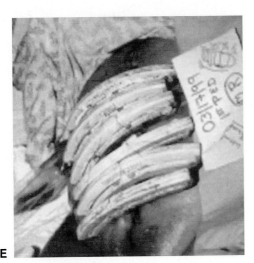

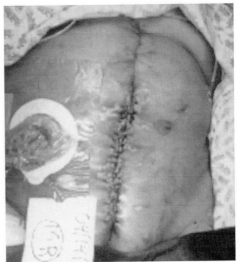

E   F

Fig. 19–16. Continued

Delayed Reconstruction (Fig. 19–18)

A 70-year-old patient, whose history included coronary artery bypass surgery 10 years previously and a left-sided mastectomy 7 years later, underwent augmentation reconstruction. The procedure, performed on an outpatient basis, consisted of four daily external expansions under local anesthesia and sedation. Preoperatively, the inframammary line was marked, after which a second line was marked 12 cm superiorly. Local anesthesia was placed along both these lines. Because of the cardiac history, ¼% xylocaine with 1/400,000 Adrenalin was used. Skin sutures were placed on the marked lines 2 to 3 cm apart and tied; the ends are left long. Four Proxiderms were applied on the marked lines and secured by the long ends of the previously tied sutures. Occlusive dressings were placed under the ends of the Proxiderms to prevent pressure on the skin, and on the sides and between the Proxiderms, and over the devices where they were secured to the patient by Elastoplast and/or adhesive tape to prevent dislodgement of the devices. A surgical brassiere and an Ace bandage were placed around the dressings and arm to prevent excessive motion.

In successive applications, needles and sutures were placed 3 to 4 mm from previous insertions so as to decrease the intensity of the skin markings and allow rapid fading. On day five, a 250-cc implant was placed under general anesthesia and the patient discharged 6 hours later. She resumed employment on the 11th postimplant day.

Immediate Reconstruction (Fig. 19–19)

A 48-year-old patient with a family history of breast cancer had undergone multiple breast biopsies over some years, the latest proved positive for cancer. Because her sister had suffered multiple complications following a Tram flap that resulted in a prolonged hospital stay, the patient underwent bilateral mastectomies followed by immediate reconstruction. At the conclusion of the mastectomies, the wound closures were observed to be under excessive tension. The following technique was adopted. A 0.2-mm silastic sheet was placed over the pectoralis major muscle as a spacer. After closure of the mastectomy wound, the inframammary line was marked, after which a second line was marked 12 cm superiorly. Four Proxiderms were placed. One tissue hook of the Proxiderm was inserted at the inframammary line as deeply as possible and the other as far superiorly as possible. Occlusive dressings were placed under the ends of the Proxiderms to prevent pressure on the skin, on the sides and between the Proxiderms, to prevent movement of the devices, and over the top of the devices, where they were secured to the patient by Elastoplast and/or adhesive tape to prevent dislodgement of the devices. A surgical brassiere and an Ace bandage were placed around the dressings. Three, 2-day applications of Proxiderms were carried out. On the 7th day, 300-cc saline implants were placed under general anesthesia. The needle marks disappeared after 2 months.

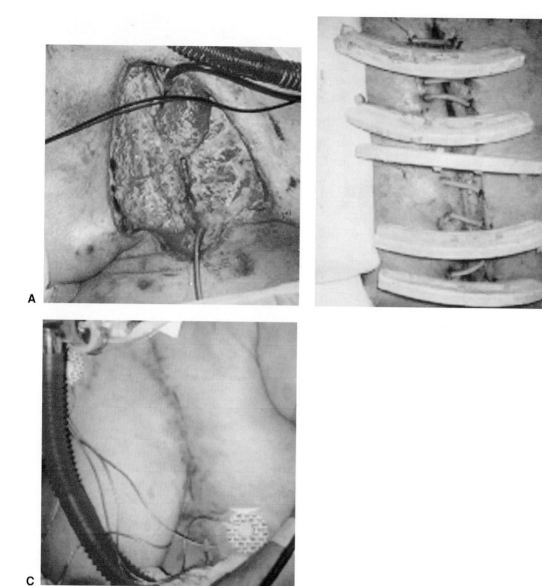

Fig. 19–17. **A.** A large presternal wound infected with antibiotic-resistant *Klebsiella* organisms is seen in an insulin-dependent 64-year-old patient, who had undergone a triple coronary artery bypass procedure. Débridement of the remains of the failed transposed pectoralis major muscle was performed. **B.** The superior portion of the wound is closed by a combination of sutures and Proxiderm devices. A tracheostomy is in place. An irrigating catheter is seen at the lower end of the wound. **C.** A well-healed wound is seen at 6 months.

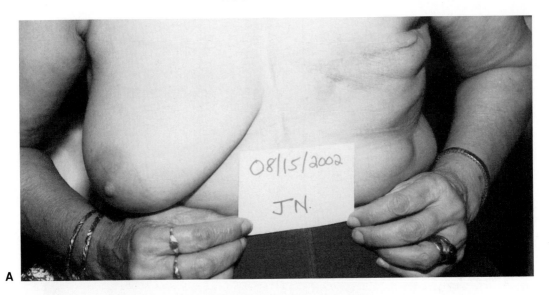

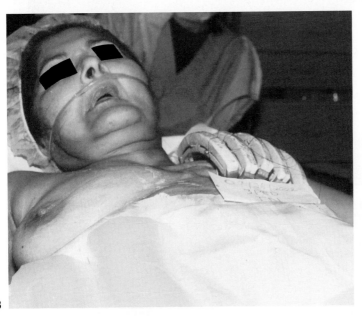

Fig. 19–18. **A.** Appearance of a 70-year-old patient, 3 years following a left mastectomy. **B.** Four Proxiderms are seen in place which are additionally secured by encircling sutures on 4th postexpansion day prior to insertion of an implant. **C.** Appearance 3 days after insertion of implant. **D.** Appearance 16 days postimplantation, illustrating the disappearance of the needle marks seen in Fig. 19-18**C**. **E.** Lateral view of breast postimplant.

HEAD AND NECK LESIONS

The head and neck is a common site for both benign and malignant lesions. In this region, it is possible to treat most patients on an outpatient basis and, in many cases, to prestretch the skin. The latter technique is particularly indicated when the postexcisional closure is difficult or might result in a visible deformity. Apart from simplifying the closure, the prestretching tends to avoid or minimize the degree of tension and the necessity for undermining of the skin. The result is an avoidance of damage to the vascular or lymphatic drainage of the skin

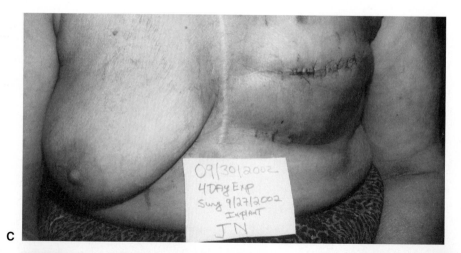

C

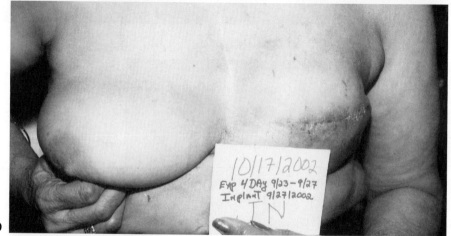

D

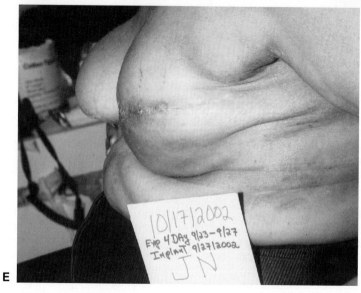

E

Fig. 19–18. Continued

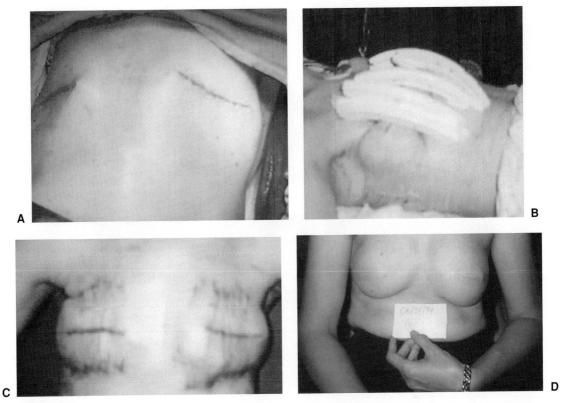

Fig. 19–19. A. Appearance of 48-year-old patient after bilateral mastectomy. **B.** Appearance after application of Proxiderm devices. **C.** Six days of Proxiderm tissue expansion. Appearance prior to implantation of breast prothesis. **D.** Appearance at 2 years. Stretch marks (seen in Fig 19 **C**) disappeared at 2 months.

with a superior cosmetic and functional result. Examples of a giant nevus (Fig. 19–20), a squamous cell carcinoma (Fig. 19–21), and a malignant lip lesion in a patient, who was considered unfit for surgery by the attending physicians (Fig. 19–22), are presented.

DISCUSSION

Special Considerations for Elderly Patients

Elderly patients in poor medical condition require special consideration. Separation of parts of the wound may exceptionally occur due to tardy healing, in which case the separation may be sutured or require another application of Proxiderms. Sutures are removed only when the margins are completely and strongly adherent. Adequate nursing care is mandatory, as these patients are prone to develop multiple pressure sores. Positional changes are important and patients are moved using an underlying turning sheet to avoid dragging across the bed, a procedure which may dislodge the devices.

Patients are placed in a 30% tilt by using supports under the shoulder blades, buttocks, and thighs, and the side is alternated every 2 hours. This degree of tilt avoids pressure on the trochanters and also facilitates turning. Elevation of the head of the bed is limited to less than 45% to avoid sliding. Finally, the closure of pressure sores with full-thickness skin and subcutaneous tissue by a minimally invasive method in patients who are generally in poor medical condition and often at an advanced age is an attractive alternative to a major surgical procedure; in most cases, the technique outlined earlier results in wound closure and healing.

Contraindications

In addition to those mentioned earlier, there are a number of special contraindications that may prevent the closure of pressure sores by means of constant-tension approximation. The presence of uncontrollable diarrhea in lesions close to the anal canal that leads to persistent soiling of the wound and the devices may preclude the use of

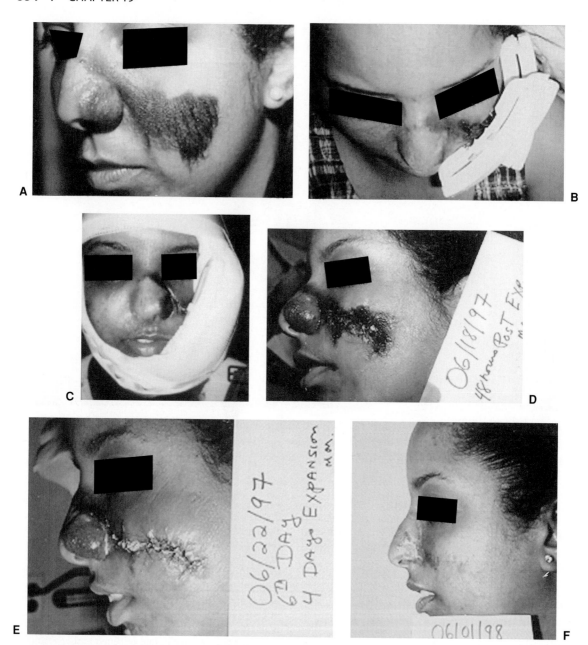

Fig. 19–20. **A.** A giant nevus involving the side of the face and nose is seen in a 22-year-old patient. **B.** Prestretching is carried out by application of Proxiderms. **C.** Method of immobilization of the devices. **D.** Appearance after 48 hours, showing inversion of the nevus. **E.** Further inversion of the lesion seen after 4 days expansion. **F.** The lesion was excised and sutured except for part of the lesion overlying the nasal cartilages, which was excised sharply and covered by a small skin graft taken from the ear. The final result is seen 1 year later.

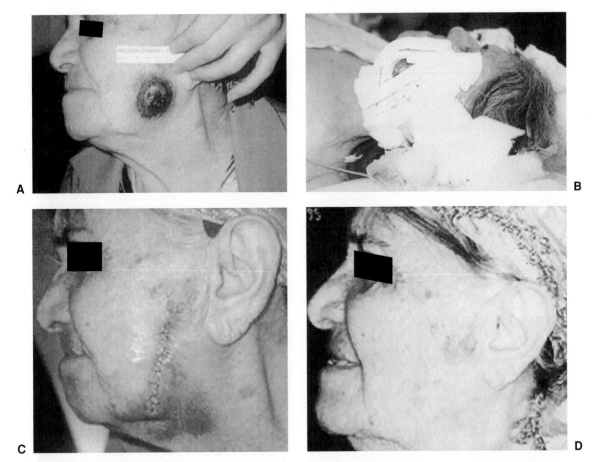

Fig. 19–21. **A.** A squamous carcinoma of the face of a 85-year-old patient. **B.** Prestretching was carried out by means of Proxiderm devices. **C.** The lesion was excised and the wound closed by primary suture. Note the absence of facial distortion. **D.** Appearance at 1 year.

this method. In lesions deeper than 6 cm in obese patients, closure of the subcutaneous cavity may be difficult; if the accurate placement of the deep sutures is not possible, this may constitute a further contraindication. With regard to foot lesions, an arterial supply with clinical signs of a marginal blood supply and an ABI below 0.7 may negate the use the constant-tension approximation.

Economic Considerations

The economic advantages of a relatively conservative and simplistic method to the patient and the health care system are derived from the earlier return of patients to their normal activities, the reduced use of the operating room, the avoidance of general anesthesia, and a reduction in the length of, or use of, hospitalization. Preoperative preparation before, and the postoperative convalescence

after, major surgery, are liable to be significant considerations in poor-risk patients. The care of a rapidly closing wound achieved by the technique described is both easier and less costly than a wound that is allowed to heal by natural means. Pressure sores, in particular, constitute a major economic problem. Costs continue to escalate as an increasing number of elderly people occupy specialized beds for longer periods. Approximately 17% of hospitalized patients develop pressure sores.[13] It is estimated that 4.5% of all elderly people in the United States reside in extended-care facilities and that, in the future, 25–40% of all elderly people will require the same extended care.[14]

In patients with lesser degrees of wound necrosis, the application of the devices 2–3 days before hospital admission for débridement and closure will allow earlier discharge of the prestretched smaller wound.

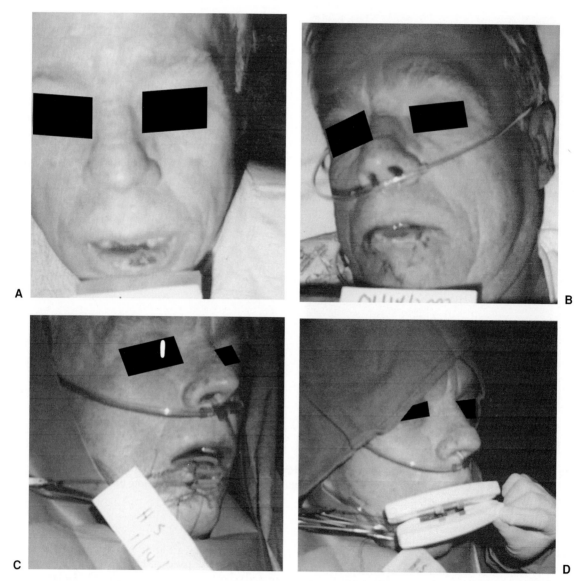

Fig. 19–22. **A.** Squamous carcinoma of the lip in a 62-year-old man is seen. **B.** Preoperative marking of lines of excision. **C.** Prestretching sutures placed through rubber booties. **D.** Application of Proxiderms for 1 day. **E.** Postexcisional defect of lip. **F.** Primary suture closure of the defect at surgery followed by 1 day of postoperative expansion. **G.** Appearance at 5 months.

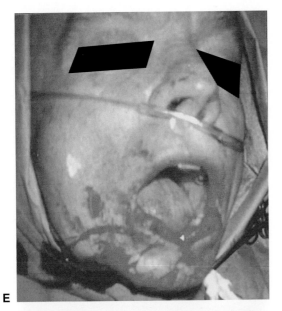

E

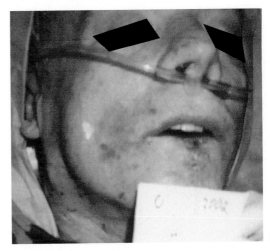

F

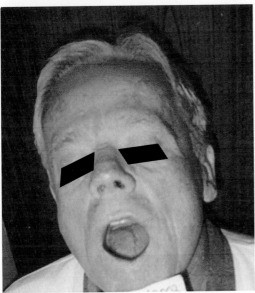

G

Fig. 19–22. Continued

REFERENCES

1. Neumann CG. Expansion of an area of skin by progressive distension of the subcutaneous balloon. *Plast Reconstruct Surg.* 1957;19:124–30.

2. Ger R. The use of external tissue expansion in the management of wounds and ulcers. *Ann Plast Surg.* 1997;38:352–357.

3. Austad ED, Thomas SB, Pasyk K. Tissue expansion: dividend or loan? *Plast Reconstruct Surg.* 1986;78:63–67.

4. Schessel ES, Lombardi CM, Dennis LN. External constant tension expansion of soft tissue for the treatment of ulceration of the foot and ankle. *J Foot Ankle Surg.* 2000;321–328.

5. Ger R. The management of neuropathic ulcers by the application of constant tension approximation: a preliminary study. *Minimally Invasive Surg.* 1996;171:179–182.

7. Ger R. Fecal diversion in management of large infected perianal lesions. *Dis Colon Thectum* 1996;39:1327–1329.

6. Schessel ES, Ger R. The management of pressure sores by constant-tension approximation. *Br J Plast Surg.* 2001;54: 439–446.

8. Schessel ES, Ger R. The management of disrupted abdominal wall wounds by constant tension approximation *Am J Surg.* 2002;184:263–268.

9. Mudge M, Hughes, LE. Incisional hernia: A 10 year prospective study of incidence and attitudes. *Br J Surg.* 1985;72: 70–71.

10. Johnson BW, Scott PG, Brunton JL, et al. Primary and secondary healing in infected wounds: an experimental study. *Arch Surg.* 1982;117:1189–1193.

11. Poole GV, Jr. Mechanical factors in abdominal wound closure; the prevention of fascial dehiscence. *Surgery* 1985;97: 631– 640.

12. Stone HH, Fabian TC, Turkleson ML, et al. Management of acute full-thickness losses of the abdominal wall. *Ann Surg.* 1981;1939:612–618.

13. Haalboom JRE. Pressure ulcers. *Lancet.* 1998;352:581.

14. Tresch DD, Simpson WM, Burton JR. Relationship of long-term and acute-care facilities: the problem of patient transfer and continuity of care. *J Am Geriatric Soc.* 1985;33: 819–826.

20 The Diabetic Foot: A Comprehensive Approach

Bok Y. Lee, Phyllis Berkowitz-Smith, V.J. Guerra, and Robert E. Madden

Introduction
Physiology
Pathophysiology
Hypercoagulable States
Role of Substance P in Diabetics with Peripheral
    Vascular Disease
Anatomy
Compartment Syndrome
Atherosclerosis
Tibial Atherosclerosis
Diabetic Peripheral Neuropathy
Perforating Ulcers of the Foot
Pathomechanics
Clinical Findings
Infections
Differential Diagnosis
Diagnostic Methods
Case Reports
    Case One
    Case Two
    Case Three

Case Four
Case Five
Case Six
Case Seven
Treatment
Antibiotic Therapy
Wound Care
Total-Contact Walking Cast
Treatment of Neurotrophic Ulcers
Amputation
    Toe Amputation
    Ray Amputation
    Transmetatarsal Amputation
    Major Amputation
Arterial Reconstructive Surgery
Lumbar Sympathectomy
Decompressive Fasciotomy
Preventive Procedures
Prognosis
References

INTRODUCTION

Diabetes mellitus is a disease characterized by hyperglycemia resulting from impaired insulin secretion and/or effectiveness. It is associated with risks for ketoacidosis or nonketotic hyperglycermia, hyperglycermic-hyperosmolar coma, and a group of late complications including retinopathy, nephropathy, atherosclerotic coronary and peripheral arterial disease, and peripheral and autonomic neuropathies. Diabetes has diverse genetic environmental and pathogenic origins.[1]

In the United States, diabetes affects approximately 12 million people of all ages. The presence of infection in the diabetic foot is an especially important clinical problem because lower-extremity infections are one of the most common reasons for hospital admission in the diabetic patient. Typically, diabetic patients with lower-extremity infections are in their fifth decade and have been diabetics for approximately 18 years, and although most are type 2 diabetics, they generally require insulin for blood glucose control. The hospital cost for amputations in the United States is over $1.2 billion, not including

Note: Chapter 20 is reproduced with permission from B.Y. Lee and B. Herz, *Surgical Management of Cutaneous Ulcers and Pressure Sores*, published by Hodder Arnold, 1998.

prostheses, rehabilitation, loss of income, and, frequently, loss of jobs. Loss of family income as a result of patient death adds to these expenses. Without doubt, the problem of foot infections in the diabetic patient population is costly to both the patient and society. Consequently, health care expenditures and medical efforts must be directed at patient education, prevention, early detection, and prompt treatment of foot infections.[2–4]

PHYSIOLOGY

Each day, during locomotion, the feet are exposed to continuous pressures and it is not surprising that foot infections are a frequent problem in the diabetic. The feet must not only support the body but must also absorb the impact forces of walking and running, adjust to uneven surfaces, provide leverage for propulsion, and accommodate the transverse rotational forces associated with knee and hip motions. A 150-pound active individual takes more than 10,000 steps per day and distributes more than 120 tons of force between his 2 feet for every mile traveled. The foot must withstand a tremendous amount of repetitive compressive, torsional, and shear forces every day. The thickened epidermis and dermis situated on loculated fatty tissue of the plantar foot pad effectively cushions these high-impact forces. The normal plantar surface can be viewed as a specialized anatomic region that absorbs the impact forces of locomotion while protecting the underlying soft tissues and bony structures. Consequently, factors that lead to alterations of the normal transmission of the forces of locomotion or to loss of sensation, as occurs in diabetic neuropathy, clearly potentiate the risk of local injury.[5,6]

PATHOPHYSIOLOGY

Diabetic foot infections often result in major (below-or above-knee) amputations (BKA; AKA). Although only 3% of diabetics are amputees, 50% of all nontraumatic major amputations of the lower extremities are performed on diabetics.[7] Previously, the natural history of the diabetic undergoing a BKA or AKA was poor, with two-thirds of the patients in some series dying within 5 years of their amputation.[8] Therefore, attention must be directed toward understanding the pathophysiological changes predisposing a diabetic patient to foot infections in order to prevent amputations and the subsequent poor prognosis. Ischemia and neuropathy are the major predisposing factors for the development of diabetic foot infections.[7,8]

In vitro and *in vivo* studies demonstrate increased tissue oxygen utilization during acute episodes of hyperglycemia.[9,10] This phenomenon appears to be due to the preferential shunting of glucose through the sorbitol instead of the glycolytic pathway, which results in decreased mitochondrial pyruvate utilization and

decreased energy production. This process has been termed hyperglycemia-induced pseudohypoxia.[10] The oxidation–reduction imbalance can be seen in poorly controlled diabetics, as well as in nondiabetics experiencing acute episodes of hyperglycemia lasting longer than 4 hours and is associated with elevated intracellular levels of fructose, sorbitol, and lactate. Increased levels of these metabolic products correlate with impaired neural, skeletal, and smooth muscle function, as well as increased capillary permeability. The potential clinical relevance of this event is that inhibitors of key enzymes of the sorbitol pathway (aldose reductase and sorbitol dehydrogenase) can limit neural, skeletal, and smooth muscle dysfunction in acute, but not chronic, hyperglycemia. This metabolic blockade of oxygen utilization in poorly controlled diabetics may explain why these patients experience a greater degree of tissue loss than nondiabetics after relatively mild ischemic episodes. These findings might also explain why diabetics are more prone to develop foot ulcerations than nondiabetics with comparable foot transcutaneous oxygen tensions. In addition, the increased capillary permeability resulting from pseudohypoxia is believed to accelerate atherogenesis by allowing atherogenic proteins and fatty acids access to the subendothelial space. This metabolic information suggests that control of hyperglycemia is important in both treatment of foot infections and the healing of ulcerations in the diabetic foot.[9-11]

The wound-healing abnormalities in patients with diabetes mellitus are the result of several factors. When carbohydrates are not available to cells for normal aerobic metabolism, oxidation of amino acids for caloric needs results in amino acid and protein depletion. When glycogenolysis and gluconeogenesis fail to provide glucose to meet the energy requirements for fibroblasts and leukocytes, they become dysfunctional and impaired wound healing results. In addition, the impaired healing appears to be related not only to an abnormal glucose mechanism but also directly to insulin. It has been demonstrated that topical application of insulin improves skin healing in mice. Other studies have shown that uncontrolled diabetic rats, exhibit improved wound healing with the administration of vitamin A.[11] Interestingly, hyperglycemia interferes with ascorbate transfer into fibroblasts and leukocytes, which also impairs the healing response. In fact, high ascorbate intake in rats increases collagen production in streptozotocin-induced diabetic rats.[11]

Impaired fibroblast and endothelial cell proliferation, epithelization, decreased collagen deposition, and reduced collagen strength are also characteristics of these streptozotocin-induced diabetic animals. In diabetic animals, beta fibroblast growth factor (β-FGF) reduces the degree of impairment of wound healing. Experimentally, many of those effects can be reversed by insulin and good glucose regulation if achieved after wound healing.[12]

Regarding increased susceptibility to infection, there has been a myriad of studies describing the poor inflammatory response in diabetic patients.[13] Abnormalities range from the inability of polymorphonuclear leukocytes to kill bacteria to T-cell defects.[13] In clinical practice, this means one must be extraordinarily aggressive surgically, excising necrotic tissue and using broad-spectrum antibiotics until the invasive organisms are identified; appropriate antibiotic therapy should then be given.

HYPERCOAGULABLE STATES

We have observed that a considerable number of diabetic patients who undergo surgery for either amputations or vascular reconstructive procedures experience a hypercoagulable state. Many patients, who have received heparin, have a poor response to heparin or have rebound phenomenon. Unfortunately, the current available laboratory techniques to determine the coagulation status or the adequacy of each patient's heparin effect are not ideal for ensuring the agent's efficacy and safety or the actual global status of the coagulation process. They are semiquantitative at best and there are inherent errors in the accuracy and specificity of their results, such as those from thromboplastin time, activated clotting time, and thrombin clotting time. In addition, the lack of a readily available, direct chemical assay for measuring heparin concentrations has limited the collection of pharmacokinetic data. Therefore, most of the patients who are given heparin are monitored using routine coagulation tests and may be under or over anticoagulated.

We have used the Surgical Analyzer, which is a hemostatic functional measurement instrument of the global coagulation process. The instrument uses an attached recorder to capture a continuous "signature" of the entire clotting process. Automated analysis shows the time of initial fibrin formation through fibrin gelation, full clot development, contraction, and lysis. The instrument is a useful tool for measuring clot formation, platelet function, and anticoagulant effect. The instrument has an axially vibrating probe immersed to a controlled depth into a cuvette containing a small measured sample of blood. The viscous drag (viscous impedance) of the probe by the blood is sensed by the transducer. The electronic circuitry quantifies the drag as a change in electrical output. The signal is transmitted to a time-based strip chart recorder, which provides a "signature" of the clot formation, clot contraction, and clot lysis processes. Two values are obtained (1) SonACT time (onset) is defined as the time for the first fibrin strands to form and is mediated by the extrinsic and intrinsic clotting mechanisms. SonACT time, normal value is 85–130 seconds. (2) Clot RATE is defined as the rate at which fibrin mass is generated and demonstrates the speed at which fibrinogen is being transformed to fibrin. The

acceptable range of rate in nonheparinized samples is 15–35%. The "signature" also permits measurement of the clot retraction time; normal values are less than 30 minutes and measures the platelet retraction process. The results obtained by the Surgical Analyzer have been compared to thromboelastography, which also evaluates the global hemodynamics of blood using three values. The direct-writing thromboelastograph is an instrument with a stylus that traces the thromboelastogram on heat-sensitive paper. The thromboelastogram is obtained by the oscillation of a cuvette containing 0.3 cc of blood. The thromboelastogram gives three main values: (a) reaction time (r time), normal: 8–12 minutes; (b) k time, normal: 4–8 min, and (c) maximum amplitude (ma), normal: 50 mm. We established normal values of the Surgical Analyzer in patients under general anesthesia (SonACT time 80–130 sec), clot RATE 15–40%). We then measured the coagulation status in patients undergoing arterial reconstructive procedures with the thromboelastograph (Fig. 20–1) and the Surgical Analyzer (Fig. 20–2).

We found that the Surgical Analyzer provides (1) improved hemostasis management in surgery, (2) reduced use of donor blood products, (3) faster identification of surgical versus nonsurgical bleeders with results are obtained in 5–10 min, (4) accurate and inexpensive heparin anticoagulation management, and (5) quick and easy screening for hypercoagulable states. Heparin has been shown to produce the following effects on the Surgical Analyzer signature: (1) the sample has a longer SonACT time, (2) the gelation phase occurs more slowly, and (3) clot retraction is very slow or not even observed, which is indicative of reduced platelet activity.

Although our purpose has been to find a reliable method to assess heparinization, we have also found the Surgical Analyzer to be useful in assessing patients with hypercoagulable states. We found that diabetic patients who undergo amputation or foot débridement for treatment of foot infections experience a transient hypercoagulable status during the operation detected in at least 30% of the cases. Therefore, it seems reasonable to find a strategy that protects these patients who have a hypercoagulable status that could cause further damage to the vascular tree.[14–21]

ROLE OF SUBSTANCE P IN DIABETICS WITH PERIPHERAL VASCULAR DISEASE

Substance P is a small peptide (Arg-Pro-Lys-Pro-Gln-Gln-Phe-Phe-Gly-Leu-Met-NH$_2$) derived from a single gene of preprotakinin A found in both unmyelinated C fibers and thinly myelinated Aδ afferent sensory fibers. *In vitro* and *in vivo* studies[23,24] have shown that substance P modulates neurogenic pain sensation and acute

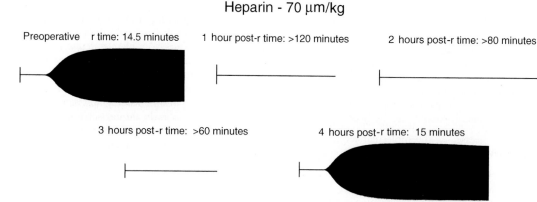

Heparin - 70 µm/kg

Preoperative   r time: 14.5 minutes   1 hour post-r time: >120 minutes   2 hours post-r time: >80 minutes

3 hours post-r time: >60 minutes   4 hours post-r time: 15 minutes

Fig. 20–1. Thromboelastograph tracings of a patient undergoing a vascular reconstructive procedure. Baseline tracing showing a normal coagulation tracing. After bolus administration of 70 units/kg of heparin there is straight line tracing at first hour and second hour showing anticoagulation effect: third hour still depicting effect and rebound phenomenon in the fourth hour.

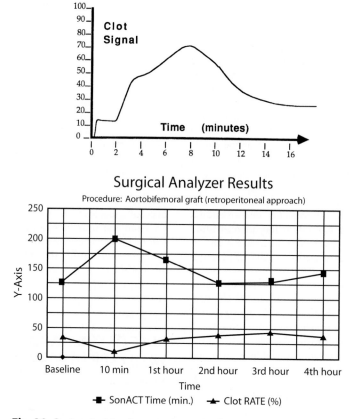

Fig. 20–2. Surgical Analyzer tracings. The first graphic shows a typical normal tracing and the results during arterial reconstructive procedure.

and delayed inflammatory reaction and stimulates proliferation of smooth muscle cells. Based on our own studies, we have identified, for the first time, substance P in the ventral root sympathetic ganglia and chain, in 20 patients with severe arterial insufficiency and/or nonhealing diabetic ulcers who underwent lumbar sympathectomy. Our data suggests that substance P is involved in the pathophysiology of chronic inflammatory reaction at the molecular level in diabetic patients with artherosclerotic occlusive disease. At the molecular level, lumbar sympathectomy may play an important role in the management of chronic inflammatory reactions, local plasma extravasation, endothelial cell proliferation, impaired wound healing, and immune response, perhaps by reducing an afferent–efferent sympathetic reflex to injury, which perpetuates the local inflammatory response.[22–24]

ANATOMY

All of the arterial supply of the foot is derived from the popliteal artery. At the lower border of the popliteus muscle, the popliteal artery divides into anterior and posterior tibial arteries. The anterior tibial artery penetrates the upper part of the interosseous membrane and enters the anterior compartment of the leg. Distally, it lies between the tibialis anterior and extensor muscles. At the ankle, the anterior tibial artery lies more medially and crosses the ankle joint anteriorly, becoming the dorsalis pedis artery. The dorsalis pedis artery usually lies laterally to the extensor hallucis longus muscle. In the space between the first and second metatarsal, the dorsalis pedis artery generally divides into a deep plantar dorsal metatarsal branch. The peroneal artery arises from the posterior tibial artery approximately 2.5 cm below the lower border of the popliteus, passes obliquely toward the fibula, and descends along its medial crest in a fibrous canal between tibialis posterior and flexor hallucis longus. It is then behind the tibiofibular syndesmosis and divides into calcanean branches, which ramify on the lateral and posterior surfaces of the calaneus. The posterior

Table 20–1. Compartments of the foot

Compartment	Muscles
1. Central	Adductor hallucis, quadratus plantae, flexor digitorum brevis, and flexor digitorum longus
2. Medial	Flexor hallucis longus, flexor hallucis brevis, and abductor hallucis
3. Lateral	Flexor digiti minimi brevis and abductor
4. Interosseous	Interossei muscles[1]

[1]From Ref. (7).

tibial artery accompanies the tibial nerve. The artery lies between the tibialis posterior and flexor digitorum muscle and the soleus muscle and tendon of the calcaneus. In the plantar space, the posterior artery divides into the medial and lateral plantar arteries. These arteries accompany the medial and lateral plantar nerves. The plantar arch is formed by anastomosis between the medial and lateral plantar arteries, with a branch of the dorsalis pedis artery at the first intermetatarsal space. Small dorsal digital arteries arise from an inconstant dorsal arcuate branch of the dorsalis pedis artery. The plantar digital vessels arise from the plantar arch. The plantar arch varies in detail, but in healthy individuals it provides abundant opportunity for collateral circulation in the distal foot. The arterioles of the skin form an internal vascular belt at the junction between subcutaneous tissue and dermis. Arising from the internal vascular belt are dermal plexi that are intimately interconnected, forming a reticular network of vessels of different sizes. From this network, arboreal terminal branches from a subpapillary plexus with capillary loops in the dermal papillae, which integrate a number of papillae into vascular districts that are also interconnected.[25]

There are four compartments of the foot: medial, central, lateral, and interosseous (Table 20–1 and Fig. 20–3). The first three are on the sole of the foot and are

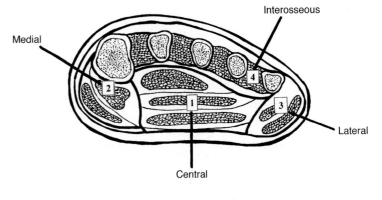

Fig. 20–3. Cross-section of the four compartments of the foot.

called the plantar compartments. The floor of the plantar compartments consists of the rigid plantar fascia and the roof is formed by the metatarsal bones and the interosseus fascia. The medial compartment is separated from the central compartment by the medial intermuscular septum, which extends from the medial calcaneal tuberosity to the head of the first metatarsal. This compartment contains the muscles associated with the great toe: the abductor hallucis, the flexor hallucis brevis, and the flexor hallucis longus. (The first limit is the shaft of the first metatarsal bone.) The medial intermuscular septum is incomplete, as it is perforated by the flexor hallucis longus passing into the central compartment. The flexor hallucis longus also has a slip connecting it to the flexor digitorum longus and the peroneus longus. The medial intermuscular septum is also breached distally where the oblique head of the abductor hallucis passes from the central to the medial compartment. Proximally, the septum is breached by the lateral plantar neurovascular bundle. Its deep attachments are the navicular bone, posterior tibial tendon, medial cuneiform bone, and lateral side of the first metatarsal bone.[26]

The central compartment contains the flexor digitorum brevis, quadratus plantae, flexor allucis longus, peroneus longus tendon, posterior tibial tendon, lumbricales, and adductor hallucis.[27,28] Jones[29] includes the lateral head of the flexor hallucis brevis in the central compartment. The medial intermuscular septum forms the medial boundary of the central compartment. Similarly, the lateral intermuscular septum forms the lateral boundary. The central component of the plantar fascia forms the superficial border and the metatarsal bones and interossei fascia provide the deep border. The central compartment is triangular in shape (its apex being proximal) and is divided into several fascial spaces. The medial intermuscular septum separates the intrinsic muscles of the great toe from the soft tissue structures of the central compartment: the extrinsic flexor tendons of the toes, medial and lateral plantar nerves and plantar vascular arches, and intrinsic muscles of the second through fourth toes.

In the lateral compartment are the muscles associated with the fifth toe: the abductor digiti quinti, the flexor digiti quinti brevi, and the adductor of the fifth toe. The medial boundary of the lateral compartment is the lateral intermuscular septum, which arises from the aponeurosis and extends from the medial tubercle of the calcaneus to the medial side of the head of the fifth metatarsal. The septum is found in the interval between the abductor digiti quinti brevis and flexor digitorum brevis. The lateral intramuscular septum is incomplete, as it is breached by the lateral plantar artery and nerve where they exit the central compartment through the second layer midway between the calcaneus and the fifth metatarsal, to enter the lateral compartment and, later, when they reenter the central compartment approxi-

mately 2.5 cm distal to the base of the fifth metatarsal entering the fourth layer.[30]

The interosseous compartment is bound by the interosseous fascia and the metatarsals and contains the seven interosseous muscles.[30,31]

Because these four deep compartments are bounded by rigid fascial and bony structures, edema associated with an acute infection may induce a rapid elevation in compartment pressures, resulting in ischemic necrosis of the confined tissues. Studies done by Goldman,[32] who injected fluid into the compartment, showed that the lateral compartment has the least potential space, the central compartment has the largest potential space, and the medial compartment has a potential space greater than that of the lateral, but less than that of the central.

In infection, bacterial spread from one compartment to another may take place at the proximal calcaneal convergence or by direct perforation through the intercompartmental septa. However, because each compartment is bound by rigid fascial separations in the medial-to-lateral and dorsal-to-plantar directions, the lateral or dorsal spread of infection is a late sign of infection. Based on the anatomy of the foot, deep space foot infections frequently show little plantar or dorsal foot abnormality. Therefore, a patient presenting with mild swelling of the foot, but toxic systemic symptoms, must be evaluated for an occult deep space infection. The deep potential spaces or compartments of the foot can allow a spread of bacteria from the plantar surface or web spaces of the foot to the ankle and lower leg region.[33–35]

COMPARTMENT SYNDROME

Compartment syndrome is a well-described clinical entity that results from increased pressure within a myofascial compartment. Mubarak and Hargens[36] introduced the concept of compartment syndrome of the foot and focused on the interossei compartment. They presented a possible treatment by decompression done with longitudinal incisions of the dorsum of the foot. Later, Whitesides[37] anecdotally described isolated compartment syndrome of the foot secondary to burns and direct trauma and recommended decompression via the medial approach of Henry. The signs and symptoms of compartment syndrome of the foot appear to be similar to that of compartment syndromes in general—a degree of pain that is out of proportion to the injury appears to be the first symptom. An early clinical sign reported by Bonutti and Gordon[38] was paresthesia in the distribution of the digital nerves of the toes, especially to pinprick, two-point discrimination, and light touch. Pain with passive dorsiflexion of the toes is also an important sign, although direct trauma may cause similar symptoms. Pallor, paresthesia, and a palpable tense compartment

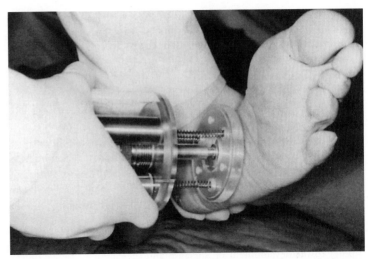

Fig. 20–4. Application of viscoelastic measurement device to the central compartment of the foot.

have also been reported. We believe that the intracompartmental pressure of the foot is important, not only because of increased interstitial pressure, but also because of the increased gravitational effect sustained by the foot.

We have measured the pressure of the foot compartments using the Stryker catheter and with a noninvasive device. We developed a noninvasive viscoelastic measurement device consisting of an instrumented hand-held probe, an electronic surface unit, and an X-Y plotter for the data display. The hand-held probe has a center indenter mounted at the end of a force transducer (Fig. 20–4). This device measures displacement and force, which gives the change in tissue volume, as muscle and fascia sheets form an enclosed space with a constant pressure and tissue compliance (Fig. 20–5). The results obtained with this device give an accurate measurement of the interstitial pressure of the compartment of the foot. The results obtained with the viscoelastic measurement device have been compared to those of the Stryker catheter and have correlated well. We believe that the compartment pressures of the foot play an important role in foot infections, reperfusion injury, and trauma, and may also be an important factor in neurotrophic ulcers.[36–38]

ATHEROSCLEROSIS

It is believed that alterations in glucose metabolism are followed by alterations in lipid metabolism. It is no wonder that a diabetic patient has his or her share of common aortoiliac and femoral popliteal atherosclerosis. The development of peripheral arterial disease can be documented in more than 50% of long-term diabetics. In a study of diabetics diagnosed within a single year, it was noted that in 22% of patients, lower-

extremity vascular calcifications were apparent in plain radiographs and that 13% lacked one or more ankle pulses. Atherosclerosis manifests at an earlier age in diabetics and tends to involve distal and smaller peripheral vessels. For example, multisegmental occlusive patterns occur more commonly below the popliteal region in diabetics than in age-matched control subjects and the metatarsal arteries are occluded in as many as 60% of diabetics. In contrast, the incidence of aortoiliac occlusive disease tends to be similar in diabetic and nondiabetic patients. Because of the frequent association of

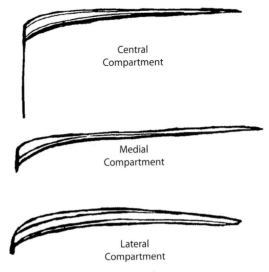

Fig. 20–5. Viscoelastic displacement curves for the three compartments of the plantar surface of the foot.

atherosclerotic peripheral disease with diabetes, as well as the increasingly encouraging results of vascular reconstruction in this patient population, the presence of reconstructable peripheral vascular disease should be considered in diabetic patients with extremity soft-tissue infections.

There are no pathognomonic capillary or arteriolar lesions associated with diabetes. Intimal thickening of the basement membrane, originally attributed to diabetics, is also found in 23% of nondiabetics. This microcapillary angiopathy seems to be variable in its tissue penetration from one patient to another, and its role in the development of foot capillary vessel alterations is questionable. Therefore, one should not assume that vascular reconstructive procedures in the diabetic are doomed to failure. In diabetics, a metabolic form of tissue ischemia related to hyperglycemia probably contributes to the development of infection and increased susceptibility to tissue injury.

TIBIAL ATHEROSCLEROSIS

The diabetic has a propensity to develop arteriosclerotic lesions in the small arteries below the knee and the foot. These lesions are not of the same microangiopathy as those associated with blindness and renal failure. Rather they are histologically typical atherosclerotic lesions involving arteries less commonly involved in patients without diabetes. If a patient presents with a necrotic forefoot and has a popliteal pulse, the chances are overwhelming that he or she is a diabetic, as other conditions such as Buerger's disease and collagen vascular diseases affecting these arteries are exceedingly rare.[35,39,40]

DIABETIC PERIPHERAL NEUROPATHY

Peripheral neuropathy clearly predisposes the patient to injury, which potentiates the risk of bacterial invasion and infection. Peripheral neuropathies are found in as many as 55% of diabetics and the incidence of neuropathies increases with the duration of the disease. The clinical spectrum and presentation of diabetic neuropathies vary greatly; initial symptoms are paresthesias, unpleasant dysesthesias, or hypersensitivity to touch. In some patients, these initial symptoms progress to complete loss of sensation. Whether the neuropathy is due to progressive distal axonopathy or focal compressive neuropathy, the results are decreased plantar sensation, intrinsic muscle atrophy, and lack of autonomic glandular and vasomotor responses. Skin insensitivity limits the patient's ability to respond to foot trauma. Intrinsic muscle atrophy produces tendon imbalances that expose the metatarsal heads to excessive trauma and shift the weight-bearing portion of the foot from protected to unprotected portions of the plantar surface. Ultimately, repetitive unprotected trauma results in bony and ligamentous rearrangements that lead to further tissue inflammation and breakdown. Autonomic dysfunction plays a significant role in diabetic foot infection, as the lack of autonomic innervation to the foot results in scaly, cracked, dry skin, decreased vasomotor tone, and edema, all of which predispose to foot infection.

The exact mechanism and relationships of the metabolic disturbances observed in diabetics to the subsequent development of neural dysfunction are still being debated.[41-46] However, an important role of linolenic acid, a prostaglandin precursor, appears likely, based on multicenter studies demonstrating that the treatment of diabetes with prostaglandin E_1 or high doses of γ-linolenic acid stabilizes and occasionally improves mild diabetic peripheral neuropathy.[46] In addition, some evidence suggests that a subgroup of diabetic patients with polyneuropathy have unsuspected concomitant compressive neuropathy that may benefit from surgical decompression. Because the development of peripheral neuropathy plays a major role in the pathogenesis of diabetic foot infections, efforts to diagnosis the type of neuropathy and therapy directed at preventing, limiting, or reversing diabetic neuropathy are of major importance. Peripheral neuropathy may be mild or severe. If mild, modification of the weight-bearing surface is effective. If severe, one should give early attention, in therapeutic attempts, to recreate a functional limb.[41-46]

PERFORATING ULCERS OF THE FOOT

Perforating ulcers of the foot are of major clinical significance, as they can lead to complications such as sepsis, protein wasting, soft tissue and bone necrosis, and eventual amputation. The management of perforating ulcers remains a complex problem. Overzealous surgical intervention has its associated complications. At times, failure of the surgery can lead to an even larger area of ulceration. Difficulty in the management of perforating ulcers is compounded by the inability to accurately assess the pathogenesis of perforating ulcers. Ulcerations on the plantar surface of the foot are usually associated with specific diseases, such as diabetes mellitus, syringomyelia, syphilis, and severe peripheral neuropathy. Perforating ulcers are associated with trauma or local pressure that initiates tissue breakdown with associated repetitive mechanical injury. In the neuropathic patient, this problem is further compounded by the relative or absolute insensitivity of the foot. As a result, small lesions in the foot may go unrecognized by the patient and become large ulcers.

Clinically, ulceration begins as a flattened callous beneath a small joint or bone, particularly in the metatarsal region, which is subject to point pressure. With repeated trauma, deformity of the bony structure, ischemia, or subcutaneous neurosis develops, clinically showing as swelling, hematoma, and inflammation. The inner portion of the ulcer may slough with or without exudates and fistulae may from. Fibrotic and sclerotic changes surrounded by a dense circumferential epidermis occur in the distal connective tissue. Subsequent soft-tissue breakdown can lead to exposure of the bone and joint surfaces, which may become secondarily infected.

Perforating ulcer was described as early as 1818 by Mott. He observed the thick, hard cuticle surrounding the plantar ulcer, as well as the insensitivity of the foot. It was not until 1852, when Nealton reported an unusual condition in the bony structure of feet leading to ulceration and when Vesignie coined the term *plantaire mal perforant*, that this ulcer received universal attention. However, it was in 1872 that Duplay and Morat reported these lesions to be neuropathic in origin and substantiated this concept by producing similar changes in the skin of denervated limbs of animals. In 1884, Treves reported ulcerations of the foot in ataxic individuals who had not experienced any alteration of sensation. Treves believed ulcer development to be secondary to the normal pressure associated with standing and movement and that once the ulcer became infected, the infection followed the course of least resistance to the bone. The following year, Kirmission reported diabetes as an associated condition with perforating ulcer of the foot. Fifty years later, Jordon described the first diabetic Charcot's joint. Ulceration was observed beneath the metatarsophalangeal joint with sensation intact at the periphery of the ulcers. Surgical dissection into deeper structures beneath the ulcer could be made without pain to the patient. In 1953, Martin reported an incidence of 22% of neurotrophic joints in diabetic patients attended at Kings College Hospital. Martin stated that diabetic neuropathy was responsible for the associated soft-tissue, joint, and bone changes leading to perforating ulceration. In such patients, it was believed, damage to nonmyelinated nerve fibers occurred earlier than to myelinated nerves, thereby lowering tissue resistance and predisposing the skin to more extensive trauma. Cutaneous ulcers associated with neuropathic arthropathies led a number of authors, notably Hodgsen, Pugh, and Young, in 1948, to suggest that infection leading to osteomyelitis was the direct cause of bone changes, independent of any associated nerve disorder.

In 1964, Classen (in Lee and Brancato[47]) presented the results of conservative and surgical treatment in 45 cases of plantar perforating ulcers of the foot. Healing was complete in those patients who had amputation of the metatarsal head, amputation of a toe with the metatarsal head, or amputation of the joint. One of eight patients who was treated conservatively, healed. In 1972, Freidman and associates (in Lee and Brancato[47]) studied the peripheral vasoconstrictor capacity in patients with diabetic neuropathy by measuring reflex skin temperature changes in the foot.[47] Skin temperature measurements showed vasomotor tone to be totally absent in only 1 of 19 patients tested. It was concluded that adrenergic sympathetic function is usually preserved in the lower extremity, even in those patients with severe diabetic neuropathy, and that most patients with this condition lack the protected effects of "autosympathectomy" for their distal cutaneous circulation. Freidman and associates recommended that neuropathic diabetics not be automatically excluded from lumbar sympathectomy when they have significant arterial occlusive disease. In 1982, Edmonds and associates (in Lee and Brancato[47]) reported blood flow to be abnormal in neurotrophic subjects, even in those limbs without ulceration. In patients with neurotrophic joints, there were marked increases in diastolic flow as well as a sharp decease in pressure from ankle to toe. Edmonds et al. concluded the neurotrophic foot to be more susceptible to abnormal mechanical stress, which eventually could lead to the neurotrophic joint and perforating ulcer. Based on the etiology and pathomechanics, and the emphasis on locating plantar perforating ulcers of the foot and the status of the peripheral circulation, surgical treatment has been redirected toward correcting the structure underlying the ulceration, using procedures that augment blood flow to the distal part of the extremity.[47]

PATHOMECHANICS

Weight distribution on the foot and the function of the great toe during pushoff are major factors in the development of ulcers on the plantar aspect of the foot. Forceplate analysis has shown that, before toe-off, weight is transferred to the medial side of the foot, which subjects the plantar surface of the great toe to heavy weight bearing and stress at the time of pushoff. Ctercteko and associates (in Lee and Brancato[47]) measured vertical forces acting on the feet of diabetic patients with neurotrophic ulceration and found proportionally less force transmitted through the toes than in normal individuals. They also showed a medial shift of the force transmitted through the metatarsal heads. All ulcers in the metatarsal region were located at the site of maximum loading. The general vertical force distribution pattern on the plantar surface of the feet of diabetics varied from normal in important aspects. The diabetic group had reduced toe loading, which was probably a reflection of neuropathic paresis of the long and short flexors and intrinsic muscles of the toes. The reduction of toe loading resulted in heavier loading in the metatarsal region. Normally 70%

of toe loading is transmitted through the hallux. Ctercteko suggested that when toe loading is reduced, the load previously taken by the hallux is transferred back onto the first metatarsal head.[47] Barret and Mooney and Stokes and associates (in Lee and Brancato[47]) reported similar results definitively showing that ulcers do occur at the site of maximum vertical force.

The relationship between pressure and plantar ulceration can be appreciated when mechanical stresses are classified in four ways: First, a necrotic blister can become an ulcer by *friction* of the skin between bone, shoe, and ground. Second, *impact* by the body's weight at heel contact produces repeated tissue damage, ulceration, and scar formation. Third, *thrust* during walking or running causes intermittent and concentrated pressures, especially under the metatarsal heads before toe-off. If sufficient, these pressures can crush cells or rupture capillaries. Because skin is more resistant to trauma, the subcutaneous tissue is more readily affected with a deep focus of necrosis or hematoma production. With repeated high pressures and an accumulation of necrotic tissue, fistula formation may ensue. Fourth, *shear* of the skin during walking, especially over the metatarsal region, can tear previously scarred tissue because of loss of elasticity. In those individuals with relative or absolute insensitivity of the foot, a long walk is more likely to produce ulceration than a number of short walks under similar conditions. When the sole of the foot is subjected to a long succession of mildly traumatic steps, the effects may be cumulative, making the tissue more susceptible to serious damage.

CLINICAL FINDINGS

More than 60 patients have been referred for perforating ulcers of the foot that had not responded to conservative treatment. Clinical findings included perforating ulceration on the plantar surface of the foot, usually under the metatarsophalangeal joints. The most frequent site was the first metatarsal. The base of the ulcerations contained dermal connective tissue with fibrotic and sclerotic changes surrounded by dense circumferential epidermis margin. Infection was characteristically low grade. Noninvasive assessment of the peripheral vascular system was measured by Doppler segmental systolic pressure profile, external magnetic flowmetry, digital photoplethysmography, and thermistor thermometry. In patients who demonstrated vascular disease, arteriography was done to locate lesions of pathological significance. Patients with impaired circulation of the distal extremities not amenable to direct arterial surgery were considered for lumbar sympathectomy using the following criteria for patient selection: an ischemic index greater than 0.35, pulsatile calf blood flow greater than 30 ml/min, with

an absence of an ankle/toe temperature gradient greater than 1.20°C. In all patients, radiographic examination of the feet were done, which demonstrated one or more of the following findings: (1) absorption of bone, (2) penciling of the metatarsal shaft, (3) fracture of the metatarsal head, (4) destruction and obliteration of joints, (5) disarticulation of phalanges, and/or (6) periosteal thickening remote from the ulcer site. The chief distinguishing difference between diabetics and nondiabetics was neuropathy. Although diabetic neuropathy was frequently accompanied by pain and paresis, the loss of pain sensation allowed the foot to endure repeated trauma. Clinical findings were, therefore, a result of complications stemming from a combination of microangiopathy and neuropathy. Commonly, these patients present with infected ulcer, either primary or superimposed on the vascular or neurotrophic lesion.[47]

INFECTIONS

In the presence of impaired blood supply or sensation, minor trauma to the foot can result in a serious foot infection. Unfortunately, in many patients, lack of meticulous attention to foot hygiene and use of poorly fitting shoes are major preventable factors in the development of foot infection. Diabetic foot infections range from local fungal infections of the nail to severe necrotizing limb or life-threatening infections. Early diagnosis and prompt definitive treatment may be delayed because of lack of foot sensation, the patient's poor eyesight, or failure of the physician, who initially sees the patient, to accurately diagnose the extent of the infectious process. Because the development of foot infection or delayed wound healing is often multifactorial, and because diabetics have a high incidence of reconstructable vascular disease, all diabetics presenting with a foot infection must be evaluated for the presence of vascular disease.[48,49]

Loss of skin integrity resulting from a puncture, laceration, or abrasion can be the initiating factor in the development of a foot infection; however, foot infections in the diabetic usually originate at the nail plates or the interdigital web spaces. In one study, 60% of foot infections started in the web spaces, 30% started around the nails, and 10% were secondary to puncture wounds.[35] The high incidence of web space and toe infections is related to the increased moisture level in the web space and the presence of excessive amounts of keratin and other debris around the nail plates. These environmental factors promote bacterial overgrowth and thereby predispose to infection. The clinical presence of a diabetic with a foot infection ranges from mild episodes of acute cellulitis to life-threatening episodes of necrotizing fasciitis.

Diabetic foot infections are classified as acute and chronic. Acute infections include localized cellulitis, septic arthritis of metatarsophalangeal joints, necrotizing cellulitis or fasciitis, deep-space infections, and gangrene (clostridial and nonclostridial). Chronic infections include neurotrophic ulcers and osteomyelitis.

Acute cellulitis beginning in the web space, if left untreated, spreads along the tendons and lumbricals associated with each toe and can quickly lead to a deep-space infection or, less commonly, to acute necrotizing cellulitis or fasciitis. In fact, toe and web space infections that progress to advanced deep-space infections are associated with the highest rate of major limb amputations. Acute necrotizing cellulitis or fasciitis and deep-compartment infections are characterized by systemic signs and symptoms of infection, including spiking fever, malaise, nausea, and the development of ketoacidosis. Clinically, necrotizing cellulitis more commonly involves the dorsum of the foot. In deep-space infections, however, a loss of the plantar surface contour and skin crease occurs, and the presence of dorsal foot swelling is variable.

Deep-space infections generally involve only the central compartment of the foot, but, because of the anatomy of these space compartments, a high index of suspicion concerning bacterial spread from the central to the lateral or medial compartment must be maintained. Destruction of the interosseous fascia allows bacteria to spread from the central to the lateral or medial compartment and the migration of the bacteria along the long flexor tendons leads to infection in the calf and lower regions. The small vessel thrombosis that accompanies deep-space infection leads to progressive tissue ischemia and necrosis. With progressive inflammation, the accumulating tissue edema results in elevation of deep-compartment pressures, contributing to ischemic necrosis of the intrinsic muscles of the foot. The development of bullous lesions on the plantar aspect of the foot is a late sign and signals the loss of the plantar vessel patency and the presence of massive plantar tissue necrosis.

The presence of gas between the tissues on x-ray can be due to clostridial infections or the milking of air into the tissues by continued walking. In this circumstance, Gram staining of the exudates or infected tissue is critical in differentiating clostridia from other bacterial pathogens and in choosing appropriate antibiotic coverage, as well as the extent and type of surgical intervention. Clostridial infection, although uncommon, tends to present with acute systemic toxicity and a rapidly cascading course.[35]

DIFFERENTIAL DIAGNOSIS

In the diabetic patient presenting with an acutely inflamed foot, a differential diagnosis must be made among gouty arthritis, Charcot's joint, and infection. Gouty arthritis causes inflammation around the metatar-

sophalangeal joint of the great toe. The lack of systemic toxicity, presence of elevated serum uric acid levels, and uric acid crystals on aspiration of the joint aid in distinguishing gouty arthritis from acute infection. Charcot's joint occurs in as many as 2.5% of diabetics and is related to repetitive traumatic injury to the insensate foot. The joints characteristically involved in this acute inflammatory process are the metatarsophalangeal, metatarsotarsal, intertarsal, and interphalangeal joints. The presence of acute erythema, edema, and joint effusions may cause a Charcot's joint to be mistaken for a foot infection, especially when a Charcot's joint is associated with a foot ulcer. However, in contrast to patients with foot infections, patients with a Charcot's joint do not show signs of systemic toxicity and white blood cell counts and erythrocyte sedimentation rates are not elevated.[49–53]

DIAGNOSTIC METHODS

A careful neurologic examination includes assessment of vibratory sense, proprioception, and light touch. The proximal extent of the neuropathy should be documented. It is common for only the forefoot to have significant neuropathy, while the hindfoot and lower leg have normal sensation.

Noninvasive vascular tests frequently underestimate the extent and severity of arterial insufficiency in diabetic patients. Bilateral ankle/brachial indices via Doppler are useful, but their accuracy in the presence of calcified vessels is severely limited. The readings can be falsely high. Other noninvasive studies include transcutaneous oximetry. These should be used only as a complement to bedside evaluation and clinical judgment. In selected patients with significant limb-threatening ischemia (ankle/brachial index <0.5, rest pain, or ischemic tissue necrosis), arteriography of the lower extremity including the foot vessels should be performed.[54]

We have used noninvasive electromagnetic flowmetry in the assessment of patients with peripheral arterial disease. This technique is capable of distinguishing three relatively discrete clinical zones (femoral, popliteal, and posterior tibial) by quantitating the peak pulsatile blood flow through the thigh and calf. As previously reported, the obtained peak pulsatile blood flow values are comparable to ischemic indices for grading the degree of ischemia. The use of electromagnetic flowmetry has enabled us to select the proper operative procedure by providing information about arterial flow (proximal, site of the lesion, and status of the runoff).[55–57]

Currently, adapted from fluid flowmetry in industrial applications, magnetic resonance flowmetry has been applied clinically. The basic principle of nuclear magnetic resonance (NMR) flowmetry can be simplified by relating the signal of blood flow as follows:

(1) magnetization is induced as the hydrogen nuclei (N) tendency in the blood to align along the direction of an applied magnetic field; (2) blood is magnetized and the amount of magnetism (M) is detected and the flow rate of magnetized blood is measured; (3) magnetization is measured by making the hydrogen nuclei resonate (R) and then applying the principle of magnetic induction: a changing resonating magnetic field creates an electric voltage in the detector, accounting for the R Blood flow measurements using NMR have been in close agreement with those obtained using other plethysmographic techniques. The examination is performed without physical contact, so evaluation of extremities having fresh or open wounds or of burn patients can be done. Perhaps more importantly, calcified vessels do not interfere with the accuracy of measurements, making MRI of particular value in diabetic patients.[58,59]

Plain radiographs of the foot are not very reliable in detecting osteomyelitis because of the high incidence of false-positive and false-negativestudies.[54] False-negative studies are relatively common for several reasons. First, lytic lesions due to infection must cause a greater than 30% bone density loss (based on the density of normal bone) to be demonstrated on plain radiographs. Furthermore, the infection must be present for longer than 7–14 days before these subtle radiographic changes can be demonstrated. The bone density of the diabetic is often reduced and the presence of osteopenic bone further decreases the ability of plain radiographs to detect osteomyelitis.[35] For this reason, radionuclide studies are often used to confirm or rule out osteomyelitis. Currently, the three-phase bone scan using technetium-99, methylene diphosphonate, and gallium-67 citrate is the most accurate and sensitive. The intense uptake of technetium-99 diphosphonate followed by an intense uptake of gallium-67 is highly suggestive for osteomyelitis. Failure to intensely localize gallium-67 suggests a localized inflammatory process. Indium-111 oxyquinolone leukocyte scan has recently been shown to detect osteomyelitis with a sensitivity of 89% and to be a reliable method for following the effectiveness of antibiotic therapy. The combined use of the three-phase bone scan and the indium-111 leukocyte scan have a sensitivity of 100% and a specificity of 81%. Computerized tomography is a superior examination for detecting the presence of sequestra. Although the MRI has been used to diagnose osteomyelitis, no comparison has been made with radionuclide scans.[60]

CASE REPORTS

Case One

A 42-year-old, insulin-dependent diabetic African American male was admitted with the chief complaint of perforating ulcer on the sole of the left foot of 1 week duration. The ulcer developed from a callus that was present 4 months prior to admission. Examination of the left foot showed a thick callus surrounding the plantar ulcer with dirty granulation and purulent discharge (Fig. 20–6). Routine noninvasive vascular studies showed normal blood flow to the lower extremities. Arteriography demonstrated no significant arterial occlusive disease. Skin thermistory thermometry evaluation, however, showed evidence of reduced tissue perfusion at the foot with a room/toe temperature gradient of 7.75°C. Radiographic examination of the left foot showed absorption and penciling of the distal two-thirds

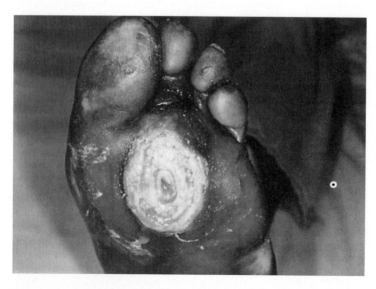

Fig. 20–6. Diabetic African American male, 42 years-old presented with perforating ulcer on the sole of the left foot with purulent discharge.

of the second and fifth metatarsal bones with disruption of the articular surface and partial dislocation of the second proximal phalanx (Fig. 20–7). To increase blood flow to the left lower extremity, a left lumbar sympathectomy was performed. A follow-up examination at 6 months demonstrated increased skin temperatures at the left calf, ankle, and toe levels, compared to those of the right extremity, with a 1.25°C improvement in the left room/toe temperature gradient. Examination of the left foot showed partial healing of the ulcer. Following this increased tissue perfusion in the sympathectomized limb, débridement of the callosity over the sole of the left foot and excision of the base of the phalanx of the left great toe through a small dorsal incision were performed to alleviate pressure necrosis. Long-term follow-up digital photoplethysmography and thermistor thermometry demonstrated a sustained increase in tissue perfusion and digital temperatures of the sympathectomized limb. At 10 years follow-up, the ulceration on the plantar surface of the foot remained healed (Fig. 20–8).

Case Two

A 53-year-old white male was admitted with cellulitis, infection, and progressive gangrene of the left foot and neurotrophic ulcers of the right foot. The patient had been diabetic for the past 15 years, which was controlled with insulin. Physical examination showed swelling of the left foot and ankle with tenderness and multiple sinuses and discharge. The distal phalangeal and metatarsal regions were deformed from a distal tendon repair done 3 years previously. Routine noninvasive external magnetic flowmetry demonstrated good pulsatile

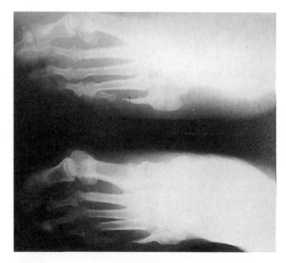

Fig. 20–7. Radiograph examination of left foot shows absorption and penciling of the distal two-thirds of the second and fifth metatarsal bones with disruption of the articular surface and partial disarticulation of the second proximal phalanx.

flow at the thigh and calf bilaterally and segmental Doppler ischemic indices were exaggerated distally (Fig. 20–9). Digital photoplethysmography demonstrated reduced blood flow waveforms at the toes bilaterally and Doppler ankle/metatarsal systolic pressure showed exaggerated pressures indicative of the presence of calcified small vessel disease (Fig. 20–10). Arteriography demonstrated good visualization of the major vessels of the lower extremities with good distal runoff

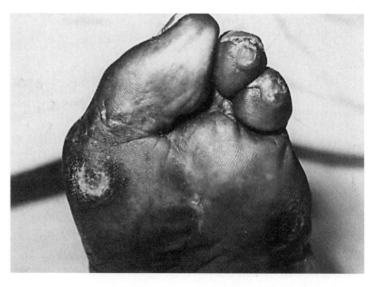

Fig. 20–8. At 10-year follow-up, perforating ulceration on the sole of the left foot remains healed.

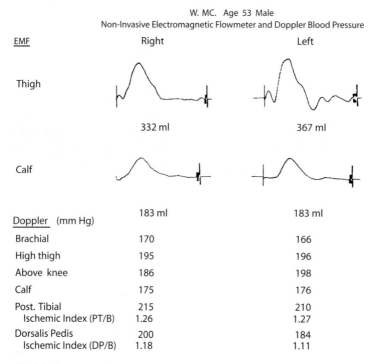

Fig. 20–9. External noninvasive electromagnetic flowmetry and Doppler segmental systolic pressures in a 53-year-old male showing no significant arterial occlusive disease to the level of the ankle. However this does indicate calcification of distal arteries.

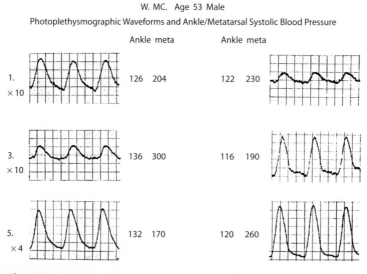

Fig. 20–10. Bilaterally reduced toe photoplethysmographic waveforms and exaggerated ankle/metatarsal pressure in a 53-year-old male demonstrate the presence of small vessel disease indicative of calcified arteries.

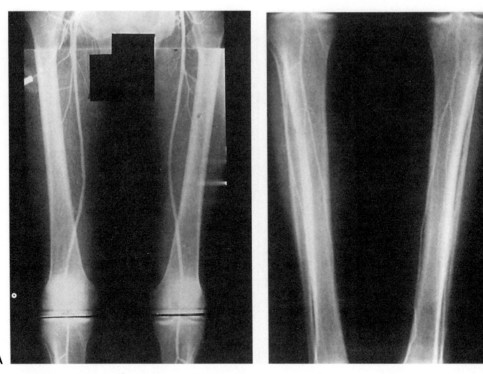

Fig. 20–11. **A** and **B.** Arteriography shows no evidence of arterial occlusive disease.

into the popliteal and tibial arteries with no significant arterial occlusive disease to the ankle level (Fig. 20–11). Radiographic study of the left foot showed osteomyelitis and advanced bony absorption, characteristic of diabetes mellitus (Fig. 20–12). Multiple débridements and incisions and drainage of the left foot did not significantly improve the foot and the patient underwent a left lumbar sympathectomy. Follow-up radiographic examination of the left foot showed actual reconstruction of the remaining bony fragment involving the phalanx of the great toe. The right foot, however, demonstrated a significant distortion of the first, second, third, and fourth toes with fusiform deformity. Active osteomyelitis involving the metatarsal bones was present (Fig. 20–13). Ulceration was present on the plantar surface of the right foot (Fig. 20–14). A right lumbar sympathectomy was recommended, but the patient refused and was discharged. The patient was readmitted 2 years later, with extensive necrosis of the sole of the right foot and extensive purulent drainage and exposure of the tarsal and metatarsal bones. He underwent a right lumbar sympathectomy and subsequent extensive débridement of the right foot with excision of the metatarsal and cuneiform bone. Following skin graft, postoperative healing was excellent (Fig. 20–15). At 8 years follow-up, thermistor thermom-

etry studies demonstrated a sustained increase in digital temperatures and tissue perfusion at the toes.

Case Three

A 38-year-old diabetic white male was admitted with neurogenic ulcerations on the plantar aspect of the great toe and sole of the left foot (Fig. 20–16). Neurological findings of the lower extremities were dissociated impairment of sensation for pain and temperature, while touch and other sensory modalities were intact. Motor power was well preserved with proprioception at the toes. Fasciculations were present in the gastrocnemius bilaterally. Electromyography demonstrated no delay in nerve conduction. The patient underwent a left lumbar sympathectomy. At the time of surgery, the blood flow in the left popliteal artery was measured using intraoperative electromagnetic flowmetry. Following sympathectomy, the mean flow increased from 42 ml/min to 110 ml/min. The pulsatile waveform pattern recorded is shown in Fig. 20–17. At 2 months postoperatively, the ulcers on the left foot were completely healed (Fig. 20–18). In this case, lumbar sympathectomy alone sufficiently augmented blood flow to promote healing of the neurogenic ulcers.

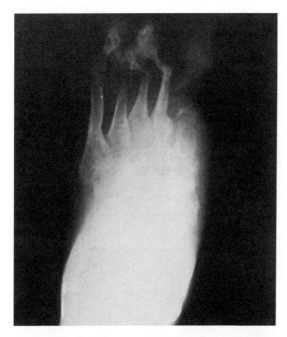

Fig. 20–12. Radiographic examination of the left foot shows osteomyelitis and advanced bony absorption characteristic of diabetes mellitus.

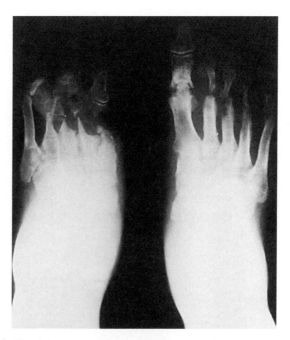

Fig. 20–13. Follow-up examination shows reconstruction of the remaining bony fragment involving the phalanx of the left great toe. Right foot shows distortion of the first, second, third, and fourth toes associated with osteomyelitis.

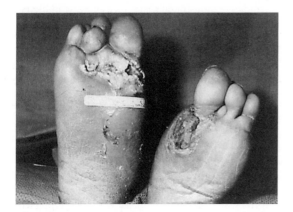

Fig. 20–14. Presence of perforating ulcers on the plantar surface of both feet (preoperatively).

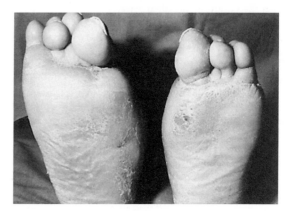

Fig. 20–15. Postoperatively both feet show excellent healing.

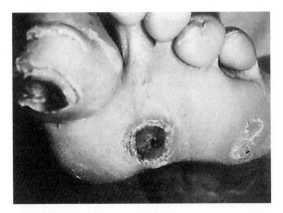

Fig. 20–16. Preoperative patient presenting with perforating ulcers on the plantar aspect of the great toe and sole of the left foot.

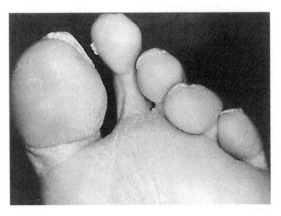

Fig. 20–18. Perforating ulcers of the left foot are completely healed, 2 months postoperatively.

Case Four

A 75-year-old male with a history of insulin-dependent diabetes for over 15 years presented with a right foot infection and complaining of severe pain. On examination, the foot appeared swollen, with increased local temperature and areas of necrosis of the dorsum of the foot. X-rays did not show the presence of gas. The ankle/brachial indices were normal, as was a computed tomography (CT) scan of the foot. The clinical diagnosis was necrotizing fasciitis. The patient underwent extensive débridement (Fig. 20–19). In the postoperative period, he received intensive local wound care including topical collagenase and local and systemic antibiotics. After resolution of infection, skin grafting was employed with early good results. At 6 months follow-up, the foot was in good condition with only a limited dorsiflexion deformity.

Case Five

A 65-year-old white male, who had been seen at another facility and was scheduled to undergo a BKA, which he refused (Fig. 20–20). He had been a diabetic for the past 10 years, which was controlled with insulin. Physical examination showed a swollen right foot with necrotic areas in the dorsolateral aspect of the foot, as well as on the fourth and fifth toes. The entire area was erythematous. X-rays did not show the presence of gas, but lytic lesions were observed in the fourth and fifth distal phalanges. Systolic segmental Doppler pressures were within the normal range. The patient underwent local wound care and received systemic antibiotics. He underwent a right lumbar sympathectomy. Intraoperative electromagnetic flow studies of the superficial femoral artery showed a 220% increase in flow immedi-

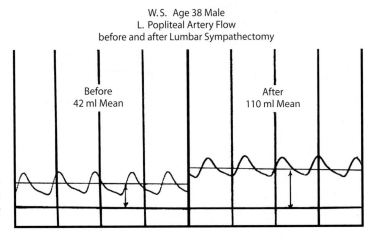

W. S. Age 38 Male
L. Popliteal Artery Flow
before and after Lumbar Sympathectomy

Before
42 ml Mean

After
110 ml Mean

Fig. 20–17. Intraoperative electromagnetic flowmetry of a 38-year-old male demonstrates an increase in blood flow during lumbar sympathectomy.

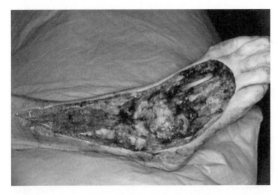

Fig. 20–19. After débridement, right foot with necrotizing fasciitis involving its dorsum.

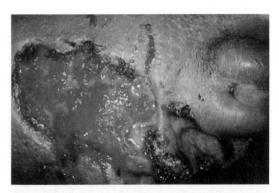

Fig. 20–20. Gangrenous changes of the right foot.

ately following the sympathectomy from 250 to 800 ml/min (Fig. 20–21). The patient underwent amputation of only two toes instead of a BKA (Fig. 20–22). At 5 years postoperative, digital temperatures showed a marked difference in the sympathectomized limb compared to the contralateral (nonsympathectomized) extremity and the Doppler systolic pressures were within normal limits. The sympathectomy effect was present 9 years later and the patient died of a myocardial infarction 10 years postsympathectomy.

Case Six

A 68-year-old male, a long-term noninsulin-dependent diabetic, presented with a gangrenous right great toe and a necrotic area on the dorsum of the foot (Fig. 20–23). Angiography showed a patent common femoral artery with occlusion of the superficial femoral artery and reconstitution of the popliteal artery with two-vessel runoff. After thorough assessment, the patient underwent a right femoropopliteal bypass using a reversed saphenous vein graft. Four months later, because of an ischemic ulcer on the anteriolateral aspect of the middle third of the leg, another angiogram was performed, which showed a patent right bypass and an occlusion of the left superficial femoral artery with a patent posterior tibial artery (Fig. 20–24). Subsequently, the patient underwent a left femoroposterior tibial bypass using an *in situ* saphenous vein graft and a concomitant ipsilateral lumbar sympathectomy. An intraoperative angiogram showed a patent graft with good visualization of the distal runoff and good communication with the dorsalis pedis artery (Fig. 20–25). Photoplethysmography results and digital temperatures improved in the sympathectomized extremity compared to the extremity with a bypass graft alone (Fig. 20–26). After débridement of the necrotic

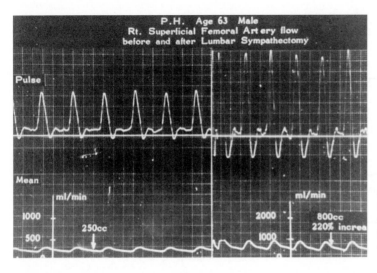

Fig. 20–21. Intraoperative electromagnetic flow studies of the superficial femoral artery showed a 220% increase in flow immediately following sympathectomy from 250 to 800 ml/min.

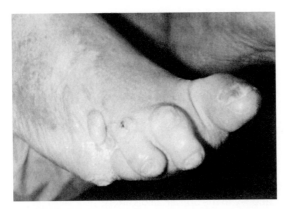

Fig. 20–22. Postoperative sympathectomy showing complete healing of huge ulcerations of dorsum of right foot.

area and a skin graft, the ulcer healed (Fig. 20–27). Twelve years later the patient had a viable left lower extremity and had undergone a right BKA (Fig. 20–28).

Case Seven

A 60-year-old white male, insulin-dependent diabetic presented complaining of severe pain with a swollen, erythematous left foot infection. Systolic Doppler pressures were within normal limits. X-rays showed neither gas nor bone involvement. The patient was placed on antibiotics, but continued to have severe pain, especially on dorsiflexion and the foot continued to be swollen and tense. The patient subsequently underwent a fasciotomy using a modified medial approach of Henry for decompression of the medial, central, interosseous, and lateral compartments of the foot (Fig. 20–29). Abundant purulent drainage was obtained from the medial and central compartments. Intensive local wound care and systemic

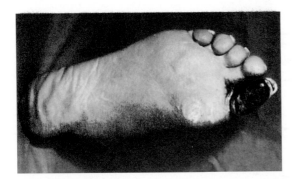

Fig. 20–23. Gangrenous right great toe and necrotic area on the dorsum of the foot.

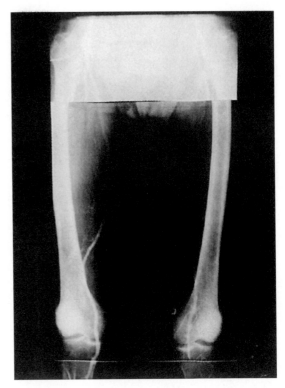

Fig. 20–24. Angiogram showing a patent right bypass and occlusion of left superficial femoral artery with a patent posterior tibial artery.

antibiotics were employed in the postoperative period. One month later, the patient received a skin graft with good healing. At 1 year follow-up, the fasciotomy wound was healed with no residual pain (Fig. 20–30).

TREATMENT

An analysis of the problem must be made and intermediate goals and outcomes must be established. Control of diabetes, which may be worsened by foot infection, is of clinical importance. Surgical intervention may be necessary for débridement of the necrotic tissue or even amputation of an irreversibly gangrenous digit. Although a major débridement followed by minor débridement at the bedside or in the clinic may be satisfactory, advanced infections will require multiple major débridements or definitive amputation. This is different than the approach required for pure ischemia.

ANTIBIOTIC THERAPY

Diabetic soft-tissue infection can spread very quickly and lead to gangrene or osteomyelitis. The infections

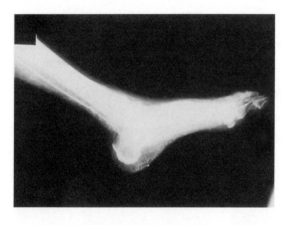

Fig. 20–25. Intraoperative angiogram showing a patent graft, adequate anastomosis, and good distal runoff in communication with the dorsalis pedis artery.

B.S. Age 67 Male
1. Fermoro-tibial Insitu saphenous Vein Bypass
   and Concomitant Left Lumbar Sympathectomy.

Intra-op administration 500cc Dextran 40 with
$^1/_2$ loading dose Heparin (2500u). Irrigation
of *insitu* saphenous vein with 500cc Dextran 40.

Doppler Ankle Ischemic Index	Pre-op	Immed. Post-op
Right	0.91	0.93
Left	0.25	0.73

Photoplethysmographic Toe Waveforms

Right

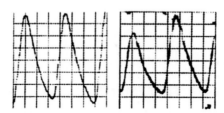

Rt. Ankle/Metatarsal Pressure (mm Hg)
              182/200   120/250

Left

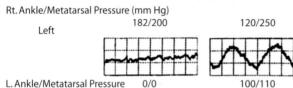

L. Ankle/Metatarsal Pressure   0/0   100/110

Room/Toe Temperature Gradient °C.

Right Toe	3.5	3.5
Left Toe	3.5	5.5

Fig. 20–26. Noninvasive vascular studies after the patient underwent a femoroposterior tibial bypass graft and concomitant sympathectomy.

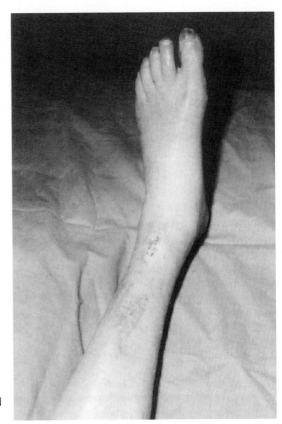

Fig. 20–27. After a skin graft, the foot lesion healed completely.

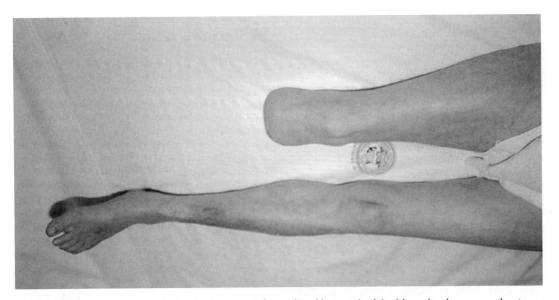

Fig. 20–28. Right lower extremity: right femoroinfrapopliteal bypass (only) without lumbar sympathectomy ended in right BKAi 5 years postoperative.

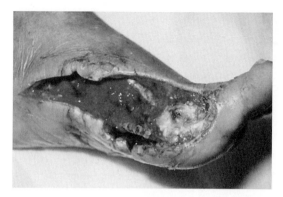

Fig. 20–29. Modified medial approach of Henry for decompression of the four compartments of the foot.

are usually mixed infections and the most severe involve a greater number and variety of Gram-negative aerobes and anaerobes. Empiric therapy for diabetic foot infections should begin with a broad-spectrum antibiotic. The microbial population is influenced by the patient's local environment (eg, home, nursing home, hospital, farm, occupation).[61] The Gram-positive cocci are primarily *Staphylococcus aureus*, as well as groups D and B streptococci. Gram-negative organisms are commonly *Escherichia coli*, *Klebsiella*, *Enterobacter aerogenes*, *Proteus mirabilis*, and *Pseudomonas aeruginosa*. Anaerobic species include *Bacteroides fragilis*, peptostreptococci, and clostridial species. The anaerobes can outnumber

the aerobes ten to one and systemic bacteremias are most commonly associated with *B. fragilis* and *S. aureus* infections.[60] Despite the polymicrobial nature of diabetic foot infections, they can be treated on an outpatient basis using short- and long-acting cephalosporins and fluorinated quinolones, such as ciprofloxacin and oral clindamycin. These have been demonstrated to be effective in diabetic foot infections. However, inpatients with diabetic foot infections are treated in a different manner, using intravenous antibiotics (Table 20–2). Ticarcillin with clavulanate as well as ampicillin with sulbactam are considered to be the first choice in the case of the superficial ulcer. Second-choice antimicrobials include cefoxitin, cephamycin, ceftizoxime, ciprofloxacin, and either clindamycin or metronidazole. For systemic sepsis, ticarcillin with clavulante, or ampicillin with sulbactam are first antibiotic choice as are cephalosporins, aztreonam, and clindamycin. An aminoglycoside can be added to a third-generation cephalosporin. As a second choice in systemic sepsis, intravenous ciprofloxacin and either metronidazole or clindamycin may be used.[61,62]

WOUND CARE

Wound care after a major surgical débridement should provide an ideal environment for tissue healing. Meticulous cleaning of the wound with normal saline or isotonic soaps is done, along with periodic sharp debridement of exudates and the application of antibiotic ointment dressings. Occlusive dressings enhance the ingrowth of delicate granulation tissues and wound closure.

There is a new semiocclusive dressing, *PolyMem*, which is permeable to the atmospheric oxygen and water vapor that has been considered as an ideal dressing choice.[63] This polymeric membrane dressing is an absorbent dressing composed of a hydrophilic polyurethane membrane matrix attached to a semipermeable thin-film backing. It is composed of four parts: (1) hydrophilic open-cell polyurethane foam, which provides the structure of the matrix; (2) poloxamer 188, a nontoxic, nonionic surfactant wound cleanser; (3) glycerol; and (4) a superabsorbent starch polymer. With the PolyMem dressing, the wound bed is not disturbed and the wound is not cleaned or flushed with saline or water unless the wound is infected or contaminated. The semipermeable film backing of the polymeric membrane wound care dressing provides a bacterial barrier while allowing gas (O_2 and CO_2) exchange and maintaining an ideal moisture vapor transmission rate.[64]

A study has shown that PolyMem, had a 78% complete ulcer healing rate compared to 0% treated with wet to dry dressings.[65] Since pain is now considered the *fifth vital sign*, the unique pain-relieving benefit of

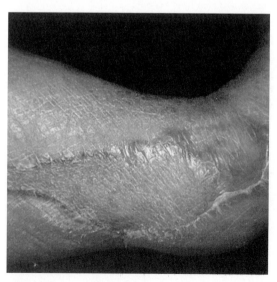

Fig. 20–30. Complete healing of fasciotomy with no residual pain at 1 year follow-up.

Table 20–2. Initial antimicrobial (empiric) therapy of diabetic foot infections

Type of infection	Common bacteria	First-choice antimicrobial therapy	Second choice of antimicrobials and/or addition
Superficial ulcer	Staphylococcus aureus, S. epidermidis, enterococci, Gram-negative aerobes, Proteus, Pseudomonas, anaerobes	Ticarcillin/clavulanate Ampicillin/sulbactam	Cefoxitin or other cephamycin, ceftizoxime, ciprofloxacin, and either clindamycin or metronidazole
Sepsis	Staphylococcus aureus, S. epidermidis, enterococci, Gram-negative aerobes, Proteus, Pseudomonas, anaerobes	Ticarcillin/clavulanate, Ampicillin/sulbactam, Imipenem/cilastatin Third-generation cephalosporin or aztreonam-with clindamycin; aminoglycoside, aztreonam, or third-generation cephalosporin with ampicillin and clindamycin	Ciprofloxacin and either clindamycin or metronidazole

PolyMem wound dressing is very important. In 2002, the United States Food and Drug Administration (FDA) permitted PolyMem wound dressings to claim that they relieve pain. In an analysis of 261 health care providers' experiences with PolyMem dressings for skin ulcers, 88% reported soothed inflamed tissues and pain relief.[66]

TOTAL-CONTACT WALKING CAST

The application of a cast over the wound aids in wound healing by (1) redistributing the weight-bearing load over the entire lower leg and plantar surface, (2) immobilizing the limb to decrease the spread of bacteria, (3) protecting the wound from further direct trauma, (4) improving the microcirculation by reducing the interstitial edema, and (5) eliminating the need for patient participation in local wound care. The total-contact plaster cast is applied with a minimum of padding around each maleolus, the anterior tibial, and the bony prominences of the first and fifth metatarsal heads. Following application of the padding, a contour plaster cast with a walking platform bottom is applied. Usually, the cast is changed weekly until the wound is healed. In patients with excessive wound exudates, the cast is changed more frequently. Using this technique, wound healing time averages 6–8 weeks.[62]

TREATMENT OF NEUROTROPHIC ULCERS

Neurotrophic ulcers can be divided into the following four clinical groups: (1) uncomplicated ulcers with a granulating bed, (2) uncomplicated ulcers with localized areas of necrotic debris, (3) locally infected ulcers, and (4) infected ulcers with extension of the infection into the deep spaces of the foot. Uncomplicated ulcers usually have minimal drainage. The treatment of an uncomplicated neurotrophic ulcer with a granulating tissue bed consists of débridement of the surrounding callus followed by the application of a total contact plaster cast. Neurotrophic ulcers with necrotic debris or local infection require more extensive surgical débridement, which commonly includes the plantar fascia, flexor tendons, the volar plate of the metatarsophalangeal joint, and the head of metatarsal bone. After the débridement of necrotic and infected tissue is complete, the metatarsophalangeal joint is open, the metatarsal head and cartilaginous surface of the proximal phalanx should be excised. Infections extending into the deep spaces of the foot require extending the incision longitudinally along the plantar surface to provide adequate drainage and debridement. During the dissection, intact vascular structures and viable muscle should be preserved. However, because tendons often undergo rapid necrosis due to their tenuous blood supply, they must be completely debrided to control the infection process. In all cases, débridement should extend down until bleeding tissue is reached.

AMPUTATION

When considering an amputation, whether it is a toe or above-knee, the goals must be to (1) control infection and remove all necrotic tissue, (2) optimize rehabilitation by performing the lowest level of amputation consistent with wound healing, (3) avoid exacerbation of other disabilities by a high-level amputation, and (4) have an adequate blood supply for wound healing.

Amputation of the lower extremity is a frequent consequence of peripheral vascular disease, peripheral neuropathy, and infection in the diabetic foot. Patients with peripheral vascular disease comprise approximately 80% of the amputees in the Western world; 75% of these amputees are diabetic.[67]

The metabolic cost of walking is increased and the self-selected walking speed decreased with more proximal level amputations. These factors become critical in diabetic patients who have concomitant multiple system disease and a limited cardiopulmonary reserve, as compared with traumatic amputees. To optimize the independence of these patients, it is essential to perform amputations at the most distal level feasible with the potential to walk after amputation.[68,69]

The *biologic amputation level* is the most distal functional amputation level with a reasonable (85–90%) potential to be healed. This is determined by clinical examination and a measure of adequate vascular flow, tissue nutrition, and immunocompetence. For amputations of the foot and ankle, the following criteria must be met: (1) the heel pad must be free of open lesions, (2) there should be no gross pus at the amputation site, and (3) there should be no local soft-tissue infection, i e, cellulitis at the level of surgery. When ascending soft-tissue cellulitis is present, this must be resolved with antibiotics, local surgery, or a combination of both, because primary wound closure will not be successful in the presence of ascending cellulitis. Impending gangrene should be evaluated by a vascular surgeon whose highest priority is limb salvage. An open partial foot amputation has frequently been performed to decompress an infection, removing gangrenous tissue prior to performing vascular reconstruction and a definitive secondary functional amputation.[35]

The Doppler-determined ankle/brachial pressure ratio (ankle/brachial index or ABI) is an important predictor of wound healing.[70] The ABI has been popularized by Wagner, who suggested that wound healing rates approach 90% when adequate inflow is present.[71] Measurement of transcutaneous oxygen partial pressure ($TcPO_2$) currently predicts a wound healing rate of approximately 90% when it is greater than 30 mm Hg,

70% when it is between 20 and 29 mm Hg, and less than 50% when it is below 20 mm Hg.[72] At present, using different light reflectance technology, the muscle oxygen of patients with peripheral vascular disease is being assessed.[73,74]

Toe Amputation

Toe amputation should be performed in diabetic patients with persistent toe ulcerations, gangrene limited to the toe, osteomyelitis of the distal and middle phalanx, or a septic interphalangeal joint. Usually, the amputation is performed after treatment has been instituted to control the infection. The level of amputation is determined by the level of infection in the phalanx and the level of involved and viable skin. The maximum amount of proximal toe that can be salvaged is to the base of the proximal phalanx. However, if the capsule of the metatarsophalangeal joint must be entered, then the amputation should be performed proximally to the neck of the metatarsal to avoid exposure of the articular cartilage. Frequently, such wounds are not closed initially but are allowed to granulate under a topical occlusive dressing or a cadaveric skin graft. Later, a split-thickness skin graft (STSG) may be used to close the wound. If the wound is primarily closed, it should be done without skin tension and a closed system drain should be used.[34,35]

Ray Amputation

When the necrotic process involves the base of the toes, a Ray amputation of the metatarsal bone is necessary. An amputation more proximal than the metatarsal neck may be performed to facilitate adequate soft-tissue coverage of the bone. If several toes are involved, they may be resected individually, either at the metatarsal necks or more proximal at the base of the metatarsals. A transmetatarsal amputation has no advantage over multiple Ray amputations. Both of these foot amputations require only a simple foam shoe insert for ambulation and differ little in their ability to preserve foot function.[34,35]

Transmetatarsal Amputation

A transmetatarsal amputation may have to be performed for foot salvage when the infection involves multiple toes or the metatarsal phalangeal joints, or when inadequate distal soft tissue is available for bony coverage. An intact plantar foot pad is necessary because the amputation will be reflected dorsally, placing the suture line on the dorsum of the foot and the thick pad on the stump end. Amputations of each metatarsal sometimes need to be varied at the osteotomy level in order to have a tension-free skin closure or to preserve sufficient tissue for wound closure over the bone. The skin incision should allow maximal preservation of excess skin and any tension on the wound closure mandates that the wound be left open to heal by secondary intention or subsequent skin grafts.[34,35]

Major Amputation

Major amputations are often necessary in patients with overwhelming sepsis or deep-compartment abscesses with extensive forefoot gangrene or impending tissue loss. Below Knee amputations (BKA) are the most commonly performed. Although through-the-knee amputations are easy to perform, they are less desirable because of the difficulty of fitting the prosthesis with an appropriate knee. The level of amputation is based on the extent of necrosis, inflammation, and infection, in addition to an evaluation of the patient's vascular status. The longer the stump, the better the anticipated rehabilitation results; therefore, every effort should be made to preserve extremity length consistent with prosthesis fitting. This may require that the amputation, whether above or below the knee with the initial operation, performed to control the infectious process and subsequent procedures be performed to achieve wound closure at a later date. In the case of a staged BKA, the posterior flap should be left as long as possible at the initial operation and then trimmed at the time of definitive closure to give a tension-free closure of the skin and a soft muscular pad at the stump end.[34]

ARTERIAL RECONSTRUCTIVE SURGERY

The decision to perform vascular surgery depends on the severity of the vascular lesions, the risk associated with surgery, and the potential for rehabilitation. Advanced age per se does not preclude surgical intervention. Modern revascularization procedures are tailored to individual requirements based on thorough preoperative assessment. With aggressive preoperative cardiovascular monitoring, revascularization can be as safe as a major amputation and less costly. At 3 years after bypass, 87% of patients with autogenous vein bypass grafts to the foot vessels continue to have patent arteries; 92% did not require amputation. In patients with extensive tissue loss or gangrene of the foot, restoration of pulsatile blood flow to the foot is required for healing. Aggressive arterial reconstruction, including bypass grafts to the foot vessels, allows débridement of soft tissue and resection of osteomyelitic bone without amputation. The attempts of revascularization for limb salvage in diabetic patients as reported by Dalsing et al.[75] have shown amputation prevention in 70% of patients for 1 year and in 60% for 3 years. This result, together with a low operative mortality rate (1.7%), justifies an aggressive attempt at limb salvage. Various factors such as outflow resistance, pedal arch anatomy, and graft material influence the results of distal bypasses. Graft material is the most important factor influencing patency. The polytetrafluoroethylene (PTFE) grafts have a higher failure rate compared to vein or composite sequential grafts. The site of distal anastomosis was not a factor influencing graft patency in some reported series.[76,77] Anastomosis to the anterior tibial, posterior tibial, or peroneal artery had the same chance for success.[78]

Endovascular techniques (balloon angioplasty and atherectomy) may restore the patency of proximal arteries with limited occlusive disease, but are generally contraindicated for limb-threatening occlusion of infrainguinal arteries.[79–81]

LUMBAR SYMPATHECTOMY

Lumbar sympathectomy has been useful in increasing blood flow in both diabetic and nondiabetic patients. We suggest resection of more than two ganglia; specifically, the second, third, and fourth, in the case of more distal atherosclerotic occlusive disease. This improves blood flow to the digits. The main indication for sympathectomy was a diffuse distribution of atherosclerotic occlusive disease not amenable to arterial reconstructive procedures. We had an 8-year cumulative limb salvage rate of 71%, with a 51% cumulative toe salvage rate. Clinical data and noninvasive vascular studies supported the role of sympathectomy in diabetic patients. Our findings suggested that sympathectomy promoted healing through increased blood flow in the presence of limited areas of pregangrene or actual gangrene of the toes, but not with extensive involvement of the toes. Lumbar sympathectomy increases skin blood flow, muscle oxygen content, improves claudication, promotes wound healing, and decreases the level of amputation.[82] There have also been reports concerning the value of sympathectomy in ischemic rest pain, ischemic ulceration, and wet gangrene, particularly digital gangrene. Lumbar sympathectomy has proved useful when performed before or during arterial reconstructive surgery.[82,83]

DECOMPRESSIVE FASCIOTOMY

The association of infection and neuropathy will lead to a delay in the diagnosis of a deep diabetic foot infection. An increase in the compartment pressure occurs with infection involving the compartment and the presence of a previously deteriorated arterial circulation. Once increased pressure has developed in the foot compartments, the only effective mode of treatment is decompression. Surgical intervention should be performed in those cases of foot infection with clinical signs of compartment syndrome, such as loss of motor power or sensation of the foot. An increase in tissue pressure above 30 mm Hg is an absolute indication for fasciotomy.

A review of the orthopedic literature reveals various recommendations regarding the surgical techniques used to decompress the osseofascial compartments of the foot. Mubarak and Hargens[36] recommended two longitudinal dorsal incisions. Hansen, Bonutti, and Bell,[84] and Wright and associates suggested a plantar medial incision. Myerson compared the use of these two approaches in experimental and clinical studies and found a double dorsal longitudinal approach to be technically easier.[85] The plantar medial approach provides a more rapid decompression of compartment pressure and can be extended proximally to allow exploration of the neurovascular bundle and its branches on the medial side of the foot and ankle. Myerson stated that the plantar medial approach is the most effective way to treat compartment syndromes not associated with fractures.[36,84,85] We believe that the medial approach to the compartments of an infected diabetic foot with increased compartment pressure is the best approach, because it allows decompression of all four compartments with a single incision and, in addition, pressure points are avoided.

PREVENTIVE PROCEDURES

Operative procedures designed to reduce mechanical trauma to the foot, wound or plantar surface reduce the risk of plantar ulcerations and the development of infections. These might include metatarsal osteotomies or removal of metatarsal heads. Bunions and clawtoe deformities should be surgically corrected before pressure-related complications occur. Fixed clawtoe deformities are corrected by resecting the base of the proximal phalanx of the great toe. Resection of the metatarsal head through a dorsal approach allows healing of the plantar ulcer by relieving the plantar prominence. Likewise, a dorsal wedge osteotomy of the adjacent metatarsal shaft near its base subsequently prevents the formation of an adjacent plantar ulcer.[86,87]

PROGNOSIS

Cutaneous ulcers are among the most common reasons for hospital admission in the diabetic patient. A diabetic foot infection represents a failure by the patient and his management team to understand and correct the multifactorial conditions that predisposed the patient to this problem. Efforts directed toward prevention of foot lesions are much more likely to meet with success than is therapy of the established foot sore. This preventive approach is likely to lead to a reduction in the incidence of major amputations and thereby improve the quality of life and life expectancy.

Understanding the pathophysiology associated with the diabetic foot is essential to the care of the diabetic patient. When there is a failure in skin integrity, prompt assessment of vascular, neural, soft tissue, and wound status enhances the possibility of a successful outcome. The complexity of the management of a diabetic requires the knowledge and skill of a multidisciplinary team—an internist, podiatrist, rehabilitation specialist, prosthetist, dietitian, and social worker in addition to a surgeon interested in caring for the complications of diabetic feet. The goals of a multidisciplinary approach are to optimize local wound care, provide corrective footwear, improve glucose control, educate the patient concerning diet and lifestyle changes, and identify the presence of peripheral neuropathies and reconstructable arterial lesions. The goals will also include improvement in circulation when necessary through arterial reconstruction and/or sympathectomy. This combined team approach has been documented to substantially reduce the incidence of major and minor amputations in the diabetic.[88,89]

REFERENCES

1. Berkow R. Disorders of carbohydrate metabolism, In: Berkow R, ed. *The Manual Merck.* Rahway, NJ: Merck Research Laboratories; 1992:1106–1107.

2. Hughes CE, Johnson CC, Bamberger DM, et al. Treatment and long-term follow-up of foot infections in patients with diabetes or ischemia: a randomized prospective, double blind comparison of cefoxitin and ceftisoxime, *Clin Ther* 1987;10 (Suppl A):36.

3. Keen H, Payan J, Allawi J, et al. Treatment of diabetic neuropathy with gammalinolenic acid. *Diabetic Care.* 1993;16:8.

4. Larson U, Anderson GBJ. Partial amputation of the foot for diabetic or arteriosclerotic gangrene. Results and factors of prognostic value. *J Bone Joint Surg.* 1978;60:126.

5. Wright DG, Desai SM, Henderson WH. Action of the subtalar and ankle joint complex during the stance phase of walking. *J Bone Joint Surg.* 1964;46:361.

6. Bojsen-Moller F. Anatomy of the forefoot: normal and pathologic. *Clin Orthop.* 1979;142:10.

7. Bouton AJM, Detecting the patient at risk for diabetic foot ulcers. *Pract Cardiol* 1983;9:135.

8. Penn I. The impact of diabetes mellitus on extremity ischemia. In: Kempczinski RF, ed. *The Ischemic Leg.* Chicago: Year Book Medical; 1985:56–69.

9. Strandness DE, Jr, Priest RE, Gibbons GE. Combined clinical and pathologic study of diabetics and nondiabetic peripheral arterial disease. *Diabetes.* 1964;13:366.

10. Tilton RG, Daughtery A, Sutera SP, et al. Myocyte contracture, vascular resistance permeability after global ischemia in isolated hearts from alloxan-induced diabetic rabbits. *Diabetes.* 1989;38:1484.

11. Cameron NE, Cotter MA. Impaired contraction and relaxation in aorta from streptozotocin-diabetic rats: the role of polyol pathway. *Diabetologia.* 1992;35:1011.

12. Kelman I, Diegelmann RF. Wound healing. In: Greenfield LJ, et al, eds. *Surgery: Scientific Principles and Practice.* Philadelphia: Lippincott; 1993:100–101.

13. Wozniak A, McLennan G, Betts WH, et al. *Immunology.* 1989; 68:359–364.

14. Tuman KJ, Spiess BD, McCarthy RJ, et al. Comparison of viscoelastic measures of coagulation after cardiopulmonary bypass. *Anesth Analg.* 1989;69:69–75.

15. Martin P, Horkay F, Rajah SM, et al. Monitoring of coagulation status using thromboelastography during pediatric open heart surgery. *Int J Clin Monit Comput.* 1991;8: 183–187.

16. Lee BY, Ostrander LE, Madden JL. Optimum heparinization during vascular reconstructive surgery. *Contemp Surg.* 1988; 33:37–41.

17. Cruickshank MK, Levine MN, Hirsh J, et al. A standard nomogram for the management of heparin therapy. *Arch Intern Med.* 1991;151:333–337.

18. Van den Besselaer AMHP, Meeuwisse-Braun J, Bertina RM. Monitoring heparin therapy: relationships between the activated partial thromboplastin time and heparin assays based on *ex vivo* heparin samples. *Thromb Haemostasis.* 1990;63: 16–23.

19. Cipolle RJ, Uden DL, Gruber SA, et al. Evaluation of rapid monitoring system to study heparin pharmacokinetics and pharmacodynamics. *Pharmacotherapy.* 1990;10: 367–372.

20. Lee BY, Thoden WR, DelGuercio LRM, et al. Monitoring coagulation dynamics with thromboelastography. *Contemp Surg.* 1984;24:19–24.

21. Lee BY, Taha S, Trainor FS, et al. Monitoring heparin therapy with thromboelastography and activated partial thromboplastin time, *World J Surg.* 1980;4: 323–330.

22. Tsigos C, Diemel LT, White A, et al. Cerebrospinal fluid levels of substance P and calcitonin-gene-related peptide: correlation with sural nerve levels and neuropathic signs in sensory diabetic polyneuropathy, *Clin Sci.* 1993;84:305–311.

23. Caufield JP, el-Lati S, Thomas G, Church MK. *Lab Invest.* 1990;63:502–510.

24. Payan DY. Neuropeptides and inflammation: the role of substance P, *Ann Rev Med.* 1989;40:341–352.

25. O'Neal LW. Surgical pathology of the foot and clinicopathological correlations. In: Levin ME, O'Neal LW. eds. *The Diabetic Foot.* St Louis: Mosby; 1983:162–200.

26. Draves DJ, Sarrafian SK. *Anatomy of the Foot and Ankle, Descriptive, Topographic, and Functional.* Philadelphia: Lippincott; 1983.

27. Draves DJ. *Anatomy of the Lower Extremity.* Baltimore: William & Wilkins; 1957.

28. Gleckman RA, Roth RR. Diabetic foot infections: prevention and treatment. *West J Med.* 1985;142:263.

29. Jones FW. *Structure and Function as Seen in the Foot.* Baltimore, MD: William & Wilkins; 1944.

30. Kamel R, Sakla BF. Anatomical compartments of the sole of the human foot. *Anat Rec* 1961;140:57–64.

31. Myerson M. Acute compartment syndromes of the foot. *Bull Hosp Dis Orthop Inst.* 1987;47:251–261.

32. Goldman FD. Deep space infections in the diabetic patient. *J Am Podiatr Med Assoc.* 1987;77:431–443.

33. Brand PW. Pressure sores. The problem. In: Kennedi RM, Cowden JM. eds. *Bedsore Biomechanics.* Baltimore, MD: University Press, 1976;19–23.

34. Griffiths HJ. Diabetic osteopathy. *Orthopedics.* 1985;8:401.

35. Bridges RM, Deitch EA. Diabetic foot infections. Pathophysiology and treatment. *Surg Clin N. Am.* 1994;74: 537–555.

36. Mubarak SJ, Hargens AR. *Compartment Syndromes and Volkmann's Contracture.* Philadelphia: Saunders; 1981.

37. Whitesides TE, In: Jahss MH. ed. *Disorders of the Foot.* Philadelphia: Saunders; 1982:1201–1203.

38. Bonutti PM, Gordon RB. Compartment syndrome of the foot. A case report, *J Bone Joint Surg.* 1986;68:1449–1451.

39. Penn I. The impact of diabetes mellitus on extremity ischemia. In: Kempczinski RF. ed. *The Ischemic Leg.* Chicago: Year Book Medical Publishers; 1985:56–69.

40. Haimovici H. Peripheral arterial disease in diabetes mellitus. In: Ellenberg M, Rifkin H. eds. *Diabetes Mellitus: Theory and Practice.* New York: McGraw-Hill, 1970;890–911.

41. Ferrier TM. Comparative study of arterial disease in amputated lower limbs from diabetics and nondiabetics (with special reference to foot arteries). *Med J. Aust.* 1967;1:5.

42. Edmonds ME, Watkins PLJ. Management of the diabetic foot. In: Dyck JP, Thomas PK, Lamberg EH, et al. eds. *Diabetic Neuropathy.* Philadelphia: Saunders, 1987;212.

43. Penn I. The impact of diabetes mellitus on extremity ischemia. In: Kempczinski RF. ed. *The Ischemic Leg.* Chicago: Year Book Medical Publishers; 1985:56–69.

44. Thomas K, Eliason SG. *Diabetic Neuropathy.* 2nd ed. Philadelphia: Saunders, 1984:1773–1810.

45. Erdman WA, Tamburro F, Jayson H, et al. Osteomyelitis: characteristics and pitfalls of diagnosis with MR imaging. *Radiology.* 1991;180:533.

46. Hoshi K, Mizushima Y, Kiyokaawa S, et al. Prostaglandin E$_1$ incorporated in lipid microspheres in the treatment of peripheral vascular disease and diabetic neuropathy. *Drugs Exp Clin Res.* 1986;12:681.

47. Lee BY, Brancato RF. Perforating ulcers of the foot. In Lee BY. ed. *Chronic Ulcers of the Skin.* New York: McGraw-Hill 1985; 111–131.

48. Leichter SB, et al. Clinical characteristics of diabetic patients with serious pedal infections, *Metabolism.* 1988;37(Suppl 1): 22.

49. Sinha S, Munichoodappa I, Kozak GP. Neuro-arthropathy (Charcot joints) in diabetes mellitus (clinical study of 101 cases). *Medicine.* 1972;51:191.

50. Dellon EL. Treatment of symptomatic diabetic neuropathy by surgical decompression of multiple peripheral nerves. *Plast Reconstr Surg.* 1992;89:689.

51. Park HM, et al. Scintigraphic evaluation of diabetic osteomyelitis. Concise communication. *J Nucl Med.* 1991;23: 1246.

52. Eisenberg B, Wrege SS, Altman MI, et al. Bone scan: Indium-WBC correlation in the diagnosis of osteomyelitis of the foot. *J Foot Surg.* 1989;28:532.

53. Erdman WA, Tamburro F, Jayson HT, et al. Osteomyelitis: characteristics and pitfalls of diagnosis with MRI imaging. *Radiology* 1991;180:536.

54. Sapico What L J, Allen SD, Henry M, et al. Diabetic foot infections: bacteriologic analysis, *Arch Intern Med.* 1986; 146:1935.

55. Lee BY, Trainor FS, Kavner D, et al. A clinical evaluation of a noninvasive electromagnetic flowmeter. *Angiology* 1975;26: 317–327.

56. Lee BY, Trainor FS, Thoden WR, et al. Use of noninvasive electromagnetic flowmetry in the assessment of peripheral arterial disease. *Surg Gynecol Obstet.* 1980; 150:342–346.

57. Lee BY, Thoden WR, Trainor FS, Kavner D. Noninvasive evaluation of peripheral arterial disease in the geriatric patient. *J Am Geriatr Soc.* 1980;28:352–360.

58. Hinton PA, Nelson JR, Kroeker R. Measuring arterial blood flow by nuclear magnetic resonance. In: Kominsky SJ. ed. *Medical and Surgical Management of the Diabetic Foot.* St. Louis: Mosby; 1994:61–70.

59. Rice KL. Magnetic resonance flowmetry: clinical applications, *J. Vasc Technol.* 1994;18:277–285.

60. Ingram C, Eron LJ, Goldberg RI, et al. Antibiotic therapy of osteomyelitis in outpatients, *Med Clin N Am.* 1988; 72:723.

61. Gibbons GW, Freeman DV. Diabetic foot infections. In: Howard RJ, Simmons RL. eds. *Surgical Infectious Diseases.* 2nd ed. Norwalk, CT: Appleton and Lang; 1988:601.

62. Williams GM. The diabetic foot. In: Cameron JL. ed. *Current Surgical Therapy.* 4th ed. St. Louis, MO: Mosby Year Book; 1992:761–765.

63. Witkowski JA, Parish LC. Cutaneous ulcer therapy. *Int J Dermatol.* 1986;25(7):420–426.

64. Bolton L, Pirone L, Chen J, et al. Dressings effects on wounds healing. *Wound.* 1990;2(4):126–134.

65. Blackman JD, Senseng D, Quinn L, et al. Clinical evaluation of semipermeable polymeric membrane dressing for the treatment of chronic diabetic foot ulcers. *Diabetes Care* 1994; 17(4):322–325.

66. Health care provider case reports of experience with Ferris Mfg. PolyMem products.

67. Skolnick AA. Foot care program for patients with leprosy may also prevent amputations in persons with diabetes. *JAMA* 1992;267:2288.

68. Pinzur MS. Amputation level selection in the diabetic foot. *Clin Orthop.* 1988;229:2236.

69. Sage R, Pinzur MS, Cronin R, et al. Complications following mid-foot amputation in neuropathic and dysvascular feet. *J Am Podiatr Med Assoc.* 1989;97:227.

70. Lee BY, McCann WJ, et al. Noninvasive assessment of wound healing potentials with determination of amputation level. *Contemp Surg.* 1980;19:20.

71. Wagner FW, Jr. Management of the diabetic neurotrophic foot: Part II. A classification and treatment program for diabetic, neuropathic, and dysvascular foot problems. In: Cooper RR, ed. *AAOS Instructional Course Lectures,* Vol 28. St. Louis, MO: Mosby; 1979.

72. Pinzur MS. Amputation level selection in the diabetic foot. *Clin Orthop.* 1993;296:68–70.

73. Ostrander LE, Cui W, Lee BY, The clinical use of green light photoplethysmography. *Surgical Forum.* 1989;520–522.

74. Cui W, Ostrander LE, Lee BY. *In vivo* reflectance of blood and tissue as function of light wavelengths. *IEEE Trans Biomed Eng.* 1990; 37:632–639.

75. Dalsing MC, White JV, Yao JST, et al. Infrapopliteal bypass for established gangrene of the forefoot or toes. *J Vasc Surg.* 1985;2:669–677.

76. O'Mara CS, Flinn WR, Neimann HL, et al. Correlation of foot arterial anatomy with early tibial bypass patency. *Surgery.* 1981;89:743–752.

77. Ascer E, Veith FJ, et al. Quantitative assessment of outflow resistance in lower extremity arterial reconstruction. *J Surg Res.* 1984;37:8–15.

78. Gibbons GW, Marcacio EJ, Jr, Burgess EM, et al. Improved quality of diabetic foot care, 1984 vs. 1990: reduced length of stay and costs, insufficient reimbursement. *Arch Surg.* 1993; 28:576–581.

79. Gupta SK, and Veith FJ. Inadequacy of diagnosis related group (DRG) reimbursements for limb salvage lower extremity arterial reconstructions. *J Vasc Surg.* 1990;11: 348–357.

80. Pomposelli FB, Jr, Jepsen SJ, Gibbons GW, et al. A flexible approach to infrapopliteal vein grafts in patients with diabetes mellitus. *Arch Surg.* 1991;126:724–729.

81. Caputo GM, Cavanagh PR, Ulbrecht PR, et al. Assessment and management of foot disease in patients with diabetes. *N Engl J Med.* 1994;331:854–860.

82. Lee BY, Madden JL, Thoden, WR, et al. Lumbar sympathectomy for toe gangrene; long-term follow-up. *Am J. Surg.* 1983; 145:398–401.

83. Lee BY, Thoden WR, Madden JL, et al. Long term follow-up of bypass procedures with and without sympathectomy. *Contemp Surg.* 1982;20:51–55.

84. Bonutti PM, Bell GR, Compartment syndrome of the foot: a case report, *J. Bone Joint Surg.* 1986;68A:1449–1451.

85. Myerson MS. Experimental decompression of fascial compartment of the foot: the basis for fasciotomy in acute compartment syndromes. *Foot Ankle.* 1988;8:308–314.

86. Jacobs RL. Hoffman procedure in the ulcerated diabetic foot. *Foot Ankle.* 1982;3:142.

87. Frykberg RG. Podiatric problems in diabetes. In: Kozac GP, Campbell CS, Hoar R, et al., eds. *Management of Diabetic Foot Problems.* Philadelphia: Saunders; 1984:S–67.

88. Edmons ME, Bludell MP, Morris M, et al. Reduction in the number of major and minor amputations: impact of a new combined foot clinic. *Diabetologia.* 1984;27:272.

89. Levin ME, O'Neal LW. *The Diabetic Foot.* 4th ed. St. Louis, MO: Mosby; 1988:1–50.

Foot Compartment Syndrome— Modified Plantar Medial Approach Fasciotomy

Bok Y. Lee, Phyllis Berkowitz-Smith, V.J. Guerra, and Irfan M. Jameel

Introduction
Anatomy of the Plantar Structures

The Operation
Position
References

INTRODUCTION

It was not until recently that the idea of acute compartment syndromes of the leg became recognized as a unified concept.[1,2] Compartment syndrome is now a well-described clinical entity that results from increased pressure within a myofascial compartment. Mubarak and Hargens[2] were pioneers of this concept in the foot. They first suggested the presence of compartment syndrome in the foot by focusing on the interosseous compartment and presenting a possible treatment by decompression performed by longitudinal incisions of the dorsum of the foot. Whitesides[3] anecdotally described isolated compartment syndrome of the foot secondary to burns and direct trauma and recommended decompression of the compartments by the plantar medial approach as described by Henry.[4]

The signs and symptoms of compartment syndrome of the foot appear to be similar to those of compartment syndromes, in general. A degree of pain that is out of proportion to the injury appears to be the first symptom. An early clinical sign reported by Bonutti and Bell[5] was paresthesia in the distribution of the digital nerves of the toes, especially to pinprick, two-point discrimination, and light touch. Pain and passive dorsiflexion of the toes are also important signs, although direct trauma may cause similar symptoms. Pallor, paresthesia, and a palpable tense compartment have also been reported.

Note: Chapter 21 is reproduced with permission from B.Y. Lee and B.Herz, *Surgical Management of Cutaneous Ulcers and Pressure Sores*, published by Hodder Arnold, 1998.

In the presence of infection, bacteria spread from one compartment to another via the proximal calcaneal convergence or by direct perforation through the intercompartment septa. However, because each compartment is bound by rigid fascial separations in the medial to lateral and dorsal to plantar directions, lateral or dorsal spread of infection is a late sign of infection. Based on the anatomy of the foot, deep-space foot infections frequently show deceptively little plantar or dorsal foot abnormality. Therefore, a patient presenting with mild swelling of the foot, but toxic systemic symptoms, must be evaluated for an occult deep-space infection. The deep potential spaces or compartments of the foot can allow spread of bacteria from the plantar surface or web spaces of the foot to the ankle and the lower leg regions.[6]

Compartment syndrome of the foot is a sequela of an overwhelming infection of the foot, such as a diabetic foot infection. This condition is caused by increased compartment pressure, producing a reduction in tissue arterial blood flow and venous return that produces a diminished local arteriovenous gradient. The sequential elevation in tissue pressure causes increased tissue anoxia and reduction in nerve and muscle function. Although the incidence of this entity is high, compartment syndrome of the foot is often overlooked or unrecognized and, if not promptly treated by reducing intracompartment pressures by fasciotomy, prognosis is poor and can lead to amputation.

Early surgical decompression of the foot by fasciotomy is the only effective means of preventing the late consequences of a compartment syndrome, such as myoneural ischemia.[1,7] If not properly treated by effective fascial decompression technique, the end result of the ischemic process is a clawfoot deformity with permanent loss of function, contracture, weakness, sensory disturbance, and gangrene formation.[8–11]

Even though surgical decompression is the only reliable method for preventing these long-term ischemic complications, the techniques of fasciotomy of the foot have not been well described. Mubarak suggested two longitudinal dorsal incisions over the metatarsals.[2] The plantar medical approach for surgical decompression of the foot was originally described by Henry, who used it for decompression of the medial and central compartments of the foot.[4] Decompression of the lateral and interosseus compartments can be achieved by a similar separate lateral approach.[12] Grodinsky[13] and Loeffler and Ballard[14] described a long medial plantar utilitarian incision for decompression of established infections of the foot. The latter approach was used more recently by Bonutti and Bell[5] for management of an isolated compartment syndrome of the foot.

We present a stepwise description of fasciotomy of the foot using a single-incision plantar medial approach. Such an approach provides for the simultaneous decompression of all four fascial compartments of the foot (Fig. 21–1). This approach involves surgical dissection mostly in nonweight-bearing regions.

ANATOMY OF THE PLANTAR STRUCTURES

There are four fascial compartments of the foot: the medial, central, lateral, and interosseous compartments. The floor of three of these compartments (medial, central and lateral) consists of the rigid plantar fascia. The

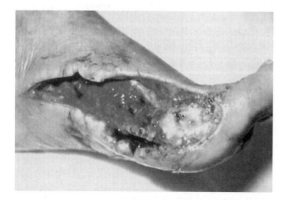

Fig. 21–1. Plantar medial incision dividing the skin and subcutaneous tissue between tuber calcanei metatarsal.

roof of these compartments is formed by the metatarsal bones and the interosseous fascia, which is the fourth fascial compartment.

The muscles are the key to surgical exposure. There are four muscle layers in the foot, starting from the skin to the bone. Layers 1 and 3 are both triads; each consist of three muscles—a central belly flanked by two companions. Layer 1 consists of the abductor hallucis, flexor digitorum brevis, and abductor digiti minimi. Similarly, layer 3 consists of the flexor hallucis, adductor hallucis, and flexor digiti minimi. Layers 2 and 4 consist of two long tendons plus short muscles. Layer 2 consists of the flexor hallucis longus, flexor digitorum longus, lumbricales, and quadratus plantae. Layer 4 consists of the peroneus longus, tibialis posterior, and interossei.

When standing on a level surface, the foot (with its skeleton) forms a vaulted cage that opens widely at the inner side. The door that keeps it closed is the abductor hallucis. If the upper fastenings of the abductor that hinge the belly of the abductor hallicus soleward are freed, then the contents of the cage (although for the moment, these may be screened by fascia) can be reached. Even when opened, the muscles are so packed and linked that until parted cleanly, the view is worthless.[11]

There are bands that hold the plantar layers close against the tarsal vault and (behind the layers) to each other. The master knot controlling this assembly is found approximately 2 cm lateral to the navicular tubercle. At this point, the flexor tendons are tied against the summit of the vault.

THE OPERATION

Position

The foot is positioned on its outer edge and the knee is partly flexed. The surgical technique of plantar medial decompression of fascial compartments of the foot involves a series of well-defined steps of dissection, as outlined in Table 21–1.

Step 1. **Incision of skin and subcutaneous tissue.** A plantar medial incision is made that divides the skin and superficial fascia at the inner side of the foot, from the ball of the great toe to the heel. This follows the length of the plantar surface of the first metatarsal and curves up to cross the tuberosity of navicular bone (Fig. 21–2). The limits of the incision are the tuber calcanei and the head of the first metatarsal. Care should be taken to avoid pressure points. Subcutaneous tissue is incised along the skin incision to visualize the medial extension of the plantar aponeurosis. Veins are identified and hemostasis is obtained using ligatures. Electrocautery use should be limited.

Table 21–1. Plantar medial fasciotomy of the foot using a single incision

Step 1	Plantar medial incision dividing the skin and subcutaneous tissue between tuber calcanei and first metatarsal
Step 2	Decompression of the medial compartment
Step 3	Dissection through the medial compartment muscles
Step 4	Identification of the plantar master knot
Step 5	Cutting off the plantar master knot and releasing the muscles
Step 6	Decompression of the central compartment
Step 7	Decompression of the interosseous compartment by several incisions in the plantar interosseous fascia
Step 8	Decompression of the lateral compartment
Step 9	Wound care after fasciotomy

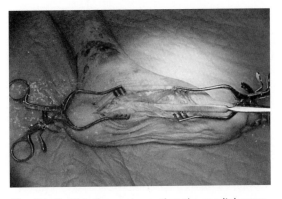

Fig. 21–3. This figure shows that the medial extension of the plantar aponeurosis is incised longitudinally to decompress the medial compartment.

Step 2. **Decompression of medial compartment.** The medial extension of the plantar aponeurosis is incised longitudinally to decompress the medial compartment (Fig. 21–3)

Step 3. **Dissection through the medial compartment.** After opening the plantar aponeurosis, the abductor hallucis tendon is identified at the inner side of the first metatarsal (Fig. 21–4). This tendon is mobilized, taking care to leave intact the adjoining fleshy fibers of flexor hallucis brevis. The tendon is used as a guide for separation of the less distinctive margins of the abductor belly. This belly is detached, first from its fascial band with the navicular tuberosity, and then from the indefinite anterior part of the vague annular ligament. The detachment is continued to the inner tuberosity of calcaneous. The muscle is then hinged soleward through a full right angle, taking care to spare the pair of small branches coming from the medial plantar nerve. Both branches lie close to the hinge, 2 and 3 cm, respectively, behind the tuberosity of the navicular.

Step 4. **Identification of the master knot.** The abductor hallucis muscle is retracted inferiorly

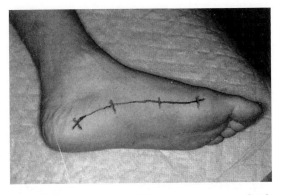

Fig. 21–2. A plantar medial incision is shown, dividing the skin and superficial fascia at the inner side of the foot from the ball of the great toe to the heel. This follows the length of the plantar surface of the first metatarsal and curves up to cross the tuberosity of navicular bone. The limits of the incision are the tuber calcanei and the head of the first metatarsal.

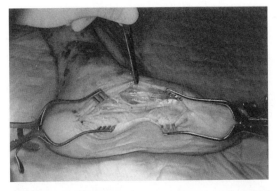

Fig. 21–4. The abductor hallucis tendon is identified at the inner side of the first metatarsal. This tendon is mobilized, taking care to leave intact adjoining fleshy fibers of flexor hallucis brevis.

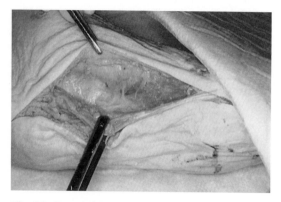

Fig. 21–5. This figure shows that the abductor hallucis muscle is retracted inferiorly. When this is done, partial screen of fascia is observed.

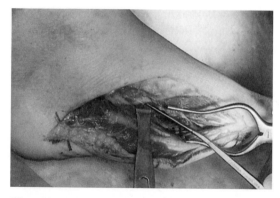

Fig. 21–7. The medial intermuscular septum is exposed and open longitudinally, decompressing the central compartment.

(Fig. 21–5). When this is done, a partial screen of fascia is observed. Located within this defective fascia are the plantar nerves and vessels. These form two bundles; the medial and lateral. These bundles first diverge approximately 3 cm behind the tuberosity of navicular.

Step 5. **Releasing the structures bound by the master knot.** Next the master knot is cut loose (Fig. 21–6). The master knot is an aponeurotic band attached 1 cm lateral to the tuberosity of the navicular, which attaches the two long second-layer tendons to the vault (flexor hallicus longus and flexor digitorum longus). This step allows for the exposure of the medial intermuscular septum.

Step 6. **Decompression of the central compartment.** The medial intermuscular septum is exposed and opened longitudinally, decompressing the central compartment (Fig. 21–7). Digital and blunt dissection are carried out, staying close to the roof formed by the metatarsals.

Step 7. **Decompression of the interosseous compartment.** The interosseous compartment is decompressed by longitudinally incising the plantar interosseous fascia superior to the quadratus plantae muscle (Fig. 21–8). The dissection between the quadratus plan-

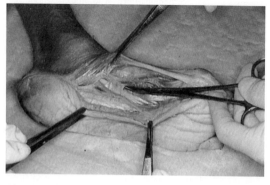

Fig. 21–6. The master knot is shown. The master knot is an aponeurotic band attached approximately 1 cm lateral to the tuberosity of the navicular.

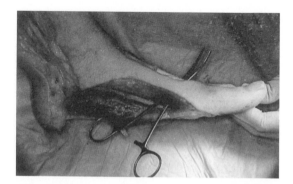

Fig. 21–8. The interosseous compartment is decompressed by longitudinally incising the plantar interosseous fascia superior to the quadratus plantae muscle. Note that in this case, additional dissection has been done to decompress the interosseous fascial compartment via the dorsum of the foot. The plantar medial incision is also extended more proximally above the level of the ankle.

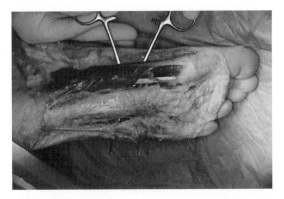

Fig. 21–9. Dissection between the lumbricales muscles and the flexor digitorum brevis muscle allows incision of the lateral intermuscular septum and decompression of the lateral compartment. In this case, an amputated foot has been dissected in which the plantar skin flap has been removed, in order to better illustrate the dissection.

tae muscle and the lumbricales muscles is deepened and the second incision in the interosseous fascia allows further decompression of the interosseous compartment. Technical considerations are the preservation of the neurovascular bundle in the posterior-medial aspect and the bifurcation of the posterior tibial artery into the medial and lateral plantar arteries, which give rise distally to the superficial arch. This travels medially and connects through the first interosseous space with the dorsalis pedis artery.

Step 8. **Decompression of the lateral compartment.** Dissection between the lumbricales muscles and the flexor digitorum brevis muscle allows incision of the lateral intermuscular septum and decompression of the lateral compartment (Fig. 21–9).

Step 9. **Wound care after fasciotomy.** After decompression of the four compartments, débride-

ment should be minimal and hemostasis established because the decompressed vessels can rebleed. The skin and all the fascial layers are left open. Steps should be taken to ensure that the wound is absolutely dry. The foot should be kept elevated. The wound is bandaged with fixed, firm sterile dressings. It has been observed in patients treated with fasciotomy, that when the drainage incision is longitudinal and opens the fascia of the infected compartment, wound healing is consistently accelerated.

REFERENCES

1. Masten FA, III. Compartment syndrome. A unified concept. *Clin Orthop.* 1975;113:8–14.
2. Mubarak SJ, Hargens AR. *Compartment Syndromes and Volkmann's Contracture.* Philadelphia: Saunders; 1981.
3. Whitesides TE. *Disorders of the Foot.* Philadelphia: Saunders; 1982.
4. Henry AK. *Extensive Exposure.* 2nd ed. New York and Edinburgh: Churchill-Livingstone; 1982.
5. Bonutti PM, Bell GR. Compartment syndrome of the foot. A case report. *J Bone Joint Surg.* 1986;68A:1449–1451.
6. Bridges RM, Deitch EA. Diabetic foot infections. Pathophysiology and treatment. *Surgical Clin N Am.* 1994;74: 537–555.
7. Whitesides TE, Jr, Harada H, Morimoto K. Compartment syndromes and the role of fasciotomy: its parameters and techniques, *AAOS Instructional Course Lectures.* Vol. 25. St. Louis; Mosby, 1977;179–196.
8. Chuinard EG, Baskin M. Claw-foot deformity. *J Bone Joint Surg.* 1973;55A:151–162.
9. Cole WH. The treatment of claw foot. *J Bone Joint Surg.* 1940;22A:895–908.
10. Jones R. An address on Volkman's ischemic contracture with special reference to treatment, *BMJ.* 1928;2:639–642.
11. Tsuge K. Treatment of established Volkman's contracture, *J Bone Joint Surg.* 1975;57A:925–929.
12. Myerson MS. Acute compartment syndrome of the foot. *Bull Hosp Dis Orthop Inst.* 1987;47:251–261.
13. Grodinsky M. A study of fascial spaces of the foot. *Surg Gynecol Obstet.* 1929;49:739–751.
14. Loeffler RD, Ballard A. Plantar fascial spaces of the foot and a proposed surgical approach. *Foot Ankle.* 1980;1:11–14.

Index

A

Abdominal wall, 327f
   contaminated wound, 328f, 329f
   wounds, 325–327
Abductor hallucis muscle, 369f
Abductor hallucis tendon, 368f
ABI, 10, 11f
Above knee amputation (AKA), 213
Acetylcholine, 174
Achilles tendon
   Integra, 272
Acute diabetic neuritis
   vascular aspects, 153–154
Acute wounds, 124
   care
      dressings, 127
      reconstructive options, 125
      special attention, 127–128
      standard management, 125
   dynamic tension, 126
   elective treatment, 301
   high static tension, 126
   management, 122–130
   principles, 126
   ritualistic teachings, 122
   skin substitutes, 300–301
   wound characteristics, 123–124
Adenosine diphosphoribose, 49
Adenosine triphosphate, 37
Adjunctive hyperbaric oxygen therapy
   indications, 59
Adjunctive systemic hyperbaric oxygen
   therapy
   contraindications, 60
African Americans
   diabetes, 349f
Age of Pericles, 74
AKA, 213
AlloDerm, 304
Allogeneic acellular dermal matrix, 30
Allogeneic keratinocyte sheets, 300,
   305–306
Alloplastic coverage
   Integra, 271
Alternating current, 90
American Diabetes Association, 7
American Physical Therapy Association, 80
Amputations
   contralateral limb
      incidences, 145
   diabetic foot, 322f, 361–362

distal tarsus, 260f
European studies, 147
Integra, 272–273
monetary costs, 147–148
partial foot
   mortality and morbidity rates, 143
ray, 361
social effects, 147–148
toe, 361
transmetatarsal, 361–362
Angioblast streaming
   healthy wound, 243f
Angiocytes
   Integra, 238f
Angiogenesis
   VAC systems, 66
   wound extracellular matrix, 20
Angiogenic growth factor combinations
   wound healing, 26
Angiotensin-converting enzyme, 51, 150
Ankle-brachial index (ABI), 10, 11f
Ankles, 315–316
   Doppler, 351f
   flowmetry, 351f
   photoplethysmographic waveforms,
      351f
Antibiotics
   advantages, 163
   diabetic foot, 161, 356–359
   infected wounds, 160
   Integra, 273, 273t
   local injections, 163
   tissue levels, 162
   topical, 163–164
Antimicrobials
   diabetic foot, 360t
Antioxidant metabolites, 92
Antithrombin III, 169
Apligraf, 10, 300, 301, 305, 306
   autologous skin graft, 32
   FDA, 32
Aristotle, 74
ArtAssist device, 213–214, 213f
   foot cuff, 214
Arterial disease
   treatment, 154
Arterial graft occlusions, 170
Arterial insufficiency, 2–3, 188
Arterial reconstructive surgery, 362
Arterial testing, 187
Arteriosclerosis obliterans, 184

Arteriosclerotic cardiovascular disease, 176
Artificial skin
   Integra, 227, 251
Assimacopoulos, 86
Atherosclerosis, 344–345
Autologous keratinocyte sheets, 299–300,
   305–306
Autologous precursor cells, 33
Autosympathectomy, 346
Axial pattern flaps, 130

B

Bacterial burden, 305
Bacterial load reduction, 66
Baroreceptors, 133
Basic fibroblast growth factor (bFGF), 223t
Becalpermin
   diabetes
      foot ulcers, 24
Behçet's syndrome, 234f
Below knee amputation (BKA), 213
Bernard, Claude, 78
Beta blockers, 150
Betaglycan, 223t
bFGF, 223t
Bilayered constructs, 300, 304–305
Bilayered skin equivalents
   wound healing, 31–32
Bilayered skin substitutes, 31–33
Biobrane, 303
Biologic amputation level, 361
Biologic coverage, 258
Biologic dressings
   grafts, 252–253
Biologic superdressing
   histoconduction and bridging,
      247–249
   Integra, 247, 251
Biomaterial wound matrix
   diabetic wound healing, 290–296
Biphasic pulsatile currents, 84
BKA, 213
Blast wounds
   gunpowder, 122
Blood sample collection, 166–167
Bone-marrow derived stem cells, 20
Boot therapy, 171
Boyle, Robert, 77
Brachial pulse volume curves, 183
Breast cancer
   immediate reconstruction, 329

Breast surgery, 327–330
Bridging
  biologic superdressing, 247–249
Buerger's disease
  inflammatory features, 157
  patients, 158
  process, 158
  smoking effects, 156
Bulk filling
  Integra, 286
Burke, John F., 228
Byzantine period, 75

C

Calciphylaxis
  Integra, 269
Callus
  formation consequences, 3
Capillaries
  functions, 132
Capillaroscopy, 156
Capillary blood flow
  blood viscosity, 132
Capillary perfusion
  physiology, 132
Cardiosynchronous external compression
  boots
  developmental considerations, 181
  external devices
    intra-aortic balloon, 181
  heart, 181
  Starling's Law
    boot hemodynamics, 181–182
Cell-activation, 110
Cell mitosis, 56
Cellular Pathology, 77
Cellulitis, 194
  toe, 196
CHF
  diabetes, 97
Cholesterol emboli, 165–166
Cholinergic nerve supply damage, 152
Cholinergic neuropathy, 153, 174
Chondroitin, 229
Chronic lymphedema
  long-lasting relief, 193
Chronic obstructive pulmonary disease
  (COPD)
  diabetes, 97
Chronic problem wound, 256–257
Chronic ulcers, 232f
  matrix macromolecules
    etiology and treatment, 109–121
Chronic wounds, 50
  etiology, 96
  life quality, 17
  skin substitutes, 300–301
Cilostazol, 149

Circulatory boots
  advantages, 163
  alternative boot differences, 177–184
  bags and boots, 191
  benefits, 180
  current illnesses, 184
  vs. ECP devices, 178–179
  FDA, 179
  historical data and occupation, 184–185
  illustrative patient examples, 192–193
  monitor settings, 192
  patient data, 184–185
  patient position, 191
  physical findings, 185–188
  pressure settings, 191–192
  pulses, 185
  PVD
    vs. invasive procedures, 179
  septic emboli block, 199
  skin and nail changes, 185
  treatment, 182, 191, 192
  ulcers, 183
Claudication
  differential diagnosis, 148
  prognosis, 148–149
  risk factors, 149
  treatment, 149
CLI
  intermittent pneumatic compression
    devices, 212–217
Clonidine, 51
Clot RATE, 340
Clotting factors, 166–175
  in vitro relationship studies, 166–167
Collagen, 46, 223t
  gene transcription, 48
    lactate, 49
  Integra, 244
  synthesis
    infection, 48
    lactate, 49
    oxygen concentration, 48
Collagenolysis, 230
Collagen VII immunostaining, 292f
Compartment syndrome, 343–344
  decompression of, 319f, 320f
Compression boots. *See*
  Cardiosynchronous external
  compression boots
Compression wraps
  wound care, 107
Conductive silicone electrodes, 95
Congestive heart failure
  diabetes, 97
Contour correction
  Integra, 286
Contralateral limb amputation
  incidences, 145

COPD
  diabetes, 97
Copper
  outer shell, 94
Costs
  amputations, 147–148
  home intravenous therapy, 162
  lower-extremity ulcers, 1
  skin substitutes, 302
  wound management, 23
Coumadin, 170
Crick, Francis HC, 79
Critical colonization
  wounds, 21
Critical limb ischemia (CLI)
  intermittent pneumatic compression
    devices, 212–217
Crohn's disease, 60
Cultured composite skin, 32–33
Cushing's syndrome, 168
Cutaneous. *See* Skin
Cutaneous blood flow
  neural control, 133
Cutaneous circulation
  noninvasive evaluation, 131–140
Cutaneous perfusion, 134–135
  fluorometry, 134–135
  laser Doppler, 134
  pressure, 135
  xenon-133 washout, 134
Cutaneous pressure
  photoplethysmography, 135–136, 137
    measurements, 137
Cutaneous vasomotor tone, 133
Cyclic-guanosine monophosphate, 173
Cytochrome, 150
Cytochrome oxidase, 45f
Cytokines
  ECM, 117
  macromolecules
    cell activation, 110–112
    matrix signaling, 112

D

Darwin, Charles Robert, 78
Debridement, 305
  leg, 317f
  necrotizing fasciitis, 355f
Decompressive fasciotomy, 362–363
Decorin, 223t
Deep vein thrombosis
  studies, 172
Dehydration
  hypoglycemia, 168
Dermagraft, 10, 219–226, 304
  clinical studies, 224
  cryopreservation of, 221
  diabetic foot ulcers, 224

histological cross section of, 221f
implantation of, 221–222
manufacture of, 220–221
mechanism of action, 222–223
storage of, 221
surgical wounds, 224
thawing of, 222
venous leg ulcers, 224
wound bed preparation for, 221–222
Dermal constructs, 300, 303–304, 306
Dermal regeneration template, 30–31
Dermis, 299
Diabetes, 7–10, 338
African Americans, 349f
amputation, 322f
CHF, 97
COPD, 97
hypercoagulable state, 167
insulin dependent, 349
hyperemia, 155
Integra, 266–267
joint replacement, 315f
pressure sores, 326f
substance P, 340–342
type 1
multiple complications, 194
Diabetic foot, 338–363
amputations, 322f, 361–362
anatomy, 342–343
antibiotic choice, 161
antibiotic treatment, 356–359
antimicrobial therapy, 360t
case reports, 349–356
clinical findings, 347
diagnosis, 348–349
differential diagnosis, 348
hypercoagulable states, 340
infection, 347–348
necrotizing cellulitis, 198
pathomechanics, 346–347
pathophysiology, 141–211, 339–340
physiology, 339
plantar wounds, 222
prevention, 363
prognosis, 363
treatment, 356
ulcers, 60, 320f, 321f, 356f
dermagraft, 224
Diabetic microcirculation, 156
Diabetic neuritis
acute
vascular aspects, 153–154
Diabetic neuropathy, 8, 151–154
foot, 153
Diabetic peripheral neuropathy, 345
Diabetic ulcers
Integra, 266
SIS, 293–295

Diabetic wound healing
biomaterial wound matrix, 290–296
Diffuse diabetic neuropathy
vascular aspects, 152–153
Diffusive vascular disease
operative risk assessment, 158–159
Direct current
wound healing, 83
Direct currents, 90
graphic representations, 84
Directional-cell migration, 110
Disease control
Integra, 273
Distal tarsus
amputation, 260f
amputations, 260f
DNA
molecular biology, 79
Doppler
ankles, 351f
cutaneous perfusion, 134
skin perfusion pressure, 135
Dorsal foot ulcer, 5f
Dorsalis pedis artery, 342
angiogram, 357f
Dressings
biologic
grafts, 252–253

E

ECM. *See* Extracellular matrix (ECM)
ECP devices
vs. circulatory boots, 178–179
Edema, 105
etiology, 106
Egyptian medicine, 73
Ehrlich, Paul, 78
Eighteenth century, 77
Eikenella corrodens, 128
Elastoplast, 329
Elderly
wound closure, 333
Electotherapeutic Terminology in Physical Therapy, 80
Electrical stimulation (ES)
antibacterial effects, 85
application guidelines, 87
chronic wounds, 88
circulatory effects, 85
clinical applications, 87–88
precautions, 87–88
wound repair, 80–89
clinical evidence, 86–87
rationale, 81–85
wound tensile strength effects, 85–86
Electric currents
electrons, 93–94

Electrode wraps
application, 96
Embryonic histogenesis
Integra, 235
End-diastolic treatments, 182
Endogenous nitric oxide, 173
Endothelial cells, 131
release of factors from, 215f
Endothelial dysfunction, 155
Endothelial progenitor cells, 34
Enterococcus, 196
Epicel, 303
Epidermis, 299
Epithelial cell migration, 109
Equinovarus deformity
foot ulcerations, 9
Equinus deformity, 6
Erythrocyte sedimentation rate, 175
ES. *See* Electrical stimulation (ES)
Essential structures
exposed, 258
Estrogen replacement therapy
risk factors, 151
European medicine, 74
Exchange vessels, 132
Excisional grafts, 299
Exposed structures
essential, 258
Integra, 270–271
External constant tension approximation
wound closure, 310
External Counterpulsation (ECP) devices
vs. circulatory boots, 178–179
External limb compression, 107
External tissue expansion
wound closure, 309–335
Extracellular matrix (ECM), 30, 109
bioactivity, 109
bioinductive activity, 118
diverse mechanisms, 111
modulation mechanisms, 117
molecule, 113
Exudate, 305

F

Fasciotomy, 359f
decompressive, 362–363
modified plantar medial approach, 366–370
operation, 367–368
plantar medial
foot, 368t
Feet. *See* Foot
Femoral artery
angiogram, 356f
intraoperative electromagnetic flow, 355f
Femoroinfrapopliteal bypass
lower extremities, 358f

Femoroposterior tibial bypass
noninvasive vascular studies, 357f
Fetal skin fibroblasts, 117
Fibrinolysis, 171
anticoagulation therapies, 169–172
biguanide therapy, 169
postoperative state, 169
Fibrinolytic activity
control group, 171
Fibrinolytic therapy, 170
Fibroblasts, 220, 220f, 223
accumulation zone
healthy wound, 243f
fetal skin, 117
Integra, 241
maturation zone
healthy wound, 243f
migration, 118
mitogenic, 115
MSF, 115
neutrophils, 82
syncytial
Integra, 235
Fibronectin, 113, 219, 223t
functional domains, 113
ion exchange, 114
modular structure, 113f
MSF, 114–116
Fibroplasia
normal wound, 246f
Fifth vital sign, 359–360
Flaps, 253–255
essential coverage, 254
ineligible, 258
reconstruction, 254
soft-tissue, 130
utilization, 254
wound closure, 254
wound healing, 254
Fleming, Alexander, 78
Flexor digitorum brevis, 370f
Flexor digitorum longus, 343
Flexor hallucis longus, 343
Fluid balance
skin substitutes, 302
Fluorometry
cutaneous perfusion, 134–135
Foot, 315–316. See also Diabetic foot
amputations, 322f, 361–362
mortality and morbidity rates, 143
central compartment, 344f
compartments of, 342–343, 342f, 342t
viscoelastic displacement curves,
344f
diabetic neuropathy, 153
gangrene, 355f
necrosis, 356f
osteomyelitis, 353f

perforating ulcers, 345–346, 353f
plantar medial fasciotomy, 368t
skin graft, 358f
Foot compartment syndrome, 366–370
Foot cuff
IPCD, 214
Foot infections
antibiotics, 161
morbidity, 160
surgery, 161
Foot ulcerations, 350f
acute wounds, 18
advance therapy prerequisites, 20–21
algorithm assessment, 14f
angiogenesis, 19–21
chronic wounds, 18
dorsal, 5f
etiology and management, 1–15
granulation, 19–21
musculoskeletal assessment and
management, 13–15
neuropathy, 13–15
non-healing developments, 2
prevention, 15
risk factors, 2–3
vascular assessment, 10–13
vascular management, 10–13
wound angiogenesis
amplification, 19
growth factors, 20
initiation, 19
vascular proliferation, 19
vascular stabilization, 20
wound assessment, 9–10
wound healing
molecular level, 18–19
wound management, 9–10
Foot X-ray admission, 199
Fournier's gangrene, 317f
Free-flap transfer, 130
Free radicals
antioxidant effects, 92
antioxidant neutralization, 100
formation, 91
mitochondria damage, 92–93
oxidation, 91
Frequency, 90
F scan, 13

G
GAG, 223, 223t, 228
Gait
biomechanics, 2
Galvanotaxis
wound healing, 83t
Gangrene, 356
foot, 355f
toe, 356f

G-CSF, 223t, 224
Gene-activated matrix, 33
Gentamicin, 163
with Integra, 273t
Giant nevus, 334f
Glutathione, 92
Glycosaminoglycans (GAG), 223, 223t,
228
Glycosylation
neuropathy, 151–152
Grafts, 252–253
biologic dressing, 252–253
specialized reconstruction, 253
thrombosis, 147
wound closure, 252
Granulation tissue, 243f, 245f
Granulocyte colony simulating factor (G-
CSF), 223t, 224
Granulomatous
Integra, 269
Greco-Roman period, 74–75
Greek medicine, 73–74
Green fluorescent protein, 33
Growth factors, 223t

H
Hallux abductovalgus, 5f
Hand dorsum
Integra, 271
Haptotaxis, 110
HBO therapy. See Hyperbaric oxygen
(HBO) therapy
HDL-cholesterol, 176
Head
Integra, 270
Head lesions, 331–333
Healing wound
metabolic wound, 46
Healthy wound, 243f, 245f
Heart disease, 194
Heel
Integra, 272
neuropathic ulcer, 293f
ulcers, 3, 5f, 323–324
debridement, 295
Hematoma, 314f
Hemodynamic booting variables
effects, 182–184
Hemodynamic forces
endothelial cell survival, 174–175
Henle, Jacob, 77
Heparin
Coumadin therapy, 169–170
Heparin binding epidermal growth factor,
223t
Hepatocyte growth factor (HGF), 173, 220
HGF, 173, 220
High risk donor sites, 258–259

High risk flaps, 258
High risk history, 257
High risk patients, 258
High risk ulcer profile, 257
High voltage pulsed current
        graphic representation, 86
        machines, 84
Hippocrates, 74
Histoconduction
        biologic superdressing, 247–249
Holstein's Isotope techniques, 135
Home intravenous therapy, 162
        cost saving, 162
Hooke, Robert, 77
Human dermal fibroblasts, 31
Hyaluronan synthesis, 117
Hydrocolloid, 294f
Hydroxylase, 45
Hyperbaric oxygen (HBO) therapy,
        34–35, 44, 51–52, 128–132, 275.
        See also Topical hyperbaric oxygen
        therapy
        adjunctive
                indications, 59
        adjunctive systemic
                contraindications, 60
        clinical research, 57
        modalities and mechanism, 58–59
        systemic, 61
                topical HBO therapy, 61
Hypercoagulable states, 167–168
        diabetes, 167
        diabetic foot, 340
        Integra, 266
Hyperglycemia
        E-selectin, 168
        neuropathy, 151–152
Hyperinsulinemia
        insulin resistance, 175–177
        weight gain, 175–177
Hyperlipidemias
        drug and diet treatment, 167
Hypertension, 176
Hypoglycemia
        excessive alcohol ingestion, 168
Hypohydrosis, 4
Hypoxia
        oxygen concentration, 52
        practical rules, 52
        truncates angiogenesis, 49
Hypoxic problems, 51

I
IGF 1, 223t
IL 6, 223t, 224
IL 8, 223t, 224
Immunopathic
        Integra, 267–268

Impaired wound healing
        etiology, 116–121
        future prospects, 116–117
Ineligible flaps, 258
Ineligible skin grafts, 258
Inert oxygen molecule
        outer shell, 91
Infarcted hand, 264f
Infected wounds, 159
        recognition, 159
        risk factors
                elderly people, 159
                tissue damage, 159
Infection
        diabetic foot, 347–348
        Integra, 269
Inflammation
        Integra, 230, 231f, 286
        persistence, 257
Inflammatory zone
        healthy wound, 243f
Injured Integra, 249f
Insulin dependent diabetes, 349
        hyperemia, 155
Insulin like growth factor 1 (IGF 1), 223t
Integra, 226–287, 227f, 304
        acute physiologic effects, 229
        acute wounds, 255
        as adjunct to surgery, 269–270
        as agent of tissue regeneration, 227
        by anatomy, 270–272
        ancillary therapies, 275
        angiocytes, 238f
        application to wound, 273
        as artificial skin, 227, 251
        biologic superdressing, 247, 251
        biology of, 228–251
        case studies, 259–263, 260f, 262f,
                263f, 265f
        chemical composition of, 228–229
        chronic wounds, 228, 256–257
                indications for, 257–273
        collagen, 244, 246f
        compliant, 246f
        complications, 275–276
        consolidation, 239
        contraction, 244
        contraindications, 276–277
        control dynamics, 241
        vs. conventional methods, 259
        conventional wound surgery, 255–256
        critical coverage, 251, 255
        diabetes, 266–267
        domain maturation, 239, 241f
        embryonic histogenesis, 235
        epidermal events, 239, 242f
        essential coverage, 251, 255
        failed, 276

fibroblasts, 241
fixation and compression, 273–274
forms and availability, 273
        at four years, 248f
granulomatous, 269
histogenesis, 237, 239–247, 239f
        cellular controllers, 239–240
        timing, 239
        vs. wound module, 239
histogenetic process, 235–239
immunopathic, 267–268
indications, 251–255
infection, 269
inflammation, 230, 231f
inflammatory wound repair
        suppression, 232–235
inpatient vs. outpatient, 285t
interim management and observation,
        274
local soft tissue pathology control,
        250–251
logistics, 275
long term management, 275
lymphatic, 267
macroarchitecture, 229
matrix filling, 237–238, 240f
matrix recognition, 235, 236f
maturation, 244–247
mechanical, anatomical, trauma and
        surgery ulcers, 268
microarchitecture, 229
micrograph, 229f
at one year, 247f
open, 276
order of events, 241
outcomes, 281–282, 281t, 282t, 283t,
        284t
overgrafts, 274
pathologic wounds, 256–257
patient profiles, 277–285, 278t
perivascular cells, 235, 238f, 239f
with platelets, 233f
preempting pathergy, 230–232
problems, 275–276
radiation and malignancy, 268–269
reconstruction, 255
recurrent disease resistance, 251
regeneration of, 244f
repair and histogenesis, 250t
scar suppression, 249–250
secondary procedures, 274–275
semibiologic non living material, 247
separated silicone, 274
similarity to normal dermis, 250
as skin regenerant, 251
structure of, 228–230
subacute physiologic effects, 232
as surgical implant, 228

Integra, *(continued)*
    syncytial transformation, 235, 237f
    technique and management,
        273–274
    transition, 235
    ulcer anatomy, 279t, 280t
    utilization, 285t
    vascular density, 241–242
    vasculogenesis, 235–236, 239f
    venous disease, 267
    wound closure, 229–230, 235
Interleukin 6 (IL 6), 223t, 224
Interleukin 8 (IL 8), 223t, 224
Intermittent claudication, 148–151
Intermittent pneumatic compression
    devices (IPCD)
    biochemical compression effects,
        214–215
    clinical results, 215–217
    critical limb ischemia, 212–217
    foot cuff, 214
    mechanical compression effects, 214
    mechanical effects, 216f
    mechanism of action, 214–215, 214f
Intermuscular septum, 343
Interosseous compartment, 369f
Interpolation flaps, 129
Intraoperative electromagnetic flow
    femoral artery, 355f
Intrinsic minus foot, 4
Inverted keratinocyte delivery system,
    303
In vitro animal studies, 86
In vitro epidermopoiesis, 35
IPCD. *See* Intermittent pneumatic
    compression devices (IPCD)
Ischemia
    classification, 191
Ischemic disease, 148
Ischemic leg
    subcutaneous changes, 178
Ischemic ulcers, 5f
    characterized, 2–3

J
Jewish period, 75
Joint replacement
    diabetes, 315f

K
Keratinocyte growth factor (KGF), 220,
    223t
Keratinocytes
    Integra, 287
Keratinocyte sheets, 303, 305–306
KGF, 220, 223t
Klebsiella, 330f
Knee joint, 312

L
Langer, Karl, 123
Large surface areas, 258
Laser Doppler
    cutaneous perfusion, 134
    skin perfusion pressure, 135
LEA. *See* Lower extremity amputations
    (LEA)
Legs, 312–313
    arteriography, 352
    compartment syndrome
        decompression of, 319f, 320f
    debridement, 317f
    veins
        emptying, 214
Lesions
    electron flow
        healing, 100
    healing process timetable, 100
    healing rates, 100
Lewis, Thomas, 78
Limb salvage
    Integra, 272–273
Lip
    squamous carcinoma, 336f, 337f
Lipid soluble antioxidants, 93
Livedoid vasculitis, 170
Lower extremities, 312–322
    femoroinfrapopliteal bypass, 358f
    Integra, 270
Lower extremity amputations (LEA)
    diabetes
        amputation incidences, 142–143
        mortality rates, 145
        proportions, 146–147
        US diagnosed population, 143
    diabetic causes, 146
    diabetics, 142
    diagnosis, 143
    hospital discharge, 144
    hospitalization length, 146
    nondiabetics, 142
    remaining leg infection risk, 144–146
    Veterans Affairs hospitals, 145
Lower-extremity ulcers
    social cost, 1–2
    treating costs, 1
Lumbar sympathectomy, 362
    electromagnetic flowmetry, 353f
Lumbricales muscles, 370f
Lymphatic
    Integra, 267
Lymphedema
    causes, 105
    chronic
        long-lasting relief, 193
    definition, 104
    healing, 106

    pneumatic pumps, 106
    secondary, 105
    wound healing, 106–107
        codependence, 104–108
        relationship, 104
Lymphoma, 60
Lysyl oxidase, 48

M
Macroarterial
    integra, 263–264
Macrophage zone
    healthy wound, 243f
Magnetic resonance angiography, 12
Major amputation, 362
Malignancy
    Integra, 268–269
Manual lymph drainage, 105
Mastectomy, 331, 332f, 333f
Master knot, 369f
Maternal blood samples
    testing of, 220
Matricryptins, 112
Matrikines, 112
    protease-generated fragments,
        112–116
Matrix fibronectin
    proteolytic degradation, 115
Matrix metalloproteinase (MMP), 22, 219
Matrix modulation cell behavior, 110–112
Matrix proteins, 223t
Mature scar, 248f
Medial intermuscular septum, 369f
Medial ischemic ulcer, 5f
Medical electricity, 80
Medieval period, 75–76
Metabolic process, 94
Metatarsal phalangeal joint, 6
Microarterial
    Integra, 265–266
Microbial invasion
    skin substitutes, 302
Microcirculation, 131
    anatomy, 131
Microcirculatory unit, 132
Microcurrents
    antioxidants, 94
Microvascular bed, 131
Microvascular composite tissue
    transplantation, 130
Migration stimulating factor (MSF), 116
    amino acid sequence, 113
    angiogenesis, 118
    expression
        venous stasis ulcer, 116
    fibroblasts, 115
    fibronectin, 114–116
    modular structure, 113f

Mitochondria
  outer and inner membranes, 93
Mitogenic factors, 110
MMP, 22, 219
Modified medial approach of Henry, 359f
Modified plantar medial approach
  fasciotomy, 366–370
  operation, 367–368
Mohammedan period, 75
Moist wound healing
  principles, 104
Molecular oxygen, 92
MSF. *See* Migration stimulating factor
  (MSF)
Murray, James, 212
Musculoskeletal deformities, 4–6
Myelinated type-A fibers, 8

N
Naughton, Gail, 219
Near-infrared reflectance oximetry,
  138–139
Neck lesions, 331–333
Necrobiosis lipoidica
  Integra, 266
Necrotizing cellulitis
  diabetic foot, 198
Necrotizing fasciitis, 60
  debridement, 355f
Negative ions
  migration, 82
Nerve compression syndrome
  neuropathy, 152
Neuropathic diseases, 151
Neuropathic ulcers, 4
  heel, 293f
Neuropathy
  bedside signs, 185
  foot ulceration, 4–5
Neurotrophic ulcers
  treatment, 360–361
Neurotropic ulcers, 8f
Nineteenth century, 77–78
Nitric oxide (NO), 173–174, 215f
Nitric oxide synthase (NOS), 173
NMR flowmetry
  diabetic foot, 348–349
NO, 173–174, 215f
Non inflammatory transition zone
  healthy wound, 243f
Nonvenous ulcers, 106
Normal reticular dermis, 248f
Normal wound
  fibroplasia, 246f
NOS, 173
Nuclear magnetic resonance (NMR)
  flowmetry
  diabetic foot, 348–349

Nuclear magnetic resonance principles,
  139

O
Oasis, 303
OrCel, 304–305
OrCel Bilayered Cellular Matrix, 32
Oriental medicine, 74
Osteomyelitis, 159–160, 194, 356
  circulatory boots, 164–165
  foot, 353f
  healed, 200
  outpatient treatment, 197
  pathophysiology diagnosis, 160
  5th toe mp joint, 195
  toe, 353f
Osteoradionecrosis, 52
Overgrafts
  Integra, 274
Oximetry, 136–137
Oxygen
  clinical wound problems, 44–51
  signaling zone, 46
  tissue, 45, 46
Oxygenase
  phagosome membrane, 47

P
Paramount, 130
Paré, Ambroise, 122
Parenteral antimicrobial-drug therapy,
  162
Partial foot amputations
  mortality and morbidity rates, 143
Partridge, Myles, 78
Pasteurella multocida, 128
Pathergy
  Integra, 230–232
Pathergy test, 234f
Pathology
  general presentation, 184
PAVAEX, 212
PDGF. *See* Platelet-derived growth factor
  (PDGF)
Penicillium notatum, 78
Pentoxifline, 150
Peptides
  and reactive hyperemia, 155
Percutaneous transluminal angioplasty
  (PTA), 13, 150
Perforating ulcers
  foot, 345–346, 353f
Peripheral nerve management
  Integra, 286–287
Peripheral neuropathy, 7
  etiologies, 7
Peripheral obstructive arterial disease,
  167

Peripheral vascular disease (PVD), 167
  circulatory boots
    invasive procedures, 179
  substance P, 340–342
Perivascular cells
  Integra, 238f, 239f
Permeable membrane
  capillaries function, 131
Peroneal artery, 342
Peroneus longus, 343
PET, 173
PGI, 172–173
Phagocytic oxygenase, 45
Phlox, 47
  congenital absence, 48
Photoelectricpletysmography probe, 179
Photoplethysmographic waveform,
  136–137
Plantaire mal perforant, 346
Plantar aponeurosis, 368f
Plantar arch, 342
Plantar diabetic foot wounds
  off weighting, 222
Plantar medial fasciotomy
  foot, 368t
Plantar structures
  anatomy of, 367
Platelet-derived growth factor (PDGF),
  22–24
  receptor, 56
  recombinant, 10
Platelet derived growth factor alpha
  (PDGF alpha), 223t, 275
Platelets
  Integra, 233f
Pleiotropic effectors, 112
Pneumatic leg devices
  differences, 178
PolyMem, 359
Popliteal artery, 342
Porcine small intestine submucosa, 31
Porter, John, 213
Position emission tomography (PET), 173
Positive ions
  migration, 82
Potential clinical utility, 117
Premarket approval application, 28
Pressure sores, 322–325, 323f
  diabetes, 326f
  sacral, 322–323
Presternal wound, 330f
Primary lymphedema, 105
Problem wound
  chronic, 256–257
Prolyl hydroxylases
  kinetics, 45f
Prophylaxis
  studies, 172

Prostacyclin (PGI), 172–173
Prostaglandin compounds, 173
    ketone, 172
Protein S deficient hypercoagulability, 232f
Proxiderm, 310, 313f, 316f, 329
Proxiderm devices, 310
Proximal phalanx
    destruction, 198
Pseudomonas, 61
Pseudomonas aeruginosa, 196
PTA, 13, 150
Pulmonary emboli
    studies, 172
Pulsed currents
    graphic representation, 84
    wound healing, 83–84
Pulse volume recordings (PVR), 11f, 12f
PVD. *See* Peripheral vascular disease (PVD)
PVR, 11f, 12f
Pyodermagangrenosum, 60

R
Radiation
    Integra, 268–269
Radiofrequency ablation, 37
Radiofrequency treatment, 38
Ray amputation, 361
Reactive hyperemia
    pneumatic boots, 154
    stimuli, 155
    vascular dysfunction, 154–156
Receptor-mediated signal-transduction
    pathways, 111
Recombinant platelet-derived growth
    factor, 10, 22–24
Reconstructive foot surgery, 13
Recurrent disease
    high risk for, 259
Regranex, 10
Renaissance period, 76
Reservoir vessels, 132
Resistance vessels, 132
Rest pain
    differential diagnosis, 148
Rheumatoid arthritis, 60
Rotation flaps, 129

S
Sacral pressure sores, 322–323, 323f
Scalp
    Integra, 271
Scar
    avoiding, 259
    contracture, 246f
        Integra, 286
    suppression
        Integra, 249–250
Schwann, Theodore, 77

Secondary lymphedema, 105
Secreted protein acidic and rich in cysteine
    (SPARC), 223t
Semmes-Weinstein monofilaments, 13
Separated silicone
    Integra, 274
Sepsis, 164
Septic shock, 164
Seventeenth Century, 76–77
Shelf life
    skin substitutes, 302
Silvadene, 9
SIS. *See* Small intestine submucosa (SIS)
Skin. *See also* Cutaneous
    artificial
        Integra, 227, 251
    cultured composite, 32–33
Skin battery potentials, 82
    human, 81
Skin equivalents, 306
    bilayered
        wound healing, 31–32
Skin flaps, 253
Skin grafts
    acute wounds
        reconstruction, 123
    foot, 358f
    full-thickness, 129
    ineligible, 258
    split-thickness, 129
Skin perfusion pressure
    laser Doppler, 135
Skin regenerant
    Integra, 251
Skin substitutes, 298–306
    acute wounds, 300–301
    adherence, 301
    bilayered, 31–33
    biodegradable, 302
    cost, 302
    defined, 299
    economics, 306
    elasticity, 301–302
    flexibility, 301–302
    fluid balance, 302
    history of, 299–301
    ideal properties, 301–302
    mechanism of action, 305–306
    microbial invasion, 302
    nontoxic/nonantigenic, 302
    pliability, 301–302
    shelf life, 302
    storage requirements, 302
Small intestine submucosa (SIS),
    291–292, 291f
    clinical evaluation, 292–293
    diabetic ulcers, 293–295
    preclinical evaluation, 292

Smoking
    pathophysiological effects, 157
    risks, 156–157
Soak solutions, 187
Sodium transport
    epithelium, 81
Soft-tissue flaps, 130
Soft-tissue infections
    circulatory boots, 164–165
    local antibiotic therapy, 164–165
SonACT, 340
SPARC, 223t
Split thickness skin grafts (STSG), 253,
    361
Squamous carcinoma, 335f
    lip, 336f, 337f
Staphylococcus aureus, 128
Staples, 127
Static electricity, 90
Stem cells
    wound angiogenesis, 33–34
    wound healing, 33–34
Storage requirements
    skin substitutes, 302
STSG, 253, 361
Subcutaneous oxygen tension, 138
Substance P
    diabetes, 340–342
    peripheral vascular disease,
        340–342
Sumerian medicine, 73
Superdressing
    biologic
        histoconduction and bridging,
            247–249
        Integra, 247, 251
Surgical Analyzer, 340, 341f
Surgical complications, 258
Surgical implant
    Integra, 228
Surgical wounds
    dermagraft, 224
Suture material, tapes , and glues, 127
Sutures, 127
Sympathetic vasoconstrictor innervation,
    131
Symptoms
    Integra controlling, 258
Syncytial fibroblasts
    Integra, 235
Syndecan, 223t
Synergistic wound healing, 69
Systematic hyperbaric oxygen therapy,
    57
Systemic calcinosis
    Integra, 269
Systemic hyperbaric oxygen therapy
    topical HBO therapy, 61

T

TAO. *See* Thromboangiitis Obliterans (TAO)
Tapes, 127
Target cells
    mitogenic response, 115
TBI. *See* Toe-brachial index (TBI)
Telangectasias, 6f
Tenascin, 223t
TFPI, 215f
TGF alpha, 223t
TGF beta, 223t, 224
Therapeutic angiogenesis, 23
Therapeutic currents
    wound healing, 83–85
Thigh, 312
Thoracic wounds, 327
Thromboangiitis Obliterans (TAO), 157–158
    inflammatory features, 157
    nature, 157
    patients, 158
    process, 158
Thromboelastogram, 340, 341f
Thrombosis, 169
Tibia, 316f
Tibial artery, 342
Tibial atherosclerosis, 345
Tibiofibular syndesmosis, 342
Tissue adhesives, 127
Tissue engineering
    Integra, 287
Tissue factor pathway inhibitor (TFPI), 215f
Tissue plasminogen activator (tPA), 215f
Tissue regeneration
    Integra, 227
TNF alpha, 223t
Toe
    amputations, 361
    cellulitis, 196
    gangrene, 356f
    osteomyelitis, 353f
Toe-brachial index (TBI), 10–11
    measurements, 11
    waveform analysis, 11
Tonic neural discharge, 133
Topical antibiotics, 163–164
Topical care
    unsuccessful, 257–258
Topical hyperbaric oxygen therapy, 59
    case studies, 62–63
    contraindication, 59
    effects, 57
    equipment, 61
    ineffectiveness, 59
    oxygen application, 58
    patient selection, 61

theorized mechanism, 59
    treatment programs, 62
    treatment protocol, 61
    VAC systems, 70
    wound
        rates, 57
    wound healing, 57
Topical oxygen bag
    application, 189
Topical oxygen therapy, 189
    results and warnings, 190
Total contact walking cast, 360
tPA, 215f
Tram flap, 329
Transcutaneous oxygen tension, 137
    measurements, 138
        distinguishing severity, 139
TransCyte, 304, 306
Transforming growth factor alpha (TGF alpha), 223t
Transforming growth factor beta (TGF beta), 223t, 224
Translucent oxygen measurement, 12
Transmetatarsal amputations, 361–362
Transposition flaps, 129
Trash feet, 165–166
Traumatic lesions, 313–314
Trochanteric lesion, 325f
Trochanteric pressure sores, 323
Trunk
    Integra, 270
Tumor necrosis factor alpha (TNF alpha), 223t
Type-A sensory fibers, 4
Type-C sensory fibers, 4

U

Ulcers. *See also* Foot ulcerations
    Charcot foot deformity, 10
    chronic, 232f
        matrix macromolecules, 109–121
    common characteristics, 4
    definition, 1
    diabetic foot, 60, 320f, 321f, 356f
        dermagraft, 224
        Integra, 266
        SIS, 293–295
    dorsal foot, 5f
    formation
        composition, 2–3
        walking biomechanics, 2–3
    ischemic, 5f
    medial ischemic, 5f
    neuropathic, 4
        heel, 293f
    neurotrophic, 8f
        treatment, 360–361
    nonvenous, 106

perforating
    foot, 345–346
pigmented legs, 195
right knee visual representation, 99
Texas University
    diabetic wound classification system, 11f
vascular insufficiency, 2–3
velocity values, 11f
visual representation, 98
wound classification systems, 11f
Yale University
    diabetic foot wound classification system, 11f
Ultra-low current electrical device, 97
    lesion, 98, 99
    wound healing treatment, 98
Ultraviolet ray machines, 90
Unmyelinated type-C fibers, 7
Unna's boot, 306
Upper extremities
    Integra, 270

V

Vacuum assisted closure, 35–36
Vacuum assisted closure (VAC), 65–66
    systems, 65
        action mechanisms, 66
        angiogenesis, 66
        application techniques, 68
        complicated wounds, 67
        contraindications, 68
        edema removal, 66
        enhanced cellular proliferation, 66
        future, 70
        indications, 68
        literature reviews, 66–67
        precautions, 68
        skin grafts, 67
        traditional wound therapy, 67
Vancomycin
    with Integra, 273t
Van Guericke, Otto, 90
Varicosities, 6f
Vascular assessments, 188
Vascular boots
    vascular test effects, 177
Vascular disease
    smoking risks, 156–157
Vascular endothelial growth factor (VEGF), 174–175, 220, 223, 223t
Vascular hormones, 166–175
    in vitro relationship studies, 166–175
Vascular impairments
    diabetic patient, 154
Vascular laboratory
    treatment, 187

Vascular migration, 22
Vascular perfusion
　critical deficiencies, 116
Vascular permeability factor, 28
Vascular tube information
　PDGF-BB, 22
VEGF, 174–175, 220, 223, 223t
Venous disease, 194
　Integra, 267
Venous disease patients, 187
Venous disease prevention, 180
Venous leg ulcers
　dermagraft, 224
Venous pressure, 183
Venous stasis ulcer, 6f
　MSF expression, 116
Venous ulcers, 106
Venous wounds
　hypoxia, 50
Versican, 223t
Vessel organization zone
　healthy wound, 243f
Viscera
　Integra, 271
VivoDerm, 303

W

Wagner classification, 191
Walking impairments
　questionnaire, 186
Water
　electricity, 95
Watson, James D., 79
Waveform
　definition, 84
Wound(s). *See also* Acute wounds
　animal studies, 48
　bolstering and dressing, 222
　chronic, 50
　　etiology, 96
　　life quality, 17
　　skin substitutes, 300–301
　molecular therapy, 17–38
Wound angiogenesis
　future directions, 37–38
Wound bed
　debridement
　　for Dermagraft, 222
　preparation, 305
Wound care, 359–360. *See also* Acute
　wounds, care
　dressing types, 126–127

Wound classification, 191
　methods, 190
Wound closure
　contraindications, 333–335
　economics, 335–336
　elderly, 333
　external tissue expansion, 309–335
　flap types, 129
　grafts, 252
　pain management, 312
　principles, 311–312
　specific procedure, 128–129
　technique, 312
Wound damage
　clinical diagnosis, 124
Wound excisions
　Integra, 273
Wound exudate, 66
Wound failure
　anticipated, 258
Wound healing, 222f
　ancient and primitive medicine, 72–73
　dermal substitutes, 29–30
　　cryopreserved dermal substitutes,
　　　29–30
　diabetic
　　biomaterial wound matrix,
　　　290–296
　direct current, 83
　electrical stimulation
　　rationale use, 81–85
　epidermal substitutes, 29
　　cultured epidermal allograft, 29
　　cultured epidermal autograft, 29
　equipment, 95
　galvanotaxis, 83t
　growth factor therapy, 21–22
　healing, 56–58
　historical aspects, 72–79
　impaired
　　etiology, 116–121
　　future prospects, 116–117
　lacerations, 124
　moist
　　principles, 104
　molecular level, 21–28
　next generation tissue engineering, 33
　other growth factors, 24–25
　oxygen, 69–70
　　angiogenesis, 49–50
　　burns, 59
　　clinical strategies, 51

　　epithelization, 50
　　immunity infection, 47–48
　　mechanisms, 47–50
　　oxidants, 50
　　theoretical and practical aspects,
　　　44–51
　prehistoric phases, 73
　pulsed current, 83–84
　research evidence, 85
　stages, 56
　therapeutic currents, 83–85
　tissue-engineered skin constructs,
　　28–34
　topical hyperbaric oxygen, 55–64
　　history, 55
　ultra-low microcurrents
　　antioxidant effects, 90–103
　wound neovascularization, 34
Wound-healing cascade, 109–110
　cell and tissue level events, 109–110
Wound management, 124, 310–311
　emergency room, 125–126
　ex vivo gene transfer, 27
　gene transfer, 26–27
　negative-pressure, 65–71
　optimizing growth factor therapy, 26
　other growth factors
　　granulocyte-macrophage colony-
　　　stimulating factor, 24
　　Keratinocyte growth factor-2, 24
　　transforming growth factor beta, 25
　stimulatory peptides, 25
　　ACT, 25
　　thymosin B-4, 25
　　TP-508, 25–26
　time-to-healing healthcare costs, 23
　in vivo gene transfer, 27–28
　　nonviral fibroblast growth
　　　factor-1, 27
　　vascular endothelial growth factor,
　　　27–28
Wound preparation
　Integra, 273
Wound repair, 251–253, 252
　electrical stimulation, 80–89
　topical care, 251–252

X

Xenografts, 302

Y

Yannas, Ioannis V., 228